Biliary Tract and Gallbladder Cancer

Biliary Tract and Gallbladder Cancer

Diagnosis and Therapy

EDITED BY

CHARLES R. THOMAS, JR.
CLIFTON DAVID FULLER

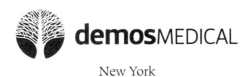

New York

Acquisitions Editor: R. Craig Percy
Cover Design: Cathleen Elliot
Copyeditor: Diane A. Lange

Visit our website at www.demosmedpub.com

Medicine is an ever-changing science undergoing continual development. Research and clinical experience are continually expanding our knowledge, in particular our knowledge of proper treatment and drug therapy. The authors, editors, and publisher have made every effort to ensure that all information in this book is in accordance with the state of knowledge at the time of production of the book.

Nevertheless, this does not imply or express any guarantee or responsibility on the part of the authors, editors, or publisher with respect to any dosage instructions and forms of application stated in the book. Every reader should examine carefully the package inserts accompanying each drug and check with a his physician or specialist whether the dosage schedules mentioned therein or the contraindications stated by the manufacturer differ from the statements made in this book. Such examination is particularly important with drugs that are either rarely used or have been newly released on the market. Every dosage schedule or every form of application used is entirely at the reader's own risk and responsibility. The editors and publisher welcome any reader to report to the publisher any discrepancies or inaccuracies noticed.

Library of Congress Cataloging-in-Publication Data

Biliary tract and gallbladder cancer : diagnosis & therapy / edited by Charles R. Thomas Jr., Clifton David Fuller.
     p. ; cm.
 Includes bibliographical references and index.
 ISBN-13: 978-1-933864-42-6 (hardcover : alk. paper)
 ISBN-10: 1-933864-42-7 (hardcover : alk. paper)
 1. Biliary tract—Cancer. I. Thomas, Charles R., 1957– II. Fuller, Clifton David.
 [DNLM: 1. Biliary Tract Neoplasms—diagnosis. 2. Biliary Tract Neoplasms—therapy. WI 735 B595 2009]
 RC280.B48B55 2009
 616.99'436—dc22
                                        2008024916

Special discounts on bulk quantities of Demos Medical Publishing books are available to corporations, professional associations, pharmaceutical companies, health care organizations, and other qualifying groups. For details, please contact:

Special Sales Department
Demos Medical Publishing
386 Park Avenue South, Suite 301
New York, NY 10016
Phone: 800–532–8663 or 212–683–0072
Fax: 212–683–0118
Email: orderdept@demosmedpub.com

Made in the United States of America

08 09 10 11   5 4 3 2 1

Dedication

To my committed and loving wife, Muriel Elleen Thomas, our two precious children, Julian Franklin Thomas and Aurielle Marie Thomas, and our parents and siblings, for their love and support of my career path.

In memory of my mother, Ruth Marie Wilson Thomas, who fought gallantly in the war against cancer and whose prayers have blessed me over the past five decades.—CT

To my wonderful and beautiful wife, Amy, our spectacular children, J.D. and Zoe, and my inspiring parents, Jeanne and Clifton, for their unparalleled love and encouragement.—CF

Contents

Preface

In an era of rapid advances in cancer therapy, biliary and gallbladder cancers remain an area in great need of attention. While these tumors are rare, the substantial and rapid mortality these tumors present with should serve as an impetus towards greater fervor in investigation into the causes and optimum treatments. However, at present, much of the knowledge regarding biliary tract and gallbladder cancers is diffusely scattered across the scientific literature, with most textbooks providing vague and cursory overviews of these rare but deadly neoplasms. Thus, we are greatly pleased to present the efforts of the investigators herein as a unified and definitive overview of the past, present, and possible future of biliary tract and gallbladder cancers.

As editors, our goal was to recruit authors who represent not only a multi-institutional, but multinational perspective. Biliary tract and gallbladder tumors are truly a global phenomenon, and the monographs presented herein reflect this global emphasis. Similarly, our desire to present a truly multidisciplinary resource is reflected in the inclusion of contributors from distinct but overlapping disciplines. In the modern setting, it is inconceivable that biliary tumors be presented with a myopic approach to diagnosis and intervention, and we are pleased to note the clear emphasis on team-based approaches to onco-logic care presented. Finally, we have sought to include segments detailing the cutting edge therapies of tomorrow, making the latest information readily available across a number of subdisciplines.

The book chapters are designed to move logically. Beginning chapters present the epidemiologic, pathologic, and pathogenetic milieu of biliary tract and gallbladder lesions, followed by excellent discussions of clinical and radiologic diagnosis and staging. The careful reader will note the emphasis on imaging techniques which has become characteristic of twenty-first-century approaches to patient care. Finally, the full armamentarium of therapeutic approaches is presented, from the local to systemic, established to experimental.

Ultimately, the true value of this book is to serve as a call for even greater large-scale collaboration. Without dedicated multi-institutional trials and protocols, the optimum therapy for gallbladder and biliary duct carcinomas will remain ill-defined. Such efforts will take years of effort and will not be "blockbuster" trials. However, the need for such evidence is indeed great for every patient with biliary tract cancer.

Finally, we wish to thank the authors of this book, whose dedication to patient care and scientific advancement are unparalleled.

Acknowledgments

The authors would like to thank all of the contributors, without whose hard work and dedicated expertise such a project would be frankly impossible. The quality of their scholarly efforts speaks for itself; nonetheless, we thank all our coauthors for their commitment to cancer patients and oncologic research.

Special thanks go to Craig Percy, senior medical acquisitions editor, Demos Medical Publishing, whose efforts to bring this book to completion required significant time and effort, and whose assistance has made the finished product a better (and more enjoyable) project than the editor's could have conceived. Many thanks go to Joe Hanson, formerly of Demos Medical Publishing, whose efforts to get this project off the ground will always be appreciated.

Finally, we wish to thank our longstanding mentors. Specifically, Dr. Fuller wishes to extend a special thanks to Charles R. Thomas, Jr., MD and Martin Fuss, MD, for their continuous encouragement and support.

Contributors

Syed A. Ahmad, MD
Associate Professor
Department of Surgery
The University of Cincinnati Medical Center
Cincinnati, Ohio

Ronald S. Arellano, MD
Instructor
Department of Radiology
Massachusetts General Hospital
Harvard Medical School
Boston, Massachusetts

Xabier de Aretxabala, MD
Professor
Department of Surgery
Clinica Alemana
Santiago, Chile

James M. Crawford, MD, PhD
Professor and Chairman
Department of Pathology, Immunology and Laboratory
    Medicine
University of Florida
Gainesville, Florida

Brian G. Czito, MD
Associate Professor
Department of Radiation Oncology
Duke University
Durham, North Carolina

Eduardo B. da Silveira, MD, MSc
Assistant Professor of Medicine
Department of Gastroenterology
Oregon Health & Science University
Staff Physician
Portland VA Medical Center
Portland, Oregon

Laura A. Dawson, MD
Associate Professor
Department of Radiation Oncology
Princess Margaret Hospital
University of Toronto
Toronto, Ontario, Canada

Andrew K. Diehl, MD, MS
O. Roger Hollan Professor and Chief
Department of Medicine
University of Texas Health Science Center at San
    Antonio
San Antonio, Texas

John DiGiovanni, PhD
Director and Professor
Department of Carcinogenesis
University of Texas M.D. Anderson Cancer Center
Smithville, Texas

Sathish Kumar Dundmadappa, MD
Assistant Professor
Department of Radiology
University of Massachusetts
Worcester, Massachusetts

Iván Roa Esterio, MD
Head, Pathology Service
Department of Pathology
Clinica Alemana de Santiago
Santiago, Chile

Douglas O. Faigel, MD
Professor of Medicine
Department of Medicine
Oregon Health & Science University
Portland, Oregon

M. Brian Fennerty, MD
Professor of Medicine
Department of Internal Medicine/Gastroenterology and
    Hepatology
Oregon Health & Science University
Portland, Oregon

Kevin Forsythe, MD
Physician
Department of Radiation Oncology
Kaiser Permanente Medical Center
Santa Clara, California

Clifton David Fuller, MD
Resident Physician
Departments of Radiation Oncology and Radiology
University of Texas Health Science Center
    at San Antonio
San Antonio, Texas

Martin Fuss, MD
Professor
Department of Radiation Medicine
Oregon Health & Science University
Portland, Oregon

John F. Gibbs, MD, MHCM
Chief, Gastrointestinal Surgery/Endoscopy
Department of Surgical Oncology
Roswell Park Cancer Institute
Buffalo, New York

Robert David Goldin, MD, FRCPath
Physician
Department of Histopathology
Imperial College London
London, United Kingdom

Manuel Gómez-Río, MD, PhD
Physician
Department of Nuclear Medicine
Virgen de las Nieves Universitary Hospital
Granada, Spain

Alessandro Guarise, MD
Chief
Department of Radiology
San Bassiano Hospital
Bassano del Grappa, Italy

Nagy Habib, ChM, FRCS
Professor
Department of Surgery
Imperial College London
London, United Kingdom

John Kaufman, MD
Chief of Vascular and Interventional Radiology
Department of Interventional Radiology
Dotter Interventional Institute
Oregon Health & Science University
Portland, Oregon

Andrew Kennedy, MD, FACR, FACRO
Radiation Oncologist
Department of Radiation Oncology
Wake Radiology Oncology Services
Cary, North Carolina

Shahid A. Khan, B Sc Hons, MBBS, PhD
Physician
Department of Hepatology and Gastroenterology
Imperial College London
London, United Kingdom

Kaoru Kiguchi, MD, PhD
Associate Professor
Co-Director of Cell and Tissue Analysis Core
Department of Carcinogenesis
University of Texas M.D. Anderson Cancer Center
Smithville, Texas

Kenneth J. Kolbeck, MD, PhD
Assistant Professor
Department of Interventional Radiology
Dotter Interventional Institute
Oregon Health & Science University
Portland, Oregon

Jerome C. Landry, MD
Professor
Department of Radiation Oncology
Emory University
Atlanta, Georgia

Joshua D. Lawson, MD
Assistant Professor
Department of Radiation Oncology
University of California, San Diego Medical Center
La Jolla, California

Chen Liu, MD, PhD
Associate Professor
Department of Pathology, Immunology and Laboratory
    Medicine
University of Florida
Gainesville, Florida

José Manuel Llamas-Elvira, MD, PhD
Physician
Department of Nuclear Medicine
Virgen de las Nieves Universitary Hospital
Granada, Spain

Andrew M. Lowy, MD
Professor of Surgery
Chief, Division of Surgical Oncology
Department of Surgery
University of California, San Diego Medical Center
Moores Cancer Center
La Jolla, California

Leonardo Marcal, MD
Assistant Professor
Department of Diagnostic Radiology
University of Texas M.D. Anderson Cancer Center
Houston, Texas

Rebecca J. McClaine, MD
Surgery Resident
Department of Surgery
University of Cincinnati Medical Center
Cincinnati, Ohio

Giovanni Morana, MD
Chief
Department of Clinical Radiology
Santa Maria dei Battuti Hospital
Treviso, Italy

Subir Nag, MD, FACR, FACRO
Director of Brachytherapy Services
Department of Radiation Oncology
Kaiser Permanente Medical Center
Santa Clara, California

Heljä Oikarinen, MD, PhD
Specialist in Radiology
Department of Diagnostic Radiology
Oulu University Hospital
Oulu, Finland

Susan L. Orloff, MD
Professor
Departments of Surgery and Molecular Microbiology
    and Immunology
Oregon Health & Science University
Director, Basic Science Research
Department of Surgery
Portland VA Medical Center
Portland, Oregon

Philip A. Philip, MD, PhD, FRCP
Professor of Medicine and Oncology
Department of Internal Medicine, Hematology/
    Oncology
Karmanos Cancer Institute
Wayne State University
Detroit, Michigan

Bassel F. El-Rayes, MD
Assistant Professor of Medicine and Oncology
Department of Internal Medicine, Hematology/
    Oncology
Karmanos Cancer Institute
Wayne State University
Detroit, Michigan

Antonio Rodríguez-Fernández, MD, PhD
Physician
Department of Nuclear Medicine
Virgen de las Nieves Universitary Hospital
Granada, Spain

Shimul Shah, MD
Assistant Professor
Department of Transplant Surgery
University of Massachusetts
Worcester, Massachusetts

Sridhar Shankar, MD
Associate Professor
Division Director, Body Imaging and Interventions
Department of Radiology
University of Massachusetts
Worcester, Massachusetts

Amar W. Sharif, MD, BSc, MBBS
Physician
Department of Hepatology and Gastroenterology
Imperial College London
London, United Kingdom

Richard R. Smith, MD
Chief, Surgical Oncology,
Tripler Army Medical Center
Tripler, Hawaii

Ross C. Smith, MD, BS, FRACS
Professor
Department of Surgery
Royal North Shore Hospital
University of Sydney
New South Wales, Australia

Janio Szklaruk, MD, PhD
Associate Professor
Department of Diagnostic Radiology
University of Texas M.D. Anderson Cancer Center
Houston, Texas

Swee H. Teh, MD, FRCSI, FACS
Director
Department of Hepatobiliary Surgery and Minimally
    Invasive Surgery
Sacred Heart Medical Center
Eugene, Oregon

Charles R. Thomas, Jr., MD
Professor and Chair
Department of Radiation Medicine
Oregon Health & Science University
Portland, Oregon

Chitra Viswanathan, MD
Assistant Professor
Department of Diagnostic Radiology
University of Texas M.D. Anderson Cancer Center
Houston, Texas

Ignacio I. Wistuba, MD
Professor
Department of Pathology
University of Texas M.D. Anderson Cancer Center
Houston, Texas

Biliary Tract and Gallbladder Cancer

I

GENERAL CONSIDERATIONS

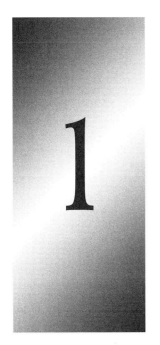

1 Epidemiology of Gallbladder and Biliary Tract Neoplasms

Clifton D. Fuller
Andrew K. Diehl

Biliary tract malignancies are numerically rare cancers that exhibit dismal long-term survival outcomes. It is estimated that 9250 cases of biliary tract cancers were diagnosed in the U.S. in 2007, with around 3250 yearly deaths annually. Early diagnosis, except as a function of serendipitous discovery upon cholecystectomy (1, 2), is rare, with the vast majority of patients presenting with either locally advanced or distant metastatic disease (3, 4). The therapeutic outcomes for advanced stage disease remain grim, raising the impetus for mortality reduction via selective screening of high-risk population in concert with primary prevention and lifestyle modification (5, 6). Such interventions are only possible by identifying specific population- level risk factors associated with biliary tract cancers, that might then be modified (7), thereby providing an important rationale for exploration of biliary tract cancer epidemiology.

Conceptually, biliary cancers may be divided topographically by anatomic site and include primary carcinomas of the gallbladder and biliary ducts. These neoplasms represent distinct epidemiologic and clinical presentations and thus should be considered separately. However, despite the clear importance of subclassifying biliary tract malignancies, the paucity of cases, and dif-ficulty in determining the primary disease site in locally advanced illness, as well as the ambiguities of both national and international registry data, impair ready analysis of extant population-based datasets. While less specific than other reports, pooled international registry data provide valuable epidemiologic information regarding biliary cancers. An example is *Cancer Incidence in Five Continents*, an open access electronic dataset by the International Agency for Research on Cancer (IARC) (8). *Cancer Incidence in Five Continents* additionally includes a dynamic statistical calculator/graph function on its website. This public database affords the ability to track differences in biliary cancer incidence between countries and subregions within countries (Figure 1.1). Though a limited number of registries are included, the range of incidence between countries is striking. Additionally, a difference is observed between the relative incidence of males and females in specific registries (Figure 1.1) (8). Broadly, these results suggest that gallbladder and other biliary tract cancers are particularly frequent in Japanese men and Eastern European women. However, as with any large registry database, care must be used in generalization of findings. Nonetheless, as both an epidemiologic resource and avenue for both comparative incidence analysis and hypothesis generation, it is an exceptionally useful tool.

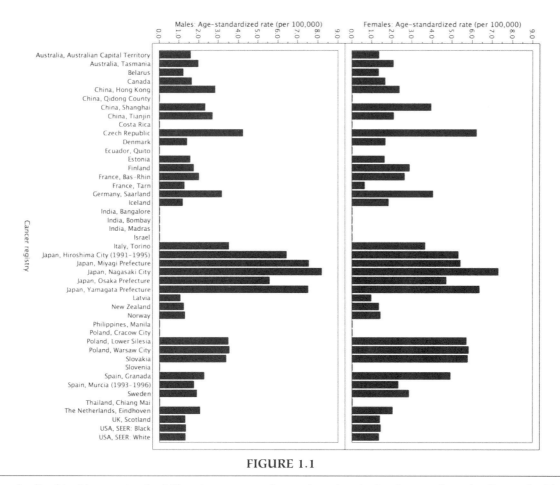

FIGURE 1.1

Age-standardized incidence rates for biliary tract cancers from selected registries, by sex, from the Cancer Incidence on Five Continents dataset (8). (From Ref. 8.)

GALLBLADDER CANCER

Incidence and Mortality

Gallbladder cancer is the fifth most common gastrointestinal malignancy in the United States (9), diagnosed in around 5000 persons in the United States each year (10). Reported data indicate that primary tumors of the gallbladder are strongly associated with age (3, 9, 11-18) and gender (9, 19-25). Incidence rates are known to increase steadily with age in both sexes (Figure 1.2). The mean age at diagnosis falls in the seventh decade, with exceedingly few tumors presenting in persons younger than 30 years. The incidence in women is markedly greater than that in men, making gallbladder cancer one of the few non-reproductive organ related cancers having a female predominant incidence pattern (22-25). Interestingly, while previously thought not to be a sex hormone-mediated process, recent findings raise the possibility that gallbladder carcinogenesis may have estrogen- or progesterone-mediated features (26-30), serving as a putative explanatory

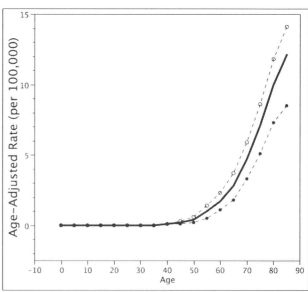

FIGURE 1.2

Age-adjusted incidence rates from the SEER dataset (1973–2004) by age at diagnosis (open circles indicate females, closed circles males; solid line indicates cumulative incidence). (From Ref. 40.)

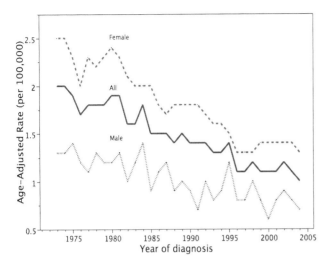

FIGURE 1.3

SEER (1973–2004) age-adjusted incidence by year of diagnosis and sex. (From Refs. 40, 275.)

mechanism for the observed male-female disparity and affording potential risk reduction via sex hormone modulation.

While the small number of cases, and dearth of rigorous histologically detailed reports, has led many authors to report gallbladder cancers as a homogenous disease entity, the relative incidence of histologic subtypes varies. In the Surveillance, Epidemiology, and

End Results (SEER) registries, adenocarcinomas exhibit an age-adjusted incidence rate of 0.9-1 per 100,000; all other histologies exhibit such low incidence rates (<0.1 per 100,000) that specific characterization of trends would be unreliable. However, some authors have posited significant differences in the epidemiologic profiles, associated risk factors, and outcomes between histologic subtypes (31-37). Accumulation of pooled datasets will in time afford confirmation using well-powered datasets. In the meantime, consideration of gallbadder cancer as a single epidemiologic grouping is an unavoidable consequence of sparse data.

Currently, gallbladder cancer accounts for an estimated 2000-3500 deaths in the United States annually. Since reliable domestic survival has been collected, starting in the late 1960s, the incidence and mortality rate from gallbladder cancers has been in substantial decline (Figures 1.3 and 1.4) (38,39). Crude annual deaths have fallen by almost one quarter, and age-adjusted mortality rate has been reduced by half (Figure 1.4) (40). There is no single explanation for this phenomenon, as there have been no substantial technical improvements in the diagnosis or treatment of gallbladder cancer during this span, and overall survival remains exceedingly poor (Figure 1.5). It has been proposed, as in international datasets, that access to and utilization of cholecystectomy for gallstones may result in reduced development of gallbladder cancers (7). As the frequency of cholecystectomy rises, the number of persons at risk to develop gallbladder cancer falls. Additionally, as gallstones are the dominant risk factor for gallbladder cancer, those at highest risk for primary gallbladder cancer are selectively removed from the risk pool by surgical intervention. Supporting data from high-risk populations in Chile (38) showed rising death

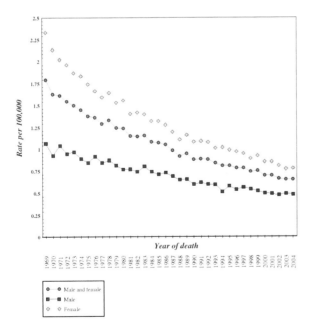

FIGURE 1.4

Age-adjusted total U.S. mortality rates for gallbladder cancer (1969–2004) by sex. (From Ref. 40.)

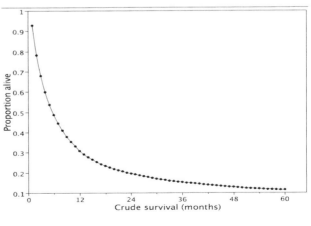

FIGURE 1.5

Crude observed survival for U.S. gallbladder carcinoma patients. (From Ref. 40.)

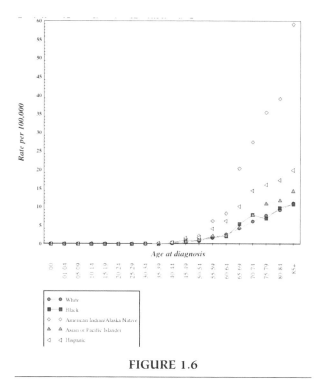

FIGURE 1.6

Age-specific crude SEER incidence rates by ethnicity for gallbladder cancer (SEER 13 Registries for 1995–2004). (From Ref. 275.)

rate from gallbladder cancer concurrent with a decline in cholecystectomies. Similarly, low-risk population data from the England, the United States, Canada (39), and Scotland (41) positively correlating cholecystectomy rates and declining cancer mortality, as well as comparison data from Sweden showing an opposite trend in the context of reduced cholecystectomy frequency, strongly support this thesis. It is estimated that one case of gallbladder cancer death is prevented for every 100 cholecystectomies performed in identified populations (38, 39). While prophylactic surgical intervention is a reasonable step in high-risk regions or population cohorts (5, 7, 18, 42), it does not represent an accepted primary indication for surgery in low-risk populations, but an unintended benefit of cholecystectomy access and utilization.

As indicated by pooled data, reliable international population-based registry reports denote substantial geographic differentials in the incidence of primary gallbladder carcinoma (Figure 1.6) (7, 43). Rates are high in Eastern Europe (7), specifically Poland (7, 44, 45), Hungary (46, 47), and the Czech Republic (46, 48), though they appear to be decreasing in some regions (47). Exceptionally high incidences have also been noted in Bolivia (49-51), Colombia (7, 52) and Chile (28, 44, 53-57). In Chile, crude incidence rates for females 0-74 years of age of 22.3 per 100,000, an astoundingly high

incidence, have been noted, in addition to a reported long-term mortality of 15.6 per 100,000 (58). Regional incidences are also notable, with northern Japan reporting markedly higher incidence than southern Japan (59). In contrast, registries in the Philippines, the United Kingdom, Spain, and Kuwait report comparatively low incidence rates (Figure 1.1).

In addition to regional variation, differences in ethnic groups within the same geographic region are noteworthy. Gallbladder cancer incidence and mortality in African American populations is approximately half that of whites in the United States. Domestically, the incidence of gallbladder neoplasms in Native American populations is exceedingly high, with a crude rate nearly five times that of Caucasian Americans in New Mexican Native American cohorts (8, 60, 61). Gallbladder cancer rates have been observed to be higher than national averages for a variety of Native American peoples residing within distinct geographic regions and with an array of dietary practices (43, 45, 62-70). For instance, while gallbladder cancer rates among Native Americans in the American Southwest are notable (7, 60, 67, 71-78), elevated rates of disease may also be seen in Alaskan natives, whose diet is substantially different (62-64, 69, 79, 80). However, a common feature for these populations is a high prevalence of cholelithiasis and an observed genetic predisposition toward increased gallstone formation (42, 45, 66).

Hispanic cultures in North and South American populations descended from New World indigenous ethnic groups have also shown an increased risk of gallbladder cancer. These groups, such as Mexican Americans in the U.S. Southwest (60, 67, 81-83) and mestizo populations in Bolivia (51, 84), have an intermediate cancer risk greater than that for non-Hispanic whites but less than that for Native American populations (67). Conversely, Hispanic Americans without direct lineage from indigenous New World ancestors do not appear to be at high risk (85). Immigrant groups also show interesting differences from their parent populations. For instance, Japanese and Korean immigrants in Los Angeles have substantially lower rates of gallbladder cancer compared to their peers from Japan and Korea (8, 86, 87). An unexplained reduction in cumulative incidence risk for both sexes was observed; however, the difference between immigrant Korean females compared to their parallel cohort in Seoul is striking-more than 50%. Additionally, several family clusters have been noted to have exceptionally high rates of gallbladder cancer (88-91), and a family history of gallbladder cancer has been correlated with increased risk (89). Cumulatively, this national, ethnic, regional, and familial incidence pattern is suggestive of multiple potential heterogeneous contributory etiologic factors of both genetic and environmental origin.

Cholelithiasis and Gallbladder Carcinoma

The central associative feature for primary carcinomas of the gallbladder appears to be comorbid gallstones (3, 19, 45, 52, 92-109). More than three quarters of gallbladder cancer patients have co-presentation of gallstones at diagnosis (102), in comparison to 25% of age-matched controls. Reported rates of incidental discovery of gallbladder carcinoma during cholecystectomy range from 0.5 to 2% in patients treated for symptomatic cholelithiasis (110). The relative risk of developing carcinoma of the gallbladder is patients with diagnosed gallstones has been estimated at between 2 and 24 times that of equivalent patients without cholelithiasis, depending on the series and population (7, 16, 18, 57, 66, 93, 105, 111). Estimates of gallbladder cancer incidence among patients with untreated stones range from 0.5 to 1% over a 20-year period (18, 66, 112-114). A Mayo Clinic-led prospective study designed to assess the epidemiologic risk of gallbladder cancer in patients with gallstones enrolled 2583 Minnesota residents with diagnosed asymptomatic cholelithiasis and subsequently followed them for more than 31,000 person-years (113). Within this series, five patients were diagnosed with gallbladder cancer after a median follow-up of slightly more than 13 years. The incidence of gallbladder cancer was significantly higher than expected for men (153 per 100,000 person-years), but not for women. However, it is difficult to justify prophylactic cholecystectomy in patients with asymptomatic gallstones in low-risk populations, since the actual incidence (9 per 10,000 person-years) and number of cancers (5/ 2583) observed was so low. Hsing et al. in a population-based series from Shanghai, found that patients with gallbladder carcinoma had significantly heavier stone burdens than control patients and estimated that 80% of all gallbladder cases in Shanghai were attributable to comorbid cholelithiasis (93). In a large population-based cohort study, Danish researchers found 42 gallbladder cancers in a total of 17,715 patients with gallstones, significantly higher than the comparison cohort with a standardized incidence ratio of 4.6 times the general population within the first 4 years of follow-up (115). A multicentric European study also showed a gallbladder cancer risk ratio of 4.7 for patients with gallstone disease (116). Nonetheless, the overall risk, excepting specific high-risk communities, is so low that in most cases prophylactic cholecystectomy is not recommended as a gallbladder cancer risk-reduction strategy. As mentioned previously, for high-risk populations there is potentially great benefit to preventative cholecystectomy; data from several nations show that access to and number of cholecystectomy procedures is associated with reduced incidence and mortality (39, 41, 58), suggesting that, in specific geographic locales of exceptional incidence, surgical prophylaxis may indeed be a reasonable option (42).

The strong association between stone formation and neoplasia appears to be the main determinant of many epidemiologic features of gallbladder cancers, such that risk factors for cholelithiasis are typically risk factors for gallbladder tumors. Illustratively, female gender (52), increased age (4, 13, 15, 19, 52, 62), fecundity (18, 30, 52), and obesity (5-7, 13, 18, 43, 52, 75, 82, 105, 116-121) are associated risk factors for both gallstones and gallbladder malignancy, as is membership in certain Native American and Hispanic ethnic groups. Patients with gallstones are also observed to develop gallbladder cancer at an earlier age than those without gallstones (97). Gallstone size has been repeatedly correlated with cancer development (7, 12, 66, 100, 108, 122, 123). Compared to patients with gallstones ≤1 cm in diameter, an odds ratio for diagnosis of gallbladder cancer of 2.4 was noted for gallstone diameters of 2-2.9 cm (123). For those with diameters ≥3 cm, the odds ratio is increased by a factor of 9.2-10.1 (66, 123). The relationship to the number of stones is less clear (12, 84, 96, 122, 124). However, correlation of number and size of the stones to cancer incidence may be reflective of age at diagnosis or long-term duration of gallstones within the gallbladder, as opposed to an independent phenomenon (12, 124). If so, this might explain why a comparatively small number of series failed to detect a relationship between stone size/number and carcinoma of the gallbladder (5, 125). With respect to the composition of gallstones, various series have noted that cholesterol stones may confer added risk of disease development (93, 94, 105, 122).

At present, the dominant mechanistic explanation for the strong and repeatedly observed association with gallstones and subsequent cancers centers on the role of chronic inflammatory conditions within the gallbladder (48, 126-128), leading eventually from metaplasia to dysplasia and, finally, malignant transformation (106, 128-132). Repeatedly, endogenous mediators of inflammatory response have been shown to colocalize with gallbladder carcinomas (126, 127, 133).

Consequently, it may be that, given confirmation of these relationships, preventive efforts with widely used anti-inflammatory pharmaceutical therapies (such as cyclooxygenase modulation [3, 26, 126, 134]) might be implemented in high-risk populations. Already, population-based data from Shanghai has suggested that utilization of aspirin is associated with decrement in gallbladder cancer incidence, without modifying risk of gallstone disease (127).

Other Associated Risk Factors

The list of identified conditions associated with primary gallbladder carcinomas is numerous and varied. Most of these putative risk factors, such as porcelain gallbladder (42, 135-140), chronic cholecystitis (141-143), and pancreatobiliary maljunction (128, 144, 145), are indicative or causative of chronic inflammatory processes and conceivably share etiologic mechanisms similar to gallstone disease-associated gallbladder cancers (128, 138), which may explain conflicting findings (136, 146, 147) regarding their association with malignant evolution. Researchers have also observed an association with several bile composition abnormalities (148-153), specifically a low ratio of bile acid/lecithin to cholesterol. Impaired contractility or motility may exacerbate risk by increasing the time of exposure to endogenous carcinogens as well (50, 149-154).

Chemical carcinogens have been proposed as cofactors for development of gallbladder cancer, primarily in animal models (155-159), but few have been

TABLE 1.1
Literature-Derived Factors Associated with Gallbladder Cancer

	RISK FACTOR	RELATED CONDITIONS	REFERENCES OF NOTE
Demographic features	Age		9, 43, 53, 62, 115, 276, 277
	Female gender		18, 20, 27, 30, 108, 278
		Early menarche	30, 279
		Early parity	30, 99, 279
		Mulitparity	30, 279
		Duration of fertility	30, 280
	Low socioeconomic status		19, 104
Comorbid conditions			
	Cholelithiasis		13, 27, 45, 66, 93, 96, 97, 104, 111–113, 115, 123, 125, 173, 81–286
		Number of stones	12
		Size of stones	7, 12, 19, 66, 93, 98, 108, 122, 123, 125, 149
		Duration of diagnosis	45, 104
	Porcelain gallbladder		128, 135, 136, 140, 146, 147
	Anomalous junction of the pancreaticobiliary duct		128, 286–294
	Chronic cholecystitis		42, 141
	Xanthogranulomatous cholecystitis		296, 297
	Obesity		5-7, 13, 18, 43, 45, 52, 75, 96, 105, 121, 297, 298
	Serum hyperlipidemia		92
	Ulcerative colitis		226, 232, 299–301
	Chronic diarrhea		45
Bacterial infections			141, 174, 302, 303
	Helicobacter sp.		173, 175, 304–307
	Salmonella typhi		52, 308–313
Dietary variables			
	High caloric intake		18, 45, 314
	Increased carbohydrates		45, 132, 298, 314
	Increased protein/meat consumption		6, 298, 314
	Low fresh fruit/fiber		6, 99, 104, 297, 298, 314
	Low vitamin/micronutrient intake		99, 298, 314–318
	Alcohol intake		30, 80, 297, 314, 319
	Chili peppers/capsicum		6, 28, 104
	Mustard oil		19
	Tea consumption		6, 107, 314
	Improperly stored ghee (clarified butter)		99
Environmental factors/ pollutants			
	Tobacco smoking/chewing		30
	Heavy metals/metallothioneins		44, 159, 320–322
	Asbestos		162, 169
	Herbicides/pesticides		158, 159, 323–326

confirmed in humans (160, 161). A relationship of gall-bladder cancer to asbestos exposure been posited, but unconfirmed (162). The few studies of occupational risk groups (163-172) that have been undertaken have been limited in size and tended to group cholangio-carcinomas and primary gallbladder cases. These studies have shown minimal reproducibility and are therefore difficult to assess (42-44, 84, 85). Factors underlying the predisposition of specific occupational groups to gallbladder cancer are thus largely unknown.

Biliary bacterial agents have been postulated to modify degradation of bile salts, with the resultant for-mation of potent carcinogens (141). Additionally, Sal-monella typhi and Helicobacter sp., as well as other bacteria, have been advocated to play a contributory role, but the impact of infectious processes remains debatable (52, 141, 173-175).

In all, a plethora of potential physiologic, dietary, and environmental cofactors have been advanced (Table 1.1). At present many are promising; however, the full relationship between these potential risk factors, possi-ble confounders (such as gallstone disease, age, and sex multicollinearity), and primary carcinomas has yet to be definitively elucidated.

Prevention

It is reasonable to assume that interventions that reduce the prevalence of cholelithiasis will lead as well to cor-responding decrement in the incidence of gallbladder neoplasms. Although effective strategies to forestall gallstone development have not yet been determined, maintenance of normal body mass index and serum lipid levels are reasonable suggestions for large-scale preventitive efforts, to dovetail with preventive efforts for cardiovascular disease and other cancers. Similarly, aspirin utilization should be considered in patients for whom such pharmacotherapy is indicated for other comorbid conditions.

In patients with an established diagnosis of cholelithiasis, the prevention of gallbladder cancer should be considered one of several potential benefits of surgical treatment. While prevention of gallbladder cancer as a single indication for cholecystectomy should be discouraged in low-risk populations, it should be recognized as a potential benefit within the milieu of considerations for surgical intervention. For patients known to be at high risk (e.g., members of high-risk regions or ethnic groups, especially those with multi-ple large stones [≥3 cm]) it may represent a reasonable option to undertake for purely prophylactic intent. The increased number of cholecystectomies may explain, at least in part, the impressive decrease in domestic mor-tality from gallbladder cancer.

BILE DUCT CANCER (CHOLANGIOCARCINOMA)

Incidence and Mortality

Cancer of the bile ducts is, like primary gallbladder car-cinoma, relatively rare, with approximately 3000 cases in the United States annually (40, 176). Strictly speak-ing, only intrahepatic bile duct cancers have tradition-ally been termed "cholangiocarcinomas" (10, 177), and thus conceptually were grouped with primary liver tumors, a practice that persists in some literature (178). However, in many locally advanced cases it is not prac-tically possible to determine whether a tumor has ini-tially arisen from the intra- or extrahepatic bile ducts. Although cholangiocarcinomas are considered a dis-tinct designation for the purposes of registry classifi-cation, they are in fact histologically indistinguishable from adenocarcinomas, and, thus, a host of different nomenclatures (bile duct cancer, ductal carcinoma, ade-nocarcinoma) are functionally synonomous. Thus, it is increasingly accepted to consider adenocarcinomas of the bile duct, regardless of location, as cholangio-carcinomas (10), as will be the case herein. Although the incidence of extrahepatic cholangiocarcinoma has remained relatively constant, the incidence of intra-hepatic cholangiocarcinoma has increased. The topo-graphic difference between intra- and extrahepatic cholangiocarcinomas is associated with distinct survival patterns and different associated risk factors. Further-more, hilar cholangiocarcinomas, or Klatskin's tumors, a topographic variant of extrahepatic carcinomas at the hepatic duct bifurcation, have a comparatively favor-able mortality profile because of their anatomic loca-tion. The differences in survival between site within the biliary tract (hilar, intrahepatic, or extrahepatic) is pri-marily presumed to be related to the time of diagnosis, stage at presentation, local invasion of adjacent struc-tures, and resectability-all shown to be predictors of posttherapy outcomes. Cancer of the extrahepatic bile ducts accounts for approximately 950-1200 deaths annually in the United States, with a crude mortality of 0.4 deaths per 100,000. SEER data suggests dismal 1- and 2-year survival rates of 24.5 and 12.8%, respec-tively, for intrahepatic lesions (179). As these large-scale domestic registry data suggest, there is little solace to be had in posttherapeutic outcomes, making primary prevention an attractive target for the reduction of dis-eased-induced morbidity and mortality. Unlike gall-bladder carcinoma, which shows a clear female pre-dominance, cholangiocarcinoma occurs as often in males as in females (180). Most patients with cholan-giocarcinomas present between the 5th and 7th decades of life, with a mean age at diagnosis of the early 60s (Figure 1.7). The international cancer registry data demonstrate comparatively modest differences in incidence between countries in light of the striking differences observed in gallbladder cancer. Nationally, registry data from Khon Kaen, northeast Thailand, reveals some of the highest incidence in the world, with age-standardized rates of 93.8-317.6 per 100,000 (181). Within this registry, cholangiocarcinoma represents the most common form of cancer. Other countries with high rates include Japan (182) and Brazil. Japanese, Filipino, and Korean immigrants in Los Angeles have rates that are among some of the highest in the world.

Several datasets have recorded an interesting phenomenon in worldwide registry data; namely, an increase in the rate of diagnoses of intrahepatic cholangiocarcinoma despite essentially static extrahepatic cholangiocarcinoma rates (Figure 1.8) (178-180, 183-187). Registries from the United Kingdom, Denmark, Japan, and the United States have exhibited the same trend (178-180, 183, 184, 186, 188-190). Recent SEER analysis shows that estimated incidence rates for intrahepatic cholangiocarcinoma progressively increased from 0.13 per 100,000 in 1973 to 0.67 per 100,000 in 1997, resulting in an estimated annual change in incidence of 9.11%. Subsequent mortality from primary intrahepatic cholangiocarcinoma similarly increased 9.4% from 1973 to 1997 (179). The age-adjusted mortality rates for this period increased from 0.4 to 0.65 per 100,000 in Caucasians, and a similar increase was seen in blacks from 0.15 to 0.58 per 100,000 (179). Further analyses have explored significant age-cohort and ethnicity differentials in intrahepatic cholangiocarcinoma incidence (178), indicating heterogeneous contributory

factors, as well as the potential confounder of registry documentation variability (191) may contribute to the degree of observed increased incidence. Nonetheless, by any measure, the approximate doubling of the incidence of intrahepatic cholangiocarcinoma is a troubling development (178, 186, 189).

Comorbid Conditions and Risk of Bile Duct Cancer

Multiple congenital abnormalities of biliary anatomy have been associated with an observed increase in risk of developing biliary duct cancers (133, 188, 189, 192-198), with particular attention having been paid to choledochal cysts (135, 189, 198) and Caroli's disease (133, 189, 199). Choledochal cysts, a congenital dilatation of the common bile duct, appear to be more common as a phenotypic presentation in Southeast Asian than in Western countries (200-202). The concurrent incidence of cholangiocarcinoma and choledochal cyst has been reported as ranging from less than 3% to 28%, a factor of 20 times that of the equivalent general population (203-206). Choledocal cysts are also associated with other malformative biliary lesions, such as anomalous union of the pancreatico-biliary ductal anatomy, which are (128, 137, 207, 208) themselves

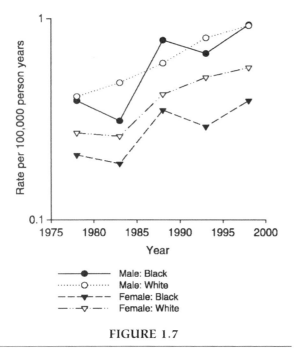

FIGURE 1.7

Age-standardized incidence rates for intrahepatic cholangiocarcinoma. (From Ref. 178.)

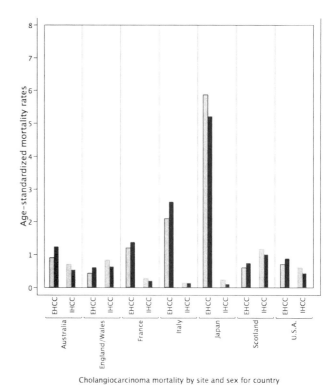

Cholangiocarcinoma mortality by site and sex for country

FIGURE 1.8

Intrahepatic and extrahepatic cholangiocarcinoma incidence by registry. (From Ref. 183.)

reported as increasing the probability of cholangiocarcinoma diagnosis (209-211). While more commonly associated with primary gallbladder cancer as opposed to cholangiocarcinoma development (195, 197, 209), it is assumed that pancreatico-biliary duct malformation shares a similar etiologic mechanism. It is hypothesized that pancreatic secretory reflux, bile stasis, ductal stone formation, and secondary chronic inflammatory processes that occur within the cyst (212) may play a role in carcinogenesis (177, 197, 213-218). Caroli's disease, a state characterized by multiple cystic dilatations of the intrahepatic segmental bile ducts, presumably has a similar mechanistic role as do choledocal cysts and pancreatico-biliary malunion and confers a risk of cholangiocarcinoma more than 100 times that estimated in patients without diagnosed biliary tract dysfunction (196, 219). Vesicular gallstone formation has been noted in several series at rates approximating those observed in age-matched populaces and has not been established as a distinctive associated risk factor with cholangiocarcinoma development. However, some series have noted comorbid bile duct or intrahepatic stones simultaneous with bile duct cancer (220-222). It is unclear whether ductal stones represent an etiologic factor, are formed as a consequence of the tumors themselves, or share a common phenomenologic raison d'etre, such as chronic cholangitis (222). Cholangitis, whether infectious or primary sclerosing, has also been repeatedly and reliably linked to disease development (133, 223-226).

Recently, in a rather interesting population analysis using SEER-Medicare linked datasets, Welzel et al. (189) identified risk features significantly associated with both extrahepatic and intrahepatic carcinomas, specifically biliary cirrhosis, cholelithiasis, alcoholic liver disease, diabetes, thyrotoxicosis, and chronic pancreatitis. Conditions associated with increased intrahepatic carcinoma included obesity, chronic nonalcoholic liver disease, hepatitis C infection, and tobacco smoking. Because obesity and nonalcoholic liver disease are increasing in incidence and are associated with intra- but not extrahepatic carcinoma, they offer a tantalizing rationale for the contrast between stable extrahepatic and advancing intrahepatic cholangiocarcinoma rates domestically. A confirmatory work using Danish registry data (180) found alcoholic liver disease, unspecified cirrhosis, cholangitis, and diabetes to be associated with carcinoma. Among other conditions, chronic inflammatory bowel disease was significantly correlated as well.

An association between cholangiocarcinoma and chronic inflammatory bowel disease, especially ulcerative colitis, is well established (224, 227-238). Further, it has been observed that the risk for development of cholangiocarcinoma is related to both duration of disease and severity of colonic involvements in patients with ulcerative colitis. Risk estimates demonstrate that approximately 0.5% of patients with ulcerative colitis can be expected to develop malignancy, a rate up to 31 times that of equivalent matched populations (228, 239). No firm association with Crohn's disease has yet been established (223). It has been observed that the onset of bile duct carcinoma is often predated by pericholangitis and sclerosing cholangitis (180). The risk of cholangiocarcinoma does not appear reduced by proctocolectomy, lending credence to the supposition that it is a primary process in the bile ducts, rather than a sequela of colonic involvement itself, is the underlying cause.

INFECTIOUS AND ENVIORNMENTAL ASSOCIATIONS

Repeated series over the last five decades have demonstrated that the high rates of intrahepatic bile duct cancer found in Southeast Asia correspond to a coincidentally high prevalence of biliary tract parasitic infections. *Clonorchis sinensis* and *Opisthorchis viverrini*, frequently encountered liver flukes in regions of China, Thailand, and Hong Kong, are strongly correlated with magnified rates of cholangiocarcinoma (181, 182, 218, 240-245). This may be accounted for by dietary practices involving the consumption of large amounts of raw and undercooked fish over the course of a lifetime. Additionally, other regions of Asia that do not share infestation rates of liver flukes as high as Northeast Thailand (181, 182, 240, 243-251) and South China (252, 253), such as Japan (182) and Korea (254-256), as well as the notably high incidence rates of South Asian immigrants in the United States (257), may also indicate contributory components from the intake of raw, dried, or fermented fish. It is also plausible that nitrosamines secondary to intake of fermented fish may act as a contributory carcinogen whose risk is either additive or synergistic with liver fluke infestation (155, 157, 243, 247, 251, 258-264).

An array of other known carcinogens have also been posited to increase risk of bile duct cancer (259, 265-270), although all require more confirmatory evidence. Thorotrast, a thorium dioxide radiologic contrast agent used in the 1950s, has been historically associated with cholangiocarcinoma (177, 188, 213). Additionally, workers in environments with heavy asbestos exposure have been postulated to have increased risk (271-273).

Prevention

Large-scale reduction in the incidence of cholangiocarcinoma in developing countries and in Southeast Asia could reasonably be achieved through large-scale reduction in liver flukes (240). Traditional single-dose antiparisitics are exceptionally effective; however, reinfection rates remain substantial. Thus, large-scale food purity controls and/or public education campaigns would be necessary to eradicate fluke infestation (177, 263). If, indeed, endogenous nitosamine carcinogenesis/cocarcinogenesis is truly a correlative risk feature, dietary supplementation with vitamin C (218) or E (274) could theoretically reduce the risk of cholangiocarcinoma. Finally, if potential noncongenital risk factors such as smoking, obesity, gallstone disease, chronic nonalcoholic liver disease, and hepatitis C infection prove to be correlates of cholangiocarcinoma, then minimization of these independent yet interactive process should be sought.

References

1. Kapoor VK. Incidental gallbladder cancer. Am J Gastroenterol 2001; 96:627-629.
2. Wagholikar GD, Behari A, Krishnani N, et al. Early gallbladder cancer. J Am Coll Surg 2002; 194:137-141.
3. Malik IA. Gallbladder cancer: current status. Expert Opin Pharmacother 2004; 5:1271-1277.
4. Misra S, Chaturvedi A, Misra NC. Gallbladder cancer. Curr Treat Options Gastroenterol 2006; 9:95-106.
5. Moerman CJ, Bueno-de-Mesquita HB. The epidemiology of gallbladder cancer: lifestyle related risk factors and limited surgical possibilities for prevention. Hepatogastroenterology 1999; 46:1533-1539.
6. Pandey M, Shukla VK. Diet and gallbladder cancer: a case-control study. Eur J Cancer Prev 2002; 11:365-368.
7. Lazcano-Ponce EC, Miquel JF, Munoz N, et al. Epidemiology and molecular pathology of gallbladder cancer. CA Cancer J Clin 2001; 51:349-364.
8. Parkin DM, Whelan SL, Ferlay J, et al. Cancer Incidence in Five Continents, Volumes I to VIII. IARC CancerBase No. 7, 2005.
9. Chaurasia P, Thakur MK, Shukla HS. What causes cancer gallbladder?: a review. HPB Surg 1999; 11:217-224.
10. de Groen PC, Gores GJ, LaRusso NF, et al. Biliary tract cancers. N Engl J Med 1999; 341:1368-1378.
11. Corrias B, Palma A. [Primitive gall bladder carcinoma in the aged. Clinical statistical contribution]. G Ital Oncol 1987; 7:25-28.
12. Csendes A, Becerra M, Rojas J, et al. Number and size of stones in patients with asymptomatic and symptomatic gallstones and gallbladder carcinoma: a prospective study of 592 cases. J Gastrointest Surg 2000; 4:481-485.
13. Ishiguro S, Inoue M, Kurahashi N, et al. Risk factors of biliary tract cancer in a large-scale population-based cohort study in Japan (JPHC study); with special focus on cholelithiasis, body mass index, and their effect modification. Cancer Causes Control 2008; 19:33-41.
14. Kaushik SP. Current perspectives in gallbladder carcinoma. J Gastroenterol Hepatol 2001; 16:848-854.
15. Kayahara M, Nagakawa T. Recent trends of gallbladder cancer in Japan: an analysis of 4,770 patients. Cancer 2007; 110:572-580.
16. Kimura W, Shimada H, Kuroda A, et al. Carcinoma of the gallbladder and extrahepatic bile duct in autopsy cases of the aged, with special reference to its relationship to gallstones. Am J Gastroenterol 1989; 84:386-390.
17. Koga A, Yamauchi S, Nakayama F. Primary carcinoma of the gallbladder. Am Surg 1985; 51:529-533.
18. Lowenfels AB, Maisonneuve P, Boyle P, et al. Epidemiology of gallbladder cancer. Hepatogastroenterology 1999; 46:1529-1532.
19. Kumar JR, Tewari M, Rai A, et al. An objective assessment of demography of gallbladder cancer. J Surg Oncol 2006; 93:610-614.
20. Saxena S, Venkatachalam U, Tandon RK. Epidemiology of gallbladder cancer: present status. J Assoc Physicians India 1995; 43:204-206.
21. Strom BL, Hibberd PL, Soper KA, et al. International variations in epidemiology of cancers of the extrahepatic biliary tract. Cancer Res 1985; 45:5165-5168.
22. Parkash O. On the relationship of cholelithiasis to carcinoma of the gall-bladder and on the sex dependency of the carcinoma of the bile ducts. A study based on the autopsy data from 1928 to 1972. Digestion 1975; 12:129-133.
23. La Vecchia C, Levi F. Sex differentials in Swiss cancer mortality. Soz Praventivmed 1988; 33:140-143.
24. Levi F, La Vecchia C, Lucchini F, et al. Trends in cancer mortality sex ratios in Europe, 1950-1989. World Health Stat Q 1992; 45:117-164.
25. Watanabe T, Omori M, Fukuda H, et al. Analysis of sex, age and disease factors contributing to prolonged life expectancy at birth, in cases of malignant neoplasms in Japan. J Epidemiol 2003; 13:169-175.
26. Baskaran V, Vij U, Sahni P, et al. Do the progesterone receptors have a role to play in gallbladder cancer? Int J Gastrointest Cancer 2005; 35:61-68.
27. Chen A, Huminer D. The role of estrogen receptors in the development of gallstones and gallbladder cancer. Med Hypotheses 1991; 36:259-260.
28. Endoh K, Nakadaira H, Yamazaki O, et al. [Risk factors for gallbladder cancer in Chilean females]. Nippon Koshu Eisei Zasshi 1997; 44:113-122.
29. Judd HL, Meldrum DR, Deftos LJ, et al. Estrogen replacement therapy: indications and complications. Ann Intern Med 1983; 98:195-205.
30. Pandey M, Shukla VK. Lifestyle, parity, menstrual and reproductive factors and risk of gallbladder cancer. Eur J Cancer Prev 2003; 12:269-272.
31. Rao S, Arya A, Aggarwal S, et al. Pure squamous cell carcinoma of the gall bladder. Indian J Pathol Microbiol 2007; 50:599-600.
32. Chan KM, Yu MC, Lee WC, et al. Adenosquamous/squamous cell carcinoma of the gallbladder. J Surg Oncol 2007; 95:129-134.
33. Mingoli A, Brachini G, Petroni R, et al. Squamous and adenosquamous cell carcinomas of the gallbladder. J Exp Clin Cancer Res 2005; 24:143-150.
34. Andrea C, Francesco C. Squamous-cell and non-squamous-cell carcinomas of the gallbladder have different risk factors. Lancet Oncol 2003; 4:393-394.
35. Willcox J, Chang FC. Squamous cell carcinoma of the gallbladder. Kans Med 1993; 94:133-134.
36. Hanada M, Shimizu H, Takami M. Squamous cell carcinoma of the gallbladder associated with squamous metaplasia and adenocarcinoma in situ of the mucosal columnar epithelium. Acta Pathol Jpn 1986; 36:1879-1886.
37. Karasawa T, Itoh K, Komukai M, et al. Squamous cell carcinoma of gallbladder-report of two cases and review of literature. Acta Pathol Jpn 1981; 31:299-308.
38. Chianale J, Valdivia G, del Pino G, et al. [Gallbladder cancer mortality in Chile and its relation to cholecystectomy rates. An analysis of the last decade]. Rev Med Chil 1990; 118:1284-1288.
39. Diehl AK, Beral V. Cholecystectomy and changing mortality from gallbladder cancer. Lancet 1981; 2:187-189.
40. Surveillance, Epidemiology, and End Results (SEER) Program (www.seer.cancer.gov) SEER*Stat Database: Incidence - SEER 17 RegsLimited Use, Nov 2006 Sub (1973-2004 varying), National Cancer Institute, DCCPS, Surveillance Research Program, Cancer Statistics Branch, released April 2003, based on the November 2006 submission. 2007.

41. Wood R, Fraser LA, Brewster DH, et al. Epidemiology of gallbladder cancer and trends in cholecystectomy rates in Scotland, 1968-1998. Eur J Cancer 2003; 39:2080-2086.

42. Sheth S, Bedford A, Chopra S. Primary gallbladder cancer: recognition of risk factors and the role of prophylactic cholecystectomy. Am J Gastroenterol 2000; 95:1402-1410.

43. Fraumeni JF, Jr. Cancers of the pancreas and biliary tract: epidemiological considerations. Cancer Res 1975; 35:3437-3446.

44. Pandey M. Risk factors for gallbladder cancer: a reappraisal. Eur J Cancer Prev 2003; 12:15-24.

45. Zatonski WA, Lowenfels AB, Boyle P, et al. Epidemiologic aspects of gallbladder cancer: a case-control study of the SEARCH Program of the International Agency for Research on Cancer. J Natl Cancer Inst 1997; 89:1132-1138.

46. Zatonski W, La Vecchia C, Levi F, et al. Descriptive epidemiology of gall-bladder cancer in Europe. J Cancer Res Clin Oncol 1993; 119:165-171.

47. Levi F, Lucchini F, Negri E, et al. The recent decline in gallbladder cancer mortality in Europe. Eur J Cancer Prev 2003; 12:265-267.

48. Wistuba, II, Gazdar AF. Gallbladder cancer: lessons from a rare tumour. Nat Rev Cancer 2004; 4:695-706.

49. Rios-Dalenz J, Correa P, Haenszel W. Morbidity from cancer in La Paz, Bolivia. Int J Cancer 1981; 28:307-314.

50. Rios-Dalenz J, Takabayashi A, Henson DE, et al. Cancer of the gallbladder in Bolivia: suggestions concerning etiology. Am J Gastroenterol 1985; 80:371-375.

51. Rios-Dalenz J, Takabayashi A, Henson DE, et al. The epidemiology of cancer of the extra-hepatic biliary tract in Bolivia. Int J Epidemiol 1983; 12:156-160.

52. Randi G, Franceschi S, La Vecchia C. Gallbladder cancer worldwide: geographical distribution and risk factors. Int J Cancer 2006; 118:1591-1602.

53. De Aretxabala X, Roa I, Araya JC, et al. Gallbladder cancer in patients less than 40 years old. Br J Surg 1994; 81:111.

54. Kirschbaum A, Pizzi A. [Which are the causes death among Chilean women?]. Rev Med Chil 1995; 123:909-915.

55. Medina E, Kaempffer AM. [Cancer mortality in Chile: epidemiological considerations]. Rev Med Chil 2001; 129:1195-1202.

56. Medina E, Kaempffer AM. [Adult mortality in Chile]. Rev Med Chil 2000; 128:1144-1149.

57. Nervi F, Duarte I, Gomez G, et al. Frequency of gallbladder cancer in Chile, a high-risk area. Int J Cancer 1988; 41:657-660.

58. Andia KM, Gederlini GA, Ferreccio RC. [Gallbladder cancer: trend and risk distribution in Chile]. Rev Med Chil 2006; 134:565-574.

59. Tominaga S, Kuroishi T, Ogawa H, et al. Epidemiologic aspects of biliary tract cancer in Japan. Natl Cancer Inst Monogr 1979; 25-34.

60. Devor EJ, Buechley RW. Gallbladder cancer in Hispanic New Mexicans: I. General population, 1957-1977. Cancer 1980; 45:1705-1712.

61. Devor EJ. Ethnogeographic patterns in gallbladder cancer. The Hague, Boston, Hingham, MA: M. Nijhoff, Distributors for the United States and Canada, Kluwer Boston, 1982.

62. Goodman MT, Yamamoto J. Descriptive study of gallbladder, extrahepatic bile duct, and ampullary cancers in the United States, 1997-2002. Cancer Causes Control 2007; 18:415-422.

63. Cobb N, Paisano RE. Patterns of cancer mortality among Native Americans. Cancer 1998; 83:2377-2383.

64. Nutting PA, Freeman WL, Risser DR, et al. Cancer incidence among American Indians and Alaska Natives, 1980 through 1987. Am J Public Health 1993; 83:1589-1598.

65. Norsted TL, White E. Cancer incidence among Native Americans of western Washington. Int J Epidemiol 1989; 18:22-27.

66. Lowenfels AB, Walker AM, Althaus DP, et al. Gallstone growth, size, and risk of gallbladder cancer: an interracial study. Int J Epidemiol 1989; 18:50-54.

67. Weiss KM, Ferrell RE, Hanis CL, et al. Genetics and epidemiology of gallbladder disease in New World native peoples.

68. Young TK, Frank JW. Cancer surveillance in a remote Indian population in northwestern Ontario. Am J Public Health 1983; 73:515-520.

69. Boss LP, Lanier AP, Dohan PH, et al. Cancers of the gallbladder and biliary tract in Alaskan natives: 1970-79. J Natl Cancer Inst 1982; 69:1005-1007.

70. Thomas DB. Epidemiologic studies of cancer in minority groups in the western United States. Natl Cancer Inst Monogr 1979:103-113.

71. Barakat J, Dunkelberg JC, Ma TY. Changing patterns of gallbladder carcinoma in New Mexico. Cancer 2006; 106:434-440.

72. Wiggins CL, Becker TM, Key CR, et al. Cancer mortality among New Mexico's Hispanics, American Indians, and non-Hispanic Whites, 1958-1987. J Natl Cancer Inst 1993; 85:1670-1678.

73. Sorem KA. Cancer incidence in the Zuni Indians of New Mexico. Yale J Biol Med 1985; 58:489-496.

74. Black WC, Key CR. Epidemiologic pathology of cancer in New Mexico's tri-ethnic population. Pathol Annu 1980; 15:181-194.

75. Morris DL, Buechley RW, Key CR, et al. Gallbladder disease and gallbladder cancer among American Indians in tricultural New Mexico. Cancer 1978; 42:2472-2477.

76. Black WC, Key CR, Carmany TB, et al. Carcinoma of the gallbladder in a population of Southwestern American Indians. Cancer 1977; 39:1267-1279.

77. Rudolph R, Cohen JJ, Gascoigne RH. Biliary cancer among Southwestern American Indians. Ariz Med 1970; 27:1-4.

78. Grimaldi CH, Nelson RG, Pettitt DJ, et al. Increased mortality with gallstone disease: results of a 20-year population-based survey in Pima Indians. Ann Intern Med 1993; 118:185-190.

79. Nielsen NH, Storm HH, Gaudette LA, et al. Cancer in Circumpolar Inuit 1969-1988. A summary. Acta Oncol 1996; 35:621-628.

80. Storm HH, Nielsen NH. Cancer of the digestive system in Circumpolar Inuit. Acta Oncol 1996; 35:553-570.

81. Diehl AK, Haffner SM, Knapp JA, et al. Dietary intake and the prevalence of gallbladder disease in Mexican Americans. Gastroenterology 1989; 97:1527-1533.

82. Diehl AK, Stern MP. Special health problems of Mexican-Americans: obesity, gallbladder disease, diabetes mellitus, and cardiovascular disease. Adv Intern Med 1989; 34:73-96.

83. Diehl AK, Stern MP, Ostrower VS, et al. Prevalence of clinical gallbladder disease in Mexican-American, Anglo, and black women. South Med J 1980; 73:438-441, 443.

84. Strom BL, Soloway RD, Rios-Dalenz JL, et al. Risk factors for gallbladder cancer. An international collaborative case-control study. Cancer 1995; 76:1747-1756.

85. Diehl AK. Epidemiology of gallbladder cancer: a synthesis of recent data. J Natl Cancer Inst 1980; 65:1209-1214.

86. Lee J, Demissie K, Lu SE, et al. Cancer incidence among Korean-American immigrants in the United States and native Koreans in South Korea. Cancer Control 2007; 14:78-85.

87. Tominaga S. Cancer incidence in Japanese in Japan, Hawaii, and western United States. Natl Cancer Inst Monogr 1985; 69:83-92.

88. Hemminki K, Li X. Familial liver and gall bladder cancer: a nationwide epidemiological study from Sweden. Gut 2003; 52:592-596.

89. Fernandez E, La Vecchia C, D'Avanzo B, et al. Family history and the risk of liver, gallbladder, and pancreatic cancer. Cancer Epidemiol Biomarkers Prev 1994; 3:209-212.

90. Trajber HJ, Szego T, de Camargo HS, Jr., et al. Adenocarcinoma of the gallbladder in two siblings. Cancer 1982; 50:1200-1203.

91. Garber JE, Shipley W. Carcinoma of the gall bladder in three members of a family. Cancer Genet Cytogenet 1989; 39:141-142.

92. Andreotti G, Chen J, Gao YT, et al. Serum lipid levels and the risk of biliary tract cancers and biliary stones: a population-based study in China. Int J Cancer 2008 May 15;122(10):

Am J Hum Genet 1984; 36:1259-1278.

2322-9.

93. Hsing AW, Gao YT, Han TQ, et al. Gallstones and the risk of biliary tract cancer: a population-based study in China. Br J Cancer 2007; 97:1577-1582.

94. Venniyoor A. Cholesterol gallstones and cancer of gallbladder (CAGB): molecular links. Med Hypotheses 2008;70(3): 646-53.

95. Hsing AW, Gao YT, McGlynn KA, et al. Biliary tract cancer and stones in relation to chronic liver conditions: a population-based study in Shanghai, China. Int J Cancer 2007; 120:1981-1985.

96. Roa I, Ibacache G, Roa J, et al. Gallstones and gallbladder cancer-volume and weight of gallstones are associated with gallbladder cancer: a case-control study. J Surg Oncol 2006; 93:624-628.

97. Dutta U, Nagi B, Garg PK, et al. Patients with gallstones develop gallbladder cancer at an earlier age. Eur J Cancer Prev 2005; 14:381-385.

98. Shi JS, Zhou LS, Han Y, et al. Expression of tumor necrosis factor and its receptor in gallstone and gallbladder carcinoma tissue. Hepatobiliary Pancreat Dis Int 2004; 3:448-452.

99. Rizvi TJ, Zuberi SJ. Risk factors for gall bladder cancer in Karachi. J Ayub Med Coll Abbottabad 2003; 15:16-18.

100. Bani-Hani KE, Yaghan RJ, Matalka, II, et al. Gallbladder cancer in northern Jordan. J Gastroenterol Hepatol 2003; 18:954-959.

101. Misra S, Chaturvedi A, Misra NC, et al. Carcinoma of the gallbladder. Lancet Oncol 2003; 4:167-176.

102. Roa I, Araya JC, Villaseca M, et al. Gallbladder cancer in a high risk area: morphological features and spread patterns. Hepatogastroenterology 1999; 46:1540-1546.

103. Scott TE, Carroll M, Cogliano FD, et al. A case-control assessment of risk factors for gallbladder carcinoma. Dig Dis Sci 1999; 44:1619-1625.

104. Serra I, Yamamoto M, Calvo A, et al. Association of chili pepper consumption, low socioeconomic status and longstanding gallstones with gallbladder cancer in a Chilean population. Int J Cancer 2002; 102:407-411.

105. Shaffer EA. Epidemiology and risk factors for gallstone disease: has the paradigm changed in the 21st century? Curr Gastroenterol Rep 2005; 7:132-140.

106. Yamamoto M, Nakajo S, Tahara E. Gallstones in gallbladder diseases. Acta Pathol Jpn 1989; 39:582-585.

107. Zhang XH, Andreotti G, Gao YT, et al. Tea drinking and the risk of biliary tract cancers and biliary stones: a population-based case-control study in Shanghai, China. Int J Cancer 2006; 118:3089-3094.

108. Zou S, Zhang L. Relative risk factors analysis of 3,922 cases of gallbladder cancer. Zhonghua Wai Ke Za Zhi 2000; 38:805-808.

109. Zou S, Zhang L, Zen G, et al. Clinical epidemiologic characteristics of 430 cases of gallbladder cancer. Chin Med J (Engl) 1998; 111:391-393.

110. Gornish AL, Averbach D, Schwartz MR. Carcinoma of the gallbladder found during laparoscopic cholecystectomy: a case report and review of the literature. J Laparoendosc Surg 1991; 1:361-367.

111. Gurleyik G, Gurleyik E, Ozturk A, et al. Gallbladder carcinoma associated with gallstones. Acta Chir Belg 2002; 102:203-206.

112. Lowenfels AB, Lindstrom CG, Conway MJ, et al. Gallstones and risk of gallbladder cancer. J Natl Cancer Inst 1985; 75:77-80.

113. Maringhini A, Moreau JA, Melton LJ, 3rd, et al. Gallstones, gallbladder cancer, and other gastrointestinal malignancies. An epidemiologic study in Rochester, Minnesota. Ann Intern Med 1987; 107:30-35.

114. Newman HF, Northup JD. Gallbladder carcinoma in cholelithiasis: a study of probability. Geriatrics 1964; 19:453-455.

115. Chow WH, Johansen C, Gridley G, et al. Gallstones, cholecystectomy and risk of cancers of the liver, biliary tract and pancreas. Br J Cancer 1999; 79:640-644.

116. Ahrens W, Timmer A, Vyberg M, et al. Risk factors for extrahepatic biliary tract carcinoma in men: medical conditions and lifestyle: results from a European multicentre case-control study. Eur J Gastroenterol Hepatol 2007; 19:623-630.

117. Kuriyama S, Tsubono Y, Hozawa A, et al. Obesity and risk of cancer in Japan. Int J Cancer 2005; 113:148-157.

118. Barnard ND, Nicholson A, Howard JL. The medical costs attributable to meat consumption. Prev Med 1995; 24:646-655.

119. Moerman CJ, Bueno de Mesquita HB, Smeets FW, et al. Consumption of foods and micronutrients and the risk of cancer of the biliary tract. Prev Med 1995; 24:591-602.

120. Diehl AK, Rosenthal M, Hazuda HP, et al. Socioeconomic status and the prevalence of clinical gallbladder disease. J Chronic Dis 1985; 38:1019-1026.

121. Engeland A, Tretli S, Austad G, et al. Height and body mass index in relation to colorectal and gallbladder cancer in two million Norwegian men and women. Cancer Causes Control 2005; 16:987-996.

122. Vitetta L, Sali A, Little P, et al. Gallstones and gall bladder carcinoma. Aust NZ J Surg 2000; 70:667-673.

123. Diehl AK. Gallstone size and the risk of gallbladder cancer. JAMA 1983; 250:2323-2326.

124. Serra I, Diehl AK. Number and size of stones in patients with asymptomatic and symptomatic gallstones and gallbladder carcinoma. J Gastrointest Surg 2002; 6:272-273; author reply 273.

125. Moerman CJ, Lagerwaard FJ, Bueno de Mesquita HB, et al. Gallstone size and the risk of gallbladder cancer. Scand J Gastroenterol 1993; 28:482-486.

126. Sakoda LC, Gao YT, Chen BE, et al. Prostaglandin-endoperoxide synthase 2 (PTGS2) gene polymorphisms and risk of biliary tract cancer and gallstones: a population-based study in Shanghai, China. Carcinogenesis 2006; 27:1251-1256.

127. Liu E, Sakoda LC, Gao YT, et al. Aspirin use and risk of biliary tract cancer: a population-based study in Shanghai, China. Cancer Epidemiol Biomarkers Prev 2005; 14:1315-1318.

128. Tazuma S, Kajiyama G. Carcinogenesis of malignant lesions of the gall bladder. The impact of chronic inflammation and gallstones. Langenbecks Arch Surg 2001; 386:224-229.

129. Lewis JT, Talwalkar JA, Rosen CB, et al. Prevalence and risk factors for gallbladder neoplasia in patients with primary sclerosing cholangitis: evidence for a metaplasia-dysplasia-carcinoma sequence. Am J Surg Pathol 2007; 31:907-913.

130. Gupta SC, Misra V, Singh PA, et al. Gall stones and carcinoma gall bladder. Indian J Pathol Microbiol 2000; 43:147-154.

131. Duarte I, Llanos O, Domke H, et al. Metaplasia and precursor lesions of gallbladder carcinoma. Frequency, distribution, and probability of detection in routine histologic samples. Cancer 1993; 72:1878-1884.

132. Strom BL, Iliopoulos D, Atkinson B, et al. Pathophysiology of tumor progression in human gallbladder: flow cytometry, CEA, and CA 19-9 levels in bile and serum in different stages of gallbladder disease. J Natl Cancer Inst 1989; 81:1575-1580.

133. Chapman RW. Risk factors for biliary tract carcinogenesis. Ann Oncol 1999; 10(suppl 4):308-311.

134. Zhi YH, Liu RS, Song MM, et al. Cyclooxygenase-2 promotes angiogenesis by increasing vascular endothelial growth factor and predicts prognosis in gallbladder carcinoma. World J Gastroenterol 2005; 11:3724-3728.

135. Kianmanesh R, Scaringi S, Castel B, et al. [Precancerous lesions of the gallbladder]. J Chir (Paris) 2007; 144:278-286.

136. Stephen AE, Berger DL. Carcinoma in the porcelain gallbladder: a relationship revisited. Surgery 2001; 129:699-703.

137. Tsai CJ. Porcelain gallbladder and cholangiocarcinoma with anomalous pancreaticobiliary union. Dig Dis Sci 2001; 46:773-775.

138. Shimizu M, Miura J, Tanaka T, et al. Porcelain gallbladder: relation between its type by ultrasound and incidence of cancer. J Clin Gastroenterol 1989; 11:471-476.

139. Gregorie HB, Jr., Robertson HC, 3rd, Treen B, et al. Porce-

lain gallbladder. J SC Med Assoc 1982; 78:48-50.

140. Berk RN, Armbuster TG, Saltzstein SL. Carcinoma in the porcelain gallbladder. Radiology 1973; 106:29-31.

141. Kumar S, Kumar S, Kumar S. Infection as a risk factor for gallbladder cancer. J Surg Oncol 2006; 93:633-639.

142. Zimnoch L, Szynaka B, Kupisz A. Study on carcinogenesis in chronic cholecystitis. Rocz Akad Med Bialymst 2004; 49(suppl 1):49-51.

143. Kanoh K, Shimura T, Tsutsumi S, et al. Significance of contracted cholecystitis lesions as high risk for gallbladder carcinogenesis. Cancer Lett 2001; 169:7-14.

144. Fumino S, Tokiwa K, Ono S, et al. Cyclooxygenase-2 expression in the gallbladder of patients with anomalous arrangement of the pancreaticobiliary duct. J Pediatr Surg 2003; 38:585-589.

145. Kimura Y, Nishikawa N, Okita K, et al. Biliary tract malignancy and chronic inflammation from the perspective of pancreaticobiliary maljunction. Oncology 2005; 69(suppl 1):41-45.

146. Cunningham SC, Alexander HR. Porcelain gallbladder and cancer: ethnicity explains a discrepant literature? Am J Med 2007; 120:e17-18.

147. Towfigh S, McFadden DW, Cortina GR, et al. Porcelain gallbladder is not associated with gallbladder carcinoma. Am Surg 2001; 67:7-10.

148. Srivastava A, Pandey SN, Choudhuri G, Mittal B. Role of genetic variant A-204C of cholesterol 7alpha-hydroxylase (CYP7A1) in susceptibility to gallbladder cancer. Mol Genet Metab. 2008 May;94(1):83-9.

149. Strom BL, Soloway RD, Rios-Dalenz J, et al. Biochemical epidemiology of gallbladder cancer. Hepatology 1996; 23:1402-1411.

150. Sugiyama Y, Kobori H, Hakamada K, et al. Altered bile composition in the gallbladder and common bile duct of patients with anomalous pancreaticobiliary ductal junction. World J Surg 2000; 24:17-20; discussion 21.

151. Peters WH, van Schaik A, Peters JH, et al. Oxidised- and total non-protein bound glutathione and related thiols in gallbladder bile of patients with various gastrointestinal disorders. BMC Gastroenterol 2007; 7:7.

152. Park JY, Park BK, Ko JS, et al. Bile acid analysis in biliary tract cancer. Yonsei Med J 2006; 47:817-825.

153. Pandey M, Shukla VK. Fatty acids, biliary bile acids, lipid peroxidation products and gallbladder carcinogenesis. Eur J Cancer Prev 2000; 9:165-171.

154. Pandey M, Sharma LB, Shukla VK. Cytochrome P-450 expression and lipid peroxidation in gallbladder cancer. J Surg Oncol 2003; 82:180-183.

155. Reznik G, Mohr U, Lijinsky W. Carcinogenic effect of N-nitroso-2,6-dimethylmorpholine in Syrian golden hamsters. J Natl Cancer Inst 1978; 60:371-378.

156. Toth B, Nagel D. Tumors induced in mice by N-methyl-N-formylhydrazine of the false morel Gyromitra esculenta. J Natl Cancer Inst 1978; 60:201-204.

157. Birt DF, Pour PM. Effects of the interaction of dietary fat and protein on N-nitrosobis(2-oxopropyl)amine-induced carcinogenesis and spontaneous lesions in Syrian golden hamsters. J Natl Cancer Inst 1985; 74:1121-1127.

158. Inomata N. Effects of ethyl 4-chloro-2-methylphenoxyacetate on bile composition in golden hamsters. Tohoku J Exp Med 1992; 166:239-249.

159. Pandey M. Environmental pollutants in gallbladder carcinogenesis. J Surg Oncol 2006; 93:640-643.

160. Paraf F, Paraf A, Barge J. [Are industrial toxic substances a risk factor in gallbladder cancer?]. Gastroenterol Clin Biol 1990; 14:877-880.

161. Mancuso TF, Brennan MJ. Epidemiological considerations of cancer of the gallbladder, bile ducts and salivary glands in the rubber industry. J Occup Med 1970; 12:333-341.

162. Marsh GM. Critical review of epidemiologic studies related to ingested asbestos. Environ Health Perspect 1983; 53:49-56.

163. Kuzmickiene I, Didziapetris R, Stukonis M. Cancer incidence in the workers cohort of textile manufacturing factory in Alytus, Lithuania. J Occup Environ Med 2004; 46:147-153.

164. Yassi A, Tate RB, Routledge M. Cancer incidence and mortality in workers employed at a transformer manufacturing plant: update to a cohort study. Am J Ind Med 2003; 44:58-62.

165. Weiderpass E, Vainio H, Kauppinen T, et al. Occupational exposures and gastrointestinal cancers among Finnish women. J Occup Environ Med 2003; 45:305-315.

166. Goldberg MS, Theriault G. Retrospective cohort study of workers of a synthetic textiles plant in Quebec: I. General mortality. Am J Ind Med 1994; 25:889-907.

167. Mironov AI, Shan'gina OV, Bul'bulian MA. [Preliminaries to a study of epidemiology of occupational cancer among workers of shoe factories]. Med Tr Prom Ekol 1994:5-7.

168. Brown DP. Mortality of workers exposed to polychlorinated biphenyls-an update. Arch Environ Health 1987; 42:333-339.

169. Malker HS, McLaughlin JK, Malker BK, et al. Biliary tract cancer and occupation in Sweden. Br J Ind Med 1986; 43:257-262.

170. Rushton L, Alderson MR, Nagarajah CR. Epidemiological survey of maintenance workers in London Transport Executive bus garages and Chiswick Works. Br J Ind Med 1983; 40:340-345.

171. Morinaga K, Oshima A, Hara I. Multiple primary cancers following exposure to benzidine and beta-naphthylamine. Am J Ind Med 1982; 3:243-246.

172. Mancuso TF. Problems and perspective in epidemiological study of occupational health hazards in the rubber industry. Environ Health Perspect 1976; 17:21-30.

173. Chen W, Li D, Cannan RJ, et al. Common presence of Helicobacter DNA in the gallbladder of patients with gallstone diseases and controls. Dig Liver Dis 2003; 35:237-243.

174. Mager DL. Bacteria and cancer: cause, coincidence or cure? A review. J Transl Med 2006; 4:14.

175. Murata H, Tsuji S, Tsujii M, et al. Helicobacter bilis infection in biliary tract cancer. Aliment Pharmacol Ther 2004; 20(suppl 1):90-94.

176. Landis SH, Murray T, Bolden S, et al. Cancer statistics, 1998. CA Cancer J Clin 1998; 48:6-29.

177. Parkin DM, Ohshima H, Srivatanakul P, et al. Cholangiocarcinoma: epidemiology, mechanisms of carcinogenesis and prevention. Cancer Epidemiol Biomarkers Prev 1993; 2:537-544.

178. McGlynn KA, Tarone RE, El-Serag HB. A comparison of trends in the incidence of hepatocellular carcinoma and intrahepatic cholangiocarcinoma in the United States. Cancer Epidemiol Biomarkers Prev 2006; 15:1198-1203.

179. Patel T. Increasing incidence and mortality of primary intrahepatic cholangiocarcinoma in the United States. Hepatology 2001; 33:1353-1357.

180. Welzel TM, Mellemkjaer L, Gloria G, et al. Risk factors for intrahepatic cholangiocarcinoma in a low-risk population: a nationwide case-control study. Int J Cancer 2007; 120:638-641.

181. Sriamporn S, Pisani P, Pipitgool V, et al. Prevalence of Opisthorchis viverrini infection and incidence of cholangiocarcinoma in Khon Kaen, Northeast Thailand. Trop Med Int Health 2004; 9:588-594.

182. Suzuki H, Isaji S, Pairojkul C, et al. Comparative clinicopathological study of resected intrahepatic cholangiocarcinoma in northeast Thailand and Japan. J Hepatobiliary Pancreat Surg 2000; 7:206-211.

183. Khan SA, Taylor-Robinson SD, Toledano MB, et al. Changing international trends in mortality rates for liver, biliary and pancreatic tumours. J Hepatol 2002; 37:806-813.

184. Patel T. Worldwide trends in mortality from biliary tract malignancies. BMC Cancer 2002; 2:10.

185. McLean L, Patel T. Racial and ethnic variations in the epidemiology of intrahepatic cholangiocarcinoma in the United States. Liver Int 2006; 26:1047-1053.

186. Shaib YH, Davila JA, McGlynn K, et al. Rising incidence of intrahepatic cholangiocarcinoma in the United States: a true increase? J Hepatol 2004; 40:472-477.

187. Taylor-Robinson SD, Toledano MB, Arora S, et al. Increase

in mortality rates from intrahepatic cholangiocarcinoma in England and Wales 1968-1998. Gut 2001; 48:816-820.

188. Shaib Y, El-Serag HB. The epidemiology of cholangiocarcinoma. Semin Liver Dis 2004; 24:115-125.

189. Welzel TM, Graubard BI, El-Serag HB, et al. Risk factors for intrahepatic and extrahepatic cholangiocarcinoma in the United States: a population-based case-control study. Clin Gastroenterol Hepatol 2007; 5:1221-1228.

190. Wood R, Brewster DH, Fraser LA, et al. Do increases in mortality from intrahepatic cholangiocarcinoma reflect a genuine increase in risk? Insights from cancer registry data in Scotland. Eur J Cancer 2003; 39:2087-2092.

191. Welzel TM, McGlynn KA, Hsing AW, et al. Impact of classification of hilar cholangiocarcinomas (Klatskin tumors) on the incidence of intra- and extrahepatic cholangiocarcinoma in the United States. J Natl Cancer Inst 2006; 98:873-875.

192. Faria G, de Aretxabala X, Sierralta A, et al. [Primary cholangiocarcinoma associated with Caroli disease]. Rev Med Chil 2001; 129:1433-1438.

193. Gupta AK, Gupta A, Bhardwaj VK, et al. Caroli's disease. Indian J Pediatr 2006; 73:233-235.

194. Jain D, Sarode VR, Abdul-Karim FW, et al. Evidence for the neoplastic transformation of Von-Meyenburg complexes. Am J Surg Pathol 2000; 24:1131-1139.

195. Okamura K, Hayakawa H, Kuze M, et al. Triple carcinomas of the biliary tract associated with congenital choledochal dilatation and pancreaticobiliary maljunction. J Gastroenterol 2000; 35:465-471.

196. Shimonishi T, Sasaki M, Nakanuma Y. Precancerous lesions of intrahepatic cholangiocarcinoma. J Hepatobiliary Pancreat Surg 2000; 7:542-550.

197. Tsuchida A, Kasuya K, Endo M, et al. High risk of bile duct carcinogenesis after primary resection of a congenital biliary dilatation. Oncol Rep 2003; 10:1183-1187.

198. Ben-Menachem T. Risk factors for cholangiocarcinoma. Eur J Gastroenterol Hepatol 2007; 19:615-617.

199. Phinney PR, Austin GE, Kadell BM. Cholangiocarcinoma arising in Caroli's disease. Arch Pathol Lab Med 1981; 105:194-197.

200. Kim HJ, Kim MH, Lee SK, et al. Normal structure, variations, and anomalies of the pancreaticobiliary ducts of Koreans: a nationwide cooperative prospective study. Gastrointest Endosc 2002; 55:889-896.

201. Juttijudata P, Palavatana C, Chiemchaisri C, et al. Choledochal cyst. J Med Assoc Thai 1984; 67:150-155.

202. Nicholl M, Pitt HA, Wolf P, et al. Choledochal cysts in western adults: complexities compared to children. J Gastrointest Surg 2004; 8:245-252.

203. Komi N, Tamura T, Miyoshi Y, et al. Nationwide survey of cases of choledochal cyst. Analysis of coexistent anomalies, complications and surgical treatment in 645 cases. Surg Gastroenterol 1984; 3:69-73.

204. Kimura K, Tsugawa C, Ogawa K, et al. Choledochal cyst. Etiological considerations and surgical management in 22 cases. Arch Surg 1978; 113:159-163.

205. Tsuchiya R, Harada N, Ito T, et al. Malignant tumors in choledochal cysts. Ann Surg 1977; 186:22-28.

206. Yeo CJ, Pitt HA, Cameron JL. Cholangiocarcinoma. Surg Clin North Am 1990; 70:1429-1447.

207. Chao TC, Jan YY, Chen MF. Primary carcinoma of the gallbladder associated with anomalous pancreaticobiliary ductal junction. J Clin Gastroenterol 1995; 21:306-308.

208. Chijiiwa K, Kimura H, Tanaka M. Malignant potential of the gallbladder in patients with anomalous pancreaticobiliary ductal junction. The difference in risk between patients with and without choledochal cyst. Int Surg 1995; 80:61-64.

209. Jung YS, Lee KJ, Kim H, et al. Risk factor for extrahepatic bile duct cancer in patients with anomalous pancreaticobiliary ductal union. Hepatogastroenterology 2004; 51:946-949.

210. Cheng SP, Yang TL, Jeng KS, et al. Choledochal cyst in adults: aetiological considerations to intrahepatic involvement. A NZ J Surg 2004; 74:964-967.

211. Komi N, Takehara H, Kunitomo K. Choledochal cyst: anom-

212. Soreide K, Soreide JA. Bile duct cyst as precursor to biliary tract cancer. Ann Surg Oncol 2007; 14:1200-1211.

213. Yamasaki K, Yamasaki A, Tosaki M, et al. Tissue distribution of Thorotrast and role of internal irradiation in carcinogenesis. Oncol Rep 2004; 12:733-738.

214. Choi BI, Han JK, Hong ST, et al. Clonorchiasis and cholangiocarcinoma: etiologic relationship and imaging diagnosis. Clin Microbiol Rev 2004; 17:540-552, table of contents.

215. Wu GS, Zou SQ, Wu XY, et al. Effects of cyclooxygenase-2 antisense vector on proliferation of human cholangiocarcinoma cells. Chin Med Sci J 2004; 19:89-92.

216. Yoon JH, Canbay AE, Werneburg NW, et al. Oxysterols induce cyclooxygenase-2 expression in cholangiocytes: implications for biliary tract carcinogenesis. Hepatology 2004; 39:732-738.

217. Wu GS, Wang JH, Liu ZR, et al. Expression of cyclooxygenase-1 and -2 in extra-hepatic cholangiocarcinoma. Hepatobiliary Pancreat Dis Int 2002; 1:429-433.

218. Holzinger F, Z'Graggen K, Buchler MW. Mechanisms of biliary carcinogenesis: a pathogenetic multi-stage cascade towards cholangiocarcinoma. Ann Oncol 1999; 10(suppl 4):122-126.

219. Dayton MT, Longmire WP, Jr., Tompkins RK. Caroli's disease: a premalignant condition? Am J Surg 1983; 145:41-48.

220. Ohta T, Nagakawa T, Konishi I, et al. Clinical experience of intrahepatic cholangiocarcinoma associated with hepatolithiasis. Jpn J Surg 1988; 18:47-53.

221. Nishihara K, Koga A, Sumiyoshi K, et al. Intrahepatic calculi associated with cholangiocarcinoma. Jpn J Surg 1986; 16:367-370.

222. Nakanuma Y, Terada T, Tanaka Y, et al. Are hepatolithiasis and cholangiocarcinoma aetiologically related? A morphological study of 12 cases of hepatolithiasis associated with cholangiocarcinoma. Virchows Arch A Pathol Anat Histopathol 1985; 406:45-58.

223. Bjornsson E, Angulo P. Cholangiocarcinoma in young individuals with and without primary sclerosing cholangitis. Am J Gastroenterol 2007; 102:1677-1682.

224. Broome U, Lofberg R, Veress B, et al. Primary sclerosing cholangitis and ulcerative colitis: evidence for increased neoplastic potential. Hepatology 1995; 22:1404-1408.

225. Fevery J, Verslype C, Lai G, et al. Incidence, diagnosis, and therapy of cholangiocarcinoma in patients with primary sclerosing cholangitis. Dig Dis Sci 2007; 52:3123-3135.

226. Yamamoto T, Uki K, Takeuchi K, et al. Early gallbladder carcinoma associated with primary sclerosing cholangitis and ulcerative colitis. J Gastroenterol 2003; 38:704-706.

227. Haworth AC, Manley PN, Groll A, et al. Bile duct carcinoma and biliary tract dysplasia in chronic ulcerative colitis. Arch Pathol Lab Med 1989; 113:434-436.

228. Mir-Madjlessi SH, Farmer RG, Sivak MV, Jr. Bile duct carcinoma in patients with ulcerative colitis. Relationship to sclerosing cholangitis: report of six cases and review of the literature. Dig Dis Sci 1987; 32:145-154.

229. Williams SM, Harned RK. Bile duct carcinoma associated with chronic ulcerative colitis. Dis Colon Rectum 1981; 24:42-44.

230. Akwari OE, van Heerden JA, Adson MA, et al. Bile duct carcinoma associated with ulcerative colitis. Rev Surg 1976; 33:289-293.

231. Akwari OE, Van Heerden JA, Foulk WT, et al. Cancer of the bile ducts associated with ulcerative colitis. Ann Surg 1975; 181:303-309.

232. Ritchie JK, Allan RN, Macartney J, et al. Biliary tract carcinoma associated with ulcerative colitis. Q J Med 1974; 43:263-279.

233. Roberts-Thomson IC, Strickland RG, Mackay IR. Bile duct carcinoma in chronic ulcerative colitis. Aust NZ J Med 1973; 3:264-267.

234. Ross AP, Braasch JW. Ulcerative colitis and carcinoma of the proximal bile ducts. Gut 1973; 14:94-97.

235. Morowitz DA, Glagov S, Dordal E, et al. Carcinoma of the biliary tract complicating chronic ulcerative colitis. Cancer 1971;

27:356-361.

236. Converse CF, Reagan JW, DeCosse JJ. Ulcerative colitis and carcinoma of the bile ducts. Am J Surg 1971; 121:39-45.

237. Babb RR, Lee RH, Peck OC. Cancer of the bile duct and chronic ulcerative colitis. Am J Surg 1970; 119:337-339.

238. Ulcerative colitis and cancer. Br Med J 1967; 1:322.

239. Yen S, Hsieh CC, MacMahon B. Extrahepatic bile duct cancer and smoking, beverage consumption, past medical history, and oral-contraceptive use. Cancer 1987; 59:2112-2116.

240. Sripa B, Kaewkes S, Sithithaworn P, et al. Liver fluke induces cholangiocarcinoma. PLoS Med 2007; 4:e201.

241. Haswell-Elkins MR, Mairiang E, Mairiang P, et al. Cross-sectional study of Opisthorchis viverrini infection and cholangiocarcinoma in communities within a high-risk area in northeast Thailand. Int J Cancer 1994; 59:505-509.

242. Parkin DM. The global health burden of infection-associated cancers in the year 2002. Int J Cancer 2006; 118:3030-3044.

243. Srivatanakul P, Ohshima H, Khlat M, et al. Opisthorchis viverrini infestation and endogenous nitrosamines as risk factors for cholangiocarcinoma in Thailand. Int J Cancer 1991; 48:821-825.

244. Srivatanakul P, Parkin DM, Jiang YZ, et al. The role of infection by Opisthorchis viverrini, hepatitis B virus, and aflatoxin exposure in the etiology of liver cancer in Thailand. A correlation study. Cancer 1991; 68:2411-2417.

245. Watanapa P. Cholangiocarcinoma in patients with opisthorchiasis. Br J Surg 1996; 83:1062-1064.

246. Mairiang E, Chaiyakum J, Chamadol N, et al. Ultrasound screening for Opisthorchis viverrini-associated cholangiocarcinomas: experience in an endemic area. Asian Pac J Cancer Prev 2006; 7:431-433.

247. Jinawath N, Chamgramol Y, Furukawa Y, et al. Comparison of gene expression profiles between Opisthorchis viverrini and non-Opisthorchis viverrini associated human intrahepatic cholangiocarcinoma. Hepatology 2006; 44:1025-1038.

248. Watanapa P, Watanapa WB. Liver fluke-associated cholangiocarcinoma. Br J Surg 2002; 89:962-970.

249. Elkins DB, Mairiang E, Sithithaworn P, et al. Cross-sectional patterns of hepatobiliary abnormalities and possible precursor conditions of cholangiocarcinoma associated with Opisthorchis viverrini infection in humans. Am J Trop Med Hyg 1996; 55:295-301.

250. Sithithaworn P, Haswell-Elkins MR, Mairiang P, et al. Parasite-associated morbidity: liver fluke infection and bile duct cancer in northeast Thailand. Int J Parasitol 1994; 24:833-843.

251. Srivatanakul P, Ohshima H, Khlat M, et al. Endogenous nitrosamines and liver fluke as risk factors for cholangiocarcinoma in Thailand. IARC Sci Publ 1991:88-95.

252. Lun ZR, Gasser RB, Lai DH, et al. Clonorchiasis: a key foodborne zoonosis in China. Lancet Infect Dis 2005; 5:31-41.

253. Schwartz DA. Cholangiocarcinoma associated with liver fluke infection: a preventable source of morbidity in Asian immigrants. Am J Gastroenterol 1986; 81:76-79.

254. Lim MK, Ju YH, Franceschi S, et al. Clonorchis sinensis infection and increasing risk of cholangiocarcinoma in the Republic of Korea. Am J Trop Med Hyg 2006; 75:93-96.

255. Choi D, Lim JH, Lee KT, et al. Cholangiocarcinoma and Clonorchis sinensis infection: a case-control study in Korea. J Hepatol 2006; 44:1066-1073.

256. Kim HJ, Yun SS, Jung KH, et al. Intrahepatic cholangiocarcinoma in Korea. J Hepatobiliary Pancreat Surg 1999; 6:142-148.

257. Jain RV, Mills PK, Parikh-Patel A. Cancer incidence in the south Asian population of California, 1988-2000. J Carcinog 2005; 4:21.

258. Honjo S, Srivatanakul P, Sriplung H, et al. Genetic and environmental determinants of risk for cholangiocarcinoma via Opisthorchis viverrini in a densely infested area in Nakhon Phanom, northeast Thailand. Int J Cancer 2005; 117:854-860.

259. Mitacek EJ, Brunnemann KD, Suttajit M, et al. Exposure to N-nitroso compounds in a population of high liver cancer regions in Thailand: volatile nitrosamine (VNA) levels in Thai food. Food Chem Toxicol 1999; 37:297-305.

260. Satarug S, Lang MA, Yongvanit P, et al. Induction of cytochrome P450 2A6 expression in humans by the carcinogenic parasite infection, opisthorchiasis viverrini. Cancer Epidemiol Biomarkers Prev 1996; 5:795-800.

261. Ikematsu Y, Tomioka T, Tajima Y, et al. Enhancement of biliary carcinogenesis in hamsters by cholecystokinin. World J Surg 1995; 19:847-850; discussion 850-841.

262. Bartsch H, Ohshima H, Pignatelli B, et al. Endogenously formed N-nitroso compounds and nitrosating agents in human cancer etiology. Pharmacogenetics 1992; 2:272-277.

263. Parkin DM, Srivatanakul P, Khlat M, et al. Liver cancer in Thailand. I. A case-control study of cholangiocarcinoma. Int J Cancer 1991; 48:323-328.

264. Schwartz DA. Helminths in the induction of cancer: Opisthorchis viverrini, Clonorchis sinensis and cholangiocarcinoma. Trop Geogr Med 1980; 32:95-100.

265. Imray CH, Newbold KM, Davis A, et al. Induction of cholangiocarcinoma in the Golden Syrian hamster using methylazoxymethyl acetate. Eur J Surg Oncol 1992; 18:373-378.

266. Brandt-Rauf PW, Fallon LF. Ampullary cancer in chemical workers. Br J Ind Med 1987; 44:569-570.

267. Anghileri LJ, Heidbreder M, Weiler G, et al. Liver tumors induced by 4-dimethylaminoazobenzene: experimental basis for a chemical carcinogenesis concept. Arch Geschwulstforsch 1976; 46:639-656.

268. Brown EV, Coleman RL. Carcinogenic activity of benzofuran and dibenzofuran analogs of p-dimethylaminoazobenzene. J Med Chem 1973; 16:717-718.

269. Byron WR, Bierbower GW, Brouwer JB, et al. Pathologic changes in rats and dogs from two-year feeding of sodium arsenite or sodium arsenate. Toxicol Appl Pharmacol 1967; 10:132-147.

270. Reddy KP, Buschmann RJ, Chomet B. Cholangiocarcinomas induced by feeding 3'-methyl-4-dimethylaminoazobenzene to rats. Histopathology and ultrastructure. Am J Pathol 1977; 87:189-204.

271. Wingren G. Mortality and cancer incidence in a Swedish art glassworks-an updated cohort study. Int Arch Occup Environ Health 2004; 77:599-603.

272. Szendroi M, Nemeth L, Vajta G. Asbestos bodies in a bile duct cancer after occupational exposure. Environ Res 1983; 30:270-280.

273. Szendroi M, Nemeth L, Vajta G. [Detection of asbestos particles in the cancerous bile duct of a patient with respiratory asbestosis]. Orv Hetil 1981; 122:1913-1915.

274. Thamavit W, Pratoomtone P, Kongtim S, et al. Inhibition by vitamin E of cholangiocarcinoma induction due to combined nitrite and aminopyrine. Asian Pac J Cancer Prev 2001; 2:69-70.

275. Fast Stats: Gallbladder Cancer- Surveillance, Epidemiology, and End Results (SEER) Program (www.seer.cancer.gov) SEER*Stat Database: Mortality - All COD, Public-Use With State, Total U.S. (1969-2004), National Cancer Institute, DCCPS, Surveillance Research Program, Cancer Statistics, released April 2007. Underlying mortality data provided by NCHS (www.cdc.gov/nchs). 2007.

276. Dhir V, Mohandas KM. Epidemiology of digestive tract cancers in India IV. Gall bladder and pancreas. Indian J Gastroenterol 1999; 18:24-28.

277. Levin B. Gallbladder carcinoma. Ann Oncol 1999; 10(suppl 4):129-130.

278. Egawa N, Tu Y, Kamisawa T. [Why is gallbladder cancer more frequent in women than in men?]. Nippon Rinsho 2006; 64(suppl 1):344-347.

279. Tavani A, Negri E, La Vecchia C. Menstrual and reproductive factors and biliary tract cancers. Eur J Cancer Prev 1996; 5:241-247.

280. Gustafsson U, Einarsson C, Eriksson LC, et al. DNA ploidy and S-phase fraction in carcinoma of the gallbladder related to histopathology, number of gallstones and survival. Anal Cell Pathol 2001; 23:143-152.

281. Hou L, Xu J, Gao YT, et al. CYP17 MspA1 polymorphism and risk of biliary tract cancers and gallstones: a population-based

study in Shanghai, China. Int J Cancer 2006; 118:2847-2853.

282. Hsing AW, Bai Y, Andreotti G, et al. Family history of gallstones and the risk of biliary tract cancer and gallstones: a population-based study in Shanghai, China. Int J Cancer 2007; 121:832-838.

283. Mano H, Roa I, Araya JC, et al. Comparison of mutagenic activity of bile between Chilean and Japanese female patients having cholelithiasis. Mutat Res 1996; 371:73-77.

284. Srivastava A, Pandey SN, Dixit M, et al. Cholecystokinin receptor A gene polymorphism in gallstone disease and gallbladder cancer. J Gastroenterol Hepatol 2007.

285. Tsuchiya Y, Serra I, Hori Y, et al. Free fatty acid concentrations in gallbladder bile collected from Chilean patients with gallstones. Clin Biochem 2006; 39:410-413.

286. Kang CM, Kim KS, Choi JS, et al. Gallbladder carcinoma associated with anomalous pancreaticobiliary duct junction. Can J Gastroenterol 2007; 21:383-387.

287. Hu B, Gong B, Zhou DY. Association of anomalous pancreaticobiliary ductal junction with gallbladder carcinoma in Chinese patients: an ERCP study. Gastrointest Endosc 2003; 57:541-545.

288. Elnemr A, Ohta T, Kayahara M, et al. Anomalous pancreaticobiliary ductal junction without bile duct dilatation in gallbladder cancer. Hepatogastroenterology 2001; 48:382-386.

289. Chao TC, Wang CS, Jan YY, et al. Carcinogenesis in the biliary system associated with APDJ. J Hepatobiliary Pancreat Surg 1999; 6:218-222.

290. Tanaka K, Ikoma A, Hamada N, et al. Biliary tract cancer accompanied by anomalous junction of pancreaticobiliary ductal system in adults. Am J Surg 1998; 175:218-220.

291. Uetsuji S, Okuda Y, Kwon AH, et al. Gallbladder cancer with a low junction of the cystic duct or an anomalous pancreaticobiliary junction. Eur J Gastroenterol Hepatol 1996; 8:1213-1217.

292. Chijiiwa K, Tanaka M, Nakayama F. Adenocarcinoma of the gallbladder associated with anomalous pancreaticobiliary ductal junction. Am Surg 1993; 59:430-434.

293. Kato T, Matsuda K, Kayaba H, et al. Pathology of anomalous junction of the pancreaticobiliary ductal system: mutagenicity of the contents of the biliary tract and nuclear atypia of the biliary epithelium. Keio J Med 1989; 38:167-176.

294. Yamauchi S, Koga A, Matsumoto S, et al. Anomalous junction of pancreaticobiliary duct without congenital choledochal cyst: a possible risk factor for gallbladder cancer. Am J Gastroenterol 1987; 82:20-24.

295. Kwon AH, Sakaida N. Simultaneous presence of xanthogranulomatous cholecystitis and gallbladder cancer. J Gastroenterol 2007; 42:703-704.

296. Takada M, Horita Y, Okuda S, et al. Genetic analysis of xanthogranulomatous cholecystitis: precancerous lesion of gallbladder cancer? Hepatogastroenterology 2002; 49:935-937.

297. Kato K, Akai S, Tominaga S, et al. A case-control study of biliary tract cancer in Niigata Prefecture, Japan. Jpn J Cancer Res 1989; 80:932-938.

298. Rai A, Mohapatra SC, Shukla HS. A review of association of dietary factors in gallbladder cancer. Indian J Cancer 2004; 41:147-151.

299. Herzog K, Goldblum JR. Gallbladder adenocarcinoma and acalculous chronic lymphoplasmacytic cholecystitis associated with ulcerative colitis [corrected]. Mod Pathol 1996; 9:194-198.

300. Dorudi S, Chapman RW, Kettlewell MG. Carcinoma of the gallbladder in ulcerative colitis and primary sclerosing cholangitis. Report of two cases. Dis Colon Rectum 1991; 34:827-828.

301. O'Connor R, Harding B, Greene D, et al. Primary carcinoma of the gall bladder associated with ulcerative colitis. Postgrad Med J 1986; 62:871-872.

302. Sharma V, Chauhan VS, Nath G, et al. Role of bile bacteria in gallbladder carcinoma. Hepatogastroenterology 2007; 54:1622-1625.

303. Pandey M, Vishwakarma RA, Khatri AK, et al. Bile, bacteria,

and gallbladder carcinogenesis. J Surg Oncol 1995; 58:282-283.

304. Bohr UR, Kuester D, Meyer F, et al. Low prevalence of Helicobacteraceae in gall-stone disease and gall-bladder carcinoma in the German population. Clin Microbiol Infect 2007; 13:525-531.

305. Pradhan SB, Dali S. Relation between gallbladder neoplasm and Helicobacter hepaticus infection. Kathmandu Univ Med J (KUMJ) 2004; 2:331-335.

306. Kobayashi T, Harada K, Miwa K, et al. Helicobacter genus DNA fragments are commonly detectable in bile from patients with extrahepatic biliary diseases and associated with their pathogenesis. Dig Dis Sci 2005; 50:862-867.

307. Messini F. [Helicobacter pylori and hepatobiliary diseases]. Clin Ter 2003; 154:55-56.

308. Shukla VK, Singh H, Pandey M, et al. Carcinoma of the gallbladder-is it a sequel of typhoid? Dig Dis Sci 2000; 45:900-903.

309. Dutta U, Garg PK, Kumar R, et al. Typhoid carriers among patients with gallstones are at increased risk for carcinoma of the gallbladder. Am J Gastroenterol 2000; 95:784-787.

310. Nath G, Singh H, Shukla VK. Chronic typhoid carriage and carcinoma of the gallbladder. Eur J Cancer Prev 1997; 6:557-559.

311. Welton JC, Marr JS, Friedman SM. Association between hepatobiliary cancer and typhoid carrier state. Lancet 1979; 1:791-794.

312. Malik IA. Clinicopathological features and management of gallbladder cancer in Pakistan: a prospective study of 233 cases. J Gastroenterol Hepatol 2003; 18:950-953.

313. Kuba K, Yamaguchi K, Nishiyama K, et al. Gallbladder carcinoma in an asymptomatic biliary typhoid carrier: report of a case. Am J Gastroenterol 1998; 93:656-657.

314. Zatonski WA, La Vecchia C, Przewozniak K, et al. Risk factors for gallbladder cancer: a Polish case-control study. Int J Cancer 1992; 51:707-711.

315. Shukla VK, Adukia TK, Singh SP, et al. Micronutrients, antioxidants, and carcinoma of the gallbladder. J Surg Oncol 2003; 84:31-35.

316. Nakadaira H, Ishizu T, Yamamoto M. Effects of selenium on gallbladder carcinogenesis induced by an intracholecystic 3-methylcholanthrene beeswax pellet in female Syrian golden hamsters. Cancer Lett 1996; 106:279-285.

317. Knekt P, Aromaa A, Maatela J, et al. Serum micronutrients and risk of cancers of low incidence in Finland. Am J Epidemiol 1991; 134:356-361.

318. Chen W, Nakadaira H, Tsunoda M, et al. Selenium contents in human gallbladder bile. Tohoku J Exp Med 1990; 161:257-259.

319. Yagyu K, Kikuchi S, Obata Y, et al. Cigarette smoking, alcohol drinking and the risk of gallbladder cancer death: a prospective cohort study in Japan. Int J Cancer 2008; 122:924-929.

320. Gupta SK, Ansari MA, Shukla VK. What makes the Gangetic belt a fertile ground for gallbladder cancers? J Surg Oncol 2005; 91:143-144.

321. Shukla VK, Prakash A, Tripathi BD, et al. Biliary heavy metal concentrations in carcinoma of the gall bladder: case-control study. Bmj 1998; 317:1288-1289.

322. Shukla VK, Aryya NC, Pitale A, et al. Metallothionein expression in carcinoma of the gallbladder. Histopathology 1998; 33:154-157.

323. Adachi Y. [Changes in the concentrations of chlornitrofen (CNP) and CNP-amino in river and faucet water in Niigata, Japan]. Nippon Eiseigaku Zasshi 1994; 48:1090-1098.

324. Takagi S. Chronic toxicity of 2-methyl-4-chlorophenoxyacetic acid (MCPA) in mice. Tohoku J Exp Med 1990; 160:97-107.

325. Shukla VK, Rastogi AN, Adukia TK, et al. Organochlorine pesticides in carcinoma of the gallbladder: a case-control study. Eur J Cancer Prev 2001; 10:153-156.

326. Suarez L, Weiss NS, Martin J. Primary liver cancer death and occupation in Texas. Am J Ind Med 1989; 15:167-175.

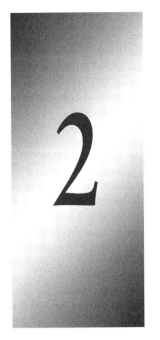

2 Role of Growth Factor–Signaling Pathways

Kaoru Kiguchi
John DiGiovanni

Biliary tract cancer (BTC), including gallbladder carcinoma (GBC), has proven challenging to treat and manage due to its poor sensitivity to conventional therapies and the inability to prevent or detect early tumor formation. To date, very few studies have attempted to decipher the molecular and cellular mechanism(s) involved in the development of GBC, and very little is known regarding the sequence of events leading to the development of GBC. A limiting factor is the lack of appropriate animal models for the development of BTC. Available animal models based on exposure to chemical carcinogens suffer from long latency between treatment and tumor development, and in most cases the tumor incidence is relatively low. We recently developed BK5.erbB2 transgenic mice in which expression of rat erbB2 cDNA is targeted to the basal layer of multiple epithelial tissues, including the biliary tract epithelium, by a bovine keratin 5 (BK5) promoter (1, 2). Adenocarcinoma of the gallbladder develops in 90% of the homozygous BK5.erbB2 transgenic mice by 2-3 months of age. The BK5.erbB2 transgenic mouse line represents the first genetically engineered mouse model for BTC. We have shown that the BK5.erbB2 transgenic line is a valid model for investigating mechanism(s) underlying the development of gallbladder carcinoma and other BTCs (2). We have found that pro-tein levels of erbB2 as well as protein levels of epidermal growth factor receptor (EGFR) are elevated in the gallbladders of BK5.erbB2 transgenic mice. In addition, we have found elevated levels of COX-2/PGE2 and elevated activity of Akt, mitogen-activated protein kinase (MAPK), and mammalian target of rapamycin (mTOR) in the GBC from these mice. These molecular alterations are similar to those reported in human GBC or BTC. In this chapter we will discuss the role of growth factors and their receptors (receptor tyrosine kinases, RTKs), downstream signaling pathways of these RTKs, and inflammatory mediators during gallbladder carcinogenesis. Understanding the growth factor-signaling pathways upregulated in GBC will provide critical clues for novel therapeutic and chemopreventive strategies using drugs and/or agents that selectively target these specific pathways.

ROLE OF GROWTH FACTORS AND RTKS IN HUMAN GALLBLADDER CARCINOGENESIS

ErbB Family

A number of RTKs have been described (3-5). Among them is the erbB family of RTKs, consisting of the epidermal growth factor receptor (EGFR/erbB1), *erb*B2 (neu), erbB3, and erbB4 (6). ErbB family RTKs have been shown to be important for normal development as well as in neoplasia (3, 7) (Figure 2.1). Although all of the erbB family members share similarities in primary structure, receptor activation mechanism, and signal transduction patterns, they bind to different ligands. EGFR binds to and can be activated by a number of different ligands of the EGF family, including EGF, transforming growth factor α (TGF-α), heparin-binding EGF-like growth factor (HB-EGF), amphiregulin (AR), betacellulin (reviewed in Refs. 8, 9), epigen, and epiregulin (10). The neuregulin subfamily consists of various isoforms referred to as 1-4 (11)which bind to erbB4 and/or erbB3 (12-16).Betacellulin, HB-EGF, and epiregulin have also been shown to bind to erbB4 (17). Ligand-dependent activation of erbB family receptors can lead to heterodimerization, particularly of EGFR, erbB3, and erbB4 with erbB2 (16). To date no ligand has been identified for erbB2 (13, 18-20). ErbB3 cannot generate signals in isolation because the kinase function of this receptor is impaired, thus relying on interaction with erbB2 for signaling. Postreceptor signaling by activated erbB family members includes signaling through the Ras/MEK/ MAPK/extracellular signal-regulated kinase (Erk), phospholipase Cγ, signal

transducer and activators of transcription (STATs), and phosphatidylinositol 3-kinase (PI3K) pathways that are common to nearly all RTKs (21) (Figure 2.1).

In terms of BTC, erbB2 overexpression has been reported in a significant percentage of GBCs (22-24) and cholangiocarcinomas (23, 25-28). Previous reports indicated that the frequency of erbB2 overexpression in BTC varied from 32.6 to 84% (22, 23, 29, 30).These differences in frequency may be due to differences in experimental method, the use of different antibodies for immunostaining, or the different criteria used for evaluation. Recently, Ogo et. al. reported that 47 out of 72 cases (65.3%) of BTC showed erbB2 overexpression detected by the Hercep Test(tm) (31). Enhanced immunoreactivity for erbB2 measured, not only in the tumors, but also in risk conditions for BTC like hepatolithiasis and primary sclerosing cholangitis (26, 27, 32-34) correlated directly with tumor differentiation and was highest in well-differentiated tumors (32-34).

Overexpression of EGFR has also been observed in BTC in the range of 30-60% (30, 35, 36). Leone et al. reported that 6 of 40 (15%) BTCs had EGFR gene mutations in the sequence coding for the tyrosine kinase domain. All of the mutations were somatic acquired point mutations, and most were found within exon 21

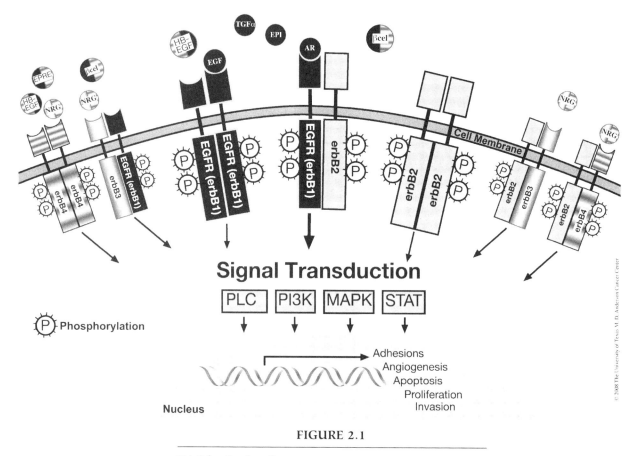

FIGURE 2.1

ErbB family signaling system.

(37). Overexpression of EGFR appears to be related to some clinical and pathological features, such as lymph node metastasis, aberrant p53 expression, proliferative activity, and differentiation (38, 39). However, neither overexpression of EFGR nor erbB2 seems to be a prognostic factor for BTC. It has been reported that bile acids activate EGFR in choloangiocytes via its ligand, TGF-α, (40) and also induce COX-2 expression via EGFR in a human BTC cell line (41).

Insulin-Like Growth Factor 1 Receptor (IGF-1R)

IGF-1R, another member of the RTK superfamily, not only plays an important role in normal growth and development, but also has been implicated in tumor development and progression (42-44). The binding of the IGF ligands (IGF-1 and IGF-2) to the extracellular subunit of IGF-IR phosphorylates the adapter proteins insulin receptor substrate (IRS)-1, IRS-2, and Shc, which serve as independent transducers. IRS1/2 mediate the antiapoptotic properties of IGF-1R through PI3K, resulting in Akt activation. Numerous Akt substrates have been identified that control key cellular processes such as apoptosis (i.e., FOXO, Bad and ASK-1), cell cycle progression (i.e., Cyclin D1, p27, and p21), transcription (i.e., IKK/NFκβ), and translation (i.e., mTOR, S6K, and eIF-4E) (45, 46) (Figure 2.2). EGFR and IGF-1R share a common molecular structure of tyrosine residues, which provide specific docking sites for the SH2 or phosphotyrosine-binding domains of adapter proteins including Grb2, Grb10, SHC, Crk, and IRS-1/2 (47) when these receptors are activated (phosphorylated). Therefore, EGFR and IGF-1R pathways utilize activation of the overlapping downstream signaling pathways (e.g., PI3K/Akt and MAPK for promoting cell growth) (Figure 2.3). Overexpression of IGF-1R has been noted in a variety of human carcinomas (48-51). Kornprat has reported that IGF-1, IGF-2, and IGF-1R were present in 55 of 57 primary GBCs and 17 of 18 metastases (52). IGF-1 and IGF-2 immunoreactivity was seen in 25 and 14, respectively, of the 55 primary tumors and in an additional 6 and 3 of the 17 metastases, respectively. No associations with tumor stage, grade or prognosis were detected. IGF-1R was expressed in 52 of 55 primary tumors and all 17 metastases. IGF-1R staining intensity decreased with tumor cell dedifferentiation. These results provide evidence for the existence of an autocrine/paracrine loop in GBC involving the IGF-1R. However, further investigation will be necessary to clarify the exact role of IGF-1R signaling in GBC.

c-MET

Hepatocyte growth factor (HGF) was discovered by Nakamura et al. (53) as a factor stimulating the DNA synthesis of cultured hepatoyctes. HGF was found to be the ligand for c-Met, an RTK that is expressed in most epithelial cells and in endothelial cells (54). The

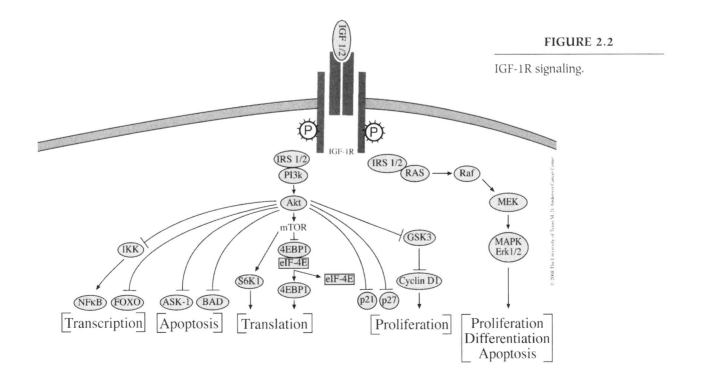

FIGURE 2.2

IGF-1R signaling.

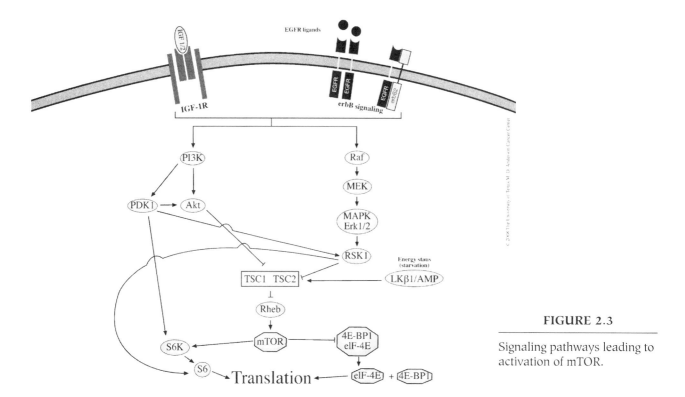

FIGURE 2.3

Signaling pathways leading to activation of mTOR.

c-Met receptor and/or its ligand HGF are often over-expressed in tumors (55, 56). Many types of malignant cells, primarily adenocarcinomas, are responsive to HGF, which stimulates cell proliferation, invasion, and metastasis via activation of c-Met (54, 55, 57). HGF is produced by nonepithelial stromal cells (58, 59), and overexpression of c-Met is a common feature of hyper-plastic biliary epithelium (27, 34). Overexpression of c-Met in human BTC has been observed most fre-quently in intrahepatic bile duct carcinoma (21.4%) and it was not associated with gene amplification (60). Overexpression of c-Met is also characteristic of the rat cholangiocarcinoma model generated by treatment with furan (61).It has also been reported that an antag-onist for HGF, NK4, inhibited the growth of human GBC cells in both a subcutaneous and a positional implantation model (62, 63).

ROLE OF MTOR AND ITS UPSTREAM REGULATORS, AKT AND MAPK, DURING HUMAN GALLBLADDER CARCINOGENESIS

The Role of mTOR in Cancer Development

Mammalian target of rapamycin (mTOR), also know as FRAP, RAFT1, and RAPT1, is a member of the phos-phoinositide kinase-related kinase (PIKK) family and is a highly conserved serine/threonine kinase (64). mTOR is a central regulator of cell growth and proliferation and functions as a biologic switch between life and death that senses changes in the cellular environment and facilitates cellular response to these changes (65). Fluxes in cellular dynamics include amino acid avail-ability (66, 67), changes in nitric oxide levels (68), and growth factor receptor signaling (69). Through its downstream effectors, mTOR relays a signal to the translational machinery leading to enhanced transla-tion of mRNAs encoding proteins that are essential for cell growth and proliferation (70, 71) (Figure 2.3).

mTOR signaling is upregulated in a significant number of human tumors either through upregulation of Akt or other regulatory pathways (65, 71-74). In many tumors, multiple alterations, both upstream and downstream of mTOR, may lead to activation of the mTOR pathway. Phosphorylation of mTOR may occur in response to signaling cues from three major pathways, namely PI3K/Akt, MAPK/Erk, and LKB1/ AMPK. Figure 2.3 shows signaling pathways leading to activation of mTOR. The mechanism of mTOR activation via the PI3K pathway is the most promi-nent and well characterized. PI3K phosphorylates the membrane-bound phosphatidylinositol 4,5-bisphos-phate at position 3 to produce phosphatidylinositol 3,4,5-trisphosphate (PIP3). PIP3 phosphorylates the serine/threonine kinases Akt and phosphatidylinosi-tol-dependent kinase 1 (PDK1). PDK1 activates Akt by phosphorylating Thr308 (75). Akt, in turn, phos-phorylates TSC2, leading to the functional inactivation of the TSC1/TSC2 complex (76-78). Mutations in either TSC1 or TSC2 result in the development of the disease tuberous sclerosis (TSC) (79). The TSC1/TSC2 complex is placed downstream from Akt and upstream from mTOR to restrict cell growth and differentiation. Akt phosphorylation of TSC2 results in mTOR activation.

Ras, through Raf kinase, activates the MAPK/Erk pathway, which interacts with a second major signaling pathway centered on mTOR via phosphorylation of RSK (80, 81). Activation of RSK requires coordinated input from the Ras/MAPK/Erk cascade and PDK1 (82, 83). RSK also provides an mTOR-independent pathway linking the Ras/Erk signaling cascade to the translational machinery through the phosphorylation of S6 ribosomal protein (84).

AMPK, through LKB1, also regulates mTOR via modulation of TSC2. AMPK is a regulator of cellular energy metabolism. In the presence of high AMP, the AMPK γ regulatory subunit binds AMP, permitting the α subunit to be phosphorylated and activated by LKB1 kinase. AMPK in turn phosphorylates TSC2, strengthening the ability of the TSC complex to block Rheb GTPase activity and lowering mTOR activity (66, 85, 86). Thus, these upstream activators of mTOR lead, in turn, to phosphorylation of two main mTOR substrates, ribosomal p70S6 kinase (S6K) and eukaryotic initiation factor 4E-binding protein-1 (4E-BP1). S6K can then phosphorylate its substrate, ribosomal protein S6. When phosphorylated, 4E-BP1 cannot bind effectively to its binding partner, eIF4E. The cumulative effect of both is to increase protein translation and, in particular, the translation of proteins that are involved in cell growth and proliferation.

The mTOR-specific inhibitor rapamycin and the recent development of rapamycin analogs has generated considerable excitement in terms of clinical trials for patients with a wide range of cancers, including rhabdosarcoma, neuroblastoma, glioblastoma, small-cell lung cancer, renal cancer osteosarcoma, pancreatic cancer, leukemia, and B-cell lymphoma (87-89).

mTOR, Akt, and MAPK Signaling in Human GBC

Recently, we reported that elevated levels of phospho-Akt and phospho-mTOR were observed in 74.1% (20 of 27) and 92.6% (25 of 27), respectively, of human gallbladder cancer specimens compared to 28.6% (2 of 7) and 28.6% (2 of 7), respectively, of normal human gallbladder specimens (90). These results suggest that activation of Akt/mTOR signaling may be an important mechanism during gallbladder carcinogenesis. However, cellular response to the upregulation of erbB2/EGFR is mediated not only by Akt signaling, but also through other downstream signaling pathways, including Raf/MAPK signaling. In fact, aberrations in MAPK signaling, which are also observed frequently in human BTC (36, 91), are commonly associated with elevations in mTOR signaling. These findings support the hypothesis that upregulation of one or more critical upstream pathways may lead to the activation of mTOR in GBC and suggest that mTOR inhibitors may have a role in the treatment of BTC.

ROLE OF INFLAMMATORY MEDIATORS DURING HUMAN GALLBLADDER CARCINOGENSIS

The Arachidonic Acid Cascade

Membrane phospholipids acted upon by phospholipase A2 (PLA2) form arachidonic acid (AA), which serves as the precursor for inflammatory mediator prostaglandins (PGs) via cyclooxygenase-2 (COX-2) (92-95) (Figure 2.4). One of the PGs, PGE_2, appears to participate in the development of inflammatory reactions and oncogenesis (96, 97). The action of PGE_2 is mediated by four G protein-coupled receptors (GPCRs): EP1, EP2, EP3, and EP4 (98) (Figure 2.4).

COX-2 Involvement in Biliary Tract Carcinogenesis

The presence of a chronic inflammatory state, usually related to gallstones, has been found to be the most significant risk factor for GBC. There is a known association between gallstones and GBC, with gallstones present in 74-92% of patients with GBC (99, 100). Pathogenic bacteria are cultured from the gallbladders of patients with GBC at a significantly greater frequency than patients with simple cholelithiasis (101). Typhoid carriers may also suffer chronic inflammation of the gallbladder and have been described to have a significantly higher risk of GBC than the rest of the population (102, 103).The presence of an anomalous pancreaticobiliary ductal junction (APDJ), which causes long-term inflammation, has also been suggested in numerous reports as a risk factor for GBC (104). In fact, a number of studies have shown that AA, PLA2, COX-2, and PGE2 are increased in BTC (105-108).Treatment of cholangiocarcinoma cells with exogenous PGE2 increases tumor cell growth and prevents apoptosis (108-114). When COX-2 was inhibited by selective COX-2 inhibitors, prevention of cholangiocarcinoma cell growth and invasion was observed in

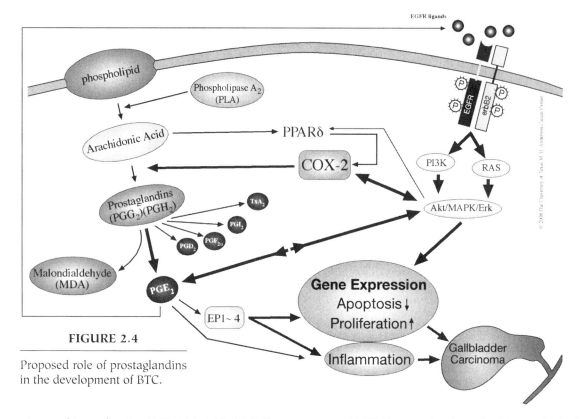

FIGURE 2.4

Proposed role of prostaglandins
in the development of BTC.

vitro and in nude mice (109-111, 113, 114).Grossman
et al. reported that a specific COX-2 inhibitor, but not
COX-1 inhibitor, decreased mitogenesis and increased
human gallbladder cell apoptosis associated with
decreased PGE$_2$ (115). These studies suggest that the
COX enzymes and the prostanoids may play a role in
the development of GBC and that COX-2 inhibitors
may have a therapeutic role in GBC (115).

Crosstalk Between COX-2 and EGFR/erbB2 in BTC

There have been several reports that show a mutual regulation between EGFR and COX-2. Bile acids, a potent
tumor promoter in the hamster model of cholangio-
genesis, were shown to induce COX-2 in cholangiocyte
cells through transactivation of EGFR (41). EGFR is
also activated by chenodeoxycholate, the primary
hydrophobic bile acid, and functions to induce COX-
2 expression through a MAPK cascade in a human
cholangiocarcinoma cell line (116). PGE$_2$ rapidly
induces phosphorylation of EGFR and triggers the
Erk2-mitogenic signaling pathway in normal gastric
epithelial and colon cancer cell lines, and PGE$_2$-induced
EGFR transactivation involves signaling transduced via
TGF-α (21). Zhang et al. reported that PGE$_2$-induced
Erk phosphorylation is abrogated by pretreatment a the
EGFR-specific tyrosine kinase inhibitor (TKI) and that
activation of the EP1 receptor is involved in PGE$_2$-stim-
ulated Erk activation in cholangiocarcinoma cells

(117).Transactivation of EGFR and Akt has been proposed as one of the important mechanisms for COX-
2- and PGE-mediated cholangiocarcinoma cell growth
(118).In addition, it has been shown that a COX-2
inhibitor blocks phosphorylation of Akt in human
cholangiocarcinoma cells (110, 119).

There is also increasing evidence that COX-2 and
PGE$_2$ may mediate some effects of erbB2 (120,
121).ErbB2 overexpression or activation increased
COX-2 gene transcription (122), and this regulation
occurred through a MAPK-dependent pathway (121).
It has also been reported that erbB2 signaling through
Akt induces COX-2 expression in breast cancer cells
(123) and that COX-2 and PGE$_2$ lead to an enhanced
expression of erbB2 (124).Co-elevation of COX-2 has
been observed not only in a rat cholangiocarcinoma
model induced by furan (125), but also in human
cholangiocarcinoma (106), supporting the possibility
that erbB2 plays a key role in regulating COX-2 expression in neoplastic and precancerous biliary tract epithelial cells. These studies suggest a link between
EGFR/erbB2 and COX-2 expression mediated by
MAPK and/or Akt activity (123, 124, 126-128) (Figure 2.4).

In addition, Xu et al reported that PPARδ, a subtype of peroxisome proliferator-activated receptors
(PPARs), induces COX-2 expression in human cholangiocarcinoma cells and that the COX-2-derived PGE$_2$
further activates PPARδ through PLA2 (129). Figure
2.4 shows the proposed crosstalk between COX-

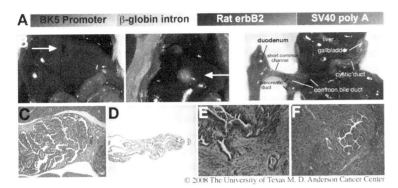

**FIGURE 2.5
GROSS APPEARANCE AND
HISTOLOGIC EVALUATIONS OF
BTC IN BK5.ERBB2 MICE.**

(A) DNA construct used to generate BK5.erbB2 mice; (B) Gallbladder (arrow) of nontransgenic littermate (left) and BK5.erbB2 mouse (middle) at 3 months of age. Gross appearance of gallbladder and adjacent biliary tract of BK5.erbB2 mouse (right). H&E staining of gallbladder in BK5.erbB2 mice (C and E) and nontransgenic mouse (D) and intrahepatic cholangiocarcinoma in BK5.erbB2 mice at 3 months of age (F).

2/PGE$_2$, erbB2/EGFR, and Akt/MAPK that may play a role in the development of BTC.

ANIMAL MODELS FOR HUMAN BTC

Spontaneous and Chemically Induced BTC

Spontaneous gallbladder cancer is rare in mice and rats (130, 131). A low incidence of gallbladder adenocarcinoma can be chemically induced in mice by continuous administration of either N-N-propyl-N-formylhydrazine (132) or 2-acetamidofluorene (133). Although spontaneous gallbladder tumors are extremely rare in hamsters (134), neoplasia can be induced by chronic exposure to 3-methylcholanthrene via slow-release capsules implanted in the gallbladder (135) or a combination of exposure to nitrosodimethylamine (in drinking water) and cholesterol pellets (implanted in gallbladder) (136).

Sirica and coworkers showed that treatment of rats with furan rapidly induced intestinal metaplasia and associated cholangiofibrosis in the right/caudate liver of rats (137) and that long-term treatment with furan (daily dose of 30 mg/kg of body weight, five times weekly by gavage for 9-13 weeks) resulted in the preferential development of cholangiocarcinoma (138). Incidence of cholangiocarcinoma was 70-90% in rats treated with furan by 16 months. The researchers demonstrated that furan-induced rat cholangiocarcinoma characteristically overexpresses erbB2, COX-2, and c-Met (61, 125, 139). In addition, they reported that emodin, a TKI, effectively inhibited the growth and tyrosine phosphorylation of erbB2 overexpressed in cultured rat C611B cholangiocarcinoma cells and in neu-transformed WB-F344 rat liver epithelial stem-like cells (WBneu). In combination, emodin (30 µM) and celecoxib (35 µM), a COX-2 inhibitor, acted synergistically to significantly suppress growth of both C611B and WBneu cells. Suppression of cell growth was associated with induction of apoptosis in the combination-

treated cells and enhanced suppression of Akt activation (113). In vivo, celecoxib also suppressed tumorigenic growth of C611B cells in vivo (111). Furthermore, they have recently shown that a rat cholangiocyte cell line infected by a retrovirus containing the transforming rat erbB2 displayed activated erbB2, Akt, and MAPK, increased telomecrase activity, and upregulated COX-2, PGE2, and vascular endothelial growth factor (140). These erbB2 transformants were tumorigenic when transplanted into isogenic rats, yielding a 100% incidence of tumors resembling human cholangiocarcinomas in their morphology (140).

BK5.erbB2 Mouse Model

Several years ago, our laboratory generated a transgenic mouse that overexpresses wild-type rat erbB2 under the control of the BK5 promoter (1) (Figure 2.5A). Overexpression of wild-type erbB2 in basal epithelial cells of gallbladder led to the development of adenocarcinoma of the gallbladder and cystic duct in 90% of these transgenic mice by 2-3 months of age. In addition, the incidence of cholangiocarcinoma was ~30%. Similarities between GBC in BK5.erbB2 mice and humans include histopathologic observation and molecular alterations such as overexpression and/or activation of erbB2, EGFR, Akt, MAPK, and COX-2. BK5.erbB2 transgenic mice appear to represent a promising tool for the development of new treatment and/or prevention modalities.

Histopathologic Features of BTC in BK5.erbB2 Mice

Necropsy of adult BK5.erbB2 mice revealed that the gallbladder was dramatically enlarged and had a white, opaque appearance (Figure 2.5B, middle). Enlarged gallbladders were often associated with a significantly dilated common bile duct (Figure 2.5B, right). This enlarged hepatic duct from the liver and the cystic duct from the gallbladder unite to form the enlarged common bile duct, which extends posteriorly through the pancreas and intestinal wall, where it opens to the mucosal surface of the duodenum as the ampulla of Vater (Figure 2.5B, right).The short common channel formed from the merging of the bile duct and the pancreatic duct was anatomically normal, as was the ampulla of Vater in these mice. The majority of the GBCs completely filled the lumen (Figure 2.5C), although some showed focal lesions (focal type). For comparison, a normal gallbladder from a nontransgenic mouse is shown in Figure 2.5D. Tumors were characterized by branching structures with finger-like projections covered with high columnar epithelium and hyperchromatic nuclei. Most of the tumors were diagnosed as well-differentiated adenocarcinomas. Carcinoma cells frequently invaded into the surrounding connective tissues (Figure 2.5E). In addition, hypervascularization was a characteristic feature of these tumors. Staining with CD31, a marker for endothelial cells, revealed extensive vascularization in an adenocarcinoma from a BK5.erbB2 mouse. Adenocarcinomas exhibited a significantly elevated labeling index (a marker of proliferation) compared to normal gallbladder epithelium as determined by staining with anti-bromodeoxyuridine (BrdU) antibody.

Tumor cells of the common bile duct often invaded into the pancreatic duct. The ampulla of Vater was dilated, and hyperplasia of the epithelium was observed in transgenic mice. Pronounced congestion of bile, inflammation, necrosis, hyperplasia of biliary duct cells, and/or tumor development was also frequently observed in intrahepatic biliary ducts of transgenic mice (Figure 2.5F).

Molecular Features of GBC in BK5.erbB2 Mice

STATUS OF EGFR AND ERBB2 IN GBC OF BK5.ERBB2 MICE

Persistent expression of the erbB2 transgene was observed in the epithelia of both gallbladder and intrahepatic biliary duct as well as in gallbladder adenocarcinomas (Figure 2.6A) and cholangiocarcinomas (Figure 2.6B). Endogenous erbB2 expression was only weakly detectable in both the intrahepatic biliary duct and gallbladder from nontransgenic mice (Figure 2.6C). Western blot analysis of gallbladder tissue lysates showed that the level of erbB2 protein was significantly elevated in BK5.erbB2 mice compared to that of nontransgenic mice, as expected (Figure 2.6D). erbB2 was also hyperphosphorylated after adjustment for total erbB2 protein level (Figure 2.6E). Interestingly, the level of EGFR protein (but not erbB3 or erbB4 protein) was elevated and hyperphosphorylated on tyrosine residues in gallbladder tissue from BK5.erbB2 mice (Figure

2.6D, E). Additional analyses by immunoprecipitation of EGFR and erbB2 followed by Western blot analysis for erbB2 and EGFR, respectively, confirmed elevated heterodimer formation between erbB2 and EGFR (data not shown) in the gallbladder tissue of BK5.erbB2 mice.

MAPK, AKT, AND MTOR IN GALLBLADDER TISSUE OF BK5.ERBB2 MICE

The status of signaling molecules downstream of erbB2/EGFR and other proteins was also examined. Although protein levels of MAPK were not changed (Figure 2.6F), both MAP kinase activity (Figure 2.6F, G) and the level of phosphorylation of Erk1 and 2 were increased in the gallbladder of transgenic mice. Furthermore, phospho-Akt, but not total Akt level, was elevated in the gallbladder of BK5.erbB2 as assessed by Western blot analysis (Figure 2.6G). We have recently reported that mTOR and signaling molecules both immediately upstream (Akt, MAPK) and downstream (p70S6K) of mTOR are hyperphosphorylated in gallbladder tissues from BK5.erbB2 mice compared with corresponding tissue from nontransgenic mice (90) (see also Figure 2.6G). We also found that cyclin D1 (Figure 2.6G), bcl-2 (Figure 2.6G), c-Met (2), E-cadherin, and β-catenin (data not shown) were upregulated in the gallbladder tissue of BK5.erbB2 compared to nontransgenic mice by Western blot analysis.

INCREASED COX-2 PROTEIN AND MRNA EXPRESSION, PGE2 SYNTHESIS, AND PHOSPHORYLATED LEVEL OF cPLA2 IN GBC OF BK5.ERBB2 MICE

The protein level (determined by immunohistochemistry and Western blot) and mRNA level (determined by RT-PCR) of COX-2 were significantly elevated in the gallbladder tissue of BK5.erbB2 mice (Figure 2.6H-J) compared to nontransgenic littermates. The level of PGE_2 was also found to be elevated in the tissue (data not shown). These results suggest that elevated prostaglandins, particularly PGE_2, may play an important role in the development of gallbladder carcinoma in BK5.erbB2 mice. Phospho-$cPLA_2$, but not total $cPLA_2$, was also elevated in the gallbladder from BK5.erbB2 mice (Figure 2.6G).

PRECLINICAL THERAPEUTIC STUDIES USING BK5.ERBB2 MICE

Orally active TKIs

We have evaluated the effect of gefitinib, a selective TKI against the EGFR, on the development of gallbladder carcinoma in BK5.erbB2 mice (141). In addition, we also assessed the effect of another quinazoline derivative,

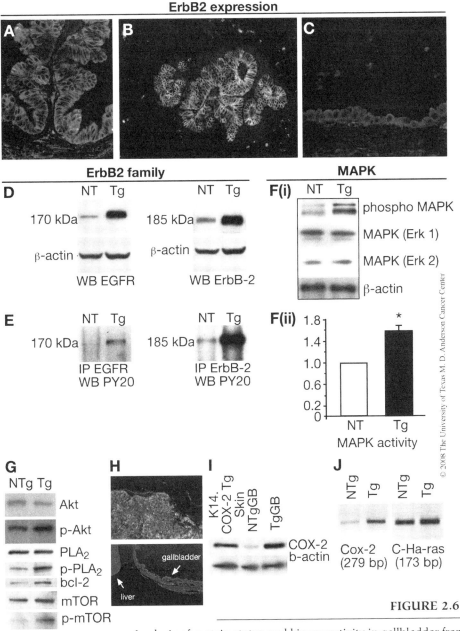

FIGURE 2.6

Analysis of protein status and kinase activity in gallbladder from 3-month-old nontransgenic and BK5.erbB2 mice. Analysis of protein status and kinase activity in gallbladder from 3-month-old nontransgenic and BK5.erbB2 mice. Immunostaining for erbB2 in gallbladder (A) and intrahepatic cholangiocarcinoma (B) from a 3-month-old BK5.erbB2 mouse and gallbladder from a nontransgenic mouse of the same age (C).(D) Whole cell lysates were analyzed by Western blot (WB) with antibodies against erbB family members. Protein was normalized to β-actin. (E) Whole cell lysates were immunoprecipitated (IP) with antibodies with the phosphotyrosine-specific antibody PY20. (F) Whole cell lysates of gallbladder were immunoprecipitated with a MAPK antibody.One half of the immunoprecipitates were subjected to WB analysis for photo-MAPK, Erk1, Erk 2, and β-actin [F(i)], and the other half were analyzed for MAPK activity [F(ii)].There was a significant increase in MAPK activity in transgenic mice (*p < 0.05, Mann-Whitney U test). (G) Whole cell lysates were analyzed by Western blot with antibodies against Akt, phospho-Akt, PLA2, phospho-PLA2, bcl-2, mTOR, phospho-mTOR, p70S60K, phospho-p70S6K, Cyclin D1 and β-actin. (H) COX-2 level determined by immunostaining in GB from BK5.erbB2 mice (upper) and nontransgenic littermate (lower). (I) Western blot analysis of COX-2 protein in gallbladder from nontransgenic mice (NTgGB) and Bk5.erbB2 mice (TgGB). Whole skin from K14.COX-2 mice (K14.COX-2) skin was used as a positive control. (J) RT-PCR analysis of COX-2 mRNA expression in gallbladder from nontransgenic (NTg) and BK5.erbB2 mice (Tg).

GW2974, which is able to block the activation of both the EGFR and erbB2. Two-month-old mice were selected for treatment as the incidence of gallbladder carcinoma reaches a plateau of ~90% by this age. BK5.erbB2 mice received either 400 ppm gefitinib or 200 ppm GW2974 in the diet for 1 month. During the course of these experiments, the status of the gallbladders in each group was monitored weekly by high-frequency ultrasound biomicroscopy (USBM) (n = 7 and 10 for gefitinib and GW2974, respectively). Treatment with either gefitinib or GW2974 resulted in a significant decrease in the incidence of gallbladder carcinoma to 17 and 3%, respectively (Figure 2.7A). These reductions corresponded to a 77% and 95% decrease in tumor incidence compared with BK5.erbB2 mice receiving the control diet, which had a GBC incidence of 72% as determined by histopathologic examination. The impact of treatment is clearly seen in the images in Figure 2.7B,

which show a gallbladder tumor prior to treatment (left panel), the same gallbladder after day 23 of treatment with GW2974, and, finally, the H&E staining, which clearly show the dramatic regression of the tumor with only hyperplasia still evident.

In the control group, adenocarcinoma cells filled the lumen, occupying at least one third of the distal portion of the gallbladder (Figure 2.7C). In most of the gallbladder adenocarcinomas that responded to either gefitinib or GW2974, we observed low-grade epithelial hyperplasia, particularly in the distal region (Figure 2.7C). Thickened connective tissue, decreased vascularization, a significantly lower labeling index as determined by BrdU incorporation, and an increase in the number of apoptotic cells as determined by TUNEL assay were also observed following treatment with either TKI (141).

Treatment with gefitinib and GW2974 resulted

FIGURE 2.7

Effects of gefitinib and GW2974 detected by histologic and ultrasound analyses. (A), Incidence of gallbladder carcinoma in BK5.erbB2 mice treated with AIN76 control diet, AIN76 diet containing 400 ppm gefitinib, and AIN76 diet containing 200 ppm GW2974. *p < 0.01. Numerator indicates number of mice found to have gallbladder tumors. Denominator indicates total number of mice treated. No mortality was observed throughout the experiment. (B) Regression of gallbladder carcinoma by GW2974 treatment as detected by ultrasound biomicroscopy. All images are from a single animal depicting the response representative of the treatment group. (Left panel) Ultrasound image of gallbladder carcinoma (maximum size: 1.35 mm) before GW2974 treatment. (Center panel) Ultrasound image of gallbladder on the 23rd day of treatment; this image indicates regression of the carcinoma (observed size: 0.46 mm). (Right panel) The lesion that remained was confirmed by H&E staining as hyperplasia. (C) Histologic evaluation of gallbladders from BK5.erbB2 mice treated with gefitinib and GW2974. (Left panel) Gallbladder of BK5.erbB2 mouse receiving AIN76 control diet. (Middle panel) Typical histologic features of the gallbladder from BK5.erbB2 mice treated with AIN76 diet containing 400 ppm gefitinib. (Right panel) Typical histologic features of the gallbladder from BK5.erbB2 mice treated with AIN76 diet containing 200 ppm GW2974.

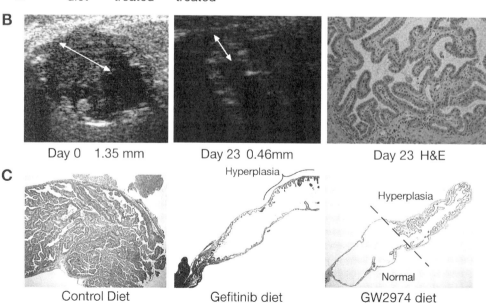

in decreased levels of both erbB2 and EGFR. Furthermore, levels of phospho-erbB2 and phospho-EGFR were markedly reduced (2). Upregulated COX-2 and activated MAPK levels were also decreased in gallbladders from BK5.erbB2 mice treated with both TKIs (2). Based on these results, targeting EGFR, and possibly erbB2, could provide a potentially new and effective therapy for patients with BTC.

CS-706, a Novel COX-2 Inhibitor

We have also examined the effects of a newly engineered COX-2 inhibitor, CS-706 (Sankyo Co.), on the development of GBC in the BK5.erbB2 mouse model (142). Two-month old mice received CS-706 (60 and 100 ppm) in the diet for one month. The therapeutic effect of CS-706 was evaluated by ultrasound images and histological analyses. (Seventy-eight percent of gallbladder tumors were diagnosed as progressive disease (PG) in the control diet group, but only 20 and 21% of the tumors displayed a progressive phenotype in 60 and 100 ppm of CS-706 treated groups, respectively. Furthermore, approximately 80% of gallbladders (80 and 79% for 60 and 100 ppm of CS-706 treatment, respectively) showed either therapeutic efficacy (partial response, PR) or prevention from progression (minimum change, MC) when treated with CS-706. The effects of both 60 and 100 ppm of CS-706 are statistically significant (Fisher's extact test) compared to the control diet (Figure 2.8A).

Both immunohistochemical and Western blot analysis (Figure 2.8B) showed that the elevated COX-2 level was markedly decreased in gallbladders from BK5.erbB2 mice treated with CS-706 compared to that from BK5.erbB2 mice on the control diet. PGE2 is the major product of COX-2-catalyzed reactiona. In addition, treatment of CS-706 strongly inhibited PGE2 production in both serum and gallbladders from BK5.erbB2 mice treated with 100 ppm of CS-706 compared to those from BK5.erbB2 mice treated with control diet (**$p < 0.05$ by two-way ANOVA test) (Figure 2.8C).

In CS-706-treated BK5.erbB2 mice, gallbladder tissue proteins showed a 1.4-fold decrease in p-EGFR and 1.5-fold decrease in p-erbB2 levels (Figure 2.8D). Furthermore, treatment with CS-706 resulted in decreased levels of both total erbB2 and EGFR. We have also found that activity of Akt, as assessed by Western blot analysis for phospho-Akt, was decreased in gallbladders from mice treated with CS-706 (Figure 2.8D). Based on these results, targeting COX-2 could provide a potentially new and effective therapy alone or in combination with other therapeutic agents for patients with BTC. One mechanism for the effects of CS-706 in this model system may be through inhibition of Akt activation.

Rapamycin

As noted above, Western blot and immunohistochemical analyses revealed elevated phosphorylation levels for Akt, mTOR, and p70S6K (Figure 2.6) in the GBC from BK5.erbB2 mice. We also analyzed the status of Akt and mTOR in human GBC (90). Immunofluorescence staining of p-Akt and p-mTOR was performed in 27 human GBC (Stage IIB diagnosed by the criteria of the American Joint Committee on Cancer) and 7 normal human gallbladders. The results showed that elevated levels of p-Akt were observed in 74.1% (20 out 27) of human GBC specimens and in only 28.6% (2 out of 7) of normal human gallbladder specimens. Elevated levels of p-mTOR were also observed in 92.6% (25 out 27) of human GBC specimens and in only 28.6% (2 out of 7) of normal human gallbladder specimens. These data reveal that human GBC has elevated p-Akt and p-mTOR levels compared to noncancerous tissue. Thus, BK5.erbB2 mice appeared appropriate for evaluating mTOR inhibitors for treatment of BTC, particularly GBC.

To evaluate the therapeutic efficacy of rapamycin, one group of BK5.erbB2 mice at ~2-3 months of age received vehicle and the other groups received 1.25, 2.5, and 5.0 mg/kg rapamycin by i.p. injection once daily for 14 days. Rapamycin reduced the incidence of GBC in a dose-dependent manner (90). Furthermore, rapamycin treatment led to decreased levels of phospho-p70S6K (Thr389) in gallbladder tissue (90). Based on these results and the fact that the Akt/mTOR pathway is activated in human gallbladder cancer, rapamycin and related drugs may be effective therapeutic agents for the treatment of human GBC.

CONCLUSION

The dismal outcomes that generally result from gallbladder carcinoma and other BTCs explain the pessimism that surrounds treatment of these cancers. Nevertheless, more aggressive surgical techniques and advanced oncologic radiation therapy have led many institutions to report an increase in long-term survival rates (143-147). Although these treatments are progressive, major improvements in patients' survival will probably result from the efforts directed toward prevention, early detection, and novel treatments derived from basic research to determine the mechanisms involved in BTC development. There is a real need to develop novel therapeutic strategies for BTC based on

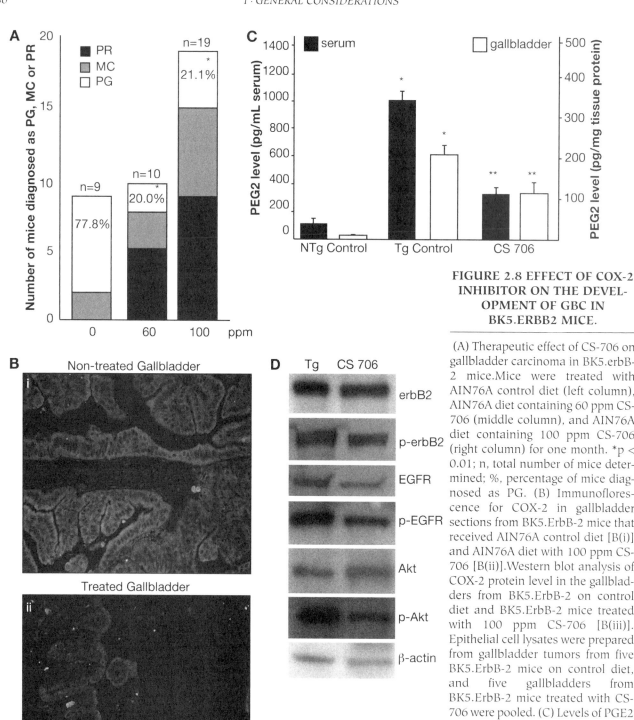

FIGURE 2.8 EFFECT OF COX-2 INHIBITOR ON THE DEVELOPMENT OF GBC IN BK5.ERBB2 MICE.

(A) Therapeutic effect of CS-706 on gallbladder carcinoma in BK5.erbB-2 mice.Mice were treated with AIN76A control diet (left column), AIN76A diet containing 60 ppm CS-706 (middle column), and AIN76A diet containing 100 ppm CS-706 (right column) for one month. *p < 0.01; n, total number of mice determined; %, percentage of mice diagnosed as PG. (B) Immunoflorescence for COX-2 in gallbladder sections from BK5.ErbB-2 mice that received AIN76A control diet [B(i)] and AIN76A diet with 100 ppm CS-706 [B(ii)].Western blot analysis of COX-2 protein level in the gallbladders from BK5.ErbB-2 on control diet and BK5.ErbB-2 mice treated with 100 ppm CS-706 [B(iii)]. Epithelial cell lysates were prepared from gallbladder tumors from five BK5.ErbB-2 mice on control diet, and five gallbladders from BK5.ErbB-2 mice treated with CS-706 were pooled. (C) Levels of PGE2 in serum and gallbladders from mice treated with CS-706. There was a statistically significant increase in PGE2 levels in both serum and gallbladders of BK5.ErbB-2 mice on the control diet (middle column) compared with nontransgenic mice (left column).*p < 0.05.Right column, there was a statistically significant decrease in PGE2 levels in both serum and gallbladders of BK5.ErbB-2 mice treated with CS-706 compared with mice treated with control diet.**p < 0.05.NTg, nontransgenic; Tg, transgenic. (D) Western blot analysis of ErbB-2, p-ErbB-2, egfr, p-EGFR, Akt, and phosphorylated Akt (p-Akt) levels in the gallbladders of BK5.ErbB-2 mice treated with 100 ppm CS-706. Epithelial cell lysates were prepared from gallbladder tumors from five BK5.ErbB-2 mice, and gallbladders from BK5.ErbB-2 mice treated with CS-706 were pooled.

the molecular mechanistic study and on exploiting select molecular targets that would significantly impact clinical studies. The animal models for human BTC appear to be a valuable tool for studying the mechanistic basis for this disease and evaluating therapeutic strategies. New drugs that selectively target specific signaling molecules that are activated in BTC, such as erbB2, EGFR, mTOR, and COX-2, and associated risk conditions may serve as potentially effective adjunct therapies or chemoprevention strategies for this cancer. A number of potential therapeutic strategies against BTC (e.g., using TKI, COX-2 inhibitor or rapamycin, alone or in combination) are worth considering based on current genomic and proteomic studies, including our results from studies with BK5.erbB2 mice.

ACKNOWLEDGMENTS

We would like to thank Shawna Johnson and Joi Holcombe for their assistance in preparing this chapter. We would also like to acknowledge Dr. Alphonse E. Sirica, Virginia Commonwealth University Medical College of Virginia Campus, for his scientific support and interactions.

References

1. Kiguchi K, Bol D, Carbajal S, et al. Constitutive expression of erbB2 in epidermis of transgenic mice results in epidermal hyperproliferation and spontaneous skin tumor development. Oncogene 2000; 19:4243-4254.
2. Kiguchi K, Carbajal S, Chan K, et al. Constitutive expression of ErbB-2 in gallbladder epithelium results in development of adenocarcinoma. Cancer Res 61:6971-6976. 2001;
3. Aaronson SA. Growth factors and cancer. Science 1991; 254:1146-1153.
4. Schlessinger J, Ullrich A. Growth factor signaling by receptor tyrosine kinases. Neuron 1992; 9:389-391.
5. Ullrich A, Schlessinger J. Signal transduction by receptors with tyrosine kinase activity. Cell 1990; 61:203-212.
6. Dougall W, Qian X, Peterson N, et al. The neu-oncogene: signal transduction pathways, transformation mechanisms and evolving therapies. Oncogene 1994; 9:2109-2123.
7. Gullick WJ. Prevalence of aberrant expression of the epidermal growth factor receptor in human cancers. Br Med Bull 1991; 47:87-98.
8. Groenen LC, Nice EC, Burgess AW. Structure-function relationships for the EGF/TGF-alpha family of mitogens. Growth Factors 1994; 11:235-257.
9. Shing Y, Christofori G, Hanahan D, et al. Betacellulin: a mitogen from pancreatic b cell tumors. Science 1993; 259:1604-1607.
10. Toyoda H, Komurasaki T, Uchida D, et al. Epiregulin. A novel epidermal growth factor with mitogenic activity for rat primary hepatocytes. J Biol Chem 1995; 270:7495-7500.
11. Holmes W, Sliwkowski M, Akita R, et al. Identification of heregulin, a specific activator of p185erbB2. Science 1992; 256:1205-1210.
12. Carraway KL, Cantley LC. A neu acquaintance for erbB3 and erbB4: a role for receptor heterodimerization in growth signaling. Cell 1994; 78:5-8.
13. Beerli RR, Hynes NE. Epidermal growth factor-related peptides activate distinct subsets of ErbB receptors and differ in their biological activities. J Biol Chem 1996; 271:6071-6076.
14. Cohen BD, Green JM, Foy L, Fell HP. HER4-mediated biological and biochemical properties in NIH 3T3 cells. Evidence for HER1-HER4 heterodimers. J Biol Chem 1996; 271:4813-4818.
15. Karunagaran D, Tzahar E, Beerli RR, et al. ErbB-2 is a common auxiliary subunit of NDF and EGF receptors: implications for breast cancer. EMBO J 1996; 15:254-264.
16. Pinkas-Kramarski R, Soussan L, Waterman H, et al. Diversification of Neu differentiation factor and epidermal growth factor signaling by combinatorial receptor interactions. EMBO J 1996; 15:2452-2467.
17. Riese DJ, Bermingham Y, Van Raaij TM., et al. Betacellulin activates the epidermal growth factor receptor and erbB-4, and induces cellular response patterns distinct from those stimulated by epidermal growth factor or neuregulin-beta. Oncogene 1996; 12:345-353.
18. King CR, Borrello I, Bellot F, Comoglio P, Schlessinger J. Egf binding to its receptor triggers a rapid tyrosine phosphorylation of the erbB-2 protein in the mammary tumor cell line SK-BR-3. EMBO J 1988; 7:1647-1651.
19. Plowman G, Culouscou J-M, Whitney G, et al. Ligand-specific activation of HER4/p180erbB4, a fourth member of the epidermal growth factor receptor family. Proc Natl Acad Sci USA 1993; 90:1746-1750.
20. Sliwkowski MX, Schaefer G, Akita RW, et al. Coexpression of erbB2 and erbB3 proteins reconstitutes a high affinity receptor for heregulin. J Biol Chem 269:14661-14665. 1994;
21. Yarden Y, Sliwkowski MX. Untangling the ErbB signalling network. Nat Rev Mol Cell Biol 2001; 2:127-137.
22. Suzuki T, Takano Y, Kakita A, Okudaira M. An immunohistochemical and molecular biological study of c-erbB-2 amplification and prognostic relevance in gallbladder cancer. Pathol Res Pract 1993; 189:283-292.
23. Chow NH, Huang SM, Chan SH, et al. Significance of c-erbB-2 expression in normal and neoplastic epithelium of biliary tract. Anticancer Res 1995; 15:1055-1059.
24. Yukawa M, Fujimori T, Hirayama D, et al. Expression of oncogene products and growth factors in early gallbladder cancer, advanced gallbladder cancer, and chronic cholecystitis [see comments]. Hum Pathol 1993; 24:37-40.
25. Suzuki H, Isaji S, Pairojkul C, Uttaravichien T. Comparative clinicopathological study of resected intrahepatic cholangiocarcinoma in northeast Thailand and Japan. J Hepatobiliary Pancreat Surg 2000; 7:206-211.
26. Ito Y, Takeda T, Sasaki Y, et al. Expression and clinical significance of the erbB family in intrahepatic cholangiocellular carcinoma. Pathol Res Pract 2001; 197:95-100.
27. Aishima S I, Taguchi K I, Sugimachi K, Shimada M, Tsuneyoshi M. c-erbB-2 and c-Met expression relates to cholangiocarcinogenesis and progression of intrahepatic cholangiocarcinoma. Histopathology 2002; 40:269-278.
28. Ukita Y, Kato M, Terada T. Gene amplification and mRNA and protein overexpression of c-erbB-2 (HER-2/neu) in human intrahepatic cholangiocarcinoma as detected by fluorescence in situ hybridization, in situ hybridization, and immunohistochemistry. J Hepatol 2002; 36:780-785.
29. Kim YW, Huh SH, Park YK, et al. Expression of the c-erb-B2 and p53 protein in gallbladder carcinomas. Oncol Rep 2001; 8:1127-1132.
30. Wiedmann M, Feisthammel J, Bluthner T, et al. Novel targeted approaches to treating biliary tract cancer: the dual epidermal growth factor receptor and ErbB-2 tyrosine kinase inhibitor NVP-AEE788 is more efficient than the epidermal growth factor receptor inhibitors gefitinib and erlotinib. Anticancer Drugs 2006; 17:783-795.
31. Oettle H, Arnold D, Hempel C, Riess H. The role of gemcitabine alone and in combination in the treatment of pancreatic cancer. Anticancer Drugs, 11:771-786. 2000;
32. Terada T, Ashida K, Endo K, et al. c-erbB-2 protein is expressed in hepatolithiasis and cholangiocarcinoma. Histopathology 1998; 33:325-331.
33. Endo K, Yoon BI, Pairojkul C, Demetris AJ, Sirica AE. ERBB-

2 overexpression and cyclooxygenase-2 up-regulation in human cholangiocarcinoma and risk conditions. Hepatology 2002; 36:439-450.

34. Terada T, Nakanuma Y, Sirica AE. Immunohistochemical demonstration of MET overexpression in human intrahepatic cholangiocarcinoma and in hepatolithiasis. Hum Pathol 1998; 29:175-180.

35. Nonomura A, Ohta G, Nakanuma Y, et al. Simultaneous detection of epidermal growth factor receptor (EGF-R), epidermal growth factor (EGF) and ras p21 in cholangiocarcinoma by an immunocytochemical method. Liver 1988;8:157-166.

36. Javle MM, Yu J, Khoury T, et al. Akt expression may predict favorable prognosis in cholangiocarcinoma. J Gastroenterol Hepatol 2006; 21:1744-1751.

37. Leone F, Cavalloni G, Pignochino Y, et al. Somatic mutations of epidermal growth factor receptor in bile duct and gallbladder carcinoma. Clin Cancer Res 2006; 12:1680-1685.

38. Ogo Y, Nio Y, Yano S, et al. Immunohistochemical expression of HER-1 and HER-2 in extrahepatic biliary carcinoma. Anticancer Res 2006; 26:763-770.

39. Lee CS, Pirdas A. Epidermal growth factor receptor immunoreactivity in gallbladder and extrahepatic biliary tract tumours. Pathol Res Pract 1995; 191:1087-1091.

40. Werneburg NW, Yoon JH, Higuchi H, Gores GJ. Bile acids activate EGF receptor via a TGF-alpha-dependent mechanism in human cholangiocyte cell lines. Am J Physiol Gastrointest Liver Physiol 2003; 285:G31-36.

41. Yoon JH., Higuchi H, Werneburg NW, Kaufmann SH, Gores GJ. Bile acids induce cyclooxygenase-2 expression via the epidermal growth factor receptor in a human cholangiocarcinoma cell line. Gastroenterology 2002; 122:985-993.

42. LeRoith D, Roberts CT, Jr. The insulin-like growth factor system and cancer. Cancer Lett 2003; 195:127-137.

43. Pollak MN, Schernhammer ES, Hankinson SE. Insulin-like growth factors and neoplasia. Nat Rev Cancer 2004; 4:505-518.

44. Foulstone E, Prince S, Zaccheo O, et al. Insulin-like growth factor ligands, receptors, and binding proteins in cancer. J Pathol 2005; 205:145-153.

45. Obenauer JC, Cantley LC, Yaffe MB. Scansite 2.0: proteome-wide prediction of cell signaling interactions using short sequence motifs. Nucleic Acids Res 2003;31:3635-3641.

46. LoPiccolo J, Granville CA, Gills JJ, Dennis PA. Targeting Akt in cancer therapy. Anticancer Drugs 2007;18:861-874.

47. Jorissen RN, Walker F, Pouliot N, et al. Epidermal growth factor receptor: mechanisms of activation and signalling. Exp Cell Res 2003; 284:31-53.

48. Ouban A, Muraca P, Yeatman T, Coppola D. Expression and distribution of insulin-like growth factor-1 receptor in human carcinomas. Hum Pathol 2003; 34:803-808.

49. Freier S, Weiss O, Eran M, et al. Expression of the insulin-like growth factors and their receptors in adenocarcinoma of the colon. Gut 1999; 44:704-708.

50. Peters G, Gongoll S, Langner C, et al. IGF-1R, IGF-1 and IGF-2 expression as potential prognostic and predictive markers in colorectal-cancer. Virchows Arch 2003; 443:139-145.

51. Schips L, Zigeuner R, Ratschek M, et al. Analysis of insulin-like growth factors and insulin-like growth factor I receptor expression in renal cell carcinoma. Am J Clin Pathol 2004; 122:931-937.

52. Kornpat P, Rehak P, Rüschoff J, Langer C. Expression of IGF-I, IGF-II, and IDF-IR in gallbladder carcinoma. A systematic analysis including primary and corresponding metastatic tumors. J Clin Pathol 2006;59:202-206.

53. Nakamura T, Nawa K, Ichihara A. Partial purification and characterization of hepatocyte growth factor from serum of hepatectomized rats. Biochem Biophys Res Commun 1984; 122:1450-1459.

54. Bottaro DP, Rubin JS, Faletto DL., et al. Identification of the hepatocyte growth factor receptor as the c-met proto-oncogene product. Science 1991; 251:802-804.

55. Di Renzo MF, Narsimhan RP, Olivero M, et al. M. Expres-

sion of the Met/HGF receptor in normal and neoplastic human tissues. Oncogene 1991; 6:1997-2003.

56. Furukawa T, Duguid WP, Kobari M, Matsuno S, Tsao MS. Hepatocyte growth factor and Met receptor expression in human pancreatic carcinogenesis. Am J Pathol 1995; 147:889-895.

57. Matsumoto K, Nakamura T. Emerging multipotent aspects of hepatocyte growth factor. J Biochem (Tokyo) 1996; 119:591-600.

58. Stoker M, Gherardi E, Perryman M, Gray J. Scatter factor is a fibroblast-derived modulator of epithelial cell mobility. Nature 1987;327:239-242.

59. Tajima H, Matsumoto K, Nakamura T. Regulation of cell growth and motility by hepatocyte growth factor and receptor expression in various cell species. Exp Cell Res 1992; 202:423-431.

60. Nakazawa K, Dobashi Y, Suzuki S, et al. Amplification and overexpression of c-erbB-2, epidermal growth factor receptor, and c-met in biliary tract cancers. J Pathol 2005; 206:356-365.

61. Radaeva S, Ferreira-Gonzalez A, Sirica AE. Overexpression of C-NEU and C-MET during rat liver cholangiocarcinogenesis: a link between biliary intestinal metaplasia and mucin-producing cholangiocarcinoma. Hepatology 1999; 29:1453-1462.

62. Tanaka T, Shimura H, Sasaki T, et al. Gallbladder cancer treatment using adenovirus expressing the HGF/NK4 gene in a peritoneal implantation model. Cancer Gene Ther 2004; 11:431-440.

63. Date K, Matsumoto K, Kuba K, et al. Inhibition of tumor growth and invasion by a four-kringle antagonist (HGF/NK4) for hepatocyte growth factor. Oncogene 1998; 17:3045-3054.

64. Abraham R T. PI 3-kinase related kinases: 'big' players in stress-induced signaling pathways. DNA Repair (Amst) 2004; 3:883-887.

65. Asnaghi L, Bruno P, Priulla M, Nicolin A. mTOR: a protein kinase switching between life and death. Pharmacol Res 2004; 50:545-549.

66. Shaw R J, Bardeesy N, Manning BD, et al. The LKB1 tumor suppressor negatively regulates mTOR signaling. Cancer Cell 2004; 6:91-99.

67. Brugarolas J, Lei K, Hurley RL., et al. Regulation of mTOR function in response to hypoxia by REDD1 and the TSC1/TSC2 tumor suppressor complex. Genes Dev 2004; 18:2893-2904.

68. Pervin S, Singh R, Hernandez E, Wu G, and Chaudhuri,G. Nitric oxide in physiologic concentrations targets the translational machinery to increase the proliferation of human breast cancer cells: involvement of mammalian target of rapamycin/eIF4E pathway. Cancer Res 2007; 67:289-299.

69. Cantley LC. The phosphoinositide 3-kinase pathway. Science 2002; 296:1655-1657.

70. Hynes NE, Boulay A. The mTOR pathway in breast cancer. J Mammary Gland Biol Neoplasia 2006; 11:53-61.

71. Wullschleger S, Loewith R, Hall MN. TOR signaling in growth and metabolism. Cell 2006; 124:471-484.

72. Hidalgo M, Rowinsky EK. The rapamycin-sensitive signal transduction pathway as a target for cancer therapy. Oncogene 2000; 19:6680-6686.

73. Richardson C J, Schalm SS., Blenis J. PI3-kinase and TOR: PIKTORing cell growth. Semin Cell Dev Biol 2004; 15:147-159.

74. Tee AR, Blenis J. mTOR, translational control and human disease. Semin Cell Dev Biol 2005; 16:29-37.

75. Alessi DR, Andjelkovic M, Caudwell B, et al. Mechanism of activation of protein kinase B by insulin and IGF-1. EMBO J 1996; 15:6541-6551.

76. Dan HC, Sun M, Yang L, et al. Phosphatidylinositol 3-kinase/Akt pathway regulates tuberous sclerosis tumor suppressor complex by phosphorylation of tuberin. J Biol Chem 2002; 277:35364-35370.

77. Inoki K, Li Y, Zhu T, Wu J, Guan KL. TSC2 is phosphorylated and inhibited by Akt and suppresses mTOR signalling. Nat Cell Biol 2002; 4:648-657.

78. Manning BD, Tee AR, Logsdon MN, Blenis J, Cantley LC. Identification of the tuberous sclerosis complex-2 tumor suppressor gene product tuberin as a target of the phosphoinositide 3-kinase/akt pathway. Mol Cell 2002; 10:151-162.

79. Gomez M, Whittemore V. Tuberous Sclerosis Complex. 3rd ed. New York: Oxford University Press, 1999.

80. Herbert TP, Tee AR, Proud CG. The extracellular signal-regulated kinase pathway regulates the phosphorylation of 4E-BP1 at multiple sites. J Biol Chem 2002; 277:11591-11596.

81. Roux PP, Blenis J. ERK and p38 MAPK-activated protein kinases: a family of protein kinases with diverse biological functions. Microbiol Mol Biol Rev 2004; 68:320-344.

82. Blenis J. Signal transduction via the MAP kinases: proceed at your own RSK. Proc Natl Acad Sci USA 1993; 90:5889-5892.

83. Jensen CJ, Buch MB, Krag TO, et al. 90-kDa ribosomal S6 kinase is phosphorylated and activated by 3-phosphoinositide-dependent protein kinase-1. J Biol Chem 1999; 274:27168-27176.

84. Roux PP, Shahbazian D, Vu H, et al. RAS/ERK signaling promotes site-specific ribosomal protein S6 phosphorylation via RSK and stimulates cap-dependent translation. J Biol Chem 2007; 282:14056-14064.

85. Inoki K, Zhu T, Guan KL. TSC2 mediates cellular energy response to control cell growth and survival. Cell 2003; 115:577-590.

86. Corradetti MN, Inoki K, Bardeesy N, DePinho RA, Guan KL. Regulation of the TSC pathway by LKB1: evidence of a molecular link between tuberous sclerosis complex and Peutz-Jeghers syndrome. Genes Dev 2004; 18:1533-1538.

87. Rowinsky EK. Targeting the molecular target of rapamycin (mTOR). Curr Opin Oncol 2004; 16:564-575.

88. Young DA, Nickerson-Nutter CL. mTOR—beyond transplantation. Curr Opin Pharmacol 2005; 5:418-423.

89. Thomas GV. mTOR and cancer: reason for dancing at the crossroads? Curr Opin Genet Dev 006; 16:78-84. 2

90. Wu Q, Kiguchi K, Kawamoto T, et al. Therapeutic effect of rapamycin on gallbladder cancer in a transgenic mouse model. Cancer Res 2007; 67:3794-3800.

91. Hori H, Ajiki T, Mita Y, et al. Frequent activation of mitogen-activated protein kinase relative to Akt in extrahepatic biliary tract cancer. J Gastroenterol 2007; 42:567-572.

92. Dubois RN, Abramson SB, Crofford L, et al. Cyclooxygenase in biology and disease. FASEB J 1998; 12:1063-1073.

93. Gupta RA, Dubois RN. Colorectal cancer prevention and treatment by inhibition of cyclooxygenase-2. Nat Rev Cancer 2001; 1:11-21.

94. Smith WL, Langenbach R. Why there are two cyclooxygenase isozymes. J Clin Invest 2001; 107:1491-1495.

95. Smith WL, DeWitt DL, Garavito RM. Cyclooxygenases: structural, cellular, and molecular biology. Annu Rev Biochem 2000; 69:145-182.

96. Stein-Werblowsky R. Prostaglandin and cancer. Oncology 1974;30:169-176.

97. Backlund MG, Mann JR, Dubois RN. Mechanisms for the prevention of gastrointestinal cancer: the role of prostaglandin E2. Oncology 2005; 69 (suppl 1):28-32.

98. Bos CL, Richel DJ, Ritsema T, Peppelenbosch MP, Versteeg HH. Prostanoids and prostanoid receptors in signal transduction. Int J Biochem Cell Biol 2004; 36:1187-1205.

99. Nagorney DM, McPherson GA. Carcinoma of the gallbladder and extrahepatic ile ducts. Semin Oncol 1988; 15:106-115.

100. Adson MA. Carcinoma of the gallbladder. Surg Clin North Am 1973;53:1203-1216.

101. Csendes A, Becerra M, Burdiles P, et al. Bacteriological studies of bile from the gallbladder in patients with carcinoma of the gallbladder, cholelithiasis, common bile duct stones and no gallstones disease. Eur J Surg 1994; 160:363-367.

102. Welton JC, Marr JS, Friedman SM. Association between hepatobiliary cancer and typhoid carrier state. Lancet 1979; 1:791-794.

103. Shukla VK, Singh H, Pandey M, Upadhyay SK, Nath G. Carcinoma of the gallbladder—is it a sequel of typhoid? Dig Dis Sci 2000; 45:900-903.

104. Chijiiwa K, Tanaka M, Nakayama F. Adenocarcinoma of the gallbladder associated with anomalous pancreaticobiliary ductal junction. Am Surg 1993; 59:430-434.

105. Koga H, Sakisaka S, Ohishi M, et al. Expression of cyclooxygenase-2 in human hepatocellular carcinoma: relevance to tumor dedifferentiation. Hepatology 1999; 29:688-696.

106. Asano T, Shoda J, Ueda T, et al. Expressions of cyclooxygenase-2 and prostaglandin E-receptors in carcinoma of the gallbladder: crucial role of arachidonate metabolism in tumor growth and progression. Clin Cancer Res 2002; 8:1157-1167.

107. Shiota G, Okubo M, Noumi T, et al. Cyclooxygenase-2 expression in hepatocellular carcinoma. Hepatogastroenterology 1999; 46:407-412.

108. Wu T, Han C, Lunz JG., et al. Involvement of 85-kd cytosolic phospholipase A(2) and cyclooxygenase-2 in the proliferation of human cholangiocarcinoma cells. Hepatology 2002; 36:363-373.

109. Han C, Leng J, Demetris AJ, Wu T. Cyclooxygenase-2 promotes human cholangiocarcinoma growth: evidence for cyclooxygenase-2-independent mechanism in celecoxib-mediated induction of p21waf1/cip1 and p27kip1 and cell cycle arrest. Cancer Res 2004; 64:1369-1376.

110. Wu T, Leng J, Han C, Demetris AJ. The cyclooxygenase-2 inhibitor celecoxib blocks phosphorylation of Akt and induces apoptosis in human cholangiocarcinoma cells. Mol Cancer Ther 2004; 3:299-307.

111. Zhang Z, Lai GH., Sirica AE. Celecoxib-induced apoptosis in rat cholangiocarcinoma cells mediated by Akt inactivation and Bax translocation. Hepatology 2004; 39:1028-1037.

112. Nzeako UC, Guicciardi ME, Yoon JH, Bronk SF, Gores G J. COX-2 inhibits Fas-mediated apoptosis in cholangiocarcinoma cells. Hepatology 2002; 35:552-559.

113. Lai GH, Zhang Z, Sirica AE. Celecoxib acts in a cyclooxygenase-2-independent manner and in synergy with emodin to suppress rat cholangiocarcinoma growth in vitro through a mechanism involving enhanced Akt inactivation and increased activation of caspases-9 and -3. Mol Cancer Ther 2003; 2:265-271.

114. Sirica AE, Lai GH, Endo K, Zhang Z, Yoon BI. Cyclooxygenase-2 and ERBB-2 in cholangiocarcinoma: potential therapeutic targets. Semin Liver Dis 2002; 22:303-313.

115. Grossman EM, Longo WE, Panesar N, Mazuski JE, Kaminski DL. The role of cyclooxygenase enzymes in the growth of human gall bladder cancer cells. Carcinogenesis 2000; 21:1403-1409.

116. Bellacosa A, Testa JR, Staal SP, Tsichlis PN. A retroviral oncogene, akt, encoding a serine-threonine kinase containing an SH2-like region. Science 1991; 254:274-277.

117. Zhang L, Jiang L, Sun Q, et al. Prostaglandin E(2) enhances mitogen-activated protein kinase/Erk pathway in human cholangiocarcinoma cells: involvement of EP1 receptor, calcium and EGF receptors signaling. Mol Cell Biochem 2007; 305:19-26.

118. Han C, Wu T. Cyclooxygenase-2-derived prostaglandin E2 promotes human cholangiocarcinoma cell growth and invasion through EP1 receptor-mediated activation of the epidermal growth factor receptor and Akt. J Biol Chem 2005; 280:24053-24063.

119. Conacci-Sorrell M, Zhurinsky J, Ben-Ze'ev A. The cadherin-catenin adhesion system in signaling and cancer. J Clin Invest 2002; 109:987-991.

120. Graus-Porta D, Beerli R, Hynes N. Single-chain antibody-mediated intracellular retention of ErbB-2 impairs Neu differentiation and epidermal growth factor signaling. Mol Cell Biol 1995; 15:1182-1191.

121. Murali R, Brennan PJ, Kieber-Emmons T, Greene MI. Structural analysis of p185c-neu and epidermal growth factor receptor tyrosine kinases: oligomerization of kinase domains. Proc Natl Acad Sci USA 1996; 93:6252-6257.

122. Vadlamudi R, Mandal M, Adam L, et al. Regulation of cyclooxygenase-2 pathway by HER2 receptor. Oncogene 1999; 18:305-314.

123. Qian X, LeVea C, Freeman J, Dougall W, Greene M. Het-

erodimerization of epidermal growth factor receptor and wild-type or kinase-deficient Neu: a mechanism of interreceptor kinase activation and transphosphorylation. Proc Natl Acad Sci USA 1994; 91:1500-1504.

124. Wada T, Qian X, Greene M. Intermolecular association of the p185neu protein and EGF receptor modulates EGF receptor function. Cell 1990; 61:1339-1347.

125. Sirica AE, Lai,GH, Zhang Z. Biliary cancer growth factor pathways, cyclo-oxygenase-2 and potential therapeutic strategies. J Gastroenterol Hepatol 2001; 16:363-372.

126. Birchmeier W, Behrens J. Cadherin expression in carcinomas: role in the formation of cell junctions and the prevention of invasiveness. Biochim Biophys Acta 1994; 1198:11-26.

127. Lawrence DS, Niu J. Protein kinase inhibitors: the tyrosine-specific protein kinases. Pharmacol Ther 1998; 77:81-114.

128. Sirotnak FM, Zakowski MF, Miller VA, Scher H I, Kris MG. Efficacy of cytotoxic agents against human tumor xenografts is markedly enhanced by coadministration of ZD1839 (Iressa), an inhibitor of EGFR tyrosine kinase. Clin Cancer Res 2000; 6:4885-4892.

129. Xu L, Han C, Wu T. A novel positive feedback loop between peroxisome proliferator-activated receptor-delta and prostaglandin E2 signaling pathways for human cholangiocarcinoma cell growth. J Biol Chem 2006; 281:33982-33996.

130. Yoshitomi K, Alison RH, Boorman GA. Adenoma and adenocarcinoma of the gall bladder in aged laboratory mice. Vet. Pathol 1986;23:523-527.

131. Haines DC, Chattopadhyay S, Ward JM. Pathology of aging B6;129 mice. Toxicol Pathol 2001; 29:653-661.

132. Toth B, Nagel D, Patil K. Tumorigenesis by N-n-propyl-N-formylhydrazine in mice. Br. J Cancer 1980; 42:922-928.

133. Enomoto M, Naoe S, Harada M, et al. Carcinogenesis in extrahepatic bile duct and gallbladder.Carcinogenic effects of N-hydroxy-2-acetamidofluorene in mice fed a "gallstone-inducing" diet. Jpn J Exp Med 1974;44:37-54.

134. Turosov VS, Gorin B. Tumours of gallbladder. In: V. Turosov and U. Mohr (eds.), Pathology of Tumours in Laboratory Animals, pp. 109-125. Lyon: IARC Scientific Publications, 1996.

135. Suzuki A, Takahashi T. Histogenesis of the gallbladder carcinoma induced by methylcholanthrene bees-wax pellets in hamsters. Jpn J Surg 1983;13:55-59.

136. Kowalewski K, Todd EF. Carcinoma of the gallbladder induced in hamsters by insertion of cholesterol pellets and feeding dimethylnitrosamine. Proc Soc Exp Biol Med 1971;136:482-486.

137. Elmore LW, Sirica AE. Phenotypic characterization of metaplastic intestinal glands and ductular hepatocytes in cholangiofibrotic lesions rapidly induced in the caudate liver lobe of rats treated with furan. Cancer Res 1991; 51:5752-5759.

138. Elmore LW, Sirica AE. "Intestinal-type" of adenocarcinoma preferentially induced in right/caudate liver lobes of rats treated with furan. Cancer Res 1993; 53:254-259.

139. Sirica AE, Radaeva S, Caran N. NEU overexpression in the furan rat model of cholangiocarcinogenesis compared with biliary ductal cell hyperplasia. Am J Pathol 1997;151:1685-1694.

140. Lai,CL, Leung N, Teo EK, et al. A. A 1-year trial of telbivudine, lamivudine, and the combination in patients with hepatitis B e antigen-positive chronic hepatitis B. Gastroenterology 2005; 129:528-536.

141. Kiguchi K, Ruffino L, Kawamoto T, Ajiki T, Digiovanni J. Chemopreventive and therapeutic efficacy of orally active tyrosine kinase inhibitors in a transgenic mouse model of gallbladder carcinoma. Clin Cancer Res 2005; 11:5572-5580.

142. Kiguchi K, Ruffino L, Kawamoto T, et al. Therapeutic effect of CS-706, a specific cyclooxygenase-2 inhibitor, on gallbladder carcinoma in BK5.ErbB-2 mice. Mol Cancer Ther 2007; 6:1709-1717.

143. Bartlett DL, Fong Y, Fortner JG, Brennan MF, Blumgart LH. Long-term results after resection for gallbladder cancer. Implications for staging and management. Ann Surg 1996; 224:639-646.

144. Shirai Y, Yoshida K, Tsukada K, Muto T, Watanabe H. Radical surgery for gallbladder carcinoma. Long-term results. Ann Surg 1992; 216:565-568.

145. Donohue JH, Nagorney DM, Grant CS, et al. Carcinoma of the gallbladder. Does radical resection improve outcome? Arch Surg 1990; 125:237-241.

146. Ogura Y, Mizumoto R, Isaji S, et al. Radical operations for carcinoma of the gallbladder: present status in Japan. World J Surg 1991; 15:337-343.

147. Curley S. Biliary tract cancer. In: Pollock RE (ed.), Surgical Oncology, pp. 273-307. Dordrecht: Kluwer Academic Publishers, 1997.

II

DIAGNOSTIC APPROACHES

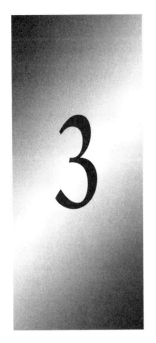

3 Histopathology and Molecular Pathogenesis of Gallbladder Cancer

Iván Roa
Xabier de Aretxabala
Ignacio I. Wistuba

Gallbladder cancer is a very rare tumor in most countries, particularly in developed countries, with the exception of certain areas of Japan (1-3). The greatest frequency is observed in the northern regions of India (4) and in Latin American countries such as Chile, Bolivia, and Mexico (5, 6).

Gallstones are one of the most important risk factors in this neoplasia (7-10). In countries like Chile, the link between mortality and the cholecystectomy rate has been proven (11, 12). Other factors such as gender, age, obesity, parity (13, 14), chronic inflammation (15, 16), gallbladder adenomas (17-19), and an anomalous pancreaticobiliary ductal junction (20, 21) have also been involved. Chronic inflammation and irritation of the gallbladder mucosa, a product of gallstones, must play an important role in the carcinogenesis; however, there are few studies linking these factors with the development of gallbladder cancer (16, 22-24).

Knowledge is limited concerning the events and genetic-molecular changes that occur during the development of gallbladder cancer (6, 15, 25, 26); however, similar to other neoplasias, initial studies have shown a series of different changes in oncogenes, tumor suppressor genes and DNA repair genes in both the early and advanced stages of the disease (27-31).

Of the most widely accepted models in gallbladder carcinogenesis, the dysplasia-carcinoma sequence is the one that has taken on the greatest significance in gallbladder cancer (15, 32, 33). Adenomas that are precursors to adenocarcinomas appear to play a secondary role (17, 32, 34). Even where there is morphologic and molecular evidence that make it possible to endorse both models, the dysplasia-carcinoma sequence seems the most plausible.

The aim of this chapter is to analyze certain aspects related to the histogenesis of gallbladder cancer as well as to point out the most frequent observations at the genetic-molecular level that have been described for this tumor.

EPITHELIAL DYSPLASIA: THE PRECURSOR TO ADENOCARCINOMA OF THE GALLBLADDER

Dysplasia Not Associated with Gallbladder Cancer

Dysplasia in the gallbladder mucosa has been defined as a change in the maturation of the glandular epithelium due to nuclear irregularity, hyperchromasia, loss of polarity, nuclear pseudostratification, a change in the

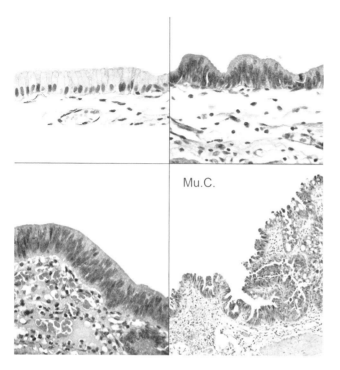

FIGURE 3.1

On the edges of the early tumor lesions studied using serial sections, adenoma foci were found only exceptionally (46, 47).

Early Gallbladder Carcinoma

CIS (pTis), mucosal carcinoma (CMu) (pT1a), and muscular carcinomas (CMp) (pT1b) are considered early gallbladder carcinomas (48-51) (Figure 3.2). Their recognition is of great significance according to the therapeutic protocols currently employed; cholecystectomy, simple or extended, would be the definitive treatment for these types of lesions (48, 52, 53).

There is little information with respect to mucosal carcinomas of the gallbladder (46, 51, 54, 55). In most countries they represent anecdotal or exceptional cases. Nevertheless, in countries with a high incidence of gallbladder cancer, like Chile, India, and Japan, mucosal carcinomas may represent up to 15-20% of all gallbladder cancers diagnosed from cholecystectomies (2, 47).

In our series (206 cases), lithiasis was present in 95% of the early carcinomas, and the actuarial survival

nucleus/cytoplasm ratio, and/or the presence of atypical mitoses (32, 35-37) (Figure 3.1). There are no consistent histologic criteria ensuring the reproducibility of the changes that characterize the dysplasia.

The frequency with which dysplasia of the gallbladder mucosa has been reported in cholecystectomies for lithiasis varies between 1 and 20% of the gallbladders with chronic cholecystitis (38-40). According to our observations, epithelial dysplasia not associated with gallbladder cancer is a rare lesion, close to 1% of cholecystectomies for lithiasis (32).

All of the dysplasias not associated with gallbladder cancer were an incidental finding during the routine histologic exam not identified macroscopically. These lesions are often multiple and are considered as precursors to gallbladder cancer (27, 35, 40, 41).

Dysplasia Associated with Gallbladder Cancer

In the mucosa adjacent to the gallbladder cancer, metaplasia, dysplasia, and carcinoma in situ (CIS) have been described at rates of 66, 81.3, and 69%, respectively (42). A close topographic relation has been shown between the infiltrating carcinoma and intraepithelial lesions, which may support its progression (35, 42-45).

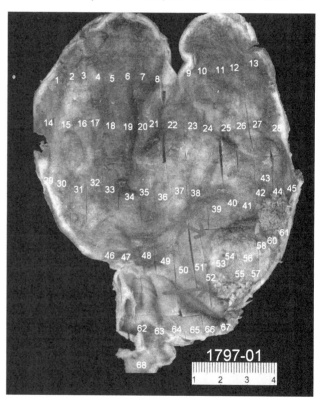

FIGURE 3.2

was 92% at 5 years. In this group, only eight patients died with evidence of progression of gallbladder cancer. In 95% of the cases, signs of chronic inflammation of the gallbladder wall were observed, with epithelial changes associated with atrophy and metaplastic foci of the mucosa (gastric and intestinal) (46).

ADENOMA AND GALLBLADDER CANCER

Solitary, sessile, and echodense gallbladder polyps greater than 1 cm are most likely to be adenomas (17, 56, 57). Despite only a small percentage of these undergoing a malignant transformation to an adenocarcinoma, until now it has not been possible to predict which ones will do so (19, 58). Gallbladder carcinomas are infrequent tumors in our series and correspond to 0.17% (44 cases) of the cholecystectomies performed for symptomatic lithiasis (18).

Most adenomas are tubular. Thirty percent of the adenomas are doubles or multiples, and 88% are located in the distal half (body and fundus) (18). The malignant transformation of gallbladder adenomas, as in the large bowel, is in proportion with the size of the adenoma (17, 59, 60). In 8 out of 32 cases of adenomas with areas of gallbladder adenocarcinomas, six were in the fundus and seven were single lesions. In six cases, the adenomas measured more than 10 mm and in two more than 5 mm in diameter (18).

DYSPLASIA-CARCINOMA SEQUENCE: THE MOST ACCEPTED MODEL IN THE DEVELOPMENT OF GALLBLADDER CANCER

Atypical epithelial lesions (dysplasias) of the gallbladder have been considered preneoplastic lesions. From them, CIS develops that evolves into a mucosal carcinoma and subsequently an infiltrating carcinoma (32, 35, 40) (Figure 3.3). In this model, the initial lesions are attributable to inflammation (16, 43). Chronic inflammation produces epithelial regeneration with adaptive changes such as metaplasias (24). Most early carcinomas show metaplastic foci and atrophy in the adjacent mucosa (42).

In the gallbladder, two types of metaplasia are observed, comparable to those observed in the stomach: the pyloric or gastric and intestinal metaplasia (40, 61, 62). Gallbladder cancers are associated with both types of metaplasia, particularly the intestinal type (33, 40, 44, 61). Dysplasia appears on these metaplasia, which progresses to a carcinoma in situ and subsequently becomes invasive (33, 63). The significance of metaplasia and its connection to dysplasia has not been completely defined in the gallbladder.

In our series of 210 completely mapped mucosal carcinoma, remnants of an adenoma were observed in only 6 cases (2.8%) (32). This finding strongly supports the notion that gallbladder carcinogenesis occurs through the transformation of the epithelium of the mucosa and not through the transformation of a pre-existing adenoma.

The difficulty in following up on dysplastic lesions in the gallbladder means that the unequivocal relationship between dysplasia and gallbladder carcinoma cannot be guaranteed. Only in exceptional circumstances can the gallbladder mucosa be examined in the absence of gallstones, which is why there is so little information with respect to the existence of epithelial dysplasia in gallbladders with no lithiasis or chronic inflammation (64).

AGE OF APPEARANCE OF THE PRECURSOR LESIONS OF THE INVASIVE CARCINOMA

The presence of gallstones, chronic inflammation, and the marked distortion of the gallbladder wall make the preoperative diagnosis of gallbladder cancer very difficult in most patients, particularly those with early cancers (65-67). In countries with a high rate of symptomatic gallstones, cholecystectomy for lithiasis is performed on thousands of patients each year (5, 68, 69). Given that there is no other selection of patients except for symptomatic lithiasis, the age at which the histologic diagnosis is established represents one of the only approximations possible for estimating the point at which these lesions occur (63).

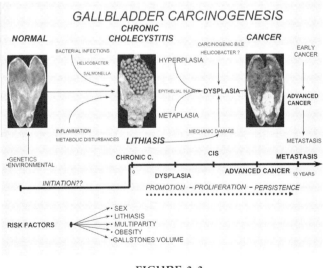

FIGURE 3.3

The average age of patients with chronic chole-cystitis in our cases was 46.5 years (SD 16.2), 51.9 years (SD 14.5) for epithelial dysplasia, and 56.8 years (SD 15.7) for mucosal carcinoma. The difference in the average ages between chronic cholecystitis and invasive cancer was 10.3 years for the general group (10.9 years for women and 9.2 years for men) (Figure 3.4). At the subserous carcinoma stage, the progression to serous carcinoma only requires a few months, suggesting that the state of subserous carcinoma is the critical point in the natural evolution of gallbladder cancer and is probably the last opportunity to modify its natural history.

MOLECULAR PATHOGENY OF GALLBLADDER CANCER

In multiple malignant neoplasias in humans, including gallbladder cancer, it has been proven that the transformation is the result of the progressive accumulation of multiple genetic alterations and that they compromise different groups of genes (oncogenes, tumor suppressor genes, and DNA repair genes) (70, 71-73).

Gallbladder cancer is one of the malignant neoplasias with the fewest published studies; therefore, information concerning the genetic molecular events that may participate in the appearance of a gallbladder cancer is limited (6, 15, 74, 75). The studies in this area suggest the presence of (1) overall genetic damage, (2) aberrant expression of genes connected to prolifer-ation and cell cycle, and (3) changes in specific genes and intracellular metabolic pathways.

It must also be mentioned that chronic inflammation of the gallbladder mucosa may play a role as capable of causing damage at the gene level and activating metabolic pathways related to the development and progression of gallbladder cancer (76-78). In this chapter we include some of the most important genetic changes described for this neoplasia.

Overall Genetic Damage in Gallbladder Cancer

Studies indicate that in gallbladder cancer there is large-scale genetic damage, demonstrated by an analysis of low-density chromosomal deletions through the entire genome and another of high density in chromosomes 3p, 8p, 9q, and 22q, where more than 30 regions with frequent deletions have been identified (29, 79), where tumor suppressor genes have been detected and studies have begun on these (30). It has also been proven that in gallbladder cancer there is a relatively high rate of genetic instability, not associated with changes in the hMSH2 and hLMH1 DNA repair genes (28). Conversely, methylation of gene promoter regions has been observed as a frequent inactivation mechanism of tumor suppressor genes and DNA repair genes (74, 80, 81). Among the genes with frequent methylation of the promoter regions are FHIT (68%), p16 (56%), PTEN

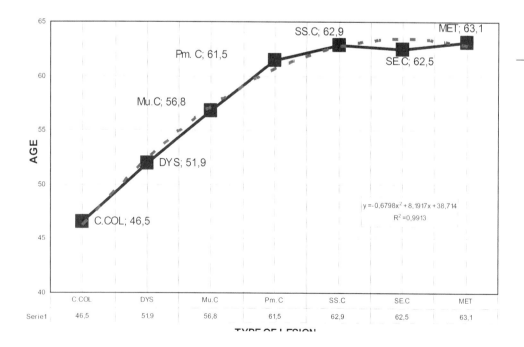

SEQUENCE AGE AND TYPE OF LESION

$$y = -0,6798x^2 + 8,1917x + 38,714$$
$$R^2 = 0,9913$$

	C.COL	DYS	Mu.C	Pm.C	SS.C	SE.C	MET
Serie1	46,5	51,9	56,8	61,5	62,9	62,5	63,1

FIGURE 3.4

(30%), p73 (28%), and APC (26%) (30) CDH1, etc. A high incidence (38%) of mitochondrial DNA mutations has also been found in gallbladder cancer, which in some way reflects the high rate of mutagenicity to which the cells of the gallbladder epithelium are subjected (82).

Study of Gene Expression in Gallbladder Cancer

Overexpression has been demonstrated in various groups of genes belonging to different metabolic pathways in gallbladder cancer (83, 84). Among other genes, the ones that stand out are of proliferation antigens and cell cycle (e.g., cyclins D2, E2, cdc/p34, geminin) (85, 86), transcription factors (e.g., homeobox B7, islet1) (87), growth factors, and growth factor receptors (e.g., hepatocyte growth factor, amphiregulin, insulin-like growth factor 1 receptor) (88, 89).

Changes in Specific Genes in Gallbladder Cancer

Changes have been proven in specific genes studied in gallbladder cancer that may play a significant role in its pathogeny. The most studied include: proto-oncogenes: K-ras (12p12.1) (90, 91), C-erbB2 (17q21.1) (92), VEGF (6p12) (93, 94), EGFR (4q25) (95, 96), and some tumor suppressor genes such as TP53 (17p13) (97, 98), p16 (9p21) (99), FHIT (3p14.2) (30, 100), CDH1 (16q22.1) (25, 80), etc.

K-ras

The main alteration of the K-ras gene observed in malignant tumors corresponds to a mutation that occurs at codon 12 and to a lesser degree at codon 13 in approximately 80% of cases. Most of these are transitions (guanine-adenine) (29, 90, 101). Most authors attribute to this gene little participation in gallbladder carcinogenesis, except for in patients with an anomalous pancreaticobiliary ductal junction, suggesting that reflux can play a role in carcinogenesis in these types of patients (102, 103).

ERBB-2

ERBB-2 codifies a tyrosine-kinase transmembrane receptor that participates in the regulation of DNA repair, cell-cycle checkpoints, and apoptosis. Its amplification and overexpression have been proven in 33-70% of gallbladder cancers (92, 104, 105). Proteic expression has not been shown in either gallbladder adenomas or dysplasias (92, 106).

Cyclooxygenase-2

The metabolism of arachidonic acid and the synthesis of prostaglandins are catalyzed by a group of cyclooxygenase (COX) enzymes. At least three isoforms have been identified (COX-1, COX-2, and COX-3) (107-109). Overexpression of COX-2 has been confirmed in many neoplasias (colon, stomach, lung, etc.) (109-112). COX-2 favors the formation of prostaglandins that inhibit apoptosis and stimulate angiogenesis and invasiveness. A relation between the expression of COX-2 and p53 has been demonstrated, suggesting that the loss of p53 function may influence the overexpression of COX-2 (113). A low proteic expression of COX-2 has been observed in nontumor gallbladder mucosa (14.3%), whereas in dysplasia and cancer, its expression is detected in 45-70%, which suggests the participation of COX-2 in the early stages of the disease.

Cyclin D1 and Cyclin E

These play a role in carcinogenesis through promotion as positive regulators of the cell-cycle progression. Overexpression of cyclins D1 and E has been detected in between 40 and 68% of gallbladder cancers (114, 115), less in dysplasias and nontumor gallbladder mucosa, which suggests that they may play a role in the initial stages of gallbladder cancer (116). Nuclear overexpression of cyclin D1 has been associated with the degree of cell proliferation and the potential for tumor infiltration, with the greatest overexpression being observed in those tumors which are poorly differentiated (86).

Vascular Endothelial Growth Factor (VEGF)

VEGF expression has been identified in 16.7% of chronic cholecystites, 35-75% of adenomas, and 38-91% of gallbladder cancers, with the greatest expression being seen in the most advanced tumors (117), suggesting a link between VEGF expression and the progression of the tumor. This coincides with the biology of most malignant tumors that require a vascular support capable of satisfying its growth needs. A connection has also been observed between the increase in VEGF expression and an abnormal expression of p53 and vice versa (117, 118).

p16/CDKN2/INK4

One of the most common changes observed in tumors is related to the inactivation of the RB-CDK-INK4A pathway, which is a frequent event in malignant neoplasias (119). The p16/CDKN2/INK4 (9p21) tumor suppressor gene participates in the cell cycle, regulating G1 progression to the S phase of the cell cycle (120, 121). The protein of the p16/INK4 gene acts as an inhibitor, avoiding pRb phosphorylation and thus avoiding progression to the S phase.

Gene inactivation has been demonstrated in half of all gallbladder carcinomas. The most frequent inactivation mechanisms are mutation, deletion, and methylation of the promoter area of the gene (79, 121-123). This contrasts with the low frequency of changes observed in the RB gene in at least 20% of gallbladder cancers (29). Some studies have shown a loss of proteic expression of p16/INK4 in around 75% of cases (120), which has been associated with a poor prognosis (117, 120).

p53

The p53 tumor suppressor gene has been extensively studied in other neoplasias, and it has been established that the point mutation occurs in specific places (so-called hot-spots) (124, 125). In more than 98% of cases, these mutations are produced in exons 5-8 (126, 127). Even when gene p53 participates in gallbladder carcinogenesis, it seems to be on the late side; its presence in preneoplastic lesions is low, and its significant increase in advanced tumor lesions has established a connection in the dysplasia-CIS-advanced carcinoma progression (128, 129). In gallbladder cancer, the immunohistochemical expression of gene p53 has been shown in more than 50% of cases (35-92%), (97, 98, 130). Most studies have confirmed point mutations in 31-70% of gallbladder cancers (97, 98, 131). The loss of heterozygocity (LOH)of the alleles in gene p53 has been proven in 92% of cases; in these cases, the LOH preceded the immunohistochemical expression of the protein (29).

FHIT

There is little information with respect to the abnormalities of this gene in gallbladder cancer (30, 80, 100, 132). The high rate of deletion of the locus at 3p14.2 (76%) and methylation (64%) of the FHIT gene in gallbladder cancer are related to a frequent loss of its immunohistochemical expression (79%) in tumor cells (100). A direct relation has also been observed between the reduction in FHIT expression and an increase in LOH. In the nontumor gallbladder epithelium, loss of FHIT expression has been observed in 9% without LOH; in dysplasia, there was a reduction in proteic expression in 55% of cases and LOH in 46% of cases and in invasive carcinoma a loss of FHIT expression in 79% and LOH in 76% (132). These studies suggest that the FHIT gene is altered sequentially and progressively in the development of gallbladder cancer.

Cadherin-Catenin Complex

Alterations in the cadherin-catenin complex are related to a loss of cell adhesion and the formation of cell populations responsible for tumor invasion (133, 134). The anomalous expression of the cadherin-catenin complex has been frequently demonstrated in a large number of neoplasias, including in the gallbladder (135-137). A reduction or absence of E-cadherin has been observed in 26% of tumors (138). Others have demonstrated a relation between the tumor grade and the expression of this molecule (139, 140). β-Catenin is a key regulator of the cadherin-catenin cell adhesion complex. The β-catenin mutation has been seen more often in gallbladder adenomas than in carcinomas (141, 142). The mutations of this gene predominantly affect exon 3 and have been observed in 10 out of 16 adenomas and in only one out of 21 carcinomas, suggesting a different carcinogenic pathway in the gallbladder (142, 143).

Other Molecular Finding

Other genes and metabolic pathways have recently been described as altered in the pathogenesis of gallbladder cancer, among which can be mentioned the loss of DCP4 expression (144, 145) and potential tumor suppressor genes located in chromosome 3p such as DUTT1 (3p12), BLU, RASSF1A, and SEMA3B (30). One recent report (Alvarez H, et al. Serial analysis of gene expression identifies novel candidate markers for gallbladder cancer. Gastrointestinal Cancers Symposium, 2007) has shown a differential expression in some genes in gallbladder cancer, such as CEACAM5, GOLPH2, LY6D, OLFM4, SSP1, CDK10, HMOX1, PEBP1, PROM1, SULF1, and CLU and some new genes-CTSD, UBD, POLD3-whose significance is still unknown in this neoplasia.

MICROSATELLITE INSTABILITY IN GALLBLADDER CANCER

Microsatellite instability has been reported in gallbladder cancer in around 10-20% of cases and also in lesions considered preneoplastic in the gallbladder (intestinal metaplasia and dysplasia) (27, 99). Microsatellite instability does not seem to be a frequent mechanism in the development of gallbladder cancer (84, 103, 146).

HTERT/TELOMERASE

Few published studies exist with respect to the role that hTERT/Telomerase may play in gallbladder cancer. Most of these studies show a minimal expression in the normal or regenerative gallbladder epithelium (4%), which increases progressively in dysplasia (25% in low-grade dysplasia, 82% in high-grade dysplasia) and in adenocarcinoma (93%) (147). Other authors have found hTERT expression in 57, 66, and 73% of the adenocarcinomas studied (148). Its eventual use as a molecular marker has been proposed for the diagnosis of gallbladder cancer, and it may have prognostic implications (147, 149).

GENETIC ANOMALIES IN THE DYSPLASIA-CARCINOMA SEQUENCE OF THE GALLBLADDER

According to the most frequently observed genetic alterations in the nontumor epithelium, dysplasia not associated with cancer and dysplasia associated with gallbladder cancer (150), initial models have appeared with changes observed in the dysplasia-carcinoma sequence (Figure 3.5). Among the genetic alterations that may be considered as early are the mutations of gene p53 (31) and the mitochondrial DNA, as well as deletions in the 17p13, 9p21 (79, 147, 151), COX-2

(16), and 3p (82) chromosome regions. The genetic alterations that appear at intermediate stages (dysplasias) see the inactivation of the FHIT gene and deletions of 22q and p16 (30, 80, 100). In advanced stages (invasive carcinoma), mutations of the ras genes and deletions of the 5q21 loci in the APC, MLH1, and VEGF genes can be found (15, 150).

A progressive increase in the frequency of allelic losses in ranges that vary between 14 and 70% in different chromosome regions (3p12-FHIT, 3p21-24, 8p21-23, 9p21-CDKN2A, 9q31-34 and 17p13-TP53) (28, 29) as well as mutations of p53 and loss of gene expression have been observed in histologically normal epithelia adjacent to areas of invasive gallbladder carcinoma, which shows that the genetic alterations in the gallbladder mucosa precede the morphologic alterations such as epithelial dysplasia, lending further support to this carcinogenetic pathway (75, 152).

INFLAMMATION AND GALLBLADDER CANCER

In a significant number of tumors of the gastrointestinal system, there is evidence that relates chronic inflam-

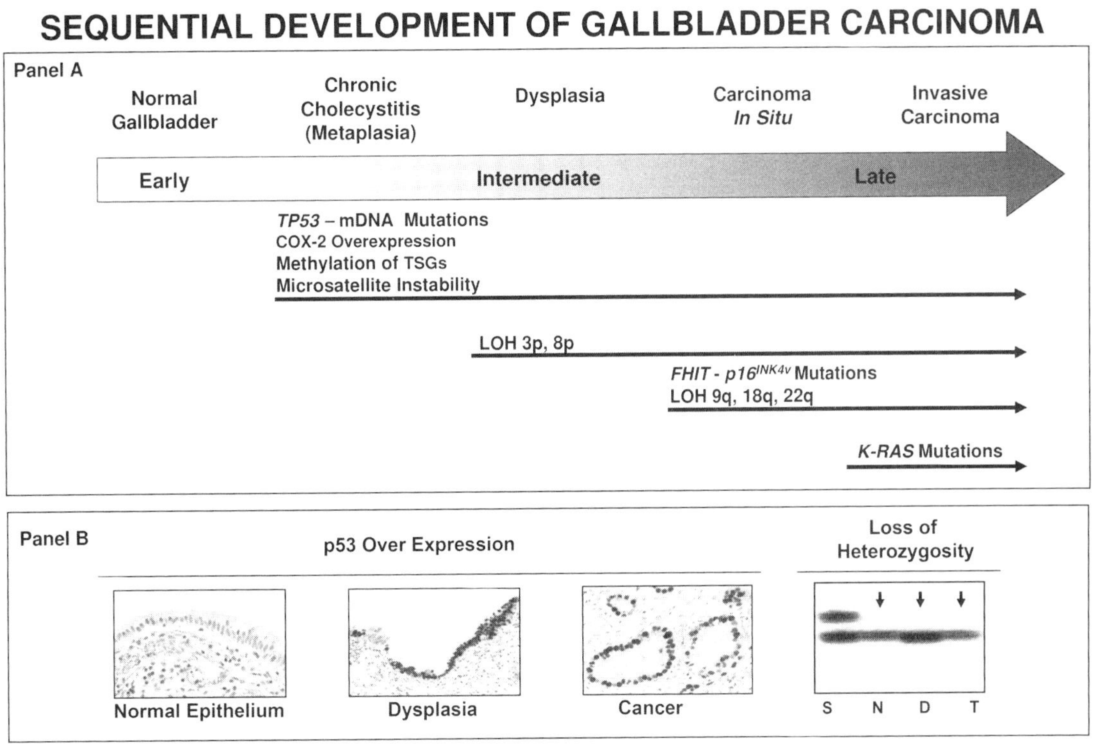

SEQUENTIAL DEVELOPMENT OF GALLBLADDER CARCINOMA

FIGURE 3.5

mation to the development of malignant tumors (77, 111). Such is the case with the adaptive changes (intestinal metaplasia) that the esophagus suffers subsequent to the damage and inflammation secondary to acid reflux. Other examples are the model of gastric carcinogenesis caused by inflammation secondary to infection by *Helicobacter pylori* (153, 154) and the tumors of the extrahepatic bile duct associated with parasitic infection by *Clonorchis sinensis* and *Opisthorchis viverrini* (155, 156).

There are still too few studies to make it possible to suggest the participation of inflammation as a significant element in the development of gallbladder carcinoma (16, 23, 77). Most morphologic studies show the presence of chronic inflammation in practically all cases of gallbladder cancer. The mechanical damage and irritation that gallstones cause to the epithelium must activate the inflammatory process and the mechanisms of regeneration and tissue repair. There is a proven link between the size and volume of gallstones and the risk of developing gallbladder cancer (7, 10). The largest gallstones are the ones that have remained the longest in the gallbladder lumen and have produced the most irritation trauma to the mucosa.

Chronic inflammation in the gallbladder is expressed morphologically in various ways. At the level of the mucosa, it is possible to observe from hyperplastic foci (infrequent) metaplasias (pyloric and intestinal) up to different degrees of atrophy, including the disappearance of the epithelium from the mucosa.

From the molecular point of view, the following has been proven: deletions from the chromosome regions in 3p, 8p, 9p (p16 locus gene), and 17p (p53 locus gene) in histologically normal epithelia of chronic cholecystitis as well as p53 mutations in 57% of normal epithelia associated with cancer (29). Most p53 gene mutations detected have been transitions, particularly C:T, which in other neoplasias has been associated with the presence of endogenous mutagens, such as those generated in inflammation (15, 157). A similar fact has been observed in mitochondrial gene mutations (25% in the gallbladder epithelium of chronic cholecystitis) (82) and a progressive increase in the intensity of the COX-2 expression, in direct relation to the progression of the histopathologic lesions proposed in the model of the sequential development of gallbladder cancer: normal epithelium-chronic cholecystitis-dysplasia-gallbladder cancer (Figure 3.4). All the evidence strongly suggests the relation existing between inflammation and gallbladder cancer; however, there is still no complete understanding of this carcinogenetic mechanism.

CONCLUSION

Like other malignant epithelial tumors, gallbladder cancer is a product of the transformation of the normal epithelium in preneoplastic and ultimately neoplastic lesions. Metaplasia is a very common finding in chronically inflamed gallbladder mucosa in over 50% of gallbladders. Gallbladder cancer is associated with both types of metaplasia, especially intestinal. On this metaplasia appears dysplasia, which progresses to carcinoma in situ and subsequently invasive carcinoma.

Recently reported molecular evidence suggests that dysplastic lesions present an altered gene expression pattern concordant with the progression to carcinoma in situ. The initial molecular characterization supports this transformation.

There is experimental and clinical evidence to support both carcinogenetic models: dysplasia-carcinoma and adenoma-carcinoma. However, the findings on the morphologic, clinical, and genetic-molecular levels suggest that these correspond to two different and independent biologic events. The low frequency of adenomas and the absence of adenomatous remains in the vicinity of early carcinomas suggest the adenoma-carcinoma sequence is of limited value in the gallbladder, with the dysplasia-carcinoma sequence being the most likely from the biologic point of view.

The dysplasia-gallbladder cancer progression is related to the ages of the patients diagnosed with these lesions. An almost exact correlation is observed between the increase in age and the intensity of the lesions, such that it has been possible to suggest a time estimate required for this transformation. According to these findings, the time required for the transformation from chronic cholecystitis to mucosal carcinoma would be 10.9 years for women and 9.2 years for men.

Gallbladder cancer represents a special model in human carcinogenesis that requires greater attention and from which valuable and important information can be obtained in the study and understanding of neoplastic processes in the human being.

ACKNOWLEDGMENTS

Study financed by Fondecyt projects #1060375 and PBC-06 CTI Salud SA.

References

1. Randi G, Franceschi S, La Vecchia C. Gallbladder cancer worldwide: geographical distribution and risk factors. Int J Cancer 2006; 118(7):1591-1602.
2. Kayahara M, Nagakawa T. Recent trends of gallbladder cancer in Japan: an analysis of 4770 patients. Cancer 2007; 110(3):572-580.

3. Lowenfels AB, Maisonneuve P, Boyle P, Zatonski WA. Epidemiology of gallbladder cancer. Hepatogastroenterology 1999; 46(27):1529-1532.

4. Kapoor VK, McMichael AJ. Gallbladder cancer: an 'Indian' disease. Natl Med J India 2003; 16(4):209-213.

5. Andia KM, Gederlini GA, Ferreccio RC. [Gallbladder cancer: trend and risk distribution in Chile]. Rev Med Chil 2006; 134(5):565-574.

6. Lazcano-Ponce EC, Miquel JF, Munoz N, et al. Epidemiology and molecular pathology of gallbladder cancer. CA Cancer J Clin 2001; 51(6):349-364.

7. Lowenfels AB, Lindström CG, Conway MJ, Hastings PR. Gallstones and risk of gallbladder cancer. JNCI 1985; 75:77-80.

8. Chow WH, Johansen C, Gridley G, Mellemkjaer L, Olsen JH, Fraumeni JF, Jr. Gallstones, cholecystectomy and risk of cancers of the liver, biliary tract and pancreas. Br J Cancer 1999; 79(3-4):640-644.

9. Lowenfels AB, Walker AM, Althaus DP, Townsend G, Domellof L. Gallstone growth, size, and risk of gallbladder cancer: an interracial study. Int J Epidemiol 1989; 18(1):50-4.

10. Roa I, Ibacache G, Roa J, Araya J, de Aretxabala X, Munoz S. Gallstones and gallbladder cancer-volume and weight of gallstones are associated with gallbladder cancer: a case-control study. J Surg Oncol 2006; 93(8):624-628.

11. Nervi F, Duarte I, Gomez G, Rodriguez G, Del Pino G, Ferrerio O, et al. Frequency of gallbladder cancer in Chile, a high-risk area. Int J Cancer 1988; 41(5):657-660.

12. Serra I, Calvo A, Maturana M, Medina E, Sharp A. Changing trends of gall-bladder cancer in Chile, a high-risk area. Int J Cancer 1990; 45(2):376-377.

13. Pandey M. Risk factors for gallbladder cancer: a reappraisal. Eur J Cancer Prev 2003; 12(1):15-24.

14. Strom BL, Soloway RD, Rios-Dalenz JL, Rodriguez-Martinez HA, West SL, Kinman JL, et al. Risk factors for gallbladder cancer. An international collaborative case-control study. Cancer 1995; 76(10):1747-1756.

15. Wistuba, II, Gazdar AF. Gallbladder cancer: lessons from a rare tumour. Nat Rev Cancer 2004; 4(9):695-706.

16. Kanoh K, Shimura T, Tsutsumi S, Suzuki H, Kashiwabara K, Nakajima T, et al. Significance of contracted cholecystitis lesions as high risk for gallbladder carcinogenesis. Cancer Lett 2001; 169(1):7-14.

17. Kozuka S, Tsubone N, Yasui A, Hachisuka K. Relation of adenoma to carcinoma in the gallbladder. Cancer 1982; 50(10):2226-2234.

18. Roa I, de Aretxabala X, Morgan R, Molina R, Araya JC, Roa J, et al. [Clinicopathological features of gallbladder polyps and adenomas]. Rev Med Chil 2004; 132(6):673-679.

19. Watanabe H, Date K, Itoi T, Matsubayashi H, Yokoyama N, Yamano M, et al. Histological and genetic changes in malignant transformation of gallbladder adenoma. Ann Oncol 1999; 10 Suppl 4:136-139.

20. Hu B, Gong B, Zhou DY. Association of anomalous pancreaticobiliary ductal junction with gallbladder carcinoma in Chinese patients: an ERCP study. Gastrointest Endosc 2003; 57(4):541-545.

21. Chijiiwa K, Kimura H, Tanaka M. Malignant potential of the gallbladder in patients with anomalous pancreaticobiliary ductal junction. The difference in risk between patients with and without choledochal cyst. Int Surg 1995; 80(1):61-64.

22. Caygill CP, Hill MJ, Braddick M, Sharp JC. Cancer mortality in chronic typhoid and paratyphoid carriers. Lancet 1994; 343(8889):83-84.

23. Kumar S. Infection as a risk factor for gallbladder cancer. J Surg Oncol 2006; 93(8):633-639.

24. Tazuma S, Kajiyama G. Carcinogenesis of malignant lesions of the gallbladder. The impact of chronic inflammation and gallstones. Langenbecks Arch Surg 2001; 386(3):224-229.

25. Takahashi T, Shivapurkar N, Riquelme E, Shigematsu H, Reddy J, Suzuki M, et al. Aberrant promoter hypermethylation of multiple genes in gallbladder carcinoma and chronic cholecystitis. Clin Cancer Res 2004; 10(18 Pt 1):6126-6133.

26. Gorunova L, Parada LA, Limon J, Jin Y, Hallen M, Hagerstrand I, et al. Nonrandom chromosomal aberrations and cytogenetic heterogeneity in gallbladder carcinomas. Genes Chromosomes Cancer 1999; 26(4):312-321.

27. Roa JC, Roa I, Correa P, Vo Q, Araya JC, Villaseca M, et al. Microsatellite instability in preneoplastic and neoplastic lesions of the gallbladder. J Gastroenterol 2005; 40(1):79-86.

28. Wistuba, II, Maitra A, Carrasco R, Tang M, Troncoso P, Minna JD, et al. High resolution chromosome 3p, 8p, 9q and 22q allelotyping analysis in the pathogenesis of gallbladder carcinoma. Br J Cancer 2002; 87(4):432-440.

29. Wistuba, II, Sugio K, Hung J, Kishimoto Y, Virmani AK, Roa I, et al. Allele-specific mutations involved in the pathogenesis of endemic gallbladder carcinoma in Chile. Cancer Res 1995; 55(12):2511-2515.

30. Riquelme E, Tang M, Baez S, Diaz A, Pruyas M, Wistuba, II, et al. Frequent epigenetic inactivation of chromosome 3p candidate tumor suppressor genes in gallbladder carcinoma. Cancer Lett 2007; 250(1):100-106.

31. Moreno M, Pimentel F, Gazdar AF, Wistuba, II, Miquel JF. TP53 abnormalities are frequent and early events in the sequential pathogenesis of gallbladder carcinoma. Ann Hepatol 2005; 4(3):192-199.

32. Roa I, de Aretxabala X, Araya JC, Roa J. Preneoplastic lesions in gallbladder cancer. J Surg Oncol 2006; 93(8):615-623.

33. Yamagiwa H, Tomiyama H. Intestinal metaplasia-dysplasia-carcinoma sequence of the gallbladder. Acta Pathol Jpn 1986; 36(7):989-997.

34. Aldridge MC, Bismuth H. Gallbladder cancer: the polyp-cancer sequence. Br J Surg 1990; 77(4):363-364.

35. Albores-Saavedra J, Alcantra-Vazquez A, Cruz-Ortiz H, Herrera-Goepfert R. The precursor lesions of invasive gallbladder carcinoma. Hyperplasia, atypical hyperplasia and carcinoma in situ. Cancer 1980; 45(5):919-927.

36. Laitio M. Histogenesis of epithelial neoplasms of human gallbladder I. Dysplasia. Pathol Res Pract 1983; 178(1):51-56.

37. Laitio M. Histogenesis of epithelial neoplasms of human gallbladder II. Classification of carcinoma on the basis of morphological features. Pathol Res Pract 1983; 178(1):57-66.

38. Mukhopadhyay S, Landas SK. Putative precursors of gallbladder dysplasia: a review of 400 routinely resected specimens. Arch Pathol Lab Med 2005; 129(3):386-390.

39. Smok G, Cervilla K, Bosch H, Csendes A. [Precancerous lesions of invasive carcinoma of the gallbladder]. Rev Med Chil 1986; 114(10):954-958.

40. Duarte I, Llanos O, Domke H, Harz C, Valdivieso V. Metaplasia and precursor lesions of gallbladder carcinoma. Frequency, distribution, and probability of detection in routine histologic samples. Cancer 1993; 72(6):1878-`884.

41. Sasatomi E, Tokunaga O, Miyazaki K. Precancerous conditions of gallbladder carcinoma: overview of histopathologic characteristics and molecular genetic findings. J Hepatobiliary Pancreat Surg 2000; 7(6):556-567.

42. Roa I, Araya JC, Wistuba I, Villaseca M, de Aretxabala X, Busel D, et al. [Epithelial lesions associated with gallbladder carcinoma. A methodical study of 32 cases]. Rev Med Chil 1993; 121(1):21-29.

43. Yamagiwa H. Mucosal dysplasia of gallbladder: isolated and adjacent lesions to carcinoma. Jpn J Cancer Res 1989; 80(3):238-243.

44. Yamamoto M, Nakajo S, Tahara E. Dysplasia of the gallbladder. Its histogenesis and correlation to gallbladder adenocarcinoma. Pathol Res Pract 1989; 185(4):454-460.

45. Albores-Saavedra J, Henson DE, Sobin LH. The WHO Histological Classification of Tumors of the Gallbladder and Extrahepatic Bile Ducts. A commentary on the second edition. Cancer 1992; 70(2):410-414.

46. Roa I, de Aretxabala X, Araya JC, Villaseca M, Roa J, Guzman P. [Incipient gallbladder carcinoma. Clinical and pathological study and prognosis in 196 cases]. Rev Med Chil 2001; 129(10):1113-1120.

47. Roa I, Araya JC, Villaseca M, Roa J, de Aretxabala X, Ibacache G. Gallbladder cancer in a high risk area: morphologi-

cal features and spread patterns. Hepatogastroenterology 1999; 46(27):1540-6.

48. de Aretxabala X, Roa I, Burgos L. Gallbladder cancer, management of early tumors. Hepatogastroenterology 1999; 46(27):1547-1551.

49. de Aretxabala X, Roa I, Araya JC, Burgos L, Flores P, Huenchullan I, et al. Operative findings in patients with early forms of gallbladder cancer. Br J Surg 1990; 77(3):291-293.

50. Shirai Y, Yoshida K, Tsukada K, Muto T, Watanabe H. Early carcinoma of the gallbladder. Eur J Surg 1992; 158(10):545-548.

51. Kapoor VK, Pradeep R, Haribhakti SP, Sikora SS, Kaushik SP. Early carcinoma of the gallbladder: an elusive disease. J Surg Oncol 1996; 62(4):284-287.

52. Reid KM, Ramos-De la Medina A, Donohue JH. Diagnosis and surgical management of gallbladder cancer: a review. J Gastrointest Surg 2007; 11(5):671-681.

53. Sikora SS, Singh RK. Surgical strategies in patients with gallbladder cancer: nihilism to optimism. J Surg Oncol 2006; 93(8):670-681.

54. Albores-Saavedra J, de Jesus Manrique J, Angeles-Angeles A, Henson DE. Carcinoma in situ of the gallbladder. A clinicopathologic study of 18 cases. Am J Surg Pathol 1984; 8(5):323-333.

55. Serra I, Sharp A, Calvo A. [Incipient cancer of the gallbladder]. Rev Med Chil 1987; 115(8):749-754.

56. Smok G, Bentjerodt R, Csendes A. [Benign polypoid lesions of the gallbladder. Their relation to gallbladder adenocarcinoma]. Rev Med Chil 1992; 120(1):31-35.

57. Csendes A, Burgos AM, Csendes P, Smok G, Rojas J. Late follow-up of polypoid lesions of the gallbladder smaller than 10 mm. Ann Surg 2001; 234(5):657-660.

58. Nakajo S, Yamamoto M, Tahara E. Morphometrical analysis of gall-bladder adenoma and adenocarcinoma with reference to histogenesis and adenoma-carcinoma sequence. Virchows Arch A Pathol Anat Histopathol 1990; 417(1):49-56.

59. Escalona A, Leon F, Bellolio F, Pimentel F, Guajardo M, Gennero R, et al. [Gallbladder polyps: correlation between ultrasonographic and histopathological findings]. Rev Med Chil 2006; 134(10):1237-1242.

60. Albores-Saavedra J, Vardaman CJ, Vuitch F. Non-neoplastic polypoid lesions and adenomas of the gallbladder. Pathol Annu 1993; 28 Pt 1:145-177.

61. Buitrago Salassa C, Javier Lespi P. [Detection of acid mucins in gastric metaplasia of the gallbladder]. Acta Gastroenterol Latinoam 2007; 37(1):11-14.

62. Albores-Saavedra J, Nadjo M, Henson D, Ziegels-Weissman J, Mones J. Intestinal metaplasia of the gallblader: A morphologic and immunocytochemical study. Hum Pathol 1986; 17:614-620.

63. Roa I, Araya JC, Villaseca M, De Aretxabala X, Riedemann P, Endoh K, et al. Preneoplastic lesions and gallbladder cancer: an estimate of the period required for progression. Gastroenterology 1996; 111(1):232-236.

64. Csendes A, Burdiles P, Smok G, Csendes P, Burgos A, Recio M. Histologic findings of gallbladder mucosa in 87 patients with morbid obesity without gallstones compared to 87 control subjects. J Gastrointest Surg 2003; 7(4):547-551.

65. Zins M, Boulay-Coletta I, Molinie V, Mercier-Pageyral B, Julles MC, Rodallec M, et al. [Imaging of a thickened-wall gallbladder]. J Radiol 2006; 87(4 Pt 2):479-493.

66. Gore RM, Yaghmai V, Newmark GM, Berlin JW, Miller FH. Imaging benign and malignant disease of the gallbladder. Radiol Clin North Am 2002; 40(6):1307-1323, vi.

67. Onoyama H, Yamamoto M, Takada M, Urakawa T, Ajiki T, Yamada I, et al. Diagnostic imaging of early gallbladder cancer: retrospective study of 53 cases. World J Surg 1999; 23(7):708-712.

68. Chianale J, Valdivia G, del Pino G, Nervi F. [Gallbladder cancer mortality in Chile and its relation to cholecystectomy rates. An analysis of the last decade]. Rev Med Chil 1990; 118(11):1284-1288.

69. Keus F, Broeders IA, van Laarhoven CJ. Gallstone disease: Surgical aspects of symptomatic cholecystolithiasis and acute cholecystitis. Best Pract Res Clin Gastroenterol 2006; 20(6):1031-1051.

70. Cahill DLC. Basic concepts in genetics. In: Vogelstein B KK, editor. The Genetic Basis of Human Cancer. New York: Mc Graw-Hill, 2002:129-130.

71. Wistuba, II, Behrens C, Milchgrub S, Bryant D, Hung J, Minna JD, et al. Sequential molecular abnormalities are involved in the multistage development of squamous cell lung carcinoma. Oncogene 1999; 18(3):643-650.

72. Maley CC. Multistage carcinogenesis in Barrett's esophagus. Cancer Lett 2007; 245(1-2):22-32.

73. El-Serag HB, Rudolph KL. Hepatocellular carcinoma: epidemiology and molecular carcinogenesis. Gastroenterology 2007; 132(7):2557-2576.

74. Pitt HA, Brenner BM. Gallbladder cancer gene hypermethylation: genetics or environment? Ann Surg Oncol 2003; 10(8):832-833.

75. Kuroki T, Tajima Y, Matsuo K, Kanematsu T. Genetic alterations in gallbladder carcinoma. Surg Today 2005; 35(2):101-105.

76. Legan M, Luzar B, Marolt VF, Cor A. Expression of cyclooxygenase-2 is associated with p53 accumulation in premalignant and malignant gallbladder lesions. World J Gastroenterol 2006; 12(21):3425-3429.

77. Thun MJ, Henley SJ, Gansler T. Inflammation and cancer: an epidemiological perspective. Novartis Found Symp 2004; 256:6-21; discussion 22-28, 49-52, 266-269.

78. Asano T, Shoda J, Ueda T, Kawamoto T, Todoroki T, Shimonishi M, et al. Expressions of cyclooxygenase-2 and prostaglandin E-receptors in carcinoma of the gallbladder: crucial role of arachidonate metabolism in tumor growth and progression. Clin Cancer Res 2002; 8(4):1157-1167.

79. Wistuba, II, Albores-Saavedra J. Genetic abnormalities involved in the pathogenesis of gallbladder carcinoma. J Hepatobiliary Pancreat Surg 1999; 6(3):237-244.

80. Roa JC, Anabalon L, Roa I, Melo A, Araya JC, Tapia O, et al. Promoter methylation profile in gallbladder cancer. J Gastroenterol 2006; 41(3):269-275.

81. House MG, Wistuba, II, Argani P, Guo M, Schulick RD, Hruban RH, et al. Progression of gene hypermethylation in gallstone gallbladder cancer. Ann Surg Oncol 2003; 10(8):882-889.

82. Tang M, Baez S, Pruyas M, Diaz A, Calvo A, Riquelme E, et al. Mitochondrial DNA mutation at the D310 (displacement loop) mononucleotide sequence in the pathogenesis of gallbladder carcinoma. Clin Cancer Res 2004; 10(3):1041-1046.

83. Jarnagin WR, Klimstra DS, Hezel M, Gonen M, Fong Y, Roggin K, et al. Differential cell cycle-regulatory protein expression in biliary tract adenocarcinoma: correlation with anatomic site, pathologic variables, and clinical outcome. J Clin Oncol 2006; 24(7):1152-1160.

84. Yoshida T, Sugai T, Habano W, Nakamura S, Uesugi N, Funato O, et al. Microsatellite instability in gallbladder carcinoma: two independent genetic pathways of gallbladder carcinogenesis. J Gastroenterol 2000; 35(10):768-774.

85. Matsubayashi H, Sato N, Fukushima N, Yeo CJ, Walter KM, Brune K, et al. Methylation of cyclin D2 is observed frequently in pancreatic cancer but is also an age-related phenomenon in gastrointestinal tissues. Clin Cancer Res 2003; 9(4):1446-1452.

86. Itoi T, Shinohara Y, Takeda K, Nakamura K, Takei K, Sanada J, et al. Nuclear cyclin D1 overexpression is a critical event proliferation and invasive growth in gallbladder. J Gastroenterol 2000; 35(2):142-149.

87. Chang YT, Hsu C, Jeng YM, Chang MC, Wei SC, Wong JM. Expression of the caudal-type homeodomain transcription factor CDX2 is related to clinical outcome in biliary tract carcinoma. J Gastroenterol Hepatol 2007; 22(3):389-394.

88. Shimura H, Date K, Matsumoto K, Nakamura T, Tanaka M. Induction of invasive growth in a gallbladder cancer cell line by hepatocyte growth factor in vitro. Jpn J Cancer Res 1995; 86(7):662-669.

89. Gohongi T, Fukumura D, Boucher Y, Yun CO, Soff GA, Compton C, et al. Tumor-host interactions in the gallbladder suppress distal angiogenesis and tumor growth: involvement of transforming growth factor beta1. Nat Med 1999; 5(10):1203-1208.

90. Roa JC, Roa I, de Aretxabala X, Melo A, Faria G, Tapia O. [K-ras gene mutation in gallbladder carcinoma]. Rev Med Chil 2004; 132(8):955-960.

91. Kim SW, Her KH, Jang JY, Kim WH, Kim YT, Park YH. K-ras oncogene mutation in cancer and precancerous lesions of the gallbladder. J Surg Oncol 2000; 75(4):246-251.

92. Kim YW, Huh SH, Park YK, Yoon TY, Lee SM, Hong SH. Expression of the c-erb-B2 and p53 protein in gallbladder carcinomas. Oncol Rep 2001; 8(5):1127-1132.

93. Giatromanolaki A, Koukourakis MI, Simopoulos C, Polychronidis A, Sivridis E. Vascular endothelial growth factor (VEGF) expression in operable gallbladder carcinomas. Eur J Surg Oncol 2003; 29(10):879-883.

94. Zhi YH, Liu RS, Song MM, Tian Y, Long J, Tu W, et al. Cyclooxygenase-2 promotes angiogenesis by increasing vascular endothelial growth factor and predicts prognosis in gallbladder carcinoma. World J Gastroenterol 2005; 11(24):3724-3728.

95. Leone F, Cavalloni G, Pignochino Y, Sarotto I, Ferraris R, Piacibello W, et al. Somatic mutations of epidermal growth factor receptor in bile duct and gallbladder carcinoma. Clin Cancer Res 2006; 12(6):1680-1685.

96. Lee CS, Pirdas A. Epidermal growth factor receptor immunoreactivity in gallbladder and extrahepatic biliary tract tumours. Pathol Res Pract 1995; 191(11):1087-1091.

97. Wistuba, II, Gazdar AF, Roa I, Albores-Saavedra J. p53 protein overexpression in gallbladder carcinoma and its precursor lesions: an immunohistochemical study. Hum Pathol 1996; 27(4):360-365.

98. Roa I, Villaseca M, Araya J, Roa J, de Aretxabala X, Melo A, et al. p53 tumour suppressor gene protein expression in early and advanced gallbladder carcinoma. Histopathology 1997; 31(3):226-230.

99. Roa JC, Vo Q, Araya JC, Villaseca M, Guzman P, Ibacache GS, et al. [Inactivation of CDKN2A gene (p16) in gallbladder carcinoma]. Rev Med Chil 2004; 132(11):1369-1376.

100. Wistuba, II, Ashfaq R, Maitra A, Alvarez H, Riquelme E, Gazdar AF. Fragile histidine triad gene abnormalities in the pathogenesis of gallbladder carcinoma. Am J Pathol 2002; 160(6):2073-2079.

101. Masuhara S, Kasuya K, Aoki T, Yoshimatsu A, Tsuchida A, Koyanagi Y. Relation between K-ras codon 12 mutation and p53 protein overexpression in gallbladder cancer and biliary ductal epithelia in patients with pancreaticobiliary maljunction. J Hepatobiliary Pancreat Surg 2000; 7(2):198-205.

102. Hanada K, Tsuchida A, Iwao T, Eguchi N, Sasaki T, Morinaka K, et al. Gene mutations of K-ras in gallbladder mucosae and gallbladder carcinoma with an anomalous junction of the pancreaticobiliary duct. Am J Gastroenterol 1999; 94(6):1638-1642.

103. Saetta AA. K-ras, p53 mutations, and microsatellite instability (MSI) in gallbladder cancer. J Surg Oncol 2006; 93(8):644-649.

104. Suzuki T, Takano Y, Kakita A, Okudaira M. An immunohistochemical and molecular biological study of c-erbB-2 amplification and prognostic relevance in gallbladder cancer. Pathol Res Pract 1993; 189(3):283-292.

105. Chow NH, Huang SM, Chan SH, Mo LR, Hwang MH, Su WC. Significance of c-erbB-2 expression in normal and neoplastic epithelium of biliary tract. Anticancer Res 1995; 15(3):1055-1059.

106. Kamel D, Paakko P, Nuorva K, Vahakangas K, Soini Y. p53 and c-erbB-2 protein expression in adenocarcinomas and epithelial dysplasias of the gallbladder. J Pathol 1993; 170(1):67-72.

107. Houston AM, Teach SJ. COX-2 inhibitors: a review. Pediatr Emerg Care 2004; 20(6):396-369; quiz 400-402.

108. Kimmey MB, Lanas A. Review article: appropriate use of proton pump inhibitors with traditional nonsteroidal anti-inflammatory drugs and COX-2 selective inhibitors. Aliment Pharmacol Ther 2004; 19(suppl 1):60-65.

109. Ota S, Bamba H, Kato A, Kawamoto C, Yoshida Y, Fujiwara K. Review article: COX-2, prostanoids and colon cancer. Aliment Pharmacol Ther 2002; 16(suppl 2):102-106.

110. Nassar A, Radhakrishnan A, Cabrero IA, Cotsonis G, Cohen C. COX-2 Expression in Invasive Breast Cancer: Correlation With Prognostic Parameters and Outcome. Appl Immunohistochem Mol Morphol 2007; 15(3):255-259.

111. Harris RE. Cyclooxygenase-2 (cox-2) and the inflammogenesis of cancer. Subcell Biochem 2007; 42:93-126.

112. Lee DS, Moss SF. COX-2 inhibition and the prevention of gastric cancer. Digestion 2006; 74(3-4):184-186.

113. Han JA, Kim JI, Ongusaha PP, Hwang DH, Ballou LR, Mahale A, et al. P53-mediated induction of Cox-2 counteracts p53- or genotoxic stress-induced apoptosis. EMBO J 2002; 21(21):5635-5644.

114. Hui AM, Li X, Shi YZ, Takayama T, Torzilli G, Makuuchi M. Cyclin D1 overexpression is a critical event in gallbladder carcinogenesis and independently predicts decreased survival for patients with gallbladder carcinoma. Clin Cancer Res 2000; 6(11):4272-4277.

115. Eguchi N, Fujii K, Tsuchida A, Yamamoto S, Sasaki T, Kajiyama G. Cyclin E overexpression in human gallbladder carcinomas. Oncol Rep 1999; 6(1):93-96.

116. Ma HB, Hu HT, Di ZL, Wang ZR, Shi JS, Wang XJ, et al. Association of cyclin D1, p16 and retinoblastoma protein expressions with prognosis and metastasis of gallbladder carcinoma. World J Gastroenterol 2005; 11(5):744-747.

117. Quan ZW, Wu K, Wang J, Shi W, Zhang Z, Merrell RC. Association of p53, p16, and vascular endothelial growth factor protein expressions with the prognosis and metastasis of gallbladder cancer. J Am Coll Surg 2001; 193(4):380-383.

118. Tian Y, Ding RY, Zhi YH, Guo RX, Wu SD. Analysis of p53 and vascular endothelial growth factor expression in human gallbladder carcinoma for the determination of tumor vascularity. World J Gastroenterol 2006; 12(3):415-419.

119. Rashid A. Cellular and molecular biology of biliary tract cancers. Surg Oncol Clin N Am 2002; 11(4):995-1009.

120. Shi YZ, Hui AM, Li X, Takayama T, Makuuchi M. Overexpression of retinoblastoma protein predicts decreased survival and correlates with loss of p16INK4 protein in gallbladder carcinomas. Clin Cancer Res 2000; 6(10):4096-4100.

121. Yoshida S, Todoroki T, Ichikawa Y, Hanai S, Suzuki H, Hori M, et al. Mutations of p16Ink4/CDKN2 and p15Ink4B/MTS2 genes in biliary tract cancers. Cancer Res 1995; 55(13):2756-2760.

122. Wistuba, II, Tang M, Maitra A, Alvarez H, Troncoso P, Pimentel F, et al. Genome-wide allelotyping analysis reveals multiple sites of allelic loss in gallbladder carcinoma. Cancer Res 2001; 61(9):3795-3800.

123. Ueki T, Hsing AW, Gao YT, Wang BS, Shen MC, Cheng J, et al. Alterations of p16 and prognosis in biliary tract cancers from a population-based study in China. Clin Cancer Res 2004; 10(5):1717-1725.

124. Vogelstein B, Kinzler KW. p53 function and dysfunction. Cell 1992; 70(4):523-6.

125. Hollstein M, Sidransky D, Vogelstein B, Harris C. p53 mutations in human cancers. Science 1991; 49:49-53.

126. Soussi T, Legros Y, Lubin R, Ory K, Schlichtholz B. Multifactorial analysis of p53 alteration in human cancer: a review. Int J Cancer 1994; 57(1):1-9.

127. Prives C, Manfredi JJ. The p53 tumor suppressor protein: meeting review. Genes Dev 1993; 7(4):529-534.

128. Downing SR, Jackson P, Russell PJ. Mutations within the tumour suppressor gene p53 are not confined to a late event in prostate cancer progression. a review of the evidence. Urol Oncol 2001; 6(3):103-110.

129. Kmet LM, Cook LS, Magliocco AM. A review of p53 expression and mutation in human benign, low malignant potential, and invasive epithelial ovarian tumors. Cancer 2003; 97(2):389-404.

130. Fujii K, Yokozaki H, Yasui W, Kuniyasu H, Hirata M, Kajiyama G, et al. High frequency of p53 gene mutation in adenocarcinomas of the gallbladder. Cancer Epidemiol Biomarkers Prev 1996; 5(6):461-466.

131. Misra S, Chaturvedi A, Goel MM, Mehrotra R, Sharma ID, Srivastava AN, et al. Overexpression of p53 protein in gallbladder carcinoma in North India. Eur J Surg Oncol 2000; 26(2):164-167.

132. Koda M, Yashima K, Kawaguchi K, Andachi H, Hosoda A, Shiota G, et al. Expression of Fhit, Mlh1, and P53 protein in human gallbladder carcinoma. Cancer Lett 2003; 199(2):131-138.

133. Beavon IR. The E-cadherin-catenin complex in tumour metastasis: structure, function and regulation. Eur J Cancer 2000; 36(13 Spec No):1607-1620.

134. Debruyne P, Vermeulen S, Mareel M. The role of the E-cadherin/catenin complex in gastrointestinal cancer. Acta Gastroenterol Belg 1999; 62(4):393-402.

135. Choi YL, Xuan YH, Shin YK, Chae SW, Kook MC, Sung RH, et al. An immunohistochemical study of the expression of adhesion molecules in gallbladder lesions. J Histochem Cytochem 2004; 52(5):591-601.

136. Tahara E. Genetic pathways of two types of gastric cancer. IARC Sci Publ 2004(157):327-349.

137. Yap AS. The morphogenetic role of cadherin cell adhesion molecules in human cancer: a thematic review. Cancer Invest 1998; 16(4):252-261.

138. Roa I, Ibacache G, Melo A, Morales E, Villaseca M, Araya J, et al. [Subserous gallbladder carcinoma: expression of cadherine-catenine complex]. Rev Med Chil 2002; 130(12):1349-1357.

139. Sasatomi E, Tokunaga O, Miyazaki K. Spontaneous apoptosis in gallbladder carcinoma. Relationships with clinicopathologic factors, expression of E-cadherin, bcl-2 protooncogene, and p53 oncosuppressor gene. Cancer 1996; 78(10):2101-2110.

140. Hirata K, Ajiki T, Okazaki T, Horiuchi H, Fujita T, Kuroda Y. Frequent occurrence of abnormal E-cadherin/beta-catenin protein expression in advanced gallbladder cancers and its association with decreased apoptosis. Oncology 2006; 71(1-2):102-110.

141. Rashid A, Gao YT, Bhakta S, Shen MC, Wang BS, Deng J, et al. Beta-catenin mutations in biliary tract cancers: a population-based study in China. Cancer Res 2001; 61(8):3406-3409.

142. Yanagisawa N, Mikami T, Saegusa M, Okayasu I. More frequent beta-catenin exon 3 mutations in gallbladder adenomas than in carcinomas indicate different lineages. Cancer Res 2001; 61(1):19-22.

143. Chang HJ, Jee CD, Kim WH. Mutation and altered expression of beta-catenin carcinogenesis. Am J Surg Pathol 2002; 26(6):758-766.

144. Parwani AV, Geradts J, Caspers E, Offerhaus GJ, Yeo CJ, Cameron JL, et al. Immunohistochemical and genetic analysis of non-small cell and small cell gallbladder carcinoma and their precursor lesions. Mod Pathol 2003; 16(4):299-308.

145. Chuang SC, Lee KT, Tsai KB, Sheen PC, Nagai E, Mizumoto K, et al. Immunohistochemical study of DPC4 and p53 proteins in gallbladder and bile duct cancers. World J Surg 2004; 28(10):995-1000.

146. Saetta AA, Gigelou F, Papanastasiou PI, Koilakou SV, Kalekou-Greca H, Miliaras D, et al. High-level microsatellite instability is not involved in gallbladder carcinogenesis. Exp Mol Pathol 2006; 80(1):67-71.

147. Luzar B, Poljak M, Cor A, Klopcic U, Ferlan-Marolt V. Expression of human telomerase catalytic protein in gallbladder carcinogenesis. J Clin Pathol 2005; 58(8):820-825.

148. Uchida N, Tsutsui K, Ezaki T, Fukuma H, Kobara H, Kamata H, et al. Combination of assay of human telomerase reverse transcriptase mRNA and cytology using bile obtained by endoscopic transpapillary catheterization into the gallbladder for diagnosis of gallbladder carcinoma. Am J Gastroenterol 2003; 98(11):2415-2419.

149. Uchida N, Tsutsui K, Ezaki T, Fukuma H, Kobara H, Kamata H, et al. Combination of assay of human telomerase reverse cytology using bile obtained by endoscopic into the gallbladder for diagnosis of gallbladder. Am J Gastroenterol 2003; 98(11):2415-2419.

150. Kim YT, Kim J, Jang YH, Lee WJ, Ryu JK, Park YK, et al. Genetic alterations in gallbladder adenoma, dysplasia and carcinoma. Cancer Lett 2001; 169(1):59-68.

151. Matsuo K, Kuroki T, Kitaoka F, Tajima Y, Kanematsu T. Loss of heterozygosity of chromosome 16q in gallbladder carcinoma. J Surg Res 2002; 102(2):133-136.

152. Roa I, Villaseca M, Araya JC, Roa J, de Aretxabala X, Fuentealba P, et al. DNA ploidy pattern and tumor suppressor gene p53 expression in gallbladder carcinoma. Cancer Epidemiol Biomarkers Prev 1997; 6(7):547-550.

153. Correa P. Chronic atrophic gastritis as precursor of cancer. In: Sherlock P, Morson BC, Barbara L, Veronesi U (ed.). Precancerous Lesions of the Gastrointestinal Tract. New York: Raven Press, 1983:145-153.

154. Correa P. Mechanism of gastric carcinogenesis. In: Joossens JV (ed.). Diet and Human Carcinogenesis. New York: Elsevier, 1985:109-115.

155. Chapman RW. Risk factors for biliary tract carcinogenesis. Ann Oncol 1999; 10 Suppl 4:308-311.

156. Watanapa P, Watanapa WB. Liver fluke-associated cholangiocarcinoma. Br J Surg 2002; 89(8):962-970.

157. Yokoyama N, Hitomi J, Watanabe H, Ajioka Y, Pruyas M, Serra I, et al. Mutations of p53 in gallbladder carcinomas in high-incidence areas of Japan and Chile. Cancer Epidemiol Biomarkers Prev 1998; 7(4):297-301.

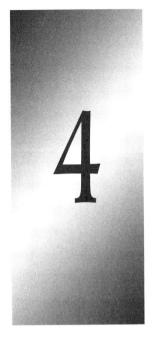

4 Histopathology and Molecular Pathogenesis of Biliary Tract Cancer

Shahid A. Khan
Robert David Goldin

Amar Sharif
Nagy Habib

Cholangiocarcinoma (CC) is a devastating malignancy arising from the ductular epithelium of the biliary tree, either within the liver parenchyma itself (intrahepatic CC), or from the extrahepatic bile ducts (extrahepatic CC). Surgery is the only known effective cure, but as CC usually presents too late for curative resection, the disease carries a dismal prognosis (1). Worldwide, CC is the second most common primary hepatic malignancy and has exhibited a striking increase in incidence and mortality rates over the past few decades (2-5). Given the paucity of effectual therapeutic options, understanding the pathogenesis of this cancer is becoming increasingly relevant. This chapter reviews the histopathology and classification of CC and explores the postulated mechanisms underlying its molecular pathogenesis.

ANATOMIC CLASSIFICATION OF CHOLANGIOCARCINOMA

Cholangiocarcinomas can be divided into intrahepatic, perihilar, and extrahepatic, depending on their location (6, 7).

Intrahepatic Cholangiocarcinomas

These make up 20-25% of all CCs and are the second most comon primary tumors of the liver.

Macroscopic features

Intrahepatic CCs are whiter and firmer than hepatocellular carcinomas as they contain more desmoplastic stroma. They more commonly occur in noncirrhotic livers than do hepatocellular carcinomas. They can be divided into three macroscopic types, which tend to carry different prognoses (8, 9):

1. Mass forming
2. Periductal-infiltrating
3. Intraductal
4. Mixed
5. Others

MASS FORMING
This is the most common type, accounting for 40-42% of this group of tumors. They are well demarcated (although unencapsulated), rounded tumors. They produce secondary obstructive changes in the surround-

ing liver. They tend not to invade the bile ducts or along the portal structures. Initially, like hepatocellular carcinomas, they invade the portal vein leading to the intrahepatic secondaries. As they grow larger they show an increasing tendency to involve Glisson's capsule and spread via the lymphatics. These tumors have a 5-year survival of approximately 20% and have a high frequency of hepatic recurrences postsurgery.

PERIDUCTAL-INFILTRATING

These are less common than the mass-forming tumors and make up 8-22% of this group of tumors. They are relatively small tumors which arise closer to the hilum. Periductal-infiltrating tumors produce thickening of the bile duct wall with varying degrees of luminal narrowing. They produce obstruction and dilatation of the associated segmental bile ducts. In contrast to mass-forming tumors, they do invade along the portal structures, often invading around the associated vessels. They involve the lymphatics and Glisson's capsule relatively early in their natural history and uncommonly invade the portal veins. These tumors have a 5-year survival of 7%. Following surgery these tumors do not often recur.

INTRADUCTAL

These are only slightly less common than the periductal-infiltrating type and account for 8-14% of this group of tumors. Theses are polypoid tumors which produce striking dilatation of the biliary tree. They have many features in common with the intraductal papillary mucinous tumors of the pancreas, which also have a relative long natural history. Characteristically they secrete large amounts of mucus and show extensive mucosal involvement. There may be invasion through the wall of the ducts. These tumors carry the best prognosis, with a 10-year survival approaching 60% (10).

MIXED

These show the features of both mass-forming and periductal-infiltrating tumors and carry a worse prognosis than do the pure mass-forming tumors; the curative resection rates are worse than for both mass-forming and periductal-infiltrating tumors.

OTHER MACROSCOPIC TYPES

These include the very uncommon multicystic variant. They are distinguished from biliary mucinous cystadenomas, which form larger cysts with thick fibrous walls that often contain ovarian-type mesenchymal stroma, particularly in women.

Microscopic features

Intrahepatic cholangiocarcinomas fall into the following histologic types (11):

1. Adenocarcinoma
2. Adeno-squamous carcinoma
3. Squamous carcinoma
4. Cholangiocellular carcinoma
5. Lymphoepithelioma-like carcinoma
6. Clear cell variant
7. Muco-epidermoid carcinoma

Over 90% of tumors are adenocarcinomas, which show a range of architectural patterns including tubular, acinar, and trabecular. The degree of differentiation also varies, with the higher grade tumors tending to be of higher stage. Cytologically the cells contain vesicular nuclei containing nucleoli which tend to be smaller and less eosinophilic than those seen in hepatocellular carcinomas. The cytoplasm may be clear, pale, or eosinophilic, and the cells may be vacuolated. Mucin almost always stains positive (Figure 4.1), although in practice this may be very focal and is not always demonstrable in needle biopsies. The intraductal tumors often form well-developed papillary structures. When the tumors are centered on large ducts, spread of tumor within them, which often takes the form of papillary structures, with well-formed fibro-vascular cores, is frequently seen. These papillae are often lined by relatively well-differentiated cells. CCs otherwise tend to be less well differentiated.

One of the characteristic features of CCs is that they induce a prominent desmoplastic stromal reaction (Figure 4.2). This feature helps distinguish them, macroscopically and microscopically, from hepatocellular carcinomas. This fibrous stroma is frequently inflamed and may even be focally calcified. Extracel-

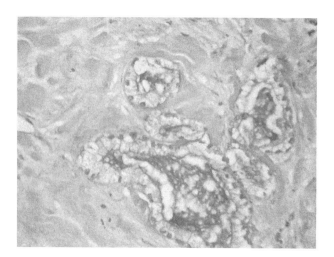

FIGURE 4.1

Cholangiocarcinomas are adenocarcinomas that usually secrete prominent mucin (diastase periodic acid Schiff stain).

lular mucin may be present within the stroma and it may even contain bile. The former feature, if marked, characterizes the tumor as a mucinous carcinoma. The tumor invades both parenchyma and portal structures. Within the latter it may closely mimic nonneoplastic bile ducts, from which it may be difficult to distinguish, especially where there is biliary obstruction (associated with bile duct proliferation and reactive nuclear atypia). On the other hand, varying degrees of true dysplasia may be seen in the bile ducts adjacent to a tumor. While this may be useful in conforming that an adenocarcinoma within the liver is in fact primary to this site (i.e., it is an intrahepatic CC) this, again, is rarely helpful in needle biopsies (12).

As described above, some intrahepatic CCs have the features of mucinous ("colloid") adenocarcinomas, although the exact percentage of mucin required to make this diagnosis (and how this should be measured) is not clearly defined. Signet ring cell cancers in which there is a noncohesive growth pattern and the cells contain prominent mucin, which displaces the nucleus to one end of the cell, are usually seen as part of tumors that also show another form of differentiation. The presence of only signet ring cells should always raise the possibility of a secondary tumor. The clear cell variant consists of tubules lined by cells that contain mucin (13). Pure squamous cell carcinomas do occur, as do mucoepidermoid carcinomas, which are composed of both malignant glandular and squamous elements. More common than the latter are adeno-squamous carcinomas in which the malignant glandular elements are associated with squamous morrules (14). Some CCs may have dedifferentiated areas composed of spindle cells.

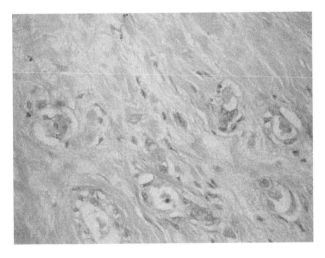

FIGURE 4.2

Cholangiocarcinomas are associated with abundant desmoplastic stroma.

These tumors may be termed sarcomatoid or spindle cell carcinomas (15). Lympho-epithelioma-like carcinomas, with the features characteristic of these tumors in other sites, including demonstrable Epstein-Barr virus-coded nuclear DNA, are very rarely seen (16).

Combined Hepatocellular-Cholangiocarcinomas

This entity needs to be distinguished from "collision tumors," in which separate CC and liver cell cancers are present in the same liver. Combined hepatocellular-cholangiocarcinomas are rare liver tumors making up less than 1% of the total. Although they have been variably classified as either variants of liver cell cancer or CC clinically, they behave more like the former, although they are genetically more similar to the latter. These tumors have, by definition, areas typical of liver cell cancer and others typical of CC. There are also areas transitional between the two composed of cells of intermediate phenotype. These tumors need to be distinguished from "stem cell tumors" which are composed entirely of cells of intermediate or progenitor cell phenotype in which there is no evidence of differentiation into either typical liver cell cancer or CC. They express the progenitor cell marker (c-kit) as well as having a phenotype intermediate between that of two more differentiated tumors they may give rise to (17-19).

DIFFERENTIAL DIAGNOSIS

Intrahepatic CCs need to be distinguished from other primary tumors of the liver, which in practice means liver cell cancers, as well as from metastatic adenocarcinomas, which are much more common than primary tumors in clinical practice.

Distinction from Liver Cell Cancer

In the distinction from liver cell cancers (20), a prominent desmoplastic stromal reaction and mucin production are key features in favor of a tumor being a cholangiocarcinoma. It should be noted that fibrolamellar carcinomas may show focal mucin production. While the growth pattern of CCs may mimic the trabecular growth pattern of liver cell cancers, the presence of fibrous tissue, rather than sinusoids between the trabeculae, helps make the distinction. The presence of definite biliary dysplasia is potentially very useful, but in practice it is rarely seen and can be very difficult to distinguish from reactive biliary changes seen as the result of obstruction due to any kind of tumor. Biliary dysplasia is characterized by nuclear stratification, micropapillary and cribiform growth patterns, nuclear hyperchromasia, and polymorphism as well as an increased mitotic rate. The presence of bile within a tumor is strongly suggestive that it is a liver cell cancer, although rarely bile may be found trapped within a CC.

Immunohistochemisry can be useful in making the distinction in difficult cases. CCs are positive for the biliary cytokeratins (CK 7 and CK19) while they are less frequently expressed by liver cell cancers, although in some series up to 50% are CK7 positive. Both types of tumor are usually CK8 positive. Liver cell cancers express HepPar1 (in over 90% of cases), whereas CD 10 (or polyclonal CEA) is useful in identifying the bile canaliculi which are present in these tumors. In situ hybridization of albumin mRNA has also been used to identify liver cell cancers. Staining for alpha-fetoprotein is infrequently of help. It has recently been suggested that the expression of claudin-4 helps in this differential diagnosis (21).

Distinction from Metastatic Adenocarcinomas

The distinction of CC from metastatic adenocarcinoma (22, 23) is one of the most common problems facing histopathologists when dealing with liver tumors. In many cases, especially in those of a foregut origin (lung, esophagus, stomach, and pancreas), a definite distinction cannot be made on pathologic grounds alone, and other clinical modalities, especially imaging, are essential. The presence of definite biliary dysplasia may be useful in making the distinction of a primary from a secondary adenocarcinoma, but for the reasons discussed above this is infrequently useful. Some kinds of metastatic adenocarcinomas have characteristic features which allow a presumptive diagnosis to be made. For example, large bowel cancer metastases are usually composed of large, well-formed glands, with prominent necrosis, which often contains calcified areas. In other cases where the primary tumor is available for examination, direct comparison is of value. Primary clear cell tumors need to be distinguished from renal or adrenal metastases. The former contain glycogen, rather than mucin.

CK7 negativity and CK20 positivity is the typical immunophenotype of metastatic large bowel cancers and indicate against a primary CC. However, other patterns of CK7 and CK20 staining are less helpful as metastatic gastric and pancreatic cancers can have the same immunophenotype as primary tumors. Metastatic breast cancers are often strongly estrogen and progesterone receptor positive. While testing prostate-specific antigen positive is valuable in identifying a metastatic tumor as being of prostatic origin, this is a very uncommon clinical problem. Metastatic lung car-

cinomas are frequently positive for thyroid transcription factor-1. Metastatic neuroendocrine tumors are positive for appropriate markers (such as synaptophyisn and chromogranin). However, focal positivity is not uncommon with CC (or hepatocellular carcinomas). Strong cytoplasmic staining for galectin 3 is a characteristic feature of intrahepatic bile ducts and of intrahepatic cholangiocarcinomas and may be useful in the differential diagnosis of these tumors.

Distinction from Benign Biliary Tumors

Although the distinction of benign from malignant bile duct tumors (24) is not a common one, it can be very difficult. Hamartomatous lesions such as microhamartomas (von Meyenberg's complexes) and peribiliary gland hamartomas (bile duct adenomas) may show marked reactive atypia when inflamed. Even normal peribilairy glands may show similar changes when inflamed. Especially in needle biopsies, even reactive bile duct proliferations may be very difficult to distinguish from a CC. However, the size of the nuclei, the degree of nuclear pleomorphism, the presence and atypicality of mitoses, and the cribiform growth pattern are usually sufficient to allow the distinction to be made between even well-differentiated adenocarcinomas and these benign lesions.

Distinction from Other Tumors

Epithelioid hemangioendotheliomas may closely resemble holangiocarcinomas in that they are both associated with abundant desmoplastic stroma, and the vascular lumina seen in the former may be confused with evidence of glandular differentiation. Immunohistochemical features of epithelioid hemangioendotheliomas include positivity for the vascular markers CD31 and C34 or, less frequently, factor VIII-related antigen (25).

Extrahepatic Cholangiocarcinomas

These can be divided into those arising close to the hilum of the liver (perihilar CC or Klatskin tumors) and those arising more distally (26, 27). The former make up approximately two thirds of this group of tumors. Three different growth patterns have been described with this group of tumors: infiltrative (75-80%), nodular (20%), and intraductal (less than 5%).

The first two groups tend to be poorly differentiated and to be associated with the marked desmoplastic reaction characteristic of typical intrahepatic CC. Intraductal tumors tend to be better differentiated and to have more delicate stroma. The large amount of stroma in the former group can make the diagnosis a very difficult one to be certain of on pathologic grounds alone. Multiple biopsies and the use of cytologic techniques are essential. Even so, it has been estimated that a diagnosis can only be made in this way in about 50% of cases. The range of histologic subtypes, and their features, is very similar to those described for intrahepatic CC described above.

Invasion of the portal vein (in approximately one third of cases) is associated with the development of lobar atrophy on the same side. Tumors arising on the background of primary sclerosing cholangitis tend to be multifocal. Lymph node metastases are common, and even in those cases selected for surgical resection they are found in up to 50% of cases. The hilar and peridochal nodes are those most frequently involved.

REPORTING RESECTION SPECIMENS

All resected tumors need to be staged using the TNM system described here (28). There are different TNM scoring systems for intrahepatic and extrahepatic tumors. A number of protocols have been developed for the cutting up and reporting of liver cancers, including intrahepatic CC. The dimensions of the tumor, a multifocal growth pattern, vascular and perineural invasion (Figure 4.3) (29), the presence of lymph node metastases (30), and the involvement of serosal surfaces of resection margins are all features that indicate a poor prognosis. The grade of the tumor is not considered an important prognostic indicator. A range of immunohistochemical markers have been reported as carrying a better prognosis. These include HLA-DR, MUC2, the overexpression of the vitamin D receptor, and the decreased expression of cyclooxygenase-2MUC1, MUC4, keratin 903, p27, tenascin, and matrix metalloproteinase-7 (Figures 4.4 and 4.5) (31-33).

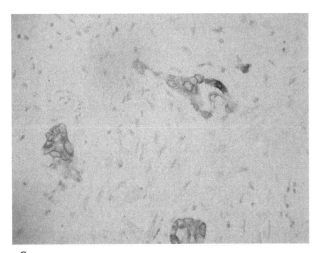

a

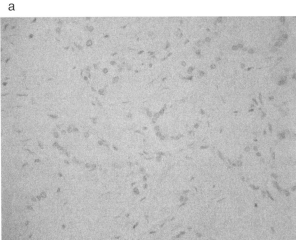

b

FIGURE 4.4

Cholangiocarcinomas are usually cytokeratin 7 positive (a) but cytokeratin 20 negative (b).

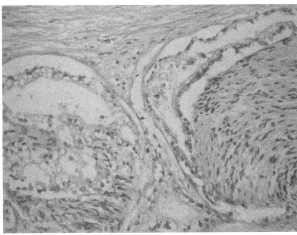

FIGURE 4.3

Marked perineural invasion is a characteristic feature of cholangiocarcinomas.

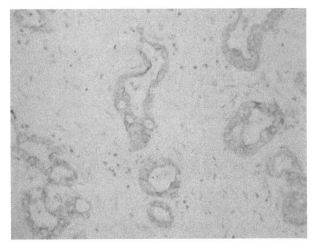

FIGURE 4.5

Intrahepatic cholangiocarcinomas: strong cytoplasmic staining for galectin 3.

TNM CLASSIFICATION

Although this classification is intended primarily for hepatocellular carcinoma, it can also be used for intrahepatic CC. TNM classification is summarized in Table 4.1.

RISK FACTORS FOR CHOLANGIOCARCINOMA

Most cases of CC are sporadic, and known risk factors account for only a minority of cases. Recognized risk factors are listed in Table 4.2 (1, 34).

Primary Sclerosing Cholangitis

Primary sclerosing cholangitis (PSC) is the most common known predisposing condition for CC in the West. Cholangiocarcinoma rates of up to 40% have been reported in PSC patients in follow-up studies and explant specimens (35). Cholangiocarcinoma in the context of PSC tends to present earlier, in 30- to 50-year age groups, compared to sporadic cases (1,36).

Liver Flukes

In East Asia, where CC is much more common than in the West, CC has been pathogenically associated with liver fluke infestation, particularly *Opisthorcis viverrini*, and less definitively *Clonorchis sinensis* (37). Most epidemiologic data, including case-control studies, are from Thailand, which has the highest incidence rates of cholangiocarcinoma worldwide (87/100,000 population) and where opisthorciasis is endemic (38). Malignant change in the biliary epithelium of Syrian hamsters occurs following infection with *O. viverrini*, particularly if fed nitrosoamines (39). These carcinogens, produced by bacteria in fish and other foods, are postulated to act as a cofactor in cholangiocarcinogenesis.

TABLE 4.1
TNM Classification and Staging for Cholangiocarcinoma

T—Primary Tumor

pTx   Primary tumor cannot be assessed
pT0   No evidence of primary tumor
pT1   Solitary tumor without vascular invasion
pT2   Solitary tumor with vascular invasion or multiple tumors , none more than cm
pT3   Multiple tumors <greater than>5 cm or tumor involving major branch of portal or hepatic vein(s)
pT4   Tumor(s) with direct invasion of adjacent organs other than the gall bladder

For hilar CC, the classification for staging extrahepatic bile duct carcinoma is appropriate.

pTx   Primary tumor cannot be assessed
pT0   No evidence of primary tumor
pTis   Carcinoma in situ
pT1a   Tumor invades subepithelial connective tissue
pT1b   Tumor invades fibromuscular layer
pT2   Tumor invades perifibromuscular connective tissue
pT3   Tumor invades adjacent structures (liver, gall bladder) and/or unilateral   tributaries of the portal vein (right or left) or hepatic artery (right or left)
pT4   Tumor invades any of the following: main portal vein or its tributaries bilaterally, common hepatic artery, or other adjacent structures

N—Regional Lymph Nodes

pNx   Regional lymph nodes cannot be assessed

pN0   No regional lymph node metastases. Histologic examination of a regional lymphadenectomy specimen will ordinarily include three or more lymph nodes. If lymph nodes are negative, but the number ordinarily examined is not met, classify as pN0.
pN1   Regional lymph node metastasis

M—Distant Metastasis

pMx Distant metastasis cannot be assessed
pM0 No distant metastasis
pM1 Distant metastasis

Stage grouping for intrahepatic tumors:

Stage I	T1	N0	M0
Stage II	T2	N0	M0
Stage IIIA	T3	N0	M0
Stage IIIB	T4	N0	M0
Stage IIIC	Any T	N1	M0
Stage IV	Any T	Any N	M1

Stage grouping for hilar cholangiocarcinoma:

Stage 0	Tis	N0	M0
Stage IA	T1	N0	M0
Stage IB	T2	N0	M0
Stage IIA	T3	N0	M0
Stage IIB	T1, T2, T3	N1	M0
Stage III	T4	Any N	M0
Stage IV	Any T	Any N	M1

TABLE 4.2
Risk Factors for Cholangiocarcinoma

Primary sclerosing cholangitis
Parasitic infection (Opisthorcis viverrini, Clonorchis sinensis)
Fibropolycystic liver disease
Intrahepatic biliary stones
Chemical carcinogen exposure
Viral hepatitis
Bile duct adenomas
Biliary papillomatosis

Source: Refs 1, 34.

Fibropolycystic Liver Disease

Congenital abnormalities of the biliary tree associated with Caroli's syndrome, congenital hepatic fibrosis, and choledochal cysts (cystic dilatations of the bile ducts) carry a 15% risk of malignant change after the second decade, the average age being 34 years (40). These biliary anomalies can lead to biliary stasis, activation of bile acids (28), and deconjugation of carcinogens. Bile duct adenomas and biliary papillomatosis are also associated with the development of cholangiocarcinoma.

Hepatolithiasis

Up to 10% of patients with intrahepatic biliary stones reportedly develop cholangiocarcinoma (41). Although rare in the West, hepatolithiasis is relatively common in parts of Asia and is associated with peripheral intrahepatic CC particularly (35). In Taiwan, up to 70% of patients undergoing surgical resection for CC have intrahepatic biliary stones, and in Japan up to 18% (42, 43). Biliary stones may lead to stasis of bile, predisposing to recurrent bacterial infections and subsequent inflammation, a potential cofactor for cholangiocarcinogenesis.

Chemical Carcinogen Exposure

Various chemical toxins have been associated with cholangiocarcinoma. Thorotrast, a radiologic contrast agent, banned several decades ago for its carcinogenic effects, has been strongly associated with the development of cholangiocarcinoma many years after exposure, increasing the risk to 300 times that of the general population (35,44). Epidemiologic associations with CC have also been made to byproducts from the rubber and chemical industries, including dioxins and nitrosamines (45) as well as to alcohol and smoking (46), but the numbers involved in these studies are generally small, results have been conflicting, and no firm conclusions can be drawn. Several novel associations with CC have been suggested in a recent case-control study from the United States. Hepatitis C virus (HCV) infection, chronic non-alcoholic liver disease, and obesity, all of which are increasing in incidence, and smoking were associated only with ICC[da1], suggesting that these conditions might explain the divergent incidence trends of the tumors (47). The mechanisms involved in chemically associated carcinogenesis are likely to involve the induction of promutagenic DNA adducts. Such adducts have been demonstrated to occur in significantly greater numbers in human CC tissue compared to controls, suggesting exposure of the biliary epithelium to DNA-toxic agents, a clear risk factor for cancerous change (48).

Viral Hepatitis

Cirrhosis, due to any underlying cause, has been associated with the risk of developing CC (47,49). A cohort study that followed up more than 11,000 patients with cirrhosis over 6 years found a 10-fold risk of CC compared to the general population (49). Hepatitis B (HBV) and HCV, the two most common causes of virally induced chronic liver disease, have also been linked to CC. A Korean case-control study found that 13% of CC cases tested positive for HCV and 14% for HBV surface antigen (HBsAg), compared to 4 and 2% of controls, respectively (50). In a similar study from Italy, 23% of CC patients were anti-HCV positive and 11.5% HBsAg positive compared with 6% and 5.5% of controls (51). A prospective control study from Japan reported the risk of developing CC in HCV-related cirrhosis at 3.5% after 10 years-1000 times greater than the general population (52). HCV is an established risk factor for hepatocellular carcinoma, and both hepatocytes and cholangiocytes have the same progenitor cell, supporting a role for HCV in cholangiocarcinogenesis. Furthermore, HCV RNA has been detected in cholangiocarcinoma tissue (53). A recent U.S. case-control study on risk factors for CC found adjusted odds ratios (OR) of 6 for HCV, and similar OR for HIV infection. Diabetes was also prevalent in CC, but thepathogenic mechanisms are unclear (54). Other infections have been implicated in CC. For example, DNA fragments from the *Helicobacter* genus have been isolated in bile from patients with biliary malignancy, although the relevance of this is as yet unclear (55). A high prevalence of *Salmonella typhi* carriage has been noted in Eastern CC patients, but this does not appear to be specific to biliary malignancy per se (56).

CHOLANGIOCARCINOGENESIS

Differences in the epidemiology, morphology, and clinical course of biliary tract cancers, along with differences in mutation and protein expression profiles, suggest that diverse carcinogenic mechanisms are likely to be involved in the development of CC (57). In keeping with the current opinion of carcinogenesis in relation to other tumors; cholangiocarcinogenesis is likely to be a multistep process. The recognized risk factors appear to have an underlying similarity in that they lead to chronic inflammation and/or cholestasis in the biliary tree. It is in this setting, in the crucial balance between inflammation/cellular repair/proliferation and normal homeostasis, that carcinogenesis appears to occur.

STEPS IN THE MOLECULAR PATHOGENESIS OF CHOLANGIOCARCINOMA

Cholangiocarcinogenesis at the molecular level is likely to be triggered by the sequelae of a highly complex cascade occurring in the aftermath of inflammation in the biliary tree. Changes in the microenvironment can lead to, for example, the proliferation of cell signaling, development of growth autonomy, avoidance of senescence, increased replication, restriction of growth inhibitory signals, and evasion of programmed cell death (34, 57). The major steps in the molecular patho-

genesis of cholangiocarcinogenesis that will be discussed are summarized in Figure 4.6 (57).

Biliary Epithelial Cell Proliferation Signaling

Biliary epithelial cell proliferation normally relies on cell surface receptor-ligand interactions, which instigate intracellular signaling cascades, leading to the activation of relevant transcription factors. In CC there is evidence to support self-sustained growth signaling related to unregulated mitogen production and/or constitutive activation of the intracellular signal transduction cascade (57).

Chronic inflammation of biliary epithelium results in the generation of cytokines and growth factors such as interleukin (IL)-6 and hepatocyte growth factor (HGF). Upregulation of gp80/gp and c-met receptors on cholangiocytes occurs, and the proliferation of cholangiocytes is promoted (58). The c-erb-2 oncogene is also expressed and dimerizes with the epidermal growth factor receptor (EGFR; transmembrane receptor), leading to constitutive activation of signal transduction pathways. Normally, antigrowth signals protect against cellular proliferation, but this control appears to be lost during cholangiocarcinogenesis. Autocrine loop signaling develops, bypassing normal cell growth regulation (57).

FIGURE 4.6

Steps in the molecular pathogenesis of cholangiocarcinoma. (From Ref. 53.)

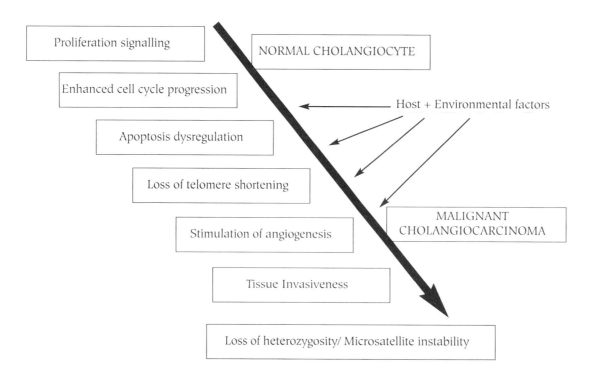

Interleukin-6

IL-6 is largely drawn from periportal stromal cells, including stellate cells. Interestingly, IL-6 is constitutively secreted by CC cells (59), which triggers pro-survival p38 mitogen-activated protein kinase. IL-6-mediated signal transducers and activators of transcription 3 (STAT-3) phosphorylation (activation) are aberrantly sustained in CC cells, resulting in enhanced expression of the antiapoptotic myeloid cell leukemia 1 (Mcl-1) (60). This sustained IL-6/STAT-3 signaling may be due to epigenetic silencing of suppressor of cytokine signaling 3 (SOCS-3), which controls the IL-6/STAT-3 signaling pathway by a classic feedback loop (61). IL-6 may also reduce cell senescence by increasing expression of telomerase (discussed further below) (62). Furthermore, IL-6 and EGFR can also influence expression of cyclooxygenase (COX)-2.

Cyclooxygenase-2

COX isoenzymes are involved in the formation of the important biologic mediators, prostaglandins (PG), from arachidonic acid. Overexpression of COX-2 by various mitogens has been implicated in cholangiocarcinogenesis, occurring in CC cells but not normal cholangiocytes (63,64). Enhanced expression of COX-2 has been shown to occur in biliary epithelia of bile duct cancer in histochemical studies (65). Exposure of biliary epithelial cells to bile acids can increase COX-2 levels via the EGFR-signaling cascade (66). Both bile acids and COX-2 upregulation have been associated with gastrointestinal luminal tumors (for example, colorectal adenomas and adenocarcinomas), e.g., by the activation of oncogenic transcription factor β-catenin (34,67). Increased COX-2 expression may have a carcinogenic role via the inhibition of Fas-mediated apoptosis (68). Another potential factor in cholangiocarcinogenesis within this complex cascade is the peroxisome proliferator activated receptor δ (PPARδ), a nuclear receptor involved in lipid oxidation. Overexpression of PPARδ was found to promote the growth of CC human cell lines via the induction of COX-2 gene expression and the production of PGE2, which in turn transactivated EGFR. COX-2-derived PGE2 further activates PPARδ through phosphorylation of cytosolic phospspholipase A2α, thus creating a positive feedback loop (69).

Inducible Nitric Oxide Synthase

Inducible nitric oxide synthase (iNOS) activation is another result of the chronic inflammatory response occurring in the biliary epithelium (70). iNOS, expressed by macrophages and epithelial cells during inflammation, generates the bioreactive molecule nitric oxide (NO), which has pleiotropic effects in carcinogenesis (71). In addition to causing DNA lesions, NO can directly interact with proteins, for example, by nitrosylation, and can increase DNA adduct formation, thus promoting DNA mutation risk. NO can also inhibit DNA repair enzymes (71). Furthermore, iNOS promotes COX-2 upregulation in murine cholangiocyte cell lines, thus stimulating further growth (72).

Augmented Cell Cycle Progression

The risk factors associated with CC produce chronic inflammation and/or cholestasis. One result of this is the exposure of biliary epithelial cells to a toxic environment that promotes DNA damage and mutation (1,34). This may overburden natural DNA repair mechanisms or directly reduce their efficacy by a nitric oxide dependent pathway (71). Mutations in key genes involved in cell cycle control, for example, k-ras and p53, may contribute to cholangiocarcinogenesis. The k-ras oncogene has a role in mitogenic signaling, and k-ras mutations have been noted in up to 39% of resected human CC specimens, particularly hilar tumors (73).

The p53 tumor suppressor gene has a key role in antigrowth signaling and regulating cell cycle progression. It controls proteins that are involved in cells entering the cell cycle as well as proteins important for apoptosis. p53 is involved in cell cycle control via regulation of the p21/WAF1/Cip1 protein. This binds to the cell division kinase (CDK) 4:cyclin D complex and stops it from phosphorylating Rb, resulting in prevention of the release of bound E2F transcription factor that normally regulates proteins critical for entrance into the S phase of the cell cycle (57,74). p53 also controls Bax, a gene product that binds to the antiapoptotic protein Bcl-2 in mitochondria and promotes apoptosis (57). p53 is mutated in the majority of human cancers, including CC, as shown in a variety of immunohistochemical and gene analysis investigations (75). Upregulation of a p53 inhibitor, such as mdm-2, has also been noted in CC as an alternative mechanism by which the normal function of p53 is compromised (76). Loss of p53 function results in uncontrolled progression through the cell cycle and reduced apoptosis. Inactivation of other tumor suppressor genes has also been implicated in CC, for example, the p16INK4A inhibitory protein, which also has a key role in controlling the CDK 4:cyclin D complex. p16INK4A gene mutations have been reported in up to 80% of human CC specimens (77,78).

In addition to p53, differential expression of several other cell-cycle regulatory proteins has been described in bile duct cancrcinoma and may correlate with tumor location, morphology, and prognosis. An immunohistochemical study of surgically resected specimens of intrahepatic, hilar, and distal CC, as well as gall bladder cancer, found that p27 expression decreased progressively from proximal to distal in the biliary tree and correlated with location-related differences in outcome. Cyclin D1 and Bcl-2 overexpression also varied according to anatomic site. Aberrant p53 staining and cyclin D1 overexpression were lower in papillary tumors compared with the more common sclerosing tumors. Following resection, overexpression of Mdm2 and absent p27 expression predicted a poorer prognosis (79).

Dysregulation of Apoptosis

Effective apoptosis, or programmed cell death, is crucial in preventing uncontrolled cell proliferation secondary to mutation and other anomalous cellular processes by removing abnormal cells including those vulnerable to malignant transformation. Immunohistochemical studies of resected human CC show a relative increase of antiapoptotic signals compared to apoptotic ones (80). Apoptosis is triggered by protein capsases resulting from ligand activation of the CD95/Fas/TRAIL/TNF receptor family and/or release of mitochondrial cytochrome c (57). Cholangiocytes express Fas receptor (Fas-R) and respond to exogenous Fas ligand (Fas-L) to undergo apoptosis. Studies on CC cell lines suggest that during cholangiocarcinogenesis, biliary epithelial cells escape apoptotic immune surveillance by disabling Fas-R signaling through the expression of FLICE inhibitor and/or increased Fas-L expression to induce apoptosis of invading T cells (81).

p53 mutations also affect transcription of the Fas gene, resulting in reduced expression of Fas on the cholangiocyte cell membrane, thus reducing susceptibility to apoptosis. A study of 30 resected human CC specimens examined the phenotypic pattern of Fas distribution and found Fas expression more common in extrahepatic compared to intrahepatic CC. Fas expression decreased from dysplastic epithelium to CC and further decreased from well to poorly differentiated tumors (82). Hence, alterations in Fas expression may be an important early event in the pathogenesis of CC. Furthermore, increases in intracellular NO in cholangiocytes, as occurs under oxidative stress, can further raise resistance to apoptosis downstream of cytochrome c release by inhibiting caspases (57,83).

Telomere Length

Telomeres have a crucial role in maintaining chromosomal stability and limiting the number of cell divisions that can occur before a cell dies. They are regions of highly repetitive 6-base-pair sequences at the end of chromosomes that conserve genetic information during cell division as DNA polymerase cannot replicate all the

way to the end of the chromosome. With every cell division, telomeres progressively shorten, eventually to a finite length when DNA polymerase can no longer bind and further DNA synthesis or cell division can no longer occur. The loss of telomere shortening is a common feature in human cancer (84). High levels of telomerase mRNA have been found in many human cancers, including CC (85). Telomere shortening has been demonstrated in metaplastic and dysplastic biliary epithelium as well as in CC, but not in normal or inflamed biliary epithelium, suggesting that telomere shortening occurs at an early stage in the carcinogenic process (86).

Stimulation of Angiogenesis

The formation of new blood vessels is necessary to feed the metabolic needs of a tumor, particularly in its early stages. CCs are greatly vascularized tumors. Studies of human CC samples and CC cell lines have detected increased levels of vascular endothelial growth factor (vEGF), possibly via stimulation by transforming growth factor (TGF) β1 (87).

Tissue Invasiveness

One reason CC presents late clinically (88) is that it is a highly infiltrative tumor with ability for local invasion. This is influenced by alterations in the expression of cellular adherence molecules. For example, immunohistochemical investigations have shown reduced expression of E-cadherin and increased expression of matrix metalloproteinases, which play a role in cancer cell invasion by degrading extracellular matrix proteins. Changes in the expression of E-cadherin were found to correlate with the tumor's histologic grade and invasiveness (89). Reduced expression of E-cadherin, α-catenin, and β-catenin have been associated with weaker intercellular adhesion (89,90).

Human aspartyl (asparaginyl) β-hydroxylase (HAAH) is a protein that is believed to play a role in malignant transformation and to favor tumor invasion (57). It is an α-ketoglutarate-dependent dioxygenase that catalyzes posttranscriptional hydroxylation of aspartate and asparagine residues in EGF-like domains of proteins. Increased expression of HAAH has been demonstrated in CC and hepatocellular carcinoma (91). Overexpression of HAAH has also been found to induce increased motility and invasion in CC cell lines, further suggesting that HAAH may contribute to the infiltrative growth pattern of CC cells (92). Apomucin (mucin core protein, MUC-1) overexpression has been demonstrated immunohistochemically in hepatocellular carcinoma and CC. High levels of expression were found to correlate with histologic differentiation, metastasis to lymph nodes, portal canal emboli, and postoperational recurrence (86).

WISP1v is an additional protein marker associated with invasive CC. It is a member of the connective tissue growth factor, cysteine-rich 61, nephroblastoma overexpressed gene (CCN) family, which encode cysteine-rich secreted proteins with roles in human fibrotic disorders and tumor progression. Genetic analysis of WISP1v on surgically resected specimens of CC found it to be overexpressed; occurring in 49% but not in normal livers (93). The WISP1v biologic effects were analyzed using the HuCCT1 human cholangiocarcinoma cell line. Expression of WISP1v was significantly associated with lymphatic and perineural invasion of tumor cells as well as a poor clinical prognosis. In vitro analysis showed that WISP1v stimulated the invasive phenotype of cholangiocarcinoma cells with activation of both p38 and p42/p44 mitogen-activated protein kinases (MAPKs) (94).

Loss of Heterozygosity and Microsatellite Instability

Loss of heterozygosity (LOH) in a cell represents the loss of one parent's contribution to part of the cell's genome. This allelic loss can arise, for example, due to deletion, chromosome loss, or gene conversion. LOH is a common finding in cancers and may signal absence of a tumor suppressor gene, leaving only one functional gene, which may be inactivated, for instance, by point mutation. An example is inactivation of the tumor suppressor gene RASSF1A in extrahepatic CC (95).

Microsatellites, or simple sequence repeats, are normal and common polymorphic loci present in DNA that consist of repeating units of 1-4 base pairs. The lengths of microsatellites are highly variable between individuals. Microsatellite instability (MSI) refers to when these sequences become unstable and can result in an increase or decrease in their length. MSI occurs secondary to damaged DNA due to defects in the DNA repair process and is postulated to be a key factor in several cancers, including colorectal, gastric, and ovarian. A study of liver fluke-related CC focusing on the chromosomal region 1p36-pter found that in 75% of cases LOH was present in one or more loci. Microsatellite instability occurred in at least one locus in 38% of cases. Fine mapping at 1p36 showed two distinctive groups of common loss. These related to lymphatic and nerve invasion and also correlated with prognosis (96).

BILE, CHOLESTASIS, AND HOST INFLUENCES

Theoretically, the reported rise in CC in the United Kingdom and other Western countries could be due either to a change in their populations' genetics, causing increased host susceptibility to CC, or to environmental changes, leading to increasing exposure to etiologic agents. Significant changes in population genetics in all the countries studied causing these findings is unlikely, particularly given the relatively short time frame. It has therefore been postulated that the environment has a role and the increase in sporadic CC may relate to the known recent increase in exposure to potentially carcinogenic environmental toxins (97-99), which are largely metabolized via the hepatobiliary system. Even if toxins have a causal role, however, as with the other recognized risk factors, only a minority of those exposed/affected will develop CC. Therefore, host genetic mechanisms that govern the metabolic response to these to pathophysiologic stimuli are likely to play a major role in determining cholangiocarcinogenesis. These metabolic responses include the detoxification of potentially carcinogenic xenobiotics, the concentration of bile constituents, such as toxic metabolites and bile acids, and the flow of bile through the bile ducts (1).

Hepatobiliary Metabolism and Transport of Xenobiotics

The issue of bile flow is particularly relevant as several proposed risk factors and mechanisms for cholangiocarcinogenesis relate to chronic cholestasis, a reduction in the flow of bile, which may result in destabilization of biliary constituents and increased exposure of cholangiocytes in the biliary epithelium to potential carcinogens.

Toxin-Metabolizing Enzymes

The hepatic enzyme systems predominantly involved in the metabolism of potentially carcinogenic xenobiotics include cytochrome P450 (CYP) and UDP-glucuronosyltransferases (UGTs). As well as being present in hepatocytes, they are also expressed and heterogeneously distributed in the biliary epithelium, thus impacting the generation and detoxification of reactive metabolites in the bile ducts (100).

CYTOCHROME P450

Environmental carcinogens are initially metabolized by cytochrome P450 (CYP) monooxygenase enzymes. There are 57 CYP proteins, most abundant in the liver, arranged into 18 families (101). Those that metabolize foreign chemicals are almost exclusively in the CYP1, CYP2, and CYP3 families. Because of their role in carcinogen metabolism and their demonstrated association with other forms of cancer (102,103), they represent candidates for susceptibility loci in cholangiocarcinogenesis. CYP isoforms of particular interest in cancer risk are summarized in Table 4.3. CYP1A2 has been implicated in the carcinogenesis of CC through the metabolism of some endogenously formed carcinogens and environmental toxins (104).

UDP GLUCORONYLTRANSFERASES

UDP glucoronyltransferases (UGTs) perform glucuronidation, a major conjugation process in the detoxification of heterocyclic amines, polyaromatic hydrocarbons, and arylamines. They are also major conjugators of bile acids. The two main families of UGTs are UGT1 and UGT2. UGT1A1 is the most abundant UGT1 isoform found in the liver and performs glucuronidation of bilirubin, and it is also selectively active towards certain phenols and 17α-ethinylestradiol. There is high interindividual variability in UGT1A1 expression. An inverse dose-response relationship was demonstrated between the detoxifying activity of the UGT1A7 genotypes and HCC (105). There are no published studies to date investigating UGT polymorphisms and CC, although preliminary proteomic studies have shown downregulation of UGTs in CCa tissue (106).

Hepatobiliary Transport

Bile flow and constituents vary between individuals. Biliary excretion of bile salts and xenobiotics is performed by transporters expressed on the apical surface of hepatocytes and cholangiocytes. These biliary transporters also govern the rate of bile flow, and dysfunc-tion of the transporters is a leading cause of cholestasis (107). The major biliary transporters include the bile salt excretory pump (BSEP), the MDR-related proteins (MRP1 and MRP3), and products of the familial intrahepatic cholestasis gene (FIC1) and multidrug resistance genes (MDR1 and MDR3) (108).

BILE ACIDS

Bile acids have long been suspected of having carcinogenic properties and have previously been implicated in colorectal cancer. The concentration of intrahepatic bile acids is tightly regulated and in normal physiology does not exceed 1-2 (M. Elevated concentrations of bile acids are toxic to the hepatocyte and cholangiocyte and have been implicated in cholestatic liver and biliary diseases (109). Bile acids stimulate cholangiocyte proliferation by the phosphatidylinositol 3-kinase pathway. Bile acids can bind to the epidermal growth factor receptor expressed on cholangiocytes in a ligand-dependent manner and transactivate it, which in turn can induce COX-2 expression (110). An alternative mechanism for cholangiocyte proliferation via EGFR is increased expression of antiapoptotic proteins, e.g., Mcl-1, which is increased in CC cell lines exposed to unconjugated bile acid. Oxysterols are oxygenated derivatives of cholesterol. These bile acid intermediates have been identified in bile from patients with biliary inflammation, known to predispose to CC. Some oxysterols are thought to further upregulate COX-2 expression via p38 MAPK activation.

TABLE 4.3

Genes Encoding Cytochrome P450 Enzymes and Functional Alleles of Potential Relevance to CC

CYTOCHROME P450	SUBSTRATE (XENOBIOTIC)	VARIANTS PROPOSED TO INFLUENCE FUNCTION	EFFECT ON ENZYME ACTIVITY
Cyp1a1	Polychlorinated hydrocarbons	Not identified	–
Cyp1a2	Polychlorinated hydrocarbons	1c	↓
		1f	↑
		Cyp1a2-7	↓ (splicing defect)
Cyp1b1	Heterocyclic amines	Not identified	–
Cyp1b2	Heterocyclic amines	Not identified	–
Cyp3a4	Polyaromatic hydrocarbons	Cyp3a4-17	↓
		Cyp3a4-18a	
Cyp2c9	Dioxins	2a, 2b, 2c, 3a, 3b,	↓
		5, 11a, 11b, 12	↓
		8	↑

* Examples of human cytochrome P450 alleles associated with cancer.

Further evidence for the carcinogenic properties of bile acids comes from studies on the farnesoid X receptor (FXR). FXR is a member of the nuclear hormone receptor superfamily and controls the synthesis and transport of bile acids. By 15 months of age, FXR-null (i.e., lacking FXR expression) male and female mice spontaneously developed hepatocellular adenomas, carcinomas, and hepatocholangiocellular carcinoma, the latter of which is rarely observed in mice (111,112). At 3 months, FXR-null mice, but not wild-type controls, had increased expression of the proinflammatory cytokine IL-1β mRNA and elevated β-catenin and its target gene c-myc. By 12 months of age, FXR-null livers displayed prominent injury and inflammation. These mice also had elevated levels of bile acids in serum and liver. Lowering the bile acid pool in FXR-null mice by a 2% cholestyramine feeding significantly reduced the malignant lesions (111, 112).

BILIARY TRANSPORTERS

Secretion of bile acids is a major determinant of bile flow (113). The bile salt export pump (BSEP, ABCB11 gene) is a canalicular transmembrane transporter gene, responsible for the active transport of bile acids across the hepatocyte canalicular membrane into bile. MDR1 mediates the canalicular excretion of xenobiotics and cytotoxins. MDR 3 encodes a phospholipid transporter protein that translocates phosphatidylcholine from the inner to the outer leaflet of the canalicular membrane. A recent study identified 45 sequence variants in the normal population (107). Children with genetic BSEP mutations develop the severe cholestatic condition progressive familial intrahepatic cholestasis type-2 (PFIC-2). Some affected individuals have developed CC in childhood (114). Loss of functional BSEP results in intrahepatocytic bile acid accumulation with consequent injury to cellular constituents, including DNA, thus potentially leading to hepatocellular carcinoma. Bile acids induce mutation via reactive oxygen and nitrogen species generated from detergent effects on membrane enzymes. Similar mechanisms may induce proliferation of abnormal stem cell elements (oval cells) that differentiate along biliary epithelium lines (114).

SUMMARY AND MODEL FOR CARCINOGENESIS IN CC

The roles of alterations in growth signaling, tumor suppressor genes, oncogenes, apoptosis, telomerase, angiogenesis, hepatic metabolizing enzymes, and hepatobiliary transport in CC have been reviewed. It is likely that the development of CC, as with probably most other tumors, is dependent on interplay between environmental factors and host genetic factors. Environmental risk factors, known and unknown, cause chronic inflammation of the biliary tree, predisposing to DNA damage in cholangiocytes. Several host factors likely affect the degree of genomic damage accumulated. These factors are likely to include genes for tumor suppression, DNA repair, cell cycle regulation, apoptosis, and oncogenes, as well as genes controlling hepato-biliary transport and the individual's environmental exposure, including the macro environment (exogenous agents such as chemicals and infection) and the micro environment (growth factors, hormones, other disease, etc.).

The likelihood that several phases are required in cholangiocarcinogenesis, suggests that a long time lag is necessary between the initiating events and eventual clinical malignancy. This is borne out by the fact that most patients are elderly. Further studies are needed to understand the relative importance of the pathways discussed and to provide molecular targets for new therapies. Given that CC appears to be increasing and kills most people affected and there have been no major advances in curative therapies, there has never been a more urgent time to investigate the etiopathogenesis behind this disease.

References

1. Khan SA, Taylor-Robinson SD, Davidson BR, et al. Cholangiocarcinoma: seminar. Lancet 2005; 366:1303-1314.
2. Khan SA, Taylor-Robinson SD, Toledano MB,, et al. Changing international trends in mortality rates for liver, biliary and pancreatic tumors. J Hepatol 2002; 37:806-813.
3. Patel T. Increasing incidence and mortality of primary intrahepatic cholangiocarcinoma in the United States. Hepatology 2001; 33:1353-1357.
4. Patel T. Worldwide trends in mortality from biliary tract malignancies. BMC Cancer 2002; 2:10.
5. Taylor-Robinson SD, Toledano MB, Arora S, Keegan TJ,, et al. Increase in mortality rates from intrahepatic cholangiocarcinoma in England and Wales 1968-1998. Gut 2001; 48:816-820.
6. Burt, Portmann, Ferrell (eds). MacSween's Pathology of the Liver. 5th ed. Amsterdam: Churchill Livingstone Elsevier, 2006:761-814.
7. Ishak, Goodman. Neoplasms of the liver. Mod Pathol. 2007; 20(suppl 1):S49-60.
8. Yamasaki S. Intrahepatic cholangiocarcinoma: macroscopic type and stage classification. J Hepatobiliary Pancreat Surg 2003;10:288-291.
9. Aishima S, Kuroda Y, Nishihara Y,, et al. Proposal of progression model for intrahepatic cholangiocarcinoma: clinicopathologic differences between hilar type and peripheral type. Am J Surg Pathol 2007; 31:1059-1067.
10. Güllüoglu MG, Ozden I, Poyanli A,, et al. Intraductal growth-type mucin-producing peripheral cholangiocarcinoma associated with biliary papillomatosis. Ann Diagn Pathol 2007; 11:34-40.
11. Hamilton, Aaltonen (eds.). World Health Organisation Classification of Tumors. Pathology and Genetics of Tumors of the Digestive System. Lyon: IARC Press, 2000:157-199.
12. Zen Y, Adsay NV, Bardadin K,, et al. Biliary intraepithelial neoplasia: an international interobserver agreement study and

proposal for diagnostic criteria. Mod Pathol 2007; 20:701-709.

13. Haas S, Gütgemann I, Wolff M,, et al. Intrahepatic clear cell cholangiocarcinoma: immunohistochemical aspects in a very rare type of cholangiocarcinoma. Am J Surg Pathol 2007; 31:902-906.

14. Tsuneyama K, Kaizaki Y, Doden K,, et al. Combined hepatocellular and cholangiocarcinoma with marked squamous cell carcinoma components arising in non-cirrhotic liver. Pathol Int 2003; 53:90-97.

15. Sumiyoshi S, Kikuyama M, Matsubayashi Y,, et al. Carcinosarcoma of the liver with mesenchymal differentiation. World J Gastroenterol 2007; 13:809-812.

16. Si MW, Thorson JA, Lauwers GY,, et al. Hepatocellular lymphoepithelioma-like carcinoma associated with Epstein Barr virus: a hitherto unrecognized entity. Diagn Mol Pathol 2004; 13:183-189.

17. Tickoo SK, Zee SY, Obiekwe S, et al. Combined hepatocellular-cholangiocarcinoma: a histopathologic, immunohistochemical, and in situ hybridization study. Am J Surg Pathol 2002; 26:989-997.

18. Zuo HQ, Yan LN, Zeng Y,, et al. Clinicopathological characteristics of 15 patients with combined hepatocellular carcinoma and cholangiocarcinoma. Hepatobiliary Pancreat Dis Int 2007; 6:161-165.

19. Kim H, Park C, Han KH, , et al. Primary liver carcinoma of intermediate (hepatocyte-cholangiocyte) phenotype. J Hepatol 2004; 40:298-304.

20. Quaglia A, Bhattacharjya S, Dhillon AP. . Limitations of the histopathological diagnosis and prognostic assessment of hepatocellular carcinoma. Histopathology 2001; 38:523-529.

21. Lódi C, Szabó E, Holczbauer A, , et al. Claudin-4 differentiates biliary tract cancers from hepatocellular carcinomas. Mod Pathol 2006; 19:460-469.

22. Dennis JL, Hvidsten TR, Wit EC, et al. Markers of adenocarcinoma characteristic of the site of origin: development of a diagnostic algorithm. Clin Cancer Res 2005; 11:3766-3772.

23. Oien P, et al. Metastatic adenocarcinoma of unknown origin. In: Kirkham N, Shepherd NA. (eds.) Progress in Pathology. Vol. 7. Cambridge: Cambridge University Press, 2007:135-162.

24. Kozaka K, Sasaki M, Fujii T,, et al. A subgroup of intrahepatic cholangiocarcinoma with an infiltrating replacement growth pattern and a resemblance to reactive proliferating bile ductules: 'bile ductular carcinoma'. Histopathology 2007; 51:390-400.

25. García-Botella A, Díez-Valladares L, Martín-Antona E, et al. Epithelioid hemangioendothelioma of the liver. J Hepatobiliary Pancreat Surg 2006; 13:167-171.

26. Burke EC, Jarnagin WR, Hochwald SN, et al. Hilar cholangiocarcinoma: patterns of spread, the importance of hepatic resection for curative operation, and a presurgical clinical staging system. Ann Surg 1998; 228:385-394.

27. Sakamoto E, Nimura Y, Hayakawa N,, et al. The pattern of infiltration at the proximal border of hilar bile duct carcinoma: a histologic analysis of 62 resected cases. Ann Surg 1998; 227:405-411.

28. Sobin, Wittekind (eds.). TNM Classification of Malignant Tumors. 6th ed. New York: Wiley-Liss, 2002.

29. Bhuiya MR, Nimura Y, Kamiya J,, et al. Clinicopathologic studies on perineural invasion of bile duct carcinoma. Ann Surg 1992; 215:344-349.

30. Tojima Y, Nagino M, Ebata T, et al. Immunohistochemically demonstrated lymph node micrometastasis and prognosis in patients with otherwise node-negative hilar cholangiocarcinoma. Ann Surg 2003; 237:201-207.

31. Tan G, Yilmaz A, De Young BR, et al. Immunohistochemical analysis of biliary tract lesions. Appl Immunohistochem Mol Morphol 2004; 12:193-197.

32. Seubwai W, Wongkham C, Puapairoj A, et al. Overexpression of vitamin D receptor indicates a good prognosis for cholangiocarcinoma: implications for therapeutics. Cancer 2007; 109:2497-2505.

33. Schmitz KJ, Lang H, Wohlschlaeger J, et al. Elevated expression of cyclooxygenase-2 is a negative prognostic factor for overall survival in intrahepatic cholangiocarcinoma. Virchows Arch 2007; 450:135-141.

34. Malhi H, Gores GJ. Cholangiocarcinoma: modern advances in understanding a deadly old disease. J Hepatol 2006; 45:856-867.

35. Shaib YH, El-Serag HB. The epidemiology of cholangiocarcinoma. Semin Liver Dis 2004; 24:115-125.

36. Broome U, Olsson R, Loof L,, et al. Natural history and prognostic factors in 305 Swedish patients with primary sclerosing cholangitis. Gut 1996; 38:610-615.

37. Watanapa P, Watanapa WB. Liver fluke-associated cholangiocarcinoma. Br J Surg 2002; 89:962-970.

38. Watanapa P. Cholangiocarcinoma in patients with opisthorchiasis. Br J Surg 1996; 83:1062-1064.

39. Thamavit W, Bhamarapravati N, Sahaphong S,, et al. Effects of dimethylnitrosamine on induction of cholangiocarcinoma in Opisthorchis viverrini-infected Syrian golden hamsters. Cancer Res 1978; 38:4634-4639.

40. Simeone. Gallbladder & biliary tree: anatomy & structural anomalies. In: Yamada, ed. Textbook of Gastroenterology. Philadelphia: Lippincott, Williams & Wilkins; 1999:2244-2257.

41. Kubo S, Kinoshita H, Hirohashi K,, et al. Hepatolithiasis associated with cholangiocarcinoma. World J Surg 1995; 19:637-641.

42. Chen MF. Peripheral cholangiocarcinoma (cholangiocellular carcinoma): clinical features, diagnosis and treatment. J Gastroenterol Hepatol 1999; 14:1144-1149.

43. Okuda K, Nakanuma Y, Miyazaki M. Cholangiocarcinoma: recent progress. Part 1: epidemiology and etiology. J Gastroenterol Hepatol 2002; 17:1049-1055.

44. Sahani D, Prasad SR, Tannabe KK,, et al. Thorotrast-induced cholangiocarcinoma. Abdom Imaging 2003; 28:72-74.

45. Hardell L, Bengtsson NO, Jonsson U, et al. Etiological aspects on primary liver cancer with special regard to alcohol, organic solvents and acute intermittent porphyria Br J Cancer 1984; 50:389-397.

46. Bergquist A, Glaumann H, Persson B, et al. Risk factors and clinical presentation of hepatobiliary carcinoma in patients with primary sclerosing cholangitis. Hepatology 1998; 27:311-316.

47. Welzel TM, Graubard BI, El-Serag HB, et al. Risk factors for intrahepatic and extrahepatic cholangiocarcinoma in the United States. Clin Gastroenterol Hepatol. 2007; 5:1221-12218.

48. Khan SA, Carmichael PL, Taylor-Robinson SD, et al. DNA adducts, detected by ^{32}P postlabelling, in human cholangiocarcinoma. Gut 2003; 52:586-591.

49. Sorensen HT, Friis S, Olsen JH, et al. Risk of liver and other types of cancer in patients with cirrhosis: a nationwide cohort study in Denmark. Hepatology 1998; 28:921-925.

50. Shin HR, Lee CU, Park HJ, et al. Hepatitis B and C virus, Clonorchis sinensis for the risk of liver cancer: a case-control study in Pusan, Korea. Int J Epidemiol 1996; 25:933-940.

51. Donato F, Gelatti U, Tagger A, et al. Intrahepatic cholangiocarcinoma and hepatitis C and B virus infection, alcohol intake, and hepatolithiasis: a case-control study in Italy. Cancer Causes Control 2001; 12:959-964.

52. Kobayashi M, Ikeda K, Saitoh S, et al. Incidence of primary cholangiocellular carcinoma of the liver in Japanese patients with hepatitis C virus-related cirrhosis. Cancer 2000; 88:2471-2477.

53. Yin F, Chen B. Detection of hepatitis C virus RNA sequences in hepatic portal cholangiocarcinoma tissue. Chin Med J 1998; 111:1068-1070.

54. Shaib YH, El-Serag HB, Davila JA, et al. Risk factors of intrahepatic cholangiocarcinoma in the United States: a case-control study. Gastroenterology 2005; 128:620-626.

55. Kobayashi M, Ikeda K, Saitoh S, et al. Helicobacter genus DNA fragments are commonly detectable in bile from patients with extrahepatic biliary diseases and associated with their pathogenesis. Dig Dis Sci 2005; 50:862-7.

56. Vaishnavi C, Kochhar R, Singh G, et al. Epidemiology of typhoid carriers among blood donors and patients with biliary, gastrointestinal and other related diseases. Microbiol Immunol. 2005; 49:107-112.

57. Berthiaume EP, Wands J. The molecular pathogenesis of cholangiocarcinoma. Semin Liver Dis 2004; 24:127-137.

58. Liu Z, Sakamoto T, Ezure T, Interleukin-6, hepatocyte growth factor, and their receptors in biliary epithelial cells during a type I ductular reaction in mice: interactions between the periductal inflammatory and stromal cells and the biliary epithelium. Hepatology 1998; 28:1260-1268.

59. Isomoto H, Kobayashi S, Werneburg NW, et al. Interleukin 6 upregulates myeloid cell leukemia-1 expression through a STAT3 pathway in cholangiocarcinoma cells. Hepatology 2005; 42:1329-1338.

60. Kobayashi S, Werneburg NW, Bronk SF, et al. IL-6 contributes to Mcl-1 up-regulation and TRAIL resistance via an Akt-signaling pathway in cholangiocarcinoma cells. Gastroenterology 2005; 128:2054-2065.

61. Isomoto H, Mott JL, Kobayashi S, et al. Sustained IL-6/STAT-3 signaling in cholangiocarcinoma cells due to SOCS-3 epigenetic silencing. Gastroenterology 2007; 132:384-396.

62. Yamagiwa Y, Meng F, Patel T.. Interleukin-6 decreases senescence and increases telomerase activity in malignant human cholangiocytes. Life Sci 2006; 78:2494-2502.

63. Chariyalertsak S, Sirikulchayanonta V, Mayer D, et al. Aberrant cyclooxygenase isozyme expression in human intrahepatic cholangiocarcinoma. Gut 2001; 48:80-86.

64. Endo K, Yoon BI, Pairojkul C, et al. ERBB-2 overexpression and cyclooxygenase-2 up-regulation in human cholangiocarcinoma and risk conditions. Hepatology 2002; 36:439-450.

65. Watanabe O, Yoshimatsu K, Shiozawa S, et al. Different expression of cyclooxygenase-2 in biliary epithelia of bile duct cancer with or without pancreaticobiliary maljunction. Anticancer Res 2004; 24:671-674.

66. Yoon JH, Higuchi H, Werneburg NW, et al. Bile acids induce cyclooxygenase-2 expression via the epidermal growth factor receptor in a human cholangiocarcinoma cell line. Gastroenterology 2002; 122:985-993.

67. Eberhart CE, Coffey RJ, Radhika A, et al. Up-regulation of cyclooxygenase 2 gene expression in human colorectal adenomas and adenocarcinomas. Gastroenterology 1994; 107:1183-1188.

68. Nzeako UC, Guicciardi ME, Yoon JH, et al. COX-2 inhibits Fas-mediated apoptosis in cholangiocarcinoma cells. Hepatology 2002; 35:552-559.

69. Xu L, Han C, Wu T. A novel positive feedback loop between peroxisome proliferator-activated receptor-delta and prostaglandin E2 signaling pathways for human cholangiocarcinoma cell growth. J Biol Chem 2006; 281:33982-33996.

70. Jaiswal M, LaRusso NF, Gores GJ. Nitric oxide in gastrointestinal epithelial cell carcinogenesis: linking inflammation to oncogenesis. Am J Physiol Gastrointest Liver Physiol 2001; 281:G626-634.

71. Jaiswal M, LaRusso NF, Burgart LJ, et al. Inflammatory cytokines induce DNA damage and inhibit DNA repair in cholangiocarcinoma cells by a NO-dependent mechanism. Cancer Res 2000; 60:184-190.

72. Ishimura N, Bronk SF, Gores GJ. Inducible nitric oxide synthase upregulates cyclooxygenase-2 in mouse cholangiocytes promoting cell growth. Am J Physiol Gastrointest Liver Physiol. 2004; 287: G88-95.

73. Isa T, Tomita S, Nakachi A, et al. Analysis of microsatellite instability, K-ras gene mutation and p53 protein overexpression in intrahepatic cholangiocarcinoma. Hepatogastroenterology 2002; 49:604-608.

74. Evan GI, Vousden KH. Proliferation, cell cycle & apoptosis in cancer. Nature 2001.17;411:342-348.

75. Khan SA, Taylor-Robinson SD, Carmichael PL, et al. Analysis of p53 mutations for a mutational signature in human intrahepatic cholangiocarcinoma. Int J Oncol 2006; 28:1269-1277.

76. Furubo S, Harada K, Shimonishi T, et al. Protein expression and genetic alterations of p53 and ras in intrahepatic cholan-

giocarcinoma. Histopathology 1999; 35:230-240.

77. Taniai M, Higuchi H, Burgart LJ, et al. p16INK4a promoter mutations are frequent in primary sclerosing cholangitis (PSC) and PSC-associated cholangiocarcinoma. Gastroenterology 2002; 123:1090-1098.

78. Tannapfel A, Sommerer F, Benicke M, et al. Genetic and epigenetic alterations of the INK4a-ARF pathway in cholangiocarcinoma. J Pathol 2002; 197:624-631.

79. Jarnagin WR, Klimstra DS, Hezel M, et al. Differential cell cycle-regulatory protein expression in biliary tract adenocarcinoma: correlation with anatomic site, pathologic variables, and clinical outcome. J Clin Oncol 2006. 24:1152-1160.

80. Okaro AC, Deery AR, Hutchins RR, et al. The expression of antiapoptotic proteins Bcl-2, Bcl-X(L), and Mcl-1 in benign, dysplastic, and malignant biliary epithelium. J Clin Pathol 2001; 54:927-932.

81. Que FG, Phan VA, Phan VH, et al. Cholangiocarcinomas express Fas ligand and disable the Fas receptor. Hepatology 1999; 30:1398-1404.

82. Jhala NC, Vickers SM, Argani P, et al. Regulators of apoptosis in cholangiocarcinoma. Arch Pathol Lab Med 2005; 129:481-486.

83. Török NJ, Higuchi H, Bronk S, et al. Nitric oxide inhibits apoptosis downstream of cytochrome C release by nitrosylating caspase 9. Cancer Res 2002; 62:1648-1653.

84. Shay JW, Bacchetti S. A survey of telomerase activity in human cancer. Eur J Cancer 1997; 33:787-791.

85. Ozaki S, Harada K, Sanzen T, et al. In situ nucleic acid detection of human telomerase in intrahepatic cholangiocarcinoma and its preneoplastic lesion. Hepatology 1999; 30:914-919.

86. Hansel DE, Meeker AK, Hicks J, et al. Telomere length variation in biliary tract metaplasia, dysplasia, and carcinoma. Mod Pathol 2006; 19:772-779.

87. Benckert C, Jonas S, Cramer T et al. Transforming growth factor beta 1 stimulates VEGF gene transcription in human cholangiocellular carcinoma cells. Cancer Res 2003; 63:1083-1092.

88. Khan SA, Davidson BR, Goldin R,et al. UK guidelines for the diagnosis and treatment of cholangiocarcinoma. Gut 2002; 51(suppl 6):VI1-VI9.

89. Endo K, Ashida K, Miyake N, et al. E-cadherin gene mutations in human intrahepatic cholangiocarcinoma. J Pathol 2001; 193:310-317.

90. Ashida K, Terada T, Kitamura Y, et al. Expression of E-cadherin, alpha-catenin, beta-catenin, and CD44 (standard and variant isoforms) in human cholangiocarcinoma: an immunohistochemical study. Hepatology 1998; 27:974-982.

91. Lavaissiere L, Jia S, Nishiyama M, et al. Overexpression of human aspartyl (asparaginyl) beta-hydroxylase in hepatocellular carcinoma and cholangiocarcinoma. J Clin Invest 1996; 98:1313-1323.

92. Maeda T, Sepe P, Lahousse S, et al. Antisense oligodeoxynucleotides directed against aspartyl (asparaginyl) beta-hydroxylase suppress migration of cholangiocarcinoma cells. J Hepatol 2003; 38:615-622.

93. Yuan SF, Li KZ, Wang L, et al. Expression of MUC1 and its significance in hepatocellular and cholangiocarcinoma tissue. World J Gastroenterol 2005; 11:4661-4666.

94. Tanaka S, Sugimachi K, Kameyama T, et al. Human WISP1v, a member of the CCN family, is associated with invasive cholangiocarcinoma. Hepatology 2003; 37:1122-1129.

95. Chen YJ, Tang QB, Zou SQ. Inactivation of RASSF1A, the tumor suppressor gene at 3p21.3 in extrahepatic cholangiocarcinoma. World J Gastroenterol 2005; 11:1333-1338.

96. Limpaiboon T, Tapdara S, Jearanaikoon P, et al. Prognostic significance of microsatellite alterations at 1p36 in cholangiocarcinoma. World J Gastroenterol 2006; 12:4377-43782.

97. Alcock RE, Bacon J, Bardget RD, et al. Persistence and fate of polychlorinated biphenyls (PCBs) in sewage sludge-amended agricultural soils. Environ Pollut. 1996;93:83-92.

98. Kjeller, K. Increase in the polychlorinated dibenzo-p-dioxin and furan content of soils and vegetation since 1840s.Environ Sci Technol 1991;25:1619-1627.

99. Dougherty CP, Henricks Holtz S, Reinert JC, et al. Dietary exposures to food contaminants across the United States. Environ Res 2000; 84:170-185.

100. Lakehal F, Wendum D, Barbu V,, et al. Phase I and phase II drug-metabolizing enzymes are expressed and heterogeneously distributed in the biliary epithelium. Hepatology 1999; 30:1498-1506.

101. Nebert DW, Russell DW. Clinical importance of the cytochromes P450. Lancet 2002; 360:1155-1162.

102. Agundez J. Cytochrome P450 gene polymorphism and cancer. Curr Drug Metab 2004; 5:211-224.

103. Silvestri L, Sonzogni L, De Silvestri A,, et al. CYP enzyme polymorphisms and susceptibility to HCV-related chronic liver disease and liver cancer. Int J Cancer 2003; 104:310-317.

104. Prawan A, Kukongviriyapan V, Tassaneeyakul W, et al. Association between genetic polymorphisms of CYP1A2, arylamine N-acetyltransferase 1, 2 and susceptibility to cholangiocarcinoma. Eur J Cancer Prev 2005; 14:245-50.

105. Tseng CS, Tang KS, Lo HW, et al. UDP-glucuronosyltransferase 1A7 genetic polymorphisms are associated with hepatocellular carcinoma risk and onset age. Am J Gastroenterol 2005; 100:1758-1763.

106. Sharif, A, Cox J, Taylor-Robinson SD, et al. Quantitative Proteomic Analysis of Intrahepatic Cholangiocarcinoma. AASLD 2006

107. Pauli-Magnus C, Stieger B, Meier Y, et al. Enterohepatic transport of bile salts and genetics of cholestasis. J Hepatol 2005; 43:342-357.

108. Trauner M, Boyer JL. Bile salt transporters. Physiol Rev 2003; 83:633-671.

109. Jansen PL. Endogenous bile acids as carcinogens. J Hepatol 2007; 47:434-435.

110. Werneburg NW, Yoon JH, Higuchi H, et al. Bile acids activate EGFreceptor via a TGF-alpha-dependent mechanism in human cholangiocyte cell lines. Am J Physiol Gastrointest Liver 2003; 285:G31-36.

111. Yang F, Huang X, Yi T, et al. Spontaneous development of liver tumors in the absence of the bile acid receptor farnesoid X receptor. Cancer Res 2007; 67:863-867.

112. Kim I, Morimura K, Shah Y, et al. Spontaneous hepatocarcinogenesis in farnesoid X receptor-null mice. Carcinogenesis 2007; 28:940-946.

113. Thompson R, Strautnieks Sl. BSEP: function and role in progressive familial intrahepatic cholestasis. Semin Liver Dis 2001; 21:545-550.

114. Scheimann AO, Strautnieks SS, Knisely AS, et al. Mutations in bile salt export pump (ABCB11) in two children with progressive familial intrahepatic cholestasis and cholangiocarcinoma. J Pediatr 2007; 150:556-559.

5 Novel Biomarkers for Biliary Tract Cancer

Ross C. Smith

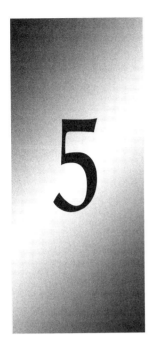

In some tumors, the understanding of abnormal biochemical pathways and genetic alteration allows for interesting new markers to establish the diagnosis and monitor treatment. Furthermore, they may lead to new and specific therapies. An example of this is the presence of c-kit staining in gastrointestinal (GI) stromal tumors, indicating that Gelvec(r) should be an efficacious treatment. This chapter reviews some of the current knowledge about our progress with cholangiocarcinoma, an uncommon cancer in the Western world. There are regional influences that increase the incidence, particularly in Southeast Asia, where chronic biliary inflammatory conditions prevaile.

Cholangiocarcinoma is generally thought to arise on a background of prolonged inflammatory events in the biliary tree. This inflammation may result from the presence of gallstones, choledochal cysts (1), a background of sclerosing cholangitis (2), or following radiotherapy. In the process of malignant transformation, hyperplasia of the biliary mucosa progresses to dysplasia and early carcinoma lesions (3), with subsequent changes in mucus production (4). The changes are considered to be sufficiently widespread to have an influence on the tissue proteome (the entire complement of proteins expressed by the genome). The frequency of such lesions in patients without underlying pathology

is less than 0.5% of cholangiocarcinomas (4).

Only cholangiocytes, the epithelial cells lining the biliary tree, are considered to have the ability to differentiate into cholangiocarcinoma. However, under severe injury or toxicity they may develop a morphology suggestive of intestinal, pancreatic acinar, hepatocyte, or ductal cell origin. If the process continues to the development of cancer, the malignant cells continue to have a phenotype related to their metaplastic origin. Small hepatocellular carcinomas may imitate cholangiocarcinoma and produce similar mucins (5). This great heterogeneity in the characteristics of cholangiocarcinoma and gallbladder carcinoma is often observed in the histology of gallbladders at the time of cholecystectomy where metaplasia similar to intestinal, gastric, or pancreatic epithelium is seen in association with dysplasia. It is therefore reasonable to expect that no one biomarker will exist which can distinguish cholangiocarcinoma from other chronic noncancerous conditions of GI ductal epithelium (6).

Biomarkers can assume many functions (Table 5.1). The ideal of having a single blood test that could establish a specific diagnosis is very difficult to achieve. This is particularly so in a rare condition because only a small false-negative rate would make the test impractical for screening purposes. In subgroups of patients at high risk of cholangiocarcinoma, such as primary sclerosing cholangitis (PSC), where there is a dominant stricture, the pretest probability of a malignant cause may be as high as 15% (http://www.gi.org/patients/gihealth/sclerosing.asp). In these cases a hypothetical test with a sensitivity and specificity of 90% would result in a posttest probability of 65%, a result of clinical value. Preliminary results using proteomic techniques are now approaching these values. Similar tests can be undertaken on bile, but difficulties exist with the preparation of the sample to give reliable results.

Biomarkers on tissue specimens (histology, fine needle aspiration biopsy, and brushings from bile duct strictures) may also be useful for improving the accuracy of diagnosis and prediction of prognosis. Identification of these biomarkers requires an understanding of the complex biology of cholangiocarcinoma.

BIOLOGIC CONSIDERATIONS FOR BIOMARKER CONCEPTS

Cholangiocytes are arranged in a single layer and have important and diverse functions, which affect bile flow and prevent the absorption of toxic substances in bile. They are also closely associated with dendritic cells as protection from bacteria and other antigens. Cholangiocytes are strongly connected by cytokeratins, and they secrete bicarbonate and a number of specialized mucins to provide protection from the bile (7). One area of importance when searching for new biomarkers is the rich mucin pool derived from cholangiocytes. The established serum biomarkers carcinoembryonic antigen (CEA) and cancer antigen (CA) 19-9 are glycoproteins and have use in the monitoring of progress of treatment, but their sensitivity and specificity (60-80%) make them poor diagnostic biomarkers, particularly because they are elevated in chronic inflamma-

---

TABLE 5.1
Aims of Biomarkers

I. Screening, diagnosis, and prognosis
   a) Discover candidate biomarkers.
   b) Qualify sensitivity and specificity of biomarkers
   c) Monitoring outcome of treatment
II. Therapy efficacy
   a) Evaluate biomarkers in clinical trials
   b) Determine dose effect of a treatment
   c) Identify new therapeutic possibilities.
III. Prediction of therapy response
   a) Identify novel targets and/or pathways
   b) Identify agents that predict clinical efficacy
   c) Develop markers that predict response to specific therapy

---

tory conditions which lead to the induction of cholangiocarcinoma. They are also frequently elevated in other malignant conditions of the GI tract, so they are poor discriminators between cancers of the GI tract.

Along with the production of mucin, cholangiocytes produce trefoil factor family (TFF) peptides, which also protect cholangiocytes and act as receptors, inducing hyperplasia or apoptosis. These proteins have intense cross-linking with sulfur bridges. The synthesis and release of TFFs are regulated by a number of environmental and local agents, estrogens, and proinflammatory and anti-inflammatory cytokines (8).

The significance of MUC mucins in developing and adult livers, various hepatobiliary diseases, and intrahepatic cholangiocarcinoma has recently been reviewed (9).

IMPORTANCE OF GLYCOPROTEINS FOR CHOLANGIOCYTES

When chronic inflammation induces metaplasia, this may take on an intestinal, gastric, or pancreatic appearance. Inflammatory biliary conditions and tumors of the biliary tree are associated with altered expression of mucins. It is interesting that alteration of mucin production begins as early as during the process of metaplasia leading to dysplasia, and this early switch is carried on through the malignant progression of cholangiocarcinomas (10). Histologic assessment of tissues may result in important diagnostic and prognostic information from the immunohistochemical study of the many mucins related to cholangiocarcinoma. When the metaplasia is of gastric cell type, it is likely to be associated with the production of MUC1, while metaplasia of intestinal cell arrangement is associated with MUC2 overproduction, implying slightly different malignant potential.

Hughes et al. (11) found that most cases of dysplastic biliary epithelium and cholangiocarcinoma display a Brunner or pyloric gland cell phenotype and a gastric foveolar cell phenotype. However, while aggressive invasive cholangiocarcinoma frequently is associated with MUC1 overexpression, altered MUC1 gene expression also occurs in inflammatory diseases and carcinomas of the GI tract and breast (12, 13), making MUC1 a poor discriminator between tumors.

Cholangiocarcinomas with a better prognosis, particularly those of the intraduct papillary type, produce large quantities of gelatinous mucin, which is predominantly MUC2. It is interesting that there is a similar progression from preinvasive lesions in the pancreas with mucin production having a dichotomy in the dysplasia-CIS-invasive carcinoma sequence. In a study of 268 pancreatic tumors, 54% of the intraductal papillary muci-nous neoplasms expressed MUC2, whereas none of the pancreatic intraepithelial neoplasms (PanINs) did. In contrast, PanINs, especially higher grade lesions, were often positive for MUC1 (61% of PanIN 3), whereas the expression of this glycoprotein was infrequent in intra-ductal papillary mucinous neoplasms (20%). This dichotomy was further accentuated in the invasive car-cinoma group (14). The MUC2 expression in the intra-hepatic biliary system, including intestinal metaplasia, intraductal papillary tumors, and mucinous carcinoma, is dependent on the CDX2 homeobox gene, which induces intestinal differentiation (15, 16).

Overexpression of mucins MUC4 and MUC5AC has also been observed in the early phase of the devel-opment of hyperplasia and dysplasia In cholangiocar-cinoma (9). MUC4 is a novel intramembrane ligand for receptor tyrosine kinase ErbB2 (HER-2) (17), which has been shown to be associated with a poorer prog-nosis in patients with mass-forming intrahepatic cholangiocarcinoma (18). The expression of MUC5AC was associated with the dysplasia-carcinoma sequence. In summary, tumors that predominantly express the gelatinous mucins-MUC2, MUC5AC, MUC5B, and MUC6-are more likely to have a good prognosis, while those associated with the transmembrane mucins-MUC1, MUC3, MUC4, MUC12, and MUC17-have a poorer prognosis.

In a study of four cases of oncocytic biliary intra-ductal papillary neoplasms (IPNs), IPNs were com-posed of distinctive oncocytic cells. The invasive carci-nomas accompanying two of the cases were also composed of oncocytes. None of the cases showed aber-rant expression of the Wnt signaling proteins, although cyclin D1 was markedly overexpressed in all four cases. Three of four cases had positive staining for MUC3, MUC4, MUC5AC, MUC5B, and MUC6. Thus the Wnt pathway proteins (especially β-catenin and E-cad-herin) are expressed normally in oncocytic variants of intraductal papillary neoplasms of the biliary tree, and the mucin profile is similar to their counterparts in the pancreas (19).

Diagnosis of cholangiocarcinoma is futher com-plicated by the presence of intrahepatic peribiliary glands, which, particularly when dysplastic, add to the complexity of the microscopic appearance of the biliary tree. These glands are present in the large intrahepatic bile ducts (20-22). The lobules of branched tubu-loalveolar seromucous glands communicate with bile ducts via conduits (23) and have serous, mucous, and endocrine cells, which stain positively for somatostatin, serotonin, and pancreatic polypeptide (24, 25) and add to the variety of cell types which may become malig-nant. These glands have been shown to secrete a sero-mucin which is rich in amylase and lipase (26, 27). Also, the bile duct wall intramural glands have sparsely branching tubular mucous glands with tall columnar cells. These glands could be confused with invasive car-cinoma.

At the ampulla of Vater the distinction between tumors arising from biliary, intestinal, or pancreatic tis-sue may be helped by a study of the mucus subtypes. Ampullary tumors can be classified histologically as either intestinal type or pancreaticobiliary type and dis-play different features according to tumor location, association with adenoma, and MUC2 expression. Fur-thermore, K-ras mutation is supposedly associated with tumors arising in the area from the ampulloduodenum to the ampullopancreatic duct, with metaplastic mucus occurring in both intestinal and pancreaticobiliary types (28).

CA 19-9 AND CEA-CURRENT MARKERS FOR CHOLANGIOCARCINOMA

CA 19-9 and CEA are the established tumor markers that have clinical utility in management of cholangio-carcinoma and gall bladder carcinoma. There are numerous studies showing that the mean values for these markers are elevated above those of patients presenting in a similar way but found to have benign pathology (29). However, there are numerous reasons why these markers are of limited value. First, they are elevated in some patients with benign conditions in whom the lev-els can be extremely high (30, 31). Both markers are ele-vated in patients with other forms of GI cancer and can-cers of the genitourinary system. Ca 19-9 is not able to be demonstrated in about 10% of the population with Lewis-negative blood factors (32). Tumor markers as a tool in diagnosing cholangiocarcinoma in patients with PSC are unfortunately not as valuable as previously reported. The serum levels of CA 19-9 frequently rise temporarily in association with a "biochemical relapse" of PSC (increased values of serum alkaline phosphatase). The marker product of CA 19-9 and CEA has a low sen-sitivity but a relatively high specificity for the detection of cholangiocarcinoma in PSC patients (33). Therefore, assessment of patients with elevated values needs to be made with an awareness of these variations. They are of most value when used in conjunction with other tests, such as radiologic findings.

In a study of 866 patients with a presentation of general biliary symptoms, CA 19-9 was investigated as a screening test for early pancreatic or biliary cancer. Of 117 subjects with an elevated level above the normal range, 115 did not develop a biliary or pancreatic malig-nancy after 2 years of follow-up and therefore had a false-positive result (34). Thus, a test with low specificity such as CA 19-9 is unacceptable as a screening test.

CA15-3 AND CA27.29 FOR SCREENING, DIAGNOSIS, AND STAGING

CA15-3 and CA27.29 are well-characterized assays for the detection of circulating MUC1 antigen in peripheral blood. This circulating marker has prognostic relevance in early-stage breast cancer (35). The production of MUC1 in breast cancer is very limited compared to that in cholangiocytes, and yet this topic has been more extensively studied in relation to breast cancer. Given the importance of mucin production by cholangiocytes, it is perhaps surprising that there is a dearth of publications studying the usefulness of such measures for the management of gallbladder carcinoma and cholangiocarcinoma. Two general types of assay measuring MUC1 gene-derived glycoprotein are used: assays for CA15-3, which are sandwich assays, and assays for CA27.29, which are competitive assays. These types of assay measure slightly different parts of this tandem-repeat molecule. As long as the tests are calibrated carefully, CA15-3 and CA27.29 measurement of MUC1 give comparable results (36). While it is likely that serum tumor markers CA15-3 and CA27.29 have prognostic value, their role in the management of early-stage breast cancer is unclear (37), and although they have value at detecting recurrence (38), there is no prospective randomized clinical trial to demonstrate survival benefit, and so their role remains uncertain (39). CA15-3 or CA27.29 can be used in conjunction with diagnostic imaging, history, and physical examination for the monitoring of patients with metastatic disease during active therapy, but they should not be used in isolation.

An interesting cross-sectional study evaluating two GI markers (CA19-9 and CEA) and four breast cancer markers (CA27.29, CA15-3, MCA, and CEA) in 213 patients demonstrated sensitivity of 90%, but specificity was 40.3% for CEA and 32.3% for CA19-9 when GI tumors were compared to benign GI disease. This was not as good as the result for breast cancer where a sensitivity of 90% and specificity of 70% was obtained for CA27.29, 67.5% for CA15-3, 52.5% for MCA, and 40% for CEA. Comparison of breast cancer and GI malignancies with other malignancies led to a marked shift of the receiver operating characteristic (ROC) curve to the right and loss of specificity. High serum antigen levels were found in late-stage tumors. Further, the presence of liver metastases in breast cancer was associated with abnormal levels of CA27-29 ($p = 0.028$). Pancreas adenocarcinomas had a higher CA19-9 antigen level (p <0.001) than other GI malignancies. None of the above markers retains its specificity when compared with a control group consisting of other malignancies (40).

MARKERS OF PROLIFERATION

Markers of cellular proliferation can be obtained from tissue samples. For many tumors such markers are predictors of a poorer prognosis. In general, markers of elevated proliferative rate correlate with a worse prognosis in untreated patients and may predict benefit from chemotherapy (41). The implementation of DNA flow cytometry as a marker of proliferative rate is complicated by the variation in methods of tissue preparation, differences in instrumentation, and methods for converting information on the histograms to the estimate of the cell cycle S-phase. In addition, interpretation of individual studies is complicated by the fact that many are too small to have statistical power, cut-offs have not been prospectively defined, and study populations have not been controlled for adjuvant systemic treatments.

There is a small number of studies examining the value of cellular proliferation in cholangiocarcinoma. The usefulness of the finding of aneuploidy has been demonstrated from samples taken from paraffin blocks, indicating that this may be a clinically useful approach in cholangiocarcinoma (42). DNA flow cytometry determination of S-phase is one of several markers of proliferative rate in tumor specimens, which is applicable to cytology specimens from biopsy of masses or brush cytology at the time of endoscopic retrograde cholangiopancreatography (ERCP). In pancreatic cancer, aneuploidy has been shown to be predictive of a poorer outcome. Aneuploidy was associated with higher than normal levels of other biologic markers of prognosis such as HER-2 (43). Despite these findings, measures of proliferation rate in cholangiocarcinoma are not routinely determined in clinical practice.

DNA analysis has been shown to add to the accuracy of CA 19-9 and CEA for the diagnosis of cholangiocarcinoma in bile duct strictures. In 57 patients with a diagnosis of PSC undergoing ERCP, brush samples were taken from strictures for cytology and DNA analysis by flow cytometry for measures of proliferation. The tumor markers CA 19-9 and CEA were determined both in serum and bile fluid. Thirty-nine patients were found to have malignant strictures (7 with PSC), and diagnostic sensitivity of 100% and specificity of 85% were reached when the results of brush cytology, DNA analysis, serum CA 19-9, and serum CEA were combined. Analyses of CA 19-9 and CEA in bile fluid had no diagnostic significance. The authors concluded that the combination of positive brush cytology at ERCP plus aneuploidy improves the results of serum CA 19-9 and CEA. The results were valuable for distinguishing between malignant and benign biliary strictures, especially in PSC patients (44). Further studies are required before these measures could be introduced into clinical practice.

P53 AS A MARKER FOR CHOLANGIOCARCINOMA

Inactivation of the tumor suppressor gene *p53* is the most common genetic abnormality in human cancer and has been implicated in the genesis of cholangiocarcinoma. It is assumed that the cause is the exposure of cholangiocytes to toxic substances being excreted in bile. P53 (protein) may be measured in paraffin-fixed tissue by immunohistochemistry (IHC) and *p53* genetic changes by gene sequencing. P53 is accumulated in the nucleus in up to 50% of cholangiocarcinoma cases, reflecting a minor abnormality of the protein and an inhibition of its natural degradation. It is interesting to note that about 90 different mutations of *p53* have been recognized and that there is little difference in the nature of these along the biliary tree. The structure and function of p53 and its role in linking cancer to specific carcinogens by way of mutational signatures has recently been reviewed (45). In a study of 36 patients with cholangiocarcinoma, clinical outcome was compared for abnormalities of sequencing of *p53* gene in the region of exon 5-8 and for P53 protein accumulation to find which measure is the better predictor of outcome. p53 gene mutations were found in 22 of 36 (61.1%) patients, and for P53 protein, expression was positive in nineteen of 36 (52.8%) patients. There were significant differences in extent of differentiation and invasion between tumors with positive and negative expression of P53 protein. However, there were no significant differences in pathologic parameters between the mutations and nonmutations. The authors concluded that the identification of alterations of the *p53* gene evaluated by DNA sequence analysis is relatively accurate, but, despite this, the overexpression of P53 protein could not act as an independent index to estimate the prognosis of cholangiocarcinoma (46). Fluke-associated cholangiocarcinoma appears more likely to overexpress *p53* than sporadic cholangiocarcinoma. This may be because of the greater likelihood of an intestinal goblet cell phenotype which overexpresses *p53* arising in fluke-associated cholangiocarcinoma. Differences in the etiopathology of the cancers may reflect different pathways to the development of cholangiocarcinoma (11).

Several studies of patients with cholangiocarcinoma suggest that high tissue P53 protein levels measured by IHC or mutations or deletions in the *p53* gene measured by single-strand conformational gel electrophoresis, manual sequencing, or allele-specific polymerase chain reaction (PCR) appear to predict poor outcome (Table 5.2). Results in studies showing no effect of p53 accumulation on survival may have been affected by small study numbers. These studies indicate that about 36% of cases accumulate P53 in the nucleus and that in these cases there is a poorer survival outcome. However, it seems unlikely that IHC for *p53* will provide sufficiently accurate results to be clinically useful, given that it detects both mutated *p53* and stabilized wild-type *p53* and conversely will miss *p53* deletions. Methods to define genetic abnormalities in *p53* more

Table 5.2			
STUDIES OF P53 IN CHOLANGIOCARCINOMA			
		P53 PROTEIN EXPRESSION	
SOURCE	NUMBER OF CASES	PERCENT	EFFECT ON SURVIVAL
Ahrendt et al., 2000 (47)	12	50	Reduced survival
Bergan et al., 2000 (48)	60 ductal type	25	Reduced survival 0.76 vs. 1.4 yr
	22 intestinal	50	
Cong et al., 2001 (49)	22	37	Reduced survival
Havlik et al., 2000 (50)	29		Reduced survival
Isa et al., 2002 (51)	23	21	No effect
Jarnagin et al., 2006 (52)	128	27	None, but effect of p27 and Mdm2 seen
Kim et al., 1999 (53)	25	37	No effect
Liu et al., 2006 (46)	36	51	Reduced survival
Kuroda et al., 2007 (54)	55	32	Reduced survival
Tannapfel et al., 1999 (55)	41	32	Reduced survival
Washington et al., 1996 (56)	41	58	No effect

precisely and conveniently might permit a more accurate analysis of the association of *p53* and clinical outcomes, either as a pure prognostic factor or as a predictor of benefit from systemic therapies. However, at present, methodologies to do so are cumbersome, expensive, and not widely available as routine clinical assays, limiting the utility of this marker in clinical practice. Furthermore, no prospective studies assessing clinical benefits using these new techniques have been published.

UROKINASE PLASMINOGEN (UPA), ITS RECEPTOR UPAR, AND PLASMINOGEN ACTIVATOR INHIBITOR 2 (PAI2) AS MARKERS OF INVASIVENESS IN CHOLANGIOCARCINOMA

The uPA system has been shown to increase invasiveness, and increased expression of these factors has been associated with poor outcome in some cancers. This system involves a cell surface receptor, uPAR, which becomes active when the uPA protein binds to it. Activation of the uPA/uPAR mechanism may be inhibited by the small proteins PAI-1 and PAI-2. Studies of pancreatico-biliary cancers indicate that poor outcome is predicted by increased expression of uPA and uPAR and further that PAI-2 is an independent predictor of improved outcome by suppression of the uPAR mechanism. Several assay formats for these markers have been evaluated, including IHC, quantitative real-time reverse transcriptase (qRT)-PCR, and enzyme-linked immunosorbent assay (ELISA) (57). Both qRT-PCR and IHC have been shown to be predictive of survival (58). Further work is required to determine the value of this measure in cholangiocarcinoma.

EXPRESSION OF CATHEPSIN AND CYCLIN PROTEINS AS MARKERS OF TUMOR PROGRESSION IN CHOLANGIOCARCINOMA

Present data are insufficient to recommend use of cathepsin measurements for management of patients with cholangiocarcinoma, although studies indicate that different cathepsins are involved in the mechanism of metastasis (59).

Similarly, the cyclin proteins which are expressed in the late G1 phase and promote the transition to the S phase of the cell cycle are abnormally expressed in some cases of cholangiocarcinoma (19, 52, 54). They can be measured by IHC in formalin-fixed paraffin-embedded (FFPE) tissue, and mRNA for cyclin E has been quantitated by RT-PCR in fresh frozen specimens

(60). Low molecular weight (LMW) forms of cyclin E have been measured by Western blot analysis of proteins in fresh frozen tissue (61). Discordance between IHC and Western blot analysis in assessment of the prognostic value of cyclin E may be related to the antibodies used for each assay, given that the reagents that detect intact cyclin E may not react with the LMW fragments. Further work is required to demonstrate the role of such in hepatobiliary tumors.

It is considered that the location of a cholangiocarcinoma may be related to the etiology of the tumor, which may influence the pathways in the dysplasia-carcinoma sequence. In a study of cell cycle proteins, tissue arrays from tumors at different sites in the biliary tree have been examined by IHC. P27, cyclin D1, and Bcl2 were more frequently overexpressed in proximal tumors, whereas P53 and Mdm2 were more frequently overexpressed in distal tumors. While cholangiocarcinomas differentially express cell cycle regulatory proteins based on tumor location and morphology, these differences were not sufficiently distinct to be of diagnostic importance. Vascular invasion, lymph node metastases, absence of p27 expression, and Mdm2 overexpression independently predicted poor outcome on multivariate analysis, and there may be prognostic roles for the proteins Mdm2 and p27. However, these measures did not provide a strong guide for prognosis (52).

PROTEOMIC ANALYSIS FOR BILIARY CARCINOMA

New technology is revealing a complex array of proteins and peptides in tissue and blood samples, and the pattern of these is distinct for different conditions. Various mixtures of truncated peptide fragments, or of modifications of proteins or peptides, such as glycosylation, cysteinylation, lipidation, and glutathionylation, require careful evaluation to determine their biologic role and the value of this new knowledge for improved diagnosis and therapeutic possibilities. It is expected that these differences, either in tissue, in the circulation, or in secreted fluids, will be sufficiently specific to evaluate many different clinical questions. For proteomic pattern analysis, computer-based algorithms have been developed to distinguish bile duct cancer from benign diseases (62). More work is required on larger numbers of samples from patients to answer specific questions such as identifying the proteins that distinguish patients with PSC from those with cholangiocarcinoma.

Protein expression in tumors reflects the activation of biologic pathways, and the degree of activation of these pathways is predictive of patient outcome (63). Furthermore, tissue may be available for proteomic assessment from samples taken at surgery and through needle biopsy and as well as from FNA or ERCP with cytology. Although cancer mechanisms are best studied in the cancer cells taken with laser dissection, many of the samples acquired include stroma. Stroma may also hold important messages about cancer biology because the migration of tumor cells relies on an interaction with the stroma and with the immune system through dendritic cells. Therefore, many opportunities exist for the discovery of new markers of different aspects of cancer biology.

Many technological advances have allowed the assessment of numerous proteins at very low concentrations. Patterns of protein expression and measurement of specific proteins open diagnostic possibilities. It is of note that the majority of serum proteins which differentiate patients with cancer from those without cancer are not derived from the neoplastic cells, but are host-specific proteins from tissues such as stroma, liver, or immunologic material (64). New methods that allow isolation of low-abundance serum proteins more likely to represent tumor markers are in development (65, 66). Alternatively, once a number of proteins have been identified and a limited number of proteins are shown to be discriminatory, they may be measured by IHC or serum-based immunoassays. Markers can then be validated individually or in combination as a profile or signature.

PROTEOMIC PATTERN ANALYSIS

Methodology

Analysis of multiple proteins or peptide fragments simultaneously can be approached in several ways, and each has positive and negative features (67). Some of these methods include multiplex ELISA, phage display, and aptamer arrays, summarized in Table 5.3 (68-70) However, the most widely studied methods involve identification of proteomic profiles as peaks on mass spectometric analysis with precise charge-to-mass ratios. In some cases, proteins have been designated by their apparent molecular weight and isoelectric point within two-dimensional (2D) gel analysis. Specific peptides can be identified further based on their amino acid sequence identity or homology to known proteins or their fragments. Some studies have used whole tumor specimens that include both epithelial cells and stroma, whereas others have used microdissected epithelial cells. If isolation of epithelial cells is not required, fine-needle aspirate can provide adequate material (71). Before mass spectroscopic analysis, preliminary separation of proteins can be performed with 2D gel analysis (72) or by binding of proteins to chips or specific sur-

faces to attract subsets of proteins called surface-enhanced laser desorption and ionization (SELDI) (70, 71, 73) and matrix-associated laser desorption and ionization (MALDI) (72), respectively. After desorption and ionization, the pattern of charged peptides generally has been analyzed by time-of-flight (TOF) mass spectroscopy. While these methods are excellent at measuring small proteins with low abundance, they are not able to identify these proteins with ease. Nonetheless, they are able to recognize patterns of proteins and demonstrate the specificity of these proteins for different conditions. The multiplex ELISAs method can also be used to detect several different proteins simultaneously (74). Multiple peptides can also be measured by phage displays or aptamers (68, 70). Indeed, screening protein arrays with sera from patients with cancer would facilitate the identification of autoantibody signatures that can be used for diagnosis and/or prognosis of patients. The usefulness of multiplexed measurements lies not only in the ability to screen many individual marker candidates, but also in evaluating the use of multiple markers in combination. The advantage of protein and serum screening of peptides and cDNA repertoires displayed on phages as well as the fabrication of protein microarrays for probing immune responses in patients has been reviewed (68).

Proteomic Pattern Analysis

This is a new field, but 362 articles listed in PubMed had the key words "proteomic analysis" and "neoplasms" addressing proteomics and cancer in 2007. SELDI-TOF has been used to profile proteins in serum and tissue from cholangiocarcinoma subjects. This demonstrated the potential of SELDI to provide serum biomarkers that differentiate cholangiocarcinoma from benign disease and/or healthy individuals (62).

In this preliminary study SELDI-TOF MS proteomic profiling differentiated cholangiocarcinoma from nonmalignant tissue, and the serum of cancer patients was differentiated from disease controls. Previous studies involving different cancer types (81-83) have shown similar findings, but the pattern of biomarkers varies between the cancer types. The most interesting discovery of the study relating to cholangiocarcinoma patients was the finding of a SELDI-derived peak (m/z 4462), demonstrated in Figure 5.1. This peak was as effective at discriminating cancer from benign serum as the tumor markers CEA or CA19-9. The relevant ROC curves are demonstrated in Figure 5.2. There was an improved diagnostic accuracy when these three serum markers were combined. Classification could be further enhanced with data generated from a panel of peaks, suggesting that analysis of pro-

TABLE 5.3
Proteomic Techniques

METHOD	DESCRIPTION	ADVANTAGE
2D gel electrophoresis	Uses isoelectric properties and SDS-PAGE to separate protein spots. Discovered proteins is biased toward abundant proteins (75, 76). 2DE does not identify proteins which are small, very basic, very acidic, or hydrophobic. 2DE is a slow process (77–80).	MS identifies proteins of interest. New software for analysis of protein spots (69).
MALDI-TOF	Matrix solution (M) + sample (S) dried on glass slide. A laser directed at surface ionizes complex, which becomes (M+S)-/+. The ionized complex is accelerated through electric potential along a flight tube to a detector. The time of flight is related to the mass to charge (m/z) of the compound.	Measures proteins up to 30 kDa. Can be helpful in sequencing of proteins and oligonucleids.
SELDI-TOF ms	Similar principles to MALDI-TOF but the glass chips have specific surfaces to select a subset of proteins. This is then covered by a matrix. The m/z of the proteins in the sample is measured by time of flight technique. The identification of unknown proteins requires further separation of the sample.	Protein pattern of low concentration. Not easy to collect proteins for identification.
Multiplex ELISA	Multiple antibodies placed in different wells, Measure by luminescence. Requires good quality antibodies to give accurate results	Small 50-μL sample is required
Phage display	Screens for protein-protein interactions and protein-DNA using genetic sequences from a DNA library of interactions. Many proteins can be tested at the same time by integrating their sequence into a suitable phage.	Suitable for testing a large number of samples.
Protein microarry	Here, different proteins are affixed in ordered fashion to a glass slide. Substrates, e.g., protein kinase, or biologically active small molecules are identified when they bind being detected by luminescence or similar technique.	Multiple interactions can be tested.
Aptomere microarray	An aptamer is a nucleic acid macromolecule that binds tightly to a specific molecular target. These are being developed as biomarkers.	Binds 1000-fold more tightly than many other reactions. It is most suited to low substrate concentrations.

teomic profiles, rather than individual proteins, may yield improved diagnostic ability. The value of this technology is in its capacity to analyze large numbers of proteins rapidly to determine which may become potential biomarkers. The low molecular weight portion of the proteome, previously hidden by the limited resolution of 2D gel electrophoresis, appears to carry an abundance of tumor-specific information with the potential to improve both diagnosis and the understanding of tumor pathogenesis.

A remarkable finding in that paper was that 14 peaks were common to both the tissue and serum groups. Of these, one peak was significantly upregulated in both cancer subgroups: *m/z* 11664, p = 0.001 (tissue), *p* <0.001 (serum). Interestingly, the 10-fold

cross validation/multivariate logistic regression models did not pick either of these proteins for any of the putative biomarker panels used above. Nonetheless, these peaks are of significant interest for future investigation.

Alterations in the serum protein profile would also seem likely both as a result of the malignant process itself and secondary to the inflammatory response, including release of cytokines and acute phase proteins from the liver. It was therefore crucial to have a control group of patients who did not have cancer but who had a variety of biliary inflammatory processes with matched liver dysfunction.

Discrimination between patients with PSC and those with the added complication of cholangiocarcinoma is perhaps one of the most difficult challenges

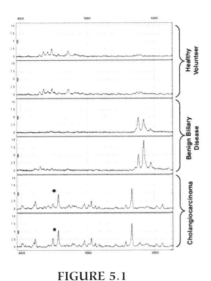

FIGURE 5.1

Printout of the protein mass profile for a small segment of the curve. Results are from the spectrum of two subjects from each of the groups: healthy controls, benign biliary disease, and cholangiocarcinoma. *m/z 4462 peak. (Modified from Ref. 62.)

because transplantation for malignancy can lead to early recurrence. In a prospective study (84) in 84 subjects, the novel tumor markers trypsinogen-1, trypsinogen-2, tumor-associated trypsin inhibitor, human chorionic gonadotropin-β and trypsin-2-α-antitrypsin were evaluated. Forty-six had transplantation for PSC, and 3 of these had an unsuspected cholangiocarcinoma. Five of the patients with cholangiocarcinoma had PSC. These

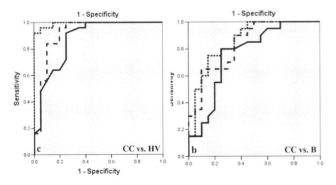

FIGURE 5.2

ROC curves for the serum results from (A) cholangiocarcinoma vs. benign disease, where the solid line is from the marker m/z 4462, the dashed line is a two-marker panel, and the dotted line includes CEA in the panel, and (B) cholangiocarcinoma vs. healthy volunteers, where the solid line represents the curve for the marker m/z 11535, the dashed line is a three-marker panel, and the dotted line is a five-marker panel including CEA and CA 19-9. (Modified from Ref. 62.)

markers were measured by the immunofluorescence technique. Serum trypsinogen-2 showed the highest accuracy in differentiating between cholangiocarcinoma and PSC. The area under the curve (AUC) value was 0.804 and 0.613 for CA19-9. Serum trypsinogen-2 also showed the highest accuracy for differentiation between PSC and PSC with simultaneous cholangiocarcinoma, with an AUC value of 0.759. This finding needs to be considered within a multimarker platform using a method such as the advanced protein microarray.

PROTEOMIC ANALYSIS OF BILE

Bile is a rich source of proteins, but the complexity of bile with its ample array of mucins and lipids, its high pH, concentrated inorganic ions, and active bile salts creates problems with analysis. Bile is freely accessible through ERCP, and it is clear that there will be important biomarkers present if some of the difficulties with analysis can be overcome. Although it is early in the discovery of the complex map of proteins in bile, there are two recent papers demonstrating that the methods are reproducible and that specific proteins can be recognized (85, 86). Two-dimensional electrophoresis (2DE) is a popular and proven separation technique for proteome analysis. One problem involves preparation of the bile sample to make it suitable for 2DE, namely, how to clean up the sample and remove lipid and carbohydrate components without destroying the proteome. Another problem relates to gaining confidence in the reproducibility and resolution of the 2D biliary maps. Only then can the protein patterns specific for potential tumor biomarker discovery be recognized. A methodologic study undertook a variety of sample preparation options to remove contaminants that affect 2DE results, including delipidation, desalination, and nucleic acid removal. A large number of protein spots was separated in 2D maps from the experimental and control groups, with means of 250 and 216 spots on pH 3-10 IPG strips, and 182 and 176 spots on pH 4-7 strips, respectively. When the authors compared bile from a patient with malignancy with bile from a patient with benign disease, approximately 16 and 23 spots were differentially expressed. This study established a reliable sample preparation process suitable for 2DE of bile fluid. By this method, 2D biliary maps with high reproducibility and resolution were obtained. The differentially displayed proteomes in the 2D biliary maps from the experimental and control groups indicated the potential application for bile fluid analysis to identify disease-associated biomarkers, especially for biliary tract tumors (87).

Human gallbladder bile from a cholesterol stone patient contained 222 different proteins, which were identified by tryptic digestion (88). However, the preparation of these samples is a laborious process requiring dialysis, precipitation, and delipidation procedures. Thus, there is a rich pool of proteins to study, but the methodology needs to be refined before the clinical utility can be realized.

One novel marker, Mac-2BP, has been found in bile using tandem mass spectrometry and demonstrated to be as frequently elevated as CA 19-9 in cholangiocarcinoma subjects. This allowed the study of bile with ELISA, and the results indicated that Mac-2BP had the ability to discriminate specimens from patients with PSC with a ROC AUC of 0.70. When both bile markers were used, the accuracy improved to an ROC-AUC of 0.75 (86). Further markers have been sought using cell culture techniques, which have suggest that CK7, CK19, U2/2, and galectin-3 may be useful markers for differential diagnosis of cholangiocarcinoma from hepatocellular carcinoma (89).

MULTIPARAMETER MARKERS

One observation that can be surmised from these results is that the cancer process is not a uniform one, otherwise the same genetic abnormalities, proteins, and peptide abnormalities would be consistently found. This heterogeneous process is the reason that a panel of biomarkers will be required to improve the discrimination power of important clinical questions. There are a number of emerging new technologies which hold promise for the future. Furthermore, correlation of protein levels with altered pathways within cancer cells may give important new insights into the causes of the differences in the proteins being expressed. Biomarkers will provide an improved understanding of the cancer mechanism and the host response to cancer.

References

1. Cullen SN, Chapman RW. Review article: current management of primary sclerosing cholangitis. Aliment Pharmacol Ther 2005; (21):933-948.
2. Zen Y, Aishima S, Ajioka Y, Haratake J, Kage M, Kondo F, et al. Proposal of histological criteria for intraepithelial atypical/proliferative biliary epithelial lesions of the bile duct in hepatolithiasis with respect to cholangiocarcinoma: preliminary report based on interobserver agreement. Pathol Int 2005; (55):180-188.
3. Terada T, Nakanuma Y. Pathological observations of intrahepatic peribiliary glands in 1,000 consecutive autopsy livers. III. Survey of necroinflammation and cystic dilatation. Hepatology 1990 Nov; (12):1229-1233.
4. Terada T, Nakanuma Y. Expression of tenascin, type IV collagen and laminin during human intrahepatic bile duct development and in intrahepatic cholangiocarcinoma. Histopathology 1994; (25):143-150.
5. Aishima S, Nishihara Y, Kuroda Y, Taguchi K, Iguchi T, Take-

tomi A, et al. Histologic characteristics and prognostic significance in small hepatocellular carcinoma with biliary differentiation: subdivision and comparison with ordinary hepatocellular carcinoma. Am J Surg Pathol 2007; (31):783-791.
6. Van Eyken P, Desmet V. Ductular metaplasia of hepatocytes. In: Sirica AE, Longnecker DS (eds.). Biliary and Pancreatic Ductal Epithelia. New York: Marcel Dekker, 2008:201-228.
7. Lazaridis KN, Gores GJ. Primary sclerosing cholangitis and cholangiocarcinoma. Semin Liver Dis 2006; (26):42-51.
8. Baus-Loncar M, Giraud AS. Multiple regulatory pathways for trefoil factor (TFF) genes. Cell Mol Life Sci 2005; (62):2921-2931.
9. Sasaki M, Ikeda H, Nakanuma Y. Expression profiles of MUC mucins and trefoil factor family (TFF) peptides in the intrahepatic biliary system: physiological distribution and pathological significance. Prog Histochem Cytochem 2007; (42):61-110.
10. Zen Y, Sasaki M, Fujii T, Chen TC, Chen MF, Yeh TS, et al. Different expression patterns of mucin core proteins and cytokeratins during intrahepatic cholangiocarcinogenesis from biliary intraepithelial neoplasia and intraductal papillary neoplasm of the bile duct-an immunohistochemical study of 110 cases of hepatolithiasis. J Hepatol 2006; (44):350-358.
11. Hughes NR, Pairojkul C, Royce SG, Clouston A, Bhathal PS. Liver fluke-associated and sporadic cholangiocarcinoma: an immunohistochemical study of bile duct, peribiliary gland and tumor cell phenotypes. J Clin Pathol 2006; (59):1073-1078.
12. Kim YS, Gum JR, Jr., Crawley SC, Deng G, Ho JJ. Mucin gene and antigen expression in biliopancreatic carcinogenesis. Ann Oncol 1999; 10(suppl 4):51-55.
13. Kim YS, Gum JR, Jr. Diversity of mucin genes, structure, function, and expression. Gastroenterology 1995; (109):999-1001.
14. Adsay NV, Merati K, Andea A, Sarkar F, Hruban RH, Wilentz RE, et al. The dichotomy in the preinvasive neoplasia to invasive carcinoma sequence in the pancreas: differential expression of MUC1 and MUC2 supports the existence of two separate pathways of carcinogenesis. Mod Pathol 2002; (15):1087-1095.
15. Ishikawa A, Sasaki M, Ohira S, Ohta T, Oda K, Nimura Y, et al. Aberrant expression of CDX2 is closely related to the intestinal metaplasia and MUC2 expression in intraductal papillary neoplasm of the liver in hepatolithiasis. Lab Invest 2004; (84):629-638.
16. Seno H, Oshima M, Taniguchi MA, Usami K, Ishikawa TO, Chiba T, et al. CDX2 expression in the stomach with intestinal metaplasia and intestinal-type cancer: Prognostic implications. Int J Oncol 2002; (21):769-774.
17. Komatsu M, Jepson S, Arango ME, Carothers Carraway CA, Carraway KL. Muc4/sialomucin complex, an intramembrane modulator of ErbB2/HER2/Neu, potentiates primary tumor growth and suppresses apoptosis in a xenotransplanted tumor. Oncogene 2001; (20):461-470.
18. Shibahara H, Tamada S, Goto M, Oda K, Nagino M, Nagasaka T, et al. Pathologic features of mucin-producing bile duct tumors: two histopathologic categories as counterparts of pancreatic intraductal papillary-mucinous neoplasms. Am J Surg Pathol 2004; (28):327-338.
19. Rouzbahman M, Serra S, Adsay NV, Bejarano PA, Nakanuma Y, Chetty R. Oncocytic papillary neoplasms of the biliary tract: a clinicopathological, mucin core and Wnt pathway protein analysis of four cases. Pathology 2007; (39):413-418.
20. Nakanuma Y, Sasaki M, Terada T, Harada K. Intrahepatic peribiliary glands of humans. II. Pathological spectrum. J Gastroenterol Hepatol 1994; (9):80-86.
21. Nakanuma Y, Katayanagi K, Terada T, Saito K. Intrahepatic peribiliary glands of humans. I. Anatomy, development and presumed functions. J Gastroenterol Hepatol 1994; (9):75-79.
22. Terada T, Nakanuma Y. Morphological examination of intrahepatic bile ducts in hepatolithiasis. Virchows Arch A Pathol Anat Histopathol 1988; (413):167-176.
23. Terada T, Nakanuma Y. Solitary cystic dilation of the intrahepatic bile duct: morphology of two autopsy cases and a

review of the literature. Am J Gastroenterol 1987; (82):1301-1305.

24. Kurumaya H, Ohta G, Nakanuma Y. Endocrine cells in the intrahepatic biliary tree in normal livers and hepatolithiasis. Arch Pathol Lab Med 1989; (113):143-147.

25. Nakanuma Y, Kurumaya H, Ohta G. Multiple cysts in the hepatic hilum and their pathogenesis. A suggestion of periductal gland origin. Virchows Arch A Pathol Anat Histopathol 1984; (404):341-350.

26. Terada T, Kida T, Nakanuma Y. Extrahepatic peribiliary glands express alpha-amylase isozymes, trypsin and pancreatic lipase: an immunohistochemical analysis. Hepatology 1993; (18):803-808.

27. Terada T, Kida T, Nakanuma Y. Extrahepatic peribiliary glands express alpha-amylase isozymes, trypsin and pancreatic lipase: an immunohistochemical analysis. Hepatology 1993; (18):803-808.

28. Matsubayashi H, Watanabe H, Yamaguchi T, Ajioka Y, Nishikura K, Kijima H, et al. Differences in mucus and K-ras mutation in relation to phenotypes of tumors of the papilla of Vater. Cancer 1999; (86):596-607.

29. Scarlett CJ, Saxby AJ, Nielsen A, Bell C, Samra JS, Hugh T, et al. Proteomic profiling of cholangiocarcinoma: diagnostic potential of SELDI-TOF MS in malignant bile duct stricture. Hepatology 2006; (44):658-666.

30. Murray MD, Burton FR, Di Bisceglie AM. Markedly elevated serum CA 19-9 levels in association with a benign biliary stricture due to primary sclerosing cholangitis. J Clin Gastroenterol 2007; (41):115-117.

31. Sanchez M, Gomes H, Marcus EN. Elevated CA 19-9 levels in a patient with Mirizzi syndrome: case report. South Med J 2006; (99):160-163.

32. Vestergaard EM, Hein HO, Meyer H, Grunnet N, Jorgensen J, Wolf H, et al. Reference values and biological variation for tumor marker CA 19-9 in serum for different Lewis and secretor genotypes and evaluation of secretor and Lewis genotyping in a Caucasian population. Clin Chem 1999; (45):54-61.

33. Bjornsson E, Kilander A, Olsson R. CA 19-9 and CEA are unreliable markers for cholangiocarcinoma in patients with primary sclerosing cholangitis. Liver 1999; (19):501-508.

34. Frebourg T, Bercoff E, Manchon N, Senant J, Basuyau JP, Breton P, et al. The evaluation of CA 19-9 antigen level in the early detection of pancreatic cancer. A prospective study of 866 patients. Cancer 1988; (62):2287-2290.

35. Martin A, Corte MD, Alvarez AM, Rodriguez JC, Andicoechea A, Bongera M, et al. Prognostic value of pre-operative serum CA 15.3 levels in breast cancer. Anticancer Res 2006; (26):3965-3971.

36. Klee GG, Schreiber WE. MUC1 gene-derived glycoprotein assays for monitoring breast cancer (CA 15-3, CA 27.29, BR): are they measuring the same antigen? Arch Pathol Lab Med 2004; (128):1131-115.

37. Molina R, Barak V, van Dalen A, Duffy MJ, Einarsson R, Gion M, et al. Tumor markers in breast cancer-European Group on Tumor Markers recommendations. Tumor Biol 2005; (26):281-293.

38. Kokko R, Holli K, Hakama M. Ca 15-3 in the follow-up of localised breast cancer: a prospective study. Eur J Cancer 2002; (38):1189-1193.

39. Khatcheressian JL, Wolff AC, Smith TJ, Grunfeld E, Muss HB, Vogel VG, et al. American Society of Clinical Oncology 2006 update of the breast cancer follow-up and management guidelines in the adjuvant setting. J Clin Oncol 2006; (24):5091-5097.

40. Frenette PS, Thirlwell MP, Trudeau M, Thomson DM, Joseph L, Shuster JS. The diagnostic value of CA 27-29, CA 15-3, mucin-like carcinoma antigen, carcinoembryonic antigen and CA 19-9 in breast and gastrointestinal malignancies. Tumor Biol 1994; (15):247-254.

41. Colozza M, Cardoso F, Sotiriou C, Larsimont D, Piccart MJ. Bringing molecular prognosis and prediction to the clinic. Clin Breast Cancer 2005; (6):61-76.

42. Bergquist A, Tribukait B, Glaumann H, Broome U. Can DNA cytometry be used for evaluation of malignancy and premalignancy in bile duct strictures in primary sclerosing cholangitis? J Hepatol 2000; (33):873-877.

43. Saxby AJ, Nielsen A, Scarlett CJ, Clarkson A, Morey A, Gill A, et al. Assessment of HER-2 status in pancreatic adenocarcinoma: correlation of immunohistochemistry, quantitative real-time RT-PCR, and FISH with aneuploidy and survival. Am J Surg Pathol 2005; (29):1125-1134.

44. Lindberg B, Arnelo U, Bergquist A, Thorne A, Hjerpe A, Granqvist S, et al. Diagnosis of biliary strictures in conjunction with endoscopic retrograde cholangiopancreaticography, with special reference to patients with primary sclerosing cholangitis. Endoscopy 2002; (34):909-916.

45. Khan SA, Thomas HC, Toledano MB, Cox IJ, Taylor-Robinson SD. p53 Mutations in human cholangiocarcinoma: a review. Liver Int 2005; (25):704-716.

46. Liu XF, Zhang H, Zhu SG, Zhou XT, Su HL, Xu Z, et al. Correlation of p53 gene mutation and expression of P53 protein in cholangiocarcinoma. World J Gastroenterol 2006; (12):4706-4709.

47. Ahrendt SA, Rashid A, Chow JT, Eisenberger CF, Pitt HA, Sidransky D. p53 overexpression and K-ras gene mutations in primary sclerosing cholangitis-associated biliary tract cancer. J Hepatobiliary Pancreat Surg 2000; (7):426-431.

48. Bergan A, Gladhaug IP, Schjolberg A, Bergan AB, Clausen OP. p53 accumulation confers prognostic information in resectable adenocarcinomas with ductal but not with intestinal differentiation in the pancreatic head. Int J Oncol 2000; (17):921-926.

49. Cong WM, Bakker A, Swalsky PA, Raja S, Woods J, Thomas S, et al. Multiple genetic alterations involved in the tumorigenesis of human cholangiocarcinoma: a molecular genetic and clinicopathological study. J Cancer Res Clin Oncol 2001; (127):187-192.

50. Havlik R, Sbisa E, Tullo A, Kelly MD, Mitry RR, Jiao LR, et al. Results of resection for hilar cholangiocarcinoma with analysis of prognostic factors 68. Hepatogastroenterology 2000; (47):927-931.

51. Isa T, Tomita S, Nakachi A, Miyazato H, Shimoji H, Kusano T, et al. Analysis of microsatellite instability, K-ras gene mutation and p53 protein overexpression in intrahepatic cholangiocarcinoma. Hepatogastroenterology 2002; (49):604-608.

52. Jarnagin WR, Klimstra DS, Hezel M, Gonen M, Fong Y, Roggin K, et al. Differential cell cycle-regulatory protein expression in biliary tract adenocarcinoma: correlation with anatomic site, pathologic variables, and clinical outcome. J Clin Oncol 2006; (24):1152-1160.

53. Kim HJ, Yun SS, Jung KH, Kwun WH, Choi JH. Intrahepatic cholangiocarcinoma in Korea. J Hepatobiliary Pancreat Surg; (6):142-148.

54. Kuroda Y, Aishima S, Taketomi A, Nishihara Y, Iguchi T, Taguchi K, et al. 14-3-3sigma negatively regulates the cell cycle, and its down-regulation is associated with poor outcome in intrahepatic cholangiocarcinoma. Hum Pathol 2007; (38):1014-1022.

55. Tannapfel A, Engeland K, Weinans L, Katalinic A, Hauss J, Mossner J, et al. Expression of p73, a novel protein related to the p53 tumor suppressor p53, and apoptosis in cholangiocellular carcinoma of the liver. Br J Cancer 1999; (80):1069-1074.

56. Washington K, Gottfried MR. Expression of p53 in adenocarcinoma of the gallbladder and bile ducts. Liver 1996; (16):99-104.

57. Duffy MJ. Urokinase-type plasminogen activator: a potent marker of metastatic potential in human cancers. Biochem Soc Trans 2002; (30):207-210.

58. Smith R, Xue A, Gill A, Scarlett C, Saxby A, Clarkson A, et al. High expression of plasminogen activator inhibitor-2 (PAI-2) is a predictor of improved survival in patients with pancreatic adenocarcinoma. World J Surg 2007; (31):493-502.

59. Terada T, Ohta T, Minato H, Nakanuma Y. Expression of pancreatic trypsinogen/trypsin and cathepsin B in human cholangiocarcinomas and hepatocellular carcinomas. Hum Pathol 1995; (26):746-752.

60. Sieuwerts AM, Look MP, Meijer-van Gelder ME, Timmermans M, Trapman AM, Garcia RR, et al. Which cyclin E prevails as prognostic marker for breast cancer? Results from a retrospective study involving 635 lymph node-negative breast cancer patients. Clin Cancer Res 2006; (12):3319-3328.

61. Keyomarsi K, Tucker SL, Buchholz TA, Callister M, Ding Y, Hortobagyi GN, et al. Cyclin E and survival in patients with breast cancer. N Engl J Med 2002; (347):1566-1575.

62. Scarlett CJ, Saxby AJ, Nielsen A, Bell C, Samra JS, Hugh T, et al. Proteomic profiling of cholangiocarcinoma: diagnostic potential of SELDI-TOF MS in malignant bile duct stricture. Hepatology 2006; (44):658-666.

63. Romani AA, Crafa P, Desenzani S, Graiani G, Lagrasta C, Sianesi M, et al. The expression of HSP27 is associated with poor clinical outcome in intrahepatic cholangiocarcinoma. BMC Cancer 2007; (7):232.

64. Bloomston M, Zhou JX, Rosemurgy AS, Frankel W, Muro-Cacho CA, Yeatman TJ. Fibrinogen gamma overexpression in pancreatic cancer identified by large-scale proteomic analysis of serum samples. Cancer Res 2006; (66):2592-2599.

65. Drake RR, Schwegler EE, Malik G, Diaz J, Block T, Mehta A, et al. Lectin capture strategies combined with mass spectrometry for the discovery of serum glycoprotein biomarkers. Mol Cell Proteomics 2006; (5):1957-1967.

66. Yang Z, Harris LE, Palmer-Toy DE, Hancock WS. Multilectin affinity chromatography for characterization of multiple glycoprotein biomarker candidates in serum from breast cancer patients. Clin Chem 2006; (52):1897-1905.

67. Mirzaei H, McBee J, Watts J, Aebersold R. Comparative evaluation of current peptide production platforms used in absolute quantification in proteomics. Mol Cell Proteomics 2007;

68. Cekaite L, Hovig E, Sioud M. Protein arrays: a versatile toolbox for target identification and monitoring of patient immune responses. Methods Mol Biol 2007; (360):335-348.

69. Elrick MM, Walgren JL, Mitchell MD, Thompson DC. Proteomics: recent applications and new technologies. Basic Clin Pharmacol Toxicol 2006; (98):432-441.

70. Fung ET, Yip TT, Lomas L, Wang Z, Yip C, Meng XY, et al. Classification of cancer types by measuring variants of host response proteins using SELDI serum assays. Int J Cancer 2005; (115):783-789.

71. Fowler LJ, Lovell MO, Izbicka E. Fine-needle aspiration in PreservCyt: a novel and reproducible method for possible ancillary proteomic pattern expression of breast neoplasms by SELDI-TOF. Mod Pathol 2004; (17):1012-1020.

72. Hudelist G, Singer CF, Pischinger KI, Kaserer K, Manavi M, Kubista E, et al. Proteomic analysis in human breast cancer: identification of a characteristic protein expression profile of malignant breast epithelium. Proteomics 2006; (6):1989-2002.

73. Hu Y, Zhang S, Yu J, Liu J, Zheng S. SELDI-TOF-MS: the proteomics and bioinformatics approaches in the diagnosis of breast cancer. Breast 2005; (14):250-255.

74. Wang X, Yu J, Sreekumar A, Varambally S, Shen R, Giacherio D, et al. Autoantibody signatures in prostate cancer. N Engl J Med 2005; (353):1224-1235.

75. Rabilloud T. Two-dimensional gel electrophoresis in proteomics: old, old fashioned, but it still climbs up the mountains. Proteomics 2002; (2):3-10.

76. Gygi SP, Corthals GL, Zhang Y, Rochon Y, Aebersold R. Evaluation of two-dimensional gel electrophoresis-based proteome analysis technology. Proc Natl Acad Sci USA 2000; (97):9390-9395.

77. Gygi SP, Corthals GL, Zhang Y, Rochon Y, Aebersold R. Evaluation of two-dimensional gel electrophoresis-based proteome analysis technology. Proc Natl Acad Sci USA 2000; (97):9390-9395.

78. Gygi SP, Rochon Y, Franza BR, Aebersold R. Correlation between protein and mRNA abundance in yeast. Mol Cell Biol 1999; (19):1720-1730.

79. Aebersold R, Goodlett DR. Mass spectrometry in proteomics. Chem Rev 2001; (101):269-295.

80. Corthals GL, Wasinger VC, Hochstrasser DF, Sanchez JC. The dynamic range of protein expression: a challenge for proteomic research. Electrophoresis 2000; (21):1104-1115.

81. Rosty C, Christa L, Kuzdzal S, Baldwin WM, Zahurak ML, Carnot F, et al. Identification of hepatocarcinoma-intestine-pancreas/pancreatitis-associated protein I as a biomarker for pancreatic ductal adenocarcinoma by protein biochip technology. Cancer Res 2002; (62):1868-1875.

82. Rai AJ, Zhang Z, Rosenzweig J, Shih I, Pham T, Fung ET, et al. Proteomic approaches to tumor marker discovery. Arch Pathol Lab Med 2002; (126):1518-1526.

83. Kozak KR, Su F, Whitelegge JP, Faull K, Reddy S, Farias-Eisner R. Characterization of serum biomarkers for detection of early stage ovarian cancer. Proteomics 2005; (5):4589-4596.

84. Lempinen M, Isoniemi H, Makisalo H, Nordin A, Halme L, Arola J, et al. Enhanced detection of cholangiocarcinoma with serum trypsinogen-2 in patients with severe bile duct strictures. J Hepatol 2007; (47):677-683.

85. Chen B, Dong JQ, Chen YJ, Wang JM, Tian J, Wang CB, et al. Two-dimensional electrophoresis for comparative proteomic analysis of human bile. Hepatobiliary Pancreat Dis Int 2007; (6):402-406.

86. Koopmann J, Thuluvath PJ, Zahurak ML, Kristiansen TZ, Pandey A, Schulick R, et al. Mac-2-binding protein is a diagnostic marker for biliary tract carcinoma. Cancer 2004; (101):1609-1615.

87. Chen B, Dong JQ, Chen YJ, Wang JM, Tian J, Wang CB, et al. Two-dimensional electrophoresis for comparative proteomic analysis of human bile. Hepatobiliary Pancreat Dis Int 2007; (6):402-406.

88. Zhou L, Lu Z, Yang A, Deng R, Mai C, Sang X, et al. Comparative proteomic analysis of human pancreatic juice: methodological study. Proteomics 2007; (7):1345-1355.

89. Srisomsap C, Sawangareetrakul P, Subhasitanont P, Panichakul T, Keeratichamroen S, Lirdprapamongkol K, et al. Proteomic analysis of cholangiocarcinoma cell line. Proteomics 2004; (4):1135-1144.

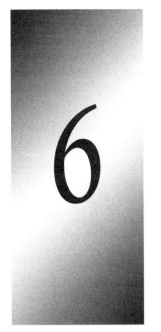

6 Pathologic Staging of Gallbladder Cancer and Biliary Tract Cancer

Chen Liu
James M. Crawford

Pathologic staging of cancer plays a critical role in the management of cancers arising from the biliary system. Cancer staging will help in the selection of adequate primary or adjuvant therapy, predict outcomes, help to evaluate the effectiveness of a given therapy, and facilitate scholarly exchange of information about cancer. Similar to other organ cancer staging systems, the TNM system (i.e., the extent of tumor invasion-T, the status of lymph nodes-N, and the distance of metastasis-M) is the most widely used staging system (1). The World Health Organization has developed a classification system based on cancer histologic types, which has not been widely used in clinical practice. The American Joint Committee on Cancer (AJCC) regularly publishes the criteria about TNM staging in all cancers. In this chapter we will outline the staging criteria for cancers arising in the gallbladder and extrahepatic biliary tract according to the guidelines in the AJCC Cancer Staging Manual, 6th ed. (2).

The premise of a cancer staging guideline is that the classification system should be able to define the tumor behavior and clinical survival. As we gain more knowledge about the biology and clinical medicine about cancers, the staging system is also evolving (3). Nevertheless, the basic tenets of cancer staging are well established.

The overall stage grouping for cancers is denoted by Roman numerals I to IV. The stage reflects the extent of tumor spreading. Stage I indicates localized cancer that is usually treatable. Stage II and Stage III indicate that the cancers are locally advanced or involve regional lymph nodes. Stage IV usually indicates the cancer is inoperable or with distant metastasis. Similar to other solid tumors, the precise overall stage of biliary tract cancer is defined by the TNM staging, which can be either clinical or pathologic.

It is necessary to emphasize that clinical staging and pathologic staging are not always identical. Clinical staging is based on findings of physical examination and imaging analysis. It is useful for planning surgical intervention, and it is particularly important for patients who have unresectable cancers. Pathologic staging is based on the examination of the resected tumor specimen. This staging system is more objective, but obviously is only able to describe the tissue that has been resected. The pathologist can make no comment about lymph nodes that have not been resected or about tumor metastasis to distant sites.

To adhere to the requirements of being a National Cancer Institute (NCI) designated cancer center, it is mandatory to record TNM pathologic staging for all resected cancer specimens. Here we want to emphasize that both clinical staging (cTNM) and pathologic staging (pTNM) should be in the patient's medical record. When referring to TNM status, one must specify whether the staging is based on clinical or pathologic data (cTNM or pTNM, respectively). Beyond NCI-designated cancer centers, it behooves all clinical care centers to record TNM staging.

To accurately report pathologic staging one must clearly understand anatomy (4). The gallbladder is located under the liver in the gallbladder fossa. The superior surface is firmly attached to the liver, while the inferior surface is covered with peritoneum. As an anatomic variation, gallbladder can be buried in the liver (intrahepatic gallbladder) or freely suspended from the liver. The gallbladder can be divided into three parts: fundus, body, and neck. Histologically (Figure 6.1), the gallbladder has four layers: (1) the mucosa (epithelium and lamina propria); (2) a smooth muscle layer; (3) a perimuscular connective tissue layer that is continuous with the interlobular connective tissue of the liver; and (4) the serosa (there is no serosa on the superior surface where it is adherent to the liver). The gallbladder is unique in the alimentary tract in that it has no muscularis mucosa and no submucosa; there is only one smooth muscle layer. Hence, invasion of gallbladder cancer through the "first" muscle layer places the cancer outside the gallbladder. Because of the immediate proximity of the gallbladder to the liver, cancer invasion along the superior portion of the gallbladder leads to direct invasion into the liver.

The extrahepatic biliary tree includes the left and right hepatic ducts, the common hepatic bile duct, and the cystic duct from the gallbladder that joins the common hepatic duct to form the common bile duct. The common bile duct travels through the head of the pancreas and the duodenal wall. It needs to be noted that the histology of the extrahepatic bile duct is unique: the wall is thin (less than 0.15 cm), consisting of mucosa, compact elastic and collagen fibers with interrupted small bundles of smooth muscles, and periductal loose connective tissue (Figure 6.2). Hence, carcinomas from the bile duct epithelial layer can easily invade through the wall and into vessels (lymphatic or vascular) and nerves in the periductal tissue. Mucous glands are also present in the wall of the distal common bile duct. In the setting of inflammation or mechanical stimulation such as stents, these glands are easily distorted and exhibit atypical cytologic features that can be mistaken for carcinoma. Therefore, caution must be exercised in interpreting biopsies of the extrahepatic biliary tree, especially on frozen sections, as inflamed mucous glands may be misinterpreted as invasive cancer.

The Vaterian system consists of the intrapancreatic common bile duct, the main pancreatic duct, the duct of Wirsung, the duodenal papilla, the ampulla of Vater (commonly referred to as ampulla), and the periampullary sphincteric smooth muscle (the sphincter of Oddi). There are common variations in the general population. Approximately 60% of the population have a true ampulla. Most of the remainder have a separate common bile duct and pancreatic duct lumena all the way to the ampullary orifice. Histologically, the ampullary region contains the abrupt transition between ductal epithelium and duodenal mucosa. In addition, mucous glands embedded in the spiral mus-

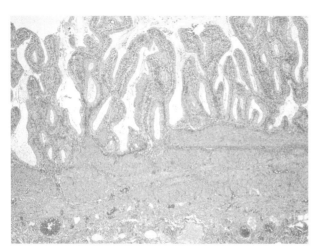

FIGURE 6.1

Normal histology of gallbladder. The image shows the mucosa, lamina propria, muscularis propria, and perimuscular connective tissue. There is no muscularis mucosa and submucosa in the gallbladder.

FIGURE 6.2

Normal histology of extrahepatic bile duct. The image of normal bile duct shows the mucosa, compact elastic and collagen fibers with interrupted small bundles of smooth muscles, and periductal loose connective tissue. Note the mucosal glands in the wall of the bile duct.

culature of the sphincter are particularly numerous in this region, which creates a problem when interpreting small biopsies. Because of this unique anatomy and histology, it is sometimes virtually impossible to ascertain the precise origin of epithelial cancers occurring in this region, i.e, from the duodenal mucosa, ampullary confluence, the common bile duct, or the pancreatic duct. For this reason, cancers in this region are usually classified as "ampullary carcinoma" and hence have their own staging system.

STAGING OF GALLBLADDER CANCER

Gallbladder carcinoma is relative rare, but it is the most common cancer of the biliary system (5). It commonly affects older patients with longstanding cholelithiasis, which afflicts 10-20% of adult populations in developed countries. Similar to cancers in the gastrointestinal tract, tumor behavior is dependent on tumor staging. Gallbladder carcinoma is relatively rare in the United States. Most such cancer cases are from Asian countries. Therefore, many clinical data used for formulating the staging criteria are from studies in these countries.

Carcinomas of gallbladder exhibit two patterns of growth: infiltrating or exophytic. The infiltrating pattern is more common. The gallbladder is usually thickened without obvious visible tumor. The exophtic tumor grows into the lumen as an irregular, cauliflower-shaped mass (Figure 6.3). Histologically, the majority of carcinomas of the gallbladder are adenocarcinoma (Figure 6.4); the other rare histologic types include squamous cell carcinoma, adenosquamous cell carcinoma, and car-

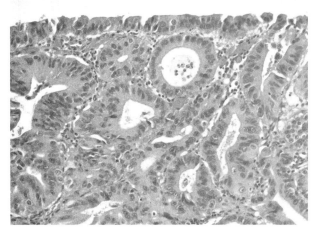

FIGURE 6.4

Histology of gallbladder carcinoma. The image demonstrates adenocarcinoma the gallbladder.

cinosarcoma. Regardless of the histologic types of the primary tumors, the same staging scheme is applied. As shown in Table 6.1, TNM information is the basis for forming the overall stage grouping of gallbladder cancers. Rarely, lymphoma, carcinoid tumors, or sarcomas are seen in the gallbladder, but the current staging system does not apply to these rare tumors.

Besides the widely used AJCC staging system, there are two clinical staging systems for gallbladder carcinoma: the Nevin system (6) and the Japanese Biliary Surgical Society system (7). However, the AJCC staging system is widely used in the United States. It has been an important tool to guide management of gallbladder carcinoma. With more available clinical data about this cancer, modification of this staging system has been recently advocated. This suggestion has been based on a comprehensive study by Fong et al (3). Using the National Cancer Database (NCDB), Fong et al. found that the current staging scheme in the AJCC Cancer Staging Handbook does not discriminate between Stage III and Stage IV in terms of

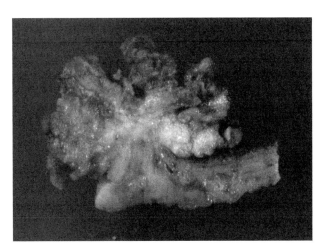

FIGURE 6.3

Gallbladder carcinoma. The exophytic growth of a gallbladder carcinoma. (Courtesy of Robin Foss at the University of Florida.)

TABLE 6.1 *Staging Gallbladder Cancer*			
STAGE	**T**	**N**	**M**
0	Tis	N0	M0
IA	T1	N0	M0
IB	T2	N0	M0
IIA	T3	N0	M0
IIB	T1-3	N1	M0
III	T4	Any N	M0
IV	Any T	Any N	M1

survival rate. As shown in Table 6.1, Stage III only includes T4NxM0 and Stage IV includes TxNxM1. The authors suggested that Stage III should include T3N0M0 and T1-T3 with any node metastasis (T1-T3N1M0) and that Stage IV should include TxN2Mx, T4N1M0, and TxNxM1. The other potential changes in gallbladder cancer staging are the inclusion of molecular prognostic markers and modern imaging findings. These two fields are advancing rapidly and a tremendous amount of information will be available in the near future. Thus, the incorporation of new information into the current staging system appears to be certain.

The foundation of the current staging scheme is pathologic staging based on an examination of resection specimens. Although gallbladder resections (cholecystectomy) are common in most hospitals, gallbladder cancer resection specimens are relatively rare. Fortunately, pathologic assessment of tumor status is readily performed, as shown in Table 6.2.

The criteria for N and M are straightforward. The T classification is dependent on the depth of the tumor invasion in the wall of the gallbladder, presence or absence of cancer invasion into the liver, hepatic artery, or portal vein, and the presence or absence in adjacent organs, which include liver, duodenum, stomach, colon, or pancreas, omentum, or extrahepatic bile ducts.

It has to be mentioned that laparoscopic cholecystectomy is more commonly used in clinical practice. Its impact on gallbladder carcinoma staging remains to be determined. It is known that approximately 50% of the gallbladder carcinomas are incidentally found during upon examination of gallbladders resected by laparoscopic cholecystectomy (8). Most of these patients have Stage I or Stage II disease. It is still questionable whether these patients should undergo immediate adjunctive radical surgical resection, though some of the studies demonstrated the survival advantage when patients had radical resection for early stage disease (9, 10). When invasive carcinoma is found during laparoscopic cholecystectomy, surgical manipulation may lead to intra-abdominal spread and endoscopic tract seeding (11, 12), which certainly complicates the staging of gallbladder cancer.

When examining gallbladders resected for cholelithiasis, it is important to thoroughly examine the mucosal surface at the time of gross inspection. The fundus must be given particular attention, since 60% of gallbladder carcinomas arise from this region. Regardless of whether a macroscopic lesion is identified, it is mandatory to take representative sections for histologic evaluation, especially when the gallbladder wall is thickened. When polyps or tumorous lesions are present, the entire lesion needs to be examined microscopically. Attention should be paid to the presence of dysplasia or carcinoma in situ and whether invasive carcinoma is present. When in situ or invasive carcinoma is identified, more tissue sections should be obtained to fully examine the extent of tumor invasion. It is also important to histologically examine any lymph nodes attached to the gallbladder specimens.

When examining gallbladder carcinoma resection specimens, it is important to maintain the anatomic orientation of the specimen and identify the cystic duct, serosal surface, or any attached liver tissue. The tumor size and location should be accurately recorded. Depending on the size of the tumor, it is advisable to submit as many sections as possible for histologic examination, because it is not uncommon for gallbladder carcinoma to be multifocal.

Tumor spread is via direct liver invasion-less commonly involvement of the hilar region and/or regional lymph node metastasis. The lymph nodes involved are often located in the retroperitoneal, right celiac, and pancreaticoduodenal regions. Thus, when more radical resection procedures are performed, careful identification of lymph nodes in the resection specimen is critical to determine the nodal status hence the tumor staging.

TABLE 6.2
Pathologic Staging of Gallbladder Carcinoma

T	**(Primary Tumor)**
TX	Primary tumor cannot be assessed
T0	No evidence of primary tumor
Tis	Carcinoma in situ
T1	Tumor invades lamina propria or muscle layer
T1a	Tumor invades lamina propria
T1b	Tumor invades muscle layer
T2	Tumor invades perimuscular connective tissue but not into serosa or into liver
T3	Tumor perforates the serosa, or directly extends to the liver, or other adjacent organs, such as stomach, duodenum, colon, pancreas, omentum, or intrahepatic bile ducts
T4	Tumor invades main portal vein, or hepatic artery, or multiple extrahepatic organs or structures

N	**(Regional Lymph Nodes)**
NX	Regional lymph nodes cannot be assessed
N0	No regional lymph node metastasis
N1	Regional lymph node metastasis.

M	**(Distant Metastasis)**
MX	Distant metastasis cannot be assessed
M0	No distant metastasis
M1	Distance metastasis

STAGING OF THE EXTRAHEPATIC BILE DUCT CANCER

Both benign and malignant tumors occur along the extrahepatic biliary system. The benign lesions include papillary adenoma and cystadenoma. The malignant tumors are predominantly adenocarcinoma with some histologic variants. Some benign inflammatory conditions may resemble malignant tumor, such as lymphoplasmacytic cholangiopathy. Differential diagnosis must be considered.

Carcinomas of the extrahepatic bile ducts exhibit multiple appearances, including an infiltrating, nodular, polypoid (Figure 6.5), or constricting pattern of growth. Dysplasia or carcinoma in situ is often seen in the setting of invasive carcinoma. In most of the surgical resection specimens, extensive cancer invasion is present, especially local spread through the wall of the bile duct into the periductal connective tissue (Figure 6.6). The tumors usually spread by direct invasion of adjacent tissue, including the portal vein, hepatic artery, liver, and pancreas. The tumors can also spread along the blood vessels, lymphatics, and small nerves.

The majority of extrahepatic biliary tract cancers (around 70%) arise from the bifurcation site of the common bile duct (i.e., the confluence site of right and left hepatic ducts). Tumors arising in this location are also referred to as Klatskin tumors. Approximately 20% of extrahepatic biliary tract cancers originate in the lower bile duct. In a small percentage of patients, cancer involves multiple segments of the extrahepatic biliary system, and it is impossible to determine the precise origin of the cancer.

Tumor staging for the extrahepatic biliary tree is only used for primary malignant tumors arising in the

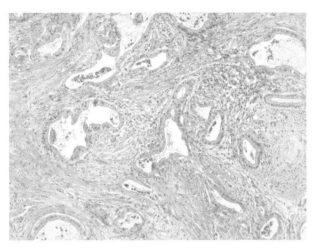

FIGURE 6.6

Adenocarcinoma of extrahepatic bile duct tumor. The image shows irregular tumor glands in the bile duct wall.

extrahepatic bile ducts above the ampulla of Vater. The staging scheme is similar to gallbladder cancer, which is based on the extent of tumor invasion, lymph node status, and distal metastasis (Tables 6.3 and 6.4). Staging correlates with overall survival. Although not included in the staging scheme, the tumor location along the extrahepatic bile ducts, certain histologic subtypes, and the histologic grade appears to influence the survival. In particular, patients with tumor arising in the distal portion of the common bile duct tend to have better survival rate than those with more proximal tumors (13). Tumors that grow in a papillary pattern to the lumen have better prognosis (14). Low-grade tumors generally have better outcome. Perineural invasion imparts a poor prognosis (15).

STAGING OF AMPULLARY CARCINOMA

As noted, the ampulla of Vater is located at the confluence of the pancreatic and common bile ducts, which forms a common channel. Both benign and malignant

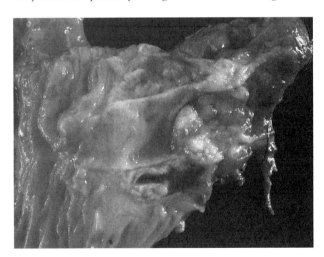

FIGURE 6.5

Extrahepatic bile duct tumor. This photograph shows an exophytic tumor mass in the lumen of common bile duct.

TABLE 6.3 *Staging Cancers of the Extrahepatic Bile Ducts*			
STAGE	**T**	**N**	**M**
0	Tis	N0	M0
IA	T1	N0	M0
IB	T2	N0	M0
IIA	T3	N0	M0
IIB	T1-3	N1	M0
III	T4	Any N	M0
IV	Any T	Any N	M1

TABLE 6.4
Pathologic Staging for Cancers of Extrahepatic Bile Ducts

T (Primary Tumor)

TX	Primary tumor cannot be assessed
T0	No evidence of primary tumor
Tis	Carcinoma in situ
T1	Tumor confined in the bile duct histologically
T2	Tumor invades beyond the wall of the bile duct
T3	Tumor invades the liver, gallbladder, pancreas, and/or unilateral branches of the portal vein (right or left) or hepatic artery (right or left)
T4	Tumor invades any of the following: main portal vein or its branches bilaterally, common hepatic artery, or other adjacent structures, such as the colon, stomach, duodenum, or abdominal wall

N (Regional Lymph Nodes)

NX	Regional lymph nodes cannot be assessed
N0	No regional lymph node metastasis
N1	Regional lymph node metastasis

M (Distant Metastasis)

MX	Distant metastasis cannot be assessed
M0	No distant metastasis
M1	Distance metastasis

tumors occur in this region. The common benign tumor is adenoma, which constitutes 80% of ampullary tumors. Adenomas can exhibit a flat, tubular, or papillary conformation. Regardless of conformation, adenomas can undergo malignant transformation.

Malignant tumors of the ampulla are predominantly adenocarcinoma. Tumors can be exophytic or infiltrative (Figure 6.6). Ampullary carcinomas tend to be associated with other primary cancers, such as colorectal carcinoma in the setting of familial adenomatosis polyposis (FAP) (16) and neurofibromas in association with Recklinghausen's disease (17).

It is difficult to distinguish ampullary carcinoma from periampullary carcinoma of the duodenum. Gross examination and histologic examination of the adjacent duodenal tissue and common bile duct tissue are critical (18). Even with rigorous effort at the time of gross dissection and histologic examination, sometimes it is still impossible to make this distinction. Fortunately, carcinomas arising both ampulla and periampulla share similar clinical and pathologic features. It is appropriate to classify the carcinoma as ampullary carcinoma even when it is difficult to know whether the tumor is from periampullary duodenal mucosa or the ampullary region proper.

The majority of ampullary carcinomas are adenocarcinoma. Multiple histologic variants occur: undifferentiated carcinoma, squamous cell carcinoma, and small cell carcinoma of the ampullary region. Although histologic subtypes of the ampullary cancers may be additional predictive factors for survival, the current staging scheme does not include the tumor histologic types. Carcinoid tumor or other neuroendocrine tumors can also occur in the ampullary region (Figure 6.7). They are clinically and histologically different from carcinoid tumors arising in the duodenum (19). The ampullary carcinoma staging system does not apply to carcinoid tumors (20).

Clinical staging of ampullary carcinoma is usually based on endoscopic ultrasonography and computed tomography. Laparoscopy is sometimes performed on patients who may have localized, potentially respectable tumors to exclude metastasis to the peritoneal surface

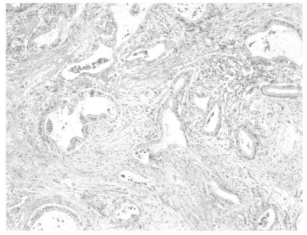

FIGURE 6.6

Adenocarcinoma of extrahepatic bile duct tumor. The image shows irregular tumor glands in the bile duct wall.

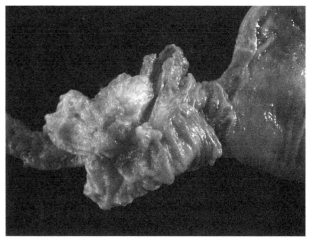

FIGURE 6.7

Ampullary cancer. This image shows an exophytic tumor mass at the ampulla of Vater.

TABLE 6.5
Staging of Ampullary Carcinoma

STAGE	T	N	M
0	Tis	N0	M0
IA	T1	N0	M0
IB	T2	N0	M0
IIA	T3	N0	M0
IIB	T1-3	N1	M0
III	T4	Any N	M0
IV	Any T	Any N	M1

and the liver. Pathologic staging is based on examination of the surgical resection specimen. The T classification depends on the extension of the primary tumor through the ampulla of Vater or the sphincter of Oddi into the duodenal wall or beyond into the head of the pancreas or contiguous soft tissue. It is worth noticing that even T4 tumors are usually locally resectable, in contrast to T staging of other solid tumors.

There is a rich lymphatic network in the peri-ampullary region. Thorough examination of all lymph nodes is required. Although the current staging schedule does not further subclassify the lymph node status (N) according to the number and location of the positive lymph nodes, studies have shown that the location and number of positive nodes does affect the survival of patients with ampullary carcinoma (21, 22). The staging system for ampullary carcinoma is given in Tables 6.5 and 6.6.

TABLE 6.6
Pathological Staging of Ampullary Carcinoma

T (Primary Tumor)

TX Primary tumor cannot be assessed
T0 No evidence of primary tumor
Tis Carcinoma in situ
T1 Tumor confined in ampulla of Vater or sphincter of Oddi
T2 Tumor invades duodenal wall
T3 Tumor invades pancreas
T4 Tumor invades peripancreatic soft tissue or other organs

N (Regional Lymph Nodes)

NX Regional lymph nodes cannot be assessed
N0 No regional lymph node metastasis
N1 Regional lymph node metastasis

M (Distant Metastasis)

MX Distant metastasis cannot be assessed
M0 No distant metastasis
M1 Distance metastasis

References

AU/PROVIDE PAGES FOR REF 4; VOL AND PAGES FOR REF 5

1. Crawford J. Principles of pathology. In: Rustgi and Cawford (eds.), Gastrointestinal Cancers. 2nd ed. Philadelphia: W.B. Saunders, 2003:133-137.
2. AJCC Cancer Staging Manual. Springer, 6th ed. New York: AJCC, 2002.
3. Fong Y, Wagman L, Gonen M, et al. Evidence-based gallbladder cancer staging: changing cancer staging by analysis of data from the National Cancer Database. Ann Surg 2006;243:767-771; discussion 771-774.
4. Crawford J. Gallbladder, extrahepatic biliary tract, and pancreas tissue processing techniques. In: Odze RD, Goldblum JR (eds.), Crawford JM (assoc. ed.), Pathology of the Gastrointestinal Tract, Pancreas, Liver and Biliary Tree. 2nd ed. Philadelphia: W.B. Saunders, 2008.
5. Miller G, Jarnagin WR. Gallbladder carcinoma. Eur J Surg Oncol 2007.
6. Donohue JH, Nagorney DM, Grant CS, Tsushima K, Ilstrup DM, Adson MA. Carcinoma of the gallbladder. Does radical resection improve outcome? Arch Surg 1990;125:237-241.
7. Onoyama H, Yamamoto M, Tseng A, Ajiki T, Saitoh Y. Extended cholecystectomy for carcinoma of the gallbladder. World J Surg 1995;19:758-763.
8. Darabos N, Stare R. Gallbladder cancer: laparoscopic and classic cholecystectomy. Surg Endosc 2004;18:144-147.
9. Sikora SS, Singh RK. Surgical strategies in patients with gallbladder cancer: nihilism to optimism. J Surg Oncol 2006;93:670-681.
10. Misra MC, Guleria S. Management of cancer gallbladder found as a surprise on a resected gallbladder specimen. J Surg Oncol 2006;93:690-698.
11. Fong Y, Brennan MF, Turnbull A, Colt DG, Blumgart LH. Gallbladder cancer discovered during laparoscopic surgery. Potential for iatrogenic tumor dissemination. Arch Surg 1993;128:1054-1056.
12. Baer HU, Metzger A, Glattli A, Klaiber C, Ruchti C, Czerniak A. Subcutaneous periumbilical metastasis of a gallbladder carcinoma after laparoscopic cholecystectomy. Surg Laparosc Endosc 1995;5:59-63.
13. Ogura Y, Mizumoto R, Tabata M, Matsuda S, Kusuda T. Surgical treatment of carcinoma of the hepatic duct confluence: analysis of 55 resected carcinomas. World J Surg 1993;17:85-92; discussion 92-93.
14. Henson DE, Albores-Saavedra J, Corle D. Carcinoma of the extrahepatic bile ducts. Histologic types, stage of disease, grade, and survival rates. Cancer 1992;70:1498-1501.
15. Bhuiya MR, Nimura Y, Kamiya J, Kondo S, Fukata S, Hayakawa N, Shionoya S. Clinicopathologic studies on perineural invasion of bile duct carcinoma. Ann Surg 1992;215:344-349.
16. Williams JA, Cubilla A, Maclean BJ, Fortner JG. Twenty-two year experience with periampullary carcinoma at Memorial Sloan-Kettering Cancer Center. Am J Surg 1979;138:662-665.
17. Klein A, Clemens J, Cameron J. Periampullary neoplasms in von Recklinghausen's disease. Surgery 1989;106:815-819.
18. Compton CC. Protocol for the examination of specimens from patients with carcinoma of the ampulla of Vater: a basis for checklists. Cancer Committee, College of American Pathologists. Arch Pathol Lab Med 1997;121:673-687.
19. Makhlouf HR, Burke AP, Sobin LH. Carcinoid tumors of the ampulla of Vater: a comparison with duodenal carcinoid tumors. Cancer 1999;85:1241-1249.
20. Hartel M, Wente MN, Sido B, Friess H, Buchler MW. Carcinoid of the ampulla of Vater. J Gastroenterol Hepatol

2005;20:676-681.
21. Sakata J, Shirai Y, Wakai T, Yokoyama N, Sakata E, Akazawa K, Hatakeyama K. Number of positive lymph nodes independently affects long-term survival after resection in patients with ampullary carcinoma. Eur J Surg Oncol 2007;33:346-351.
22. Roder JD, Schneider PM, Stein HJ, Siewert JR. Number of lymph node metastases is significantly associated with survival in patients with radically resected carcinoma of the ampulla of Vater. Br J Surg 1995;82:1693-1696.

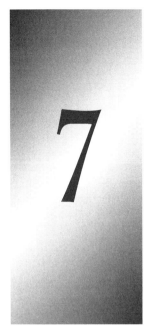

7 Overview of Current Diagnostic Imaging Strategies

Heljä Oikarinen

arcinoma of the gallbladder is the fifth most common malignant tumor of the gastrointestinal tract. Cancers of the bile ducts are less common, but their incidence has been increasing (1). Bile duct tumors can be classified as intrahepatic (or peripheral) cholangio-carcinomas (ICC), hilar (or Klatskin) tumors, and extrahepatic tumors. Klatskin tumors are the most common (2). Most biliary tumors (tumors of the gallbladder and the bile ducts) are malignant adenocarcinomas, the prognosis for which has been dismal. Other malignant biliary neoplasms are anaplastic or squamous cell carcinomas of the gallbladder, anaplastic carcinomas and cystadenocarcinomas of the bile ducts, and carcinomas of the ampulla of Vater. Metastases, carcinoid tumors, lymphomas, and sarcomas of the biliary tract also occur.

Early diagnosis of biliary tumors would be important to improve their prognosis, and accurate staging would help to choose the best possible treatment. However, biliary tumors present specific diagnostic challenges. Their symptoms may be mild or unspecific, such as malaise, mild fever, weight loss, or a sensation of fullness. In the case of bile duct obstruction, jaundice may be the presenting sign. The differences in the clinical behavior of bile duct cancers are due to variation in the location and size of the tumor at the time of diag-

nosis. A tumor of the papilla of Vater or the distal common bile duct may cause jaundice at an early stage, while ICC-or gallbladder carcinomas-are often advanced before causing symptoms of obstruction. Gallbladder carcinoma is often found incidentally in a resected cholecystectomy specimen. Gallstones are present in most of the affected patients.

Imaging modalities, imaging-guided fine-needle aspiration (FNA), and endoscopic brush samples play a crucial role in the diagnostic work-up, although laboratory findings or tumor markers may also be suggestive of a tumor. However, there is no single modality capable of reliably detecting and accurately staging biliary cancers, hence, complementary modalities are usually needed.

This chapter will concentrate on the potential of different imaging modalities to respond to the challenge of how to diagnose and stage biliary cancers. The current state-of-the-art strategies are also discussed. Subsequent chapters in book will go into greater depth.

Similar imaging modalities and diagnostic strategies are mainly used for both carcinoma of the gallbladder and carcinoma of the bile ducts. Therefore, the possibilities of each imaging method in both cancer types are presented under the subheadings of the modalities. Although jaundice with bile duct obstruction is typical for cancer of the bile ducts, it is also common in advanced gallbladder cancer.

It is, however, somewhat problematic to give detailed, up-to-date information about the diagnostic possibilities of the modern imaging modalities and strategies in biliary cancers, in part due to the rapid emergence of novel technology. We lack new large-scale studies of the sensitivities of modern magnetic resonance imaging (MRI) with magnetic resonance cholangiography (MRC) or multidetector computed tomography (MDCT) in biliary cancers. The studies are mostly about older techniques, e.g., computed tomography (CT) without a multidetector technique with high-resolution images and multiplanar reconstructions of good quality. The classification and nomenclature of bile duct tumors is also variable and confusing, and original studies are often about tumors from only one location, e.g., Klatskin tumors. Also, the studies are often retrospective, the size of the study population can be small, and there are differences in study design, algorithms, and equipment, which makes it difficult to compare different papers. Nevertheless, the conclusions of the pertinent literature are highlighted and discussed.

SPREAD, STAGING, AND TREATMENT OF BILIARY CANCERS

With the exception of ampullary carcinoma, the prognosis of biliary carcinomas is poor. In biliary cancers, the histologic type, the staging, and, in the case of carcinoma of the bile ducts, the location of the tumor are the most important prognostic factors. Resection provides the only chance of cure, and since advanced surgical techniques are increasingly used, there is a need for accurate preoperative staging and determination of the best therapeutic option.

Gallbladder carcinoma spreads early in its course. It invades the wall of the gallbladder and spreads into the regional lymph nodes (the cystic duct node and the pericholedochal, hilar, peripancreatic, periduodenal, periportal, celiac, and superior mesenteric nodes). Spread into the liver segments IV and V, duodenum, colon, abdominal wall, and common hepatic duct may also occur. ICC may spread directly into the surrounding hepatic parenchyma, portal pedicle, and bile duct. It may also spread into the regional lymph nodes, and late intrahepatic and pulmonary metastases occur. Ampullary carcinoma infiltrates locally, sometimes involving the regional lymph nodes. In the case of other bile duct carcinomas, in addition to the location, length, and local invasion of the tumor, spread into the liver, hepatic artery, portal vein, gallbladder, regional lymph nodes (as in gallbladder carcinoma), and adjacent organs and tissues should be evaluated. The TNM classifications of biliary tumors are used for staging. There are separate staging schemes for gallbladder carcinoma, ICC, and tumors arising more distally in the biliary tract (2, 3).

There are various practices for the treatment of biliary cancers. In gallbladder carcinomas, surgery is the only curative therapy in properly selected patients. The presence of major vascular encasement or metastases leads to a nonoperative approach. Simple cholecystectomy is feasible at an early stage (stage I, T1N0M0; Table 7.1). The debate over how aggressive the surgery for more advanced cancers should be continues. Patients with advanced cancer or significant comorbidities are candidates for biliary enteric bypass or biliary drainage, and chemotherapy and radiotherapy are also possible (4).

ICC is managed with liver resection, but early detection of ICC is difficult, and fewer than 10% of patients with ICC have resectable disease. Lymph node spread, vascular invasion, positive margins, and bilobar distribution are associated with a poor prognosis. There is no universally accepted surgical approach for tumors of the perihilar area, and variable practices are employed. Surgical resectability is shown by about one third of patients. Bismuth staging is often used to describe the extent of tumor involvement within the ductal system (Table 7.2). Criteria for unresectability have been published and are presented in Table 7.3 and will be discussed in greater detail elsewhere. The operative goal is complete resection with a negative histologic margin. The operative procedure for distal bile duct cancers consists of pancreaticoduodenectomy or local bile duct excision. Hepaticojejunostomy and regional lymph node dissection may also be required. Ampullary carcinoma is usually treated by pancreaticoduodenectomy. Endoscopic treatment or transduodenal excision is reserved for high-risk patients (4, 5).

TABLE 7.1
T-Classification of Gallbladder Carcinoma

T1	Tumor invades lamina propria or muscle layer
T2	Tumor invades perimuscular connective tissue, no extension beyond serosa or into liver
T3	Tumor perforates serosa and/or directly invades the liver and/or one other adjacent organ or structure, e.g., stomach, duodenum, colon, pancreas, omentum, extrahepatic bile ducts
T4	Tumor invades main portal vein or hepatic artery, or invades two or more extrahepatic organs or structures

Source: Ref. 3.

Table 7.2

Bismuth Classification of Hilar Carcinoma

Type I	Confluence of the right and left hepatic ducts not involved
Type II	Tumor involves the confluence of the hepatic ducts
Type III	Tumor involves the confluence of the hepatic ducts and extends into the right (IIIA) or left duct (IIIB)
Type IV	Tumor extends into both hepatic ducts and the confluence

Source: Ref. 4.

Patients with unresectable bile duct carcinoma may need palliative treatment for jaundice, which can be accomplished by biliary enteric bypass, percutaneous biliary drainage, or by inserting a plastic or metallic stent percutaneously or endoscopically. Catheters suffer from the risk of infection or dislodgement, and the major problems with plastic stents are displacement and occlusion with sludge. Self-expandable metallic stents inserted by radiologists have advantages over plastic stents in they can be introduced on a small delivery catheter, have a large inner diameter, and remain in a fixed position after release. However, they may also cause infections or become occluded by tumor ingrowth or overgrowth. Radiotherapy or chemotherapy is used as adjuvant therapy or palliation, and arterial chemoembolization and photodynamic therapy are also possible (6, 7). Subsequent chapters on therapeutic approaches will discuss therapy in greater detail.

TABLE 7.3
Criteria for Unresectability in Patients with Hilar Cancers

Medical comorbidities limiting the patient's ability to undergo major surgery

Significant underlying liver disease prohibiting liver resection necessary for curative surgery based on preoperative imaging

Bilateral tumor extension to secondary biliary radicals

Encasement or occlusion of the main portal vein

Lobar atrophy with contralateral portal vein involvement

Contralateral tumor extension to secondary biliary radicals

Evidence of metastases to N2 level lymph nodes

Presence of distant metastases

Source: Ref. 5.

A few biostatistical terms will be defined here, as they are used widely in the literature and in subsequent chapters. Sensitivity is the proportion of true positives (TP) that are correctly identified by the test, and specificity is the proportion of true negatives (TN) that are correctly identified by the test. Positive predictive value is the proportion of patients with positive test results who are correctly diagnosed, and negative predictive value is the proportion of patients with negative test results who are correctly diagnosed. Accuracy is the proportion of true results in the population. It is defined as a ratio of TP + TN and TP + FP + FN + TN.

ULTRASOUND

Transabdominal ultrasound (US) is often the first imaging modality applied to patients with nonspecific gastrointestinal complaints or jaundice. It is a suitable method for even mild symptoms, and it is commonly available. US does not include any radiation, the examination can be performed bedside, and it is relatively inexpensive. However, the value of US depends on the experience of the operator and the quality of the equipment. It may also be problematic in the case of obese patients and in the presence of bowel gas. The sensitivity of US to reveal a primary tumor of the gallbladder or the bile ducts has increased to over 90% with technical development of the equipment, although problems do occur, especially with small bile duct tumors (8, 9).

Carcinoma of the Gallbladder

A tumor of the gallbladder may appear on US as a mass of variable echogenicity filling the entire lumen of the gallbladder (exophytic type) (Figure 7.1). There may be tumor necrosis, and echogenic foci may be related to gallstones, air, or calcification of the wall of the tumor itself. Other manifestations are focal or diffuse thickening of the gallbladder wall, which can be hypo- or hyperechoic and often irregular (infiltrating type) (Figure 7.2), or an intraluminal fungate mass with a nodular or smooth contour and variable echogenicity (polypoid type). The mass type (exophytic) is the most common, and the infiltrating type has been the most difficult to detect by US. Gallstones may disturb the visualization of tumors (10-12).

US- or CT-guided FNA is necessary to reveal the malignant nature of the tumor. This technique has a diagnostic accuracy of 95%. For differential diagnosis, tumorous sludge, other causes of wall thickening (e.g., cholecystitis), benign polyps, and other malignancies should be noticed.

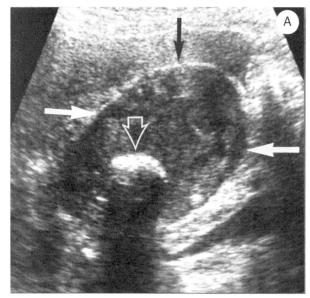

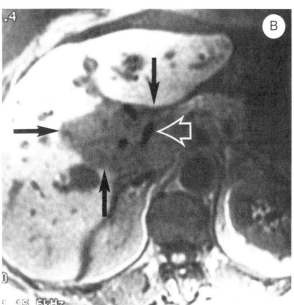

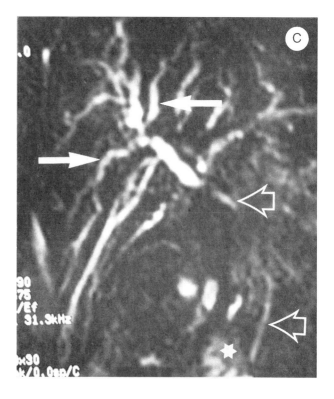

FIGURE 7.1

Figure 7.1 Gallbladder carcinoma. (A) Sonography reveals tumorous tissue replacing the gallbladder (arrows). A gallstone is also seen (open arrow). (B) MRI (T1 fat-saturated gradient echo) shows tumorous tissue even in the hilar area (arrows). There are vessels inside the tumorous area (open arrow). (C) MRC reveals intrahepatic bile duct dilatation (arrows). Extrahepatic bile ducts are seen only partly (open arrows) because of the strictures caused by tumorous tissue. Duodenum (asterisk). (From Ref. 2.)

Early-stage cancers have been difficult to detect sonographically. However, it has been reported that most early cancerous lesions appear polypoid at US, and high-resolution US can detect even small lesions. Lesions larger than 1 cm are more likely to be malignant. There have been efforts to differentiate benign from malignant lesions with Doppler, and the results are suggestive at best (13, 14).

For detailed analysis, endoscopic US (EUS) or intraductal US (IDUS) have also been promising (15, 16). Laparoscopic US may help to detect unsuspected cancer during laparoscopic cholecystectomy. High-frequency EUS can provide high-resolution images, and it can reveal the layered structure of the gallbladder and gallbladder masses. It has been useful in differentiating polyps or wall thickening. In the presence of polyps, the internal echogenicity and contour of polypoid lesions is analyzed. EUS is also used to guide FNA procedures. However, EUS and IDUS are more invasive, less widely available, and more examiner-dependent (15, 16).

Carcinoma of the Bile Ducts

The most frequently seen abnormality due to carcinoma of the bile ducts at US is dilatation of the intrahepatic bile ducts, which may also accompany advanced gallbladder carcinoma. In fact, such dilatation can be an

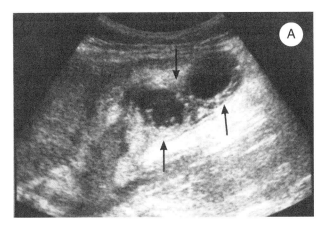

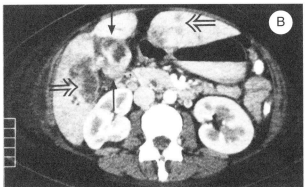

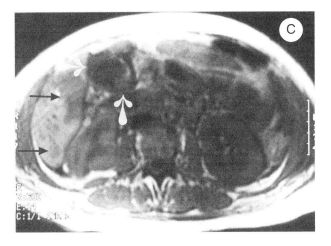

FIGURE 7.2

Gallbladder carcinoma. (A) The gallbladder is thick-walled and deformed (arrows) due to carcinoma (sonography). (B) CT (arterial phase) also reveals a tumorous gallbladder (arrows) and metastases of the liver (open arrows). (C) The thickened gallbladder wall (white arrows) seen in MRI (T1 spin echo). Liver metastases are also visible (black arrows). (From Ref. 2.)

indirect sign of a biliary tumor. The accuracy of US to define the level and cause of obstruction with surgical obstructive jaundice has been 95% and 88%, respec-

tively. Malignancies are found especially in obstructions at the intra- or suprapancreatic level or at or proximal to the porta hepatis. The zone of transition from a dilated to a nondilated or nonvisualized duct should be evaluated regardless of the imaging modality. Bile duct carcinoma can also be visible as a mass (exophytic, nodular), an infiltrating tumor (sclerosing, periductally infiltrating), or a polypoid growth (papillary, intra-ductal growth). The infiltrating type has been especially difficult to detect. The polypoid type is rare and of low-grade malignancy (17-20).

The mass-forming type of ICC, Klatskin tumor, or extrahepatic carcinoma may present as a tumor mass with variable echogenicity (Figure 7.3). Carcinomas of the distal common bile duct are often small. The archi-tecture is also dependent on the amount of fibrous tis-sue, mucin, calcification, and necrosis. An infiltrating tumor may show a diffusely abnormal liver echo pat-tern or focal irregularity of the ducts. However, in these two types, US may only reveal bile duct dilatation-a small mass or bile duct wall thickening may not be depicted. A polypoid tumor may be single or multiple with variable echoes, and a mucin-secreting tumor (intraductal papillary mucinous tumor) may present as a cystic mass and sometimes severe bile duct dilatation. With bile duct cancers, peripheral bile duct dilatation, necrosis, satellite nodules, calcification, lobar atrophy, pressure effects, and, in the case of Klatskin tumors, segmental dilatation and nonunion of the right and left ducts may also be seen. Lobar atrophy may be caused by vascular or biliary obstruction (18, 21).

Contrast-enhanced US has been introduced to characterize focal liver lesions and has shown hyper-perfusion in the arterial phase and punched-out defects in the late portal venous phase with ICC. It has also improved the detection and staging of malignant hilar obstruction (mostly caused by biliary malignancies) compared with unenhanced sonography (22, 23).

US- or CT-guided FNA may reveal the malignant nature of the tumor. However, FNA can be hazardous in the case of hilar tumors due to the adjacent big ves-sels. Differential diagnosis of bile duct cancer includes other malignant diseases (e.g., liver and lymph node metastases, hepatocellular carcinoma, pancreatic can-cer, or gallbladder carcinoma), bile duct stones, and benign tumors or strictures (e.g., primary sclerosing cholangitis). Extrinsic tumors may displace, encircle, obstruct, or invade the bile ducts visualized by differ-ent modalities.

To get detailed information, laparoscopic US or EUS may show the presence and origin of a small hilar or com-mon bile duct tumor. IDUS has also been valuable in bil-iary strictures, and it can show tumor extension. EUS-guided FNA is useful in bile duct tumors, too (16, 24).

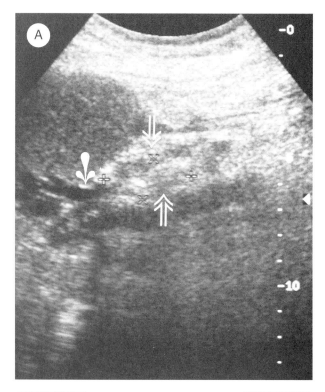

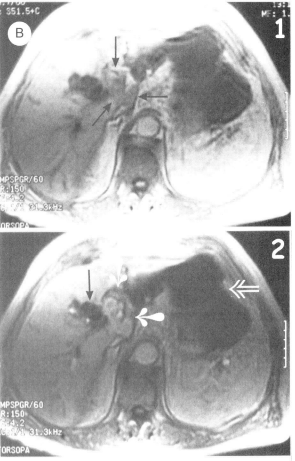

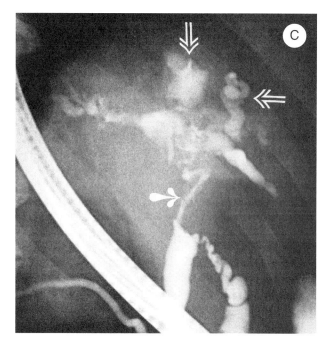

FIGURE 7.3

Figure 7.3 Klatskin tumor. (A) Intrahepatic biliary dilatation (white arrow) ends in the hilar area, where sonography shows an unclear heterogeneous mass (open arrows). (B) (1) MRI (T1 gradient echo) reveals slightly different tissue in the hilar area (arrows). (2) Gadolinium-enhanced MRI (T1 gradient echo) shows nonhomogeneously enhanced tissue in the hilar area (white arrows). Intrahepatic bile duct dilatation (black arrow) and a biloma (open arrow) are also shown. (C) ERC shows a long stricture of the common hepatic duct (arrow) and intrahepatic bile duct dilatation (open arrows). (From Ref. 2.)

In the case of an ampullary tumor, transabdominal US may only reveal the double-duct sign (dilatation of the bile duct and the pancreatic duct). Endoscopy with a biopsy, EUS, or IDUS may show the tumor itself, and EUS and IDUS are able to define the size and invasion of the tumor (25).

Staging of Biliary Cancers by US

US may help to reveal the spread of a suspected malignancy. Doppler can be used to analyze hepatic vessels. In gallbladder carcinoma or Klatskin tumors, US with Doppler can detect spread into the liver, the portal vein, and the bile ducts rather well, but it is not equally good in the detection of lymph node and especially peritoneal metastases. Advanced gallbladder carcinoma has been understaged by US. There are also controversial results about US in liver and lymph node invasion in gallbladder carcinoma. At any rate, other imaging modalities are also involved in the difficult analysis of pathologic, but normal-sized lymph nodes (8, 11, 21).

More invasive EUS, IDUS, or laparoscopic or intraoperative US has improved staging. EUS and IDUS are useful especially in evaluating the distal common bile duct and the regional lymph nodes, but they are not suitable for the detection of distant metastases (9).

COMPUTED TOMOGRAPHY

Further investigations after US are usually desirable in ambiguous cases or if there is any suspicion of a resectable biliary tumor after US. Recent technological developments have led to improvements in CT and MRI. As previously mentioned, we lack comparative reports of MDCT and modern MRI with MRC on the sensitivity of finding and staging biliary cancers, which makes it difficult to rank these two methods. The choice of modality also depends on local expertise, capacity, and facilities. Sometimes both modalities are needed.

With MDCT, the liver can be imaged in a single breathhold, which eliminates artifacts from respiratory motion and slice misregistration. Thin, high-resolution images and high-quality multiplanar reformations of even curved structures are produced. The arterial and portovenous phases can be separated, and vascular structures can be displayed. CT angiography (CTA) with high-resolution three-dimensional (3D) angiograms and virtual CT cholangioscopy are also possible. There are not yet many reports of the utility of CT cholangiography with cholangiographic contrast medium. In biliary tumors, the CT protocol should include biphasic CT acquisition with the arterial and portovenous phases in gallbladder tumors and triphasic acquisition with an additional delayed phase in tumors of the bile ducts (26). In spite of the marked improvement of image quality, modern MDCT continues to suffer from the increasingly high levels of radiation and possible allergy to the iodinated contrast medium.

Carcinoma of the Gallbladder

The sensitivity of CT in the detection of gallbladder carcinoma has been about 90%. Helical CT has been accurate in the diagnosis of T2 and more advanced lesions (Table 7.1). The findings of gallbladder carcinoma may include a heterogeneous mass replacing the gallbladder, wall thickening (Figure 7.2), or a fungate (polypoid) tumor. The mass may have variable enhancement, an ill-defined contour, and low-attenuation areas of necrosis or calcification. Wall thickening and a polypoid

tumor may enhance, and the adjacent gallbladder wall may be thickened with a polypoid change. There have been differences in the enhancement of the wall thickening between carcinoma and chronic cholecystitis. Protrusion of the quadrate lobe with lymphadenopathy has been reported to be unique to gallbladder carcinoma (10, 27, 28).

Carcinoma of the Bile Ducts

Bile duct carcinoma often shows abrupt termination of bile duct dilatation at CT, which can be a finding in advanced gallbladder carcinoma as well. The accuracy of CT to determine the level and cause of obstruction has been 97% and 94%, respectively. The sensitivity of CT to find bile duct carcinoma has been about 90% (29). However, CT may not readily detect a small mass or bile duct wall thickening.

A mass-type tumor (Figure 7.4) manifests as a low-attenuation mass, which may show peripheral enhancement during the arterial and portal venous phases. Delayed images with concentric retention of contrast are typical of highly fibrous content, and some tumors may only visualize on delayed images. This feature may help to differentiate them from hepatocellular carcinoma. Focal, eccentric wall thickening may have various enhancement patterns (Figure 7.5). A polypoid-type tumor can be a single or multiple intraductal lesion with increased enhancement on delayed scans. In the case of excessive amounts of mucin, accumulated mucin can cause significant ductal dilatation, direct continuity of a cystic tumor to the ducts, and increased attenuation of the ducts caused by tumor casts or by diffuse spreading of the tumor. CT may have an important role in the diagnosis of papillary tumors (17, 18, 30-33).

In the case of an ampullary tumor, CT may reveal both the double-duct sign and the tumor itself (Figure 7.6) (25). Bile duct carcinoma may also show calcification, biliary dilatation, nonunion of the right and left hepatic ducts, satellite lesions, lobar atrophy, and capsular retraction. Stents inserted to relieve jaundice may limit the usefulness of CT in diagnosis and staging.

Staging of Biliary Cancers by CT

CT has been quite sensitive in assessing liver, vascular, and bile duct invasion of gallbladder carcinoma (Figure 7.2) or bile duct tumor (Figure 7.4), but not carcinomatous spread into lymph nodes, some adjacent organs, omentum, and peritoneum (27, 29, 34). In practice, however, CT seems to be the best modality for assessing peritoneal spread. As mentioned earlier, helical CT has provided good accuracy in the diagnosis of

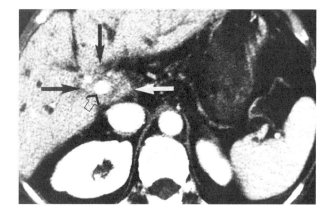

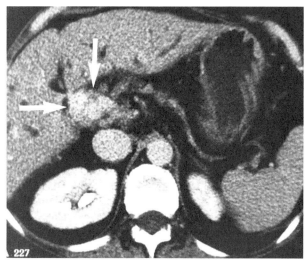

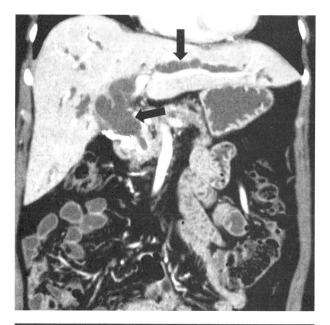

FIGURE 7.4

Bile duct carcinoma. (top) CT in the venous phase shows a heterogeneous mass (arrows) in the hilar area around the portal vein (open arrow). The common bile duct is not seen because of obliteration caused by the tumor. (bottom) In the delayed phase the mass shows enhancement (arrows). (From Ref. 2.)

the local extent of carcinomas of the gallbladder in T2 (Table 7.1) and more advanced lesions (28). Infiltrating gallbladder carcinoma may show irregular enhancement with regions of necrosis. The accuracy for local staging has been better for intraluminal mass types than for thickened wall type tumors. Dual-phase helical CT has been reported to be a useful tool in assessing the resectability of gallbladder cancers (35).

The accuracy of MDCT has been 77% in T staging of extrahepatic bile duct carcinoma, 63% in N staging, and 97% in M staging (Table 7.4) (36). In one report, 3D MDCT angiography and cholangiography with biliary contrast agent through a transhepatic drainage catheter showed the degree of vascular and biliary involvement of a Klatskin tumor. The diagnostic accuracy of portal vein and hepatic artery invasion was 94% and 89%, respectively (37).

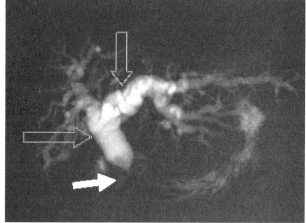

FIGURE 7.5

Carcinoma of the common bile duct. (top) Coronal view reconstruction of contrast-enhanced CT reveals enhancement of the thickened wall of a 2-cm stricture in the distal common bile duct (arrow) and marked intra- and extrahepatic bile duct dilatation (thick arrows). (bottom) MRCP (4-cm-thick slab) visualizes a stricture in the distal common bile duct (arrow) and marked intra- and extrahepatic bile duct dilatation (open arrows).

MAGNETIC RESONANCE IMAGING AND MAGNETIC RESONANCE CHOLANGIOGRAPHY

Fast-imaging techniques have made MRI more useful in biliary imaging. T1- and T2- weighted images of the liver can be obtained within a single breathhold. Using gadolinium chelate, it is possible to obtain images in the arterial, portal venous, and delayed phases. MRC is the least invasive mode of cholangiography, and it can

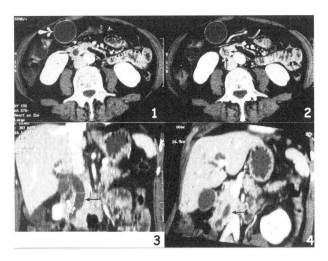

FIGURE 7.6

Carcinoma of the papilla of Vater. Enhanced CT reveals a dilated gallbladder (white arrow) and a common bile duct (black arrow) (1) with an enhancing small mass in the ampullary area (arrows) (2). The coronary reconstructions show similar findings: the mass (white arrow) and the dilated common bile duct (black arrow) (3, 4). (From Ref. 2.)

show a detailed map of the biliary tree. Many studies consider MRC to be equally diagnostic as direct cholangiography in biliary diseases (38). It is often a noninvasive alternative to endoscopic retrograde cholangiopancreatography (ERCP) or percutaneous transhepatic cholangiography (PTC), or when traditional cholangiography fails. MR imaging also has multiplanar capability, and it does not cause any radiation. However, there are certain contraindications to MRI as well, and interventions are usually not available.

Intrahepatic segmentary ducts are visible up to the first-order branches at MRC, and more peripheral ducts are seen in the case of dilatation. The accuracy of MRC to diagnose the presence and level of obstruction approaches 100%, and it can show the bile ducts

---

TABLE 7.4
T-Classification of Carcinoma of Extrahepatic Bile Ducts

T1	Tumor confined to the wall of the bile duct
T2	Tumor invades beyond the wall of the bile duct
T3	Tumor invades the liver, gallbladder, pancreas, and/or unilateral tributaries of the portal vein or hepatic artery
T4	Tumor invades any of the following: main portal vein or its tributaries bilaterally, common hepatic artery, or other adjacent structures, e.g., colon, stomach, duodenum, abdominal wall

Source: Ref. 3.

both above and below the obstruction as well as the severity of dilatation (Figure 7.1). Information on adjacent organs or extrinsic masses is also provided by MRC. However, the evaluation of obstruction in the case of bile duct carcinoma or advanced gallbladder carcinoma requires not only MRC, but also T1 and T2 images with gadolinium and magnetic angiography (MRA). Combined MRI/MRC has been superior to MRC or endoscopic retrograde cholangiography (ERC) alone in identifying malignant strictures in Klatskin tumors, and MRA is able to provide images that resemble standard angiography (26, 39, 40).

Carcinoma of the Gallbladder

There are only a few reports of MRI in the diagnosis of gallbladder carcinoma, but it has been considered a promising method. The tumor has been hypointense on T1 images (Figure 7.2) and hyperintense or heterogeneous on T2 images compared with the liver. With gadolinium, there may be early irregular enhancement, which persists throughout the dynamic study. Dynamic MRI has been used to differentiate different malignant gallbladder lesions from benign changes based on the enhancement pattern. The method has been promising (41-43).

Carcinoma of the Bile Ducts

At MRC, bile duct carcinoma may typically show an irregular, asymmetric biliary stricture or obstruction with a dilatation above it (Figures 7.5 and 7.7). The morphology and length of the stricture can be evaluated by MRC. The accuracy of magnetic resonance cholangiopancreatography (MRCP) to differentiate extrahepatic bile duct cancer from benign stricture has been comparable with that of ERCP. However, differential diagnosis of a stricture may be difficult with MRC alone, and the discovery of a tumor at MRI may help to suspect a malignancy. MRC/MRI may show a mass- or a polyp-type tumor, and advanced gallbladder malignancy may also be revealed (32, 44, 45). Single-shot thick-slab MRCP has been superior to multisection thin-slice MRCP in hilar carcinomas both in image quality and in ductal visualization. However, the latter facilitated the visualization of periductal lesions and adjacent structures. A combination of these techniques with MRI has been recommended in malignant hilar obstruction (46). However, in view of recent technical improvements, thin-slice MRCP with MIP is the best choice today. Biliary drainage can make bile duct assessment difficult, and MRC should hence be performed before biliary drainage.

ICC and hilar tumors have been hypo- or isointense on T1 images (Figure 7.3), while the former have

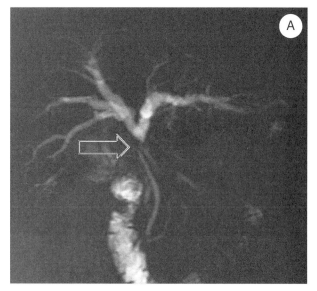

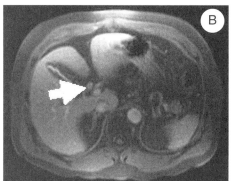

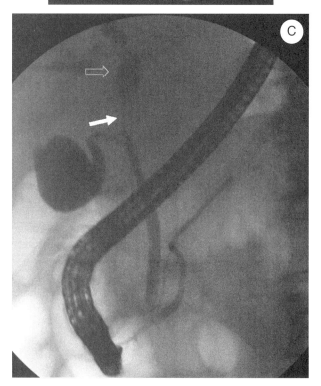

FIGURE 7.7

Klatskin tumor. (A) MRCP (2-cm-thick slab) shows intra-hepatic bile duct dilatation and a short, tight stricture in the common hepatic duct next to the bifurcation (arrow). (B) Gadolinium-enhanced MRI (T1 fat-saturated gradient echo) reveals enhancement of the wall thickening of the stricture (arrow). (C) ERC shows a short stricture in the common hepatic duct (arrow) and dilated intrahepatic bile ducts (open arrow).

been hyperintense and the latter variable on T2 images. ICC may also have a hypointense central scar. There may be peripheral enhancement by gadolinium and concentric enhancement in the delayed phase. A high mucin content can cause high signal intensity on T2 images. Dilated ducts (Figure 7.3), capsular retraction, satellite lesions, and lobar atrophy may also be seen, and segmental cholestasis may cause segmental hyper-intensity on T1 images (30, 31).

An extrahepatic mass is often hypointense in both T1 and T2 images, and the malignancy may show strong enhancement in the delayed phase. A papillary tumor is less enhanced. Ampullary carcinomas have had low signal intensity on T1 and T2 images and have enhanced less than the pancreas. MRCP may reveal the double-duct sign. MRI with MRC is also useful in the differential diagnosis of periampullary carcinomas (32, 45, 47).

Staging of Biliary Cancers by MRI

There is only scant information about the sensitivity of MRI/MRC in the staging of biliary cancers. MRI with MRC and MRA has revealed liver invasion and spread into the bile ducts, vessels, lymph nodes, peritoneum, or pancreas and liver metastases in bile duct cancers. In gallbladder carcinoma, it has been sensitive in at least the first three groups of spread (Figures 7.1 and 7.2), but its status in for instance lymph node spread is still unclear. The accuracy of MRI in the assessment of lymph node metastases in malignant hilar obstruction-mostly caused by hilar carcinomas-has been 66%. Dynamic MRI has been used to assess the depth of carcinoma invasion in gallbladder carcinoma. The signal intensity of the tumor in the liver is similar to that of the primary tumor. The T1 signal intensity contrast between the tumor and the surrounding tissues also facilitates the detection of tumor extension into surrounding structures. When MRA and digital sub-traction angiography have been compared for their ability to reveal arterial and venous invasion in bile duct carcinoma, similar diagnostic accuracies have been obtained (45, 46, 48-50).

CHOLANGIOGRAPHY

Traditionally, tumors causing biliary obstruction have been evaluated with cholangiography, ERC, or PTC. This technique provides a detailed view of the anatomy of the biliary tree and detects the level of obstruction in 100% of cases. It may provide the most accurate anatomic information because of its better spatial resolution compared to MRC. Brushings, biopsies, or bile cytology may also be simultaneously obtained to facilitate the final diagnosis. Cholangiography is performed for therapeutic purposes as well: a plastic or metallic stent may be inserted either endoscopically or percutaneously, or percutaneous biliary drainage can be accomplished (51). Traditional cholangiography is still one of the main alternatives for single examination after US, especially in the case of bile duct obstruction, but it may also be performed in combination with CT and/or MRI with MRC.

At cholangiography, bile duct carcinoma may appear as an irregular stricture of variable length, a diffuse sclerosing change, or polypoid filling defects, or it may obstruct the duct (Figures 7.3 and 7.7). Luminal narrowing is usually abrupt, irregular, or uneven. Cholangiography can be essential to evaluate the disease extent. Advanced gallbladder malignancy may show bile duct changes or cause external bile duct compression. In ampullary carcinoma, PTC may show stenosis, obstruction, or an irregular polypoid filling defect, and ERCP may reveal the double-duct sign and the tumor itself. In a very small ampullary tumor, ERCP with its dynamic capability may be more diagnostic than MRCP (25, 51, 52).

However, traditional cholangiography has its drawbacks. In cases of total obstruction, ERC does not show the cranial extent of the stricture, and PTC does not show the caudal extent. They are invasive procedures, not always possible, and carry the risk of complications. ERCP is associated with significant morbidity-pancreatitis, cholangitis, hemorrhage, perforation, sepsis-and a mortality of 0.2-1%. Cholangiography requires contrast medium and ionizing radiation, the technique is operator dependent, and it only provides information on the bile ducts.

OTHER MODALITIES

Angiography has had a major role in revealing encasement of the portal vein and hepatic artery by the malignancy. The recent improved versions of helical CT and MRI are increasingly replacing traditional angiography, unless there is a lack of capacity and facilities. Similar diagnostic accuracies were obtained when MRA was compared with digital subtraction angiography for arterial or venous tumor invasion in hilar cancers (53).

The FDG-PET (2-fluoro-2-deoxy-D-glucose-positron emission tomography) technique is based on the uptake of a radioactive-labeled glucose analogue by rapidly metabolizing tumors. The sensitivity of FDG-PET in revealing gallbladder or bile duct carcinoma has been quite high. However, its sensitivity in bile duct carcinoma has been dependent on the tumor subtype, being higher for the mass type than the infiltrating type. FDG-PET can reveal distant metastases, but there have been problems with carcinomatosis and regional lymph nodes. Unfortunately, it has only limited spatial resolution and is not widely available (26, 49).

PET-CT (positron emission tomography-computed tomography) combines functional and structural imaging. It may help to visualize non-FDG-accumulating tumors, carcinomatosis, or metastatic lymph nodes. It has been sensitively able to reveal gallbladder or bile duct carcinomas and distant metastases, but it has also been insensitive for regional lymph node metastases (54, 55).

Cholangioscopy with biopsies may reveal a small tumor or the longitudinal extent of a bile duct tumor. In the case of an ampullary tumor, endoscopy and biopsy may significantly contribute to the diagnosis. Sometimes even laparoscopy and biopsies are necessary to reveal the extent of the biliary malignancy, e.g., to detect occult lymph node and peritoneal metastases.

STRATEGIES OF IMAGING

A flow diagram of imaging strategies in a typical case of a suspected biliary malignancy is shown in Figure 7.8.

The prognosis of biliary cancers has been mainly dismal. However, recent advances in surgical techniques have led to a need for improved detection and staging of these cancers. There has also been rapid development of radiologic techniques, which has improved the diagnostic possibilities. Early diagnosis would be important in improving the prognosis, and careful staging would help in choosing the best possible treatment. All this still remains a challenge. There is no single modality capable of reliably detecting and especially staging biliary cancers. In spite of these major advances, each modality seems to have its restrictions, and there are variable capacities and practices. Detailed recommendations cannot be given, and continuing advances will still modify the practice.

Transabdominal US is often the first imaging modality applied to patients with jaundice or nonspecific gastrointestinal complaints. It is noninvasive, nonradiative, and commonly available, and it is a suitable method for assessing even mild symptoms. US visualizes

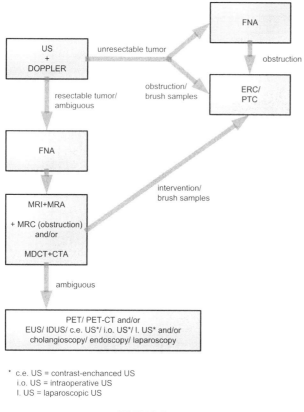

```
                              ┌──────────┐
                              │   FNA    │
                              └──────────┘
┌──────────┐   unresectable tumor            │ obstruction
│   US     │ ──────────────────┐              ▼
│    +     │                   ├──────►  ┌──────────┐
│ DOPPLER  │ ──┐   obstruction/           │  ERC/    │
└──────────┘   │   brush samples          │  PTC     │
      │        └──────────────────────►   └──────────┘
      │ resectable tumor/                       ▲
      │ ambiguous                               │
      ▼                                         │
┌──────────┐                                    │
│   FNA    │                                    │
└──────────┘            intervention/           │
      │                 brush samples           │
      ▼                                         │
┌──────────┐ ──────────────────────────────────┘
│ MRI+MRA  │
│+ MRC     │
│(obstruction)│
│  and/or  │
│ MDCT+CTA │
└──────────┘
      │ ambiguous
      ▼
┌─────────────────────────────────────┐
│   PET/ PET-CT and/or                 │
│ EUS/ IDUS/ c.e. US*/ i.o. US*/ l. US*│
│ and/or cholangioscopy/ endoscopy/    │
│ laparoscopy                          │
└─────────────────────────────────────┘
```

* c.e. US = contrast-enchanced US
  i.o. US = intraoperative US
  l. US = laparoscopic US

FIGURE 7.8

bile duct obstruction accurately, and it is able to reveal a gallbladder or bile duct tumor in about 90% of cases, but less well able to reveal especially small bile duct lesions. If a biliary malignancy is suspected, US-guided FNA is often able to confirm the final diagnosis. US with Doppler is helpful, but of limited value, in staging.

Further investigations are usually desirable in ambiguous cases or if US suggests a resectable tumor. Technological developments have led to improvements especially in MRI and CT. Both methods may yield additional information of the tumor and/or its extent. Fast-imaging techniques have made MRI potentially more valuable, and MRC is the least invasive mode of cholangiography, which is useful with MRI in the case of biliary obstruction. It is practical especially in patients who are unlikely to require any therapeutic intervention. The technique should include T1 and T2 sequences and gadolinium, often with MRC and MRA. There is ongoing discussion about the ranking of MRI and modern CT. The advantage of MRI is the absence of radiation.

Modern MDCT can produce multiplanar reconstructions of good quality, but the increased x-ray dose makes it problematic. MDCT with CT cholangiography has been as reliable as MRC in assessing the level

of obstruction and ductal extension of Klatskin tumors. The protocol should include biphasic or triphasic CT acquisition, and vascular structures can also be displayed. Simultaneously, CT of the thorax may reveal metastases of the lungs. Since we lack new large-scale comparative reports of MRI and MDCT and their respective sensitivities, it is difficult to rank these methods. The choice also depends on the contraindications, local expertise, facilities, relative cost, and capacity. In ambiguous cases, both methods may be needed.

Traditional cholangiography (PTC or ERCP) is still often necessary and may provide the most accurate anatomic information. It is also needed for therapeutic purposes in the case of bile duct obstruction. Brushings, biopsies, or bile cytology may be obtained simultaneously, unless imaging-guided FNA is available. However, cholangiography is invasive, includes radiation, and carries the risk of complications.

Further, EUS and IDUS might help in the diagnosis and staging of the tumor as well, but they are invasive and not widely available and do not reveal distant metastases. PET and especially PET-CT have been promising ways to reveal the tumor and distant metastases, and cholangioscopy may determine the longitudinal extent of a bile duct change. Sometimes even laparoscopy with biopsies or laparoscopic or intraoperative US, when available, may be needed.

Detection of preneoplastic lesions of the gallbladder and microscopic tumor extension is a big challenge for the future. Again, large-scale comparison studies of the sensitivities of MRI/MRC and MDCT in biliary cancers and their staging would be helpful. And the development of even better spatial resolution of MRC and intervention-compatible MRI scanners and instruments would also be welcome.

References

1. Ward EM, Fulcher AS, Pereles FS, Gore RM. Neoplasms of the gallbladder and biliary tract. In: Gore RM, Levine MS, eds. Textbook of Gastrointestinal Radiology. Philadelphia: W.B. Saunders Company; 2000:1360-1374.
2. Oikarinen H. Dignostic imaging of carcinomas of the gallbladder and the bile ducts. Acta Radiol 2006; 47:345-358.
3. Wittekind C, Greene FL, Hutter RVP, Klimpfinger M, Sobin LH, eds. Digestive system tumors. In: TNM Atlas. Heidelberg: Springer; 2005:73-154.
4. Choi H, Loyer EM, Charnsangavej C. Neoplasms of the liver and the bile ducts. Semin Roentgenol 2004; 39:412-427.
5. Chamberlain RS, Blumgart LH. Hilar cholangiocarcinoma: a review and commentary. Ann Surg Oncol 2000; 7:55-66.
6. Lee K-H, Lee DY, Kim KW. Biliary intervention for cholangiocarcinoma. Abdom Imaging 2004; 29:581-589.
7. Oikarinen H, Leinonen S, Karttunen A, Tikkakoski T, Hetemaa T, Mäkelä J, et al. Patency and complications of percutaneously inserted metallic stents in malignant biliary obstruction. J Vasc Interv Radiol 1999; 10:1387-1393.
8. Bach AM, Loring LA, Hann LE, Illescas FF, Fong Y, Blumgart LH. Gallbladder cancer: can ultrasonography evaluate extent

of disease? J Ultrasound Med 1998; 17:303-309.

9. Yarmenitis SD. Ultrasound of the gallbladder and the biliary tree. Eur Radiol 2002; 12:270-282.

10. Levy AD, Murkata LA, Rohrmann CA. Gallbladder carcinoma: radiologic-pathologic correlation. Radiographics 2001; 21:295-314.

11. Oikarinen H, Päivänsalo M, Lähde S, Tikkakoski T, Suramo I. Radiological findings in cases of gallbladder carcinoma. Eur J Radiol 1993; 17:179-183.

12. Rooholamini SA, Tehrani NS, Razavi MK, Au AH, Hansen GC, Ostrzega N, et al. Imaging of gallbladder carcinoma. Radiographics 1994; 14:291-306.

13. Chijiiwa K, Sumiyoshi K, Nakayama F. Impact of recent advances in hepatobiliary imaging techniques on the preoperative diagnosis of carcinoma of the gallbladder. World J Surg 1991; 15:322-327.

14. Gore RM, Yaghmai V, Newmark GM, Berlin JW, Miller FH. Imaging benign and malignant disease of the gallbladder. Radiol Clin North Am 2002; 40:1307-1323.

15. Matsumoto J. Endoscopic ultrasonography diagnosis of gallbladder lesions. Endoscopy 1998; 30(suppl 1):A124-127.

16. Meara RS, Jhala D, Eloubeidi MA, Eltoum I, Chhieng DC, Crowe DR, et al. Endoscopic ultrasound-guided FNA biosy of bile duct and gallbladder: analysis of 53 cases. Cytopathology 2006; 17:42-49.

17. Baron LR, Tublin ME, Peterson MS. Imaging the spectrum of biliary tract disease. Radiol Clin North Am 2002; 40:1325-1354.

18. Lim JH. Cholangiocarcinoma: morphologic classification according to growth pattern and imaging findings. Am J Roentgenol 2003; 181:819-827.

19. Mittelstaedt CA. Ultrasound of the bile ducts. Semin Roentgenol 1997; 32:161-171.

20. Päivänsalo M, Oikarinen H, Tikkakoski T, Puumala K, Suramo I. Radiological findings in bile duct carcinoma. Fortschr Röntgenstr 1993; 159:4-9.

21. Hann LE, Greatrex KV, Bach AM, Fong Y, Blumgart LH. Cholangiocarcinoma at the hepatic hilus: sonographic findings. Am J Roentgenol 1997; 168:985-989.

22. Dietrich CF. Characterisation of focal liver lesions with contrast enhanced ultrasonography. Eur J Radiol 2004; 51S: S9-17.

23. Khalili K, Metser U, Wilson SR. Hilar biliary obstruction: preliminary results with Levovist-enhanced sonography. Am J Roentgenol 2003; 180:687-693.

24. Inui K, Miyoshi H. Cholangiocarcinoma and intraductal sonography. Gastrointest Endosc Clin North Am 2005; 15:143-155.

25. Buck JL, Elsayed AM. From the archives of the AFIP. Ampullary tumors: radiologic-pathologic correlation. Radiographics 1993; 13:193-212.

26. Zech CJ, Schoenberg SO, Reiser M, Helmberger T. Cross-sectional imaging of biliary tumors: current clinical status and future developments. Eur Radiol 2004; 14:1174-1187.

27. Ohtani T, Shirai Y, Tsukada K, Muto T, Hatakeyama K. Spread of gallbladder carcinoma: CT evaluation with pathologic correlation. Abdom Imaging 1996; 21:195-201.

28. Yoshimitsu K, Honda H, Shinozaki K, Aibe H, Kuroiwa T, Irie H, et al. Helical CT of the local spread of carcinoma of the gallbladder: evaluation according to the TNM system in patients who underwent surgical resection. Am J Roentgenol 2002; 179:423-428.

29. Feydy A, Vilgrain V, Denys A, Sibert A, Belghiti J, Vullierme M-P, et al. Helical CT assessment in hilar cholangiocarcinoma: correlation with surgical and pathologic findings. Am J Roentgenol 1999; 172:73-77.

30. Choi BI, Lee JM, Han JK. Imaging of intrahepatic and hilar cholangiocarcinoma. Abdom Imaging 2004; 29:548-557.

31. Han JK, Lee JM. Intrahepatic intraductal cholangiocarcinoma. Abdom Imaging 2004; 29:558-564.

32. Lim JH, Lee WJ, Takehara Y, Lim HK. Imaging of extrahepatic cholangiocarcinoma. Abdom Imaging 2004; 29:565-571.

33. Tillich M, Mischinger H-J, Preisegger K-H, Rabl H, Szolar DH. Multiphasic helical CT in diagnosis and staging of hilar cholangiocarcinoma. Am J Roentgenol 1998; 171:651-658.

34. Kalra N, Suri S, Gupta R, Natarajan SK, Khandelwal N, Wig JD, et al. MDCT in the staging of gallbladder carcinoma. Am J Roentgenol 2006; 186:758-762.

35. Kumaran V, Gulati S, Paul B, Pande K, Sahni P, Chattopadhyay K. The role of dual-phase helical CT in assessing resectability of carcinoma of the gallbladder. Eur Radiol 2002; 12:1993-1999.

36. Park M-S, Lee DK, Kim M-J, Lee WJ, Yoon D-S, Lee SJ, et al. Preoperative staging accuracy of multidetector row computed tomography for extrahepatic bile duct carcinoma. J Comp Ass Tomogr 2006; 30:362-367.

37. Chen HW, Pan AZ, Zhen ZJ, Su SY, Wang JH, Yu SCH, et al. Preoperative evaluation of resectability of Klatskin tumor with 16-MDCT angiography and cholangiography. Am J Roentgenol 2006; 186:1580-1586.

38. Varghese JC, Farrell MA, Courtney G, Osborne H, Murray FE, Lee MJ. A prospective comparison of magnetic resonance cholangiopancreatography with endoscopic retrograde cholangiopancreatography in the evaluation of patients with suspected biliary tract disease. Clin Radiol 1999; 54:513-520.

39. Holzknecht N, Gauger J, Sackmann M, Thoeni RF, Schurig J, Holl J, et al. Breath-hold MR cholangiography with snapshot techniques: prospective comparison with endoscopic retrograde cholangiography. Radiology 1998; 206:657-664.

40. Vogl TJ, Schwarz WO, Heller M, Herzog C, Zangos S, Hintze RE, et al. Staging of Klatskin tumours (hilar cholangiocarcinomas): comparison of MR cholangiography, MR imaging, and endoscopic retrograde cholangiography. Eur Radiol 2006; 16:2317-2325.

41. Sagoh T, Itoh K, Togashi K, Shibata T, Minami S, Noma S, et al. Gallbladder carcinoma: evaluation with MR imaging. Radiology 1990; 174:131-136.

42. Tseng JH, Wan YL, Hung CF, Ng KK, Pan KT, Chou AS, et al. Diagnosis and staging of gallbladder carcinoma. Evaluation with dynamic MR imaging. Clin Imaging 2002; 26:177-182.

43. Yoshimitsu K, Honda H, Kaneko K, Kuroiwa T, Irie H, Ueki T, et al. Dynamic MRI of the gallbladder lesions: differentiation of benign from malignant. J Magn Reson Im 1997; 7:696-701.

44. Park M-S, Kim TK, Kim KW, Park SW, Lee JK, Kim J-S, et al. Differentiation of extrahepatic bile duct cholangiocarcinoma from benign stricture: findings at MRCP versus ERCP. Radiology 2004; 233:234-240.

45. Takehara Y. Preoperative assessment of extrahepatic cholangiocarcinoma with imaging. Abdom Imaging 2004; 29:572-580.

46. Hänninen EL, Pech M, Jonas S, Ricke J, Thelen A, Langrehr J, et al. Magnetic resonance imaging including magnetic resonance cholangiopancreatography for tumor localization and therapy planning in malignant hilar obstructions. Acta Radiol 2005; 46:462-470.

47. Semelka RC, Kelekis NL, John G, Ascher SM, Burdeny D, Siegelman ES. Ampullary carcinoma: demonstration by current MR techniques. J Magn Reson Im 1997; 7:153-156.

48. Kaza RK, Gulati M, Wig JD, Chawla YK. Evaluation of gallbladder carcinoma with dynamic magnetic resonance imaging and magnetic resonance cholangiopancreatography. Australasian Radiol 2006; 50:212-217.

49. Rodriguez-Fernandez A, Gomez-Rio M, Medina-Benitez A, Villar-Del Moral J, Ramos-Font C, Ramia-Angel JM, et al. Application of modern imaging methods in diagnosis of gallbladder cancer. J Surg Oncol 2006; 93:650-664.

50. Schwartz LH, Black J, Fong Y, Jarnagin W, Blumgart L, Gruen D, et al. Gallbladder carcinoma: findings at MR imaging with MR cholangiopancreatography. J Comp Ass Tomogr 2002; 26:405-410.

51. Brugge WR. Endoscopic techniques to diagnose and manage biliary tumors. J Clin Oncol 2005; 23:4561-4565.

52. Geier A, Nguyen HN, Gartung C, Matern S. MRCP and ERCP to detect small ampullary carcinoma. Lancet 2000; 356:1607-1608.

53. Misra S, Chaturvedi A, Misra NC, Sharma ID. Carcinoma of the gallbladder. The Lancet Oncology 2003; 4:167-176.

54. Petrowsky H, Wildbrett P, Husarik DB, Hany TF, Tam S, Jochum W, et al. Impact of integrated positron emission tomography and computed tomography on staging and management of gallbladder cancer and cholangiocarcinoma. J Hepatol 2006; 45:43-50.

55. Rosenbaum SJ, Stergar H, Antoch G, Veit P, Bockisch A, Kuhl H. Staging and follow-up of gastrointestinal tumors with PET/CT. Abdom Imaging 2006; 31:25-35.

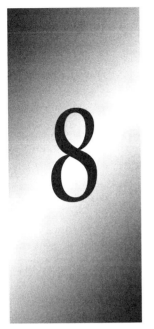

8 Imaging of Hepatic Transplantation for Biliary Tract Cancer

Sridhar Shankar
Sathish Kumar Dundmadappa
Shimul Shah

Cholangiocarcinoma (CCA) accounts for 2% of all malignancies in the United States, and 40-60% are considered hilar, arising at the hepatic duct bifurcation (1). Complete operative resection may be curative, but local extension of disease often precludes complete resection. Less than 20% of patients with hilar cholangiocarcinoma are amenable to a potentially curative resection (2). Even with complete resection, local recurrence is common with most series reporting 5-year survival of 25-35% (3).

The major factors that preclude curative resection are:

1. Hilar tumor extending to both lobes of the liver remains unresectable despite the fact that they may not have other extrahepatic disease.
2. Patients with primary sclerosing cholangitis (PSC) tolerate resection poorly because of the underlying liver impairment.
3. Invasion of the main portal vein (PV) or common hepatic artery, tumor extension into lobe with invasion of the contralateral branch of the PV, and/or hepatic artery render the tumor unresectable.
4. Dissection in the hepatic hilum has the potential to cause tumor spillage

Liver transplantation (LT) may yield a solution for the clinical scenarios outlined above. LT has several benefits over conventional resection for hilar cholangiocarcinoma. It is not limited by the traditional criteria of unresectability. Without the need to dissect the porta hepatis in the region of tumor, there is decreased possibility of tumor spillage and a higher chance of achieving a clear margin (longitudinal and circumferential). In addition, patients with hilar cholangiocarcinoma with underlying PSC tolerate resection poorly, and LT is an attractive option as it aims at the treatment of the tumor as well as the underlying liver disease (4).

Several reports historically have shown poor outcomes after liver transplantation for CCA, with poorer outcomes following liver transplantation when compared to other diagnoses (5). Unfavorable mortality in these earlier reports was due to a high risk for recurrence. The stage of disease in these cases was often advanced. Two centers have subsequently demonstrated that with selection of patients with only earlier stage disease and the addition of neoadjuvant therapy, the survival after liver transplantation for CCA approaches the outcomes for other diseases (6, 7). Both centers utilized a new paradigm for CCA involving a formal staging procedure carried out after completion of neoadjuvant therapy before proceeding to transplantation to ensure the disease is confined to the liver and does not involve perihilar lymph nodes.

Traditionally, neoadjuvant chemoradiation for hilar CCA has been limited by its toxicity, particularly to the liver (see Chapters 18 and 21). Major liver resections may be challenging after such treatment, as the remnant radiated liver is likely to be functionally suboptimal. LT following neoadjuvant chemoradiation is not limited by hepatotoxicity as the diseased and radiated liver is replaced by a new liver (4).

The most important disadvantage of the LT protocol for hilar CCA is the limited availability of cadaveric donor organs. The remarkable progress of living donor liver transplant (LDLT) in recent years has made the long waiting lists for transplantation redundant in centers actively engaged in LDLT. Liver transplantation without neoadjuvant therapy should probably be avoided in patients with hilar CCA, with long-term patient survival in the range of 28% at 5 years and a prohibitively high recurrence rate.

Patients with CCA experience a set of complications attributable to neoadjuvant therapy, including higher rates of hepatic arterial thrombosis and PV stenosis. Hepatic artery thrombosis is avoided (in deceased donor recipients) by use of donor iliac artery grafts between the donor hepatic artery and the recipient infrarenal aorta. PV stenosis is amenable to percutaneous transhepatic angioplasty and stent placement (3).

ROLE OF IMAGING

Multiphasic computed tomography (CT) and magnetic resonance imaging (MRI) are the cornerstones of imaging, both pre- and postoperatively, with ultrasound (US) being utilized intraoperatively and in the immediate postoperative period.

EVALUATION IN TRANSPLANT RECIPIENTS

Liver Parenchyma and the Malignancy

Evaluation of the local extent of tumor is critical because the CCA must be above the cystic duct and be unresectable as assessed by an experienced hepatobiliary surgeon. Patients with intrahepatic metastasis, uncontrolled infection, prior attempts at resection, prior irradiation or chemotherapy for this disease, or evidence of extrahepatic disease including lymph node metastasis would be excluded.

The caudate lobe can become enlarged and surround the inferior vena cava (IVC). Exposure of the IVC and removal of the liver from the retrohepatic portion of the IVC can be a technical challenge in such cases. This situation becomes relevant in cases of living donor transplantation in which the cava is preserved.

Splenoportal Venous Axis

Diffuse thrombosis of the PV and superior mesenteric vein remains a contraindication to liver transplantation. However, if there is focal or a lesser degree of involvement, a variety of surgical techniques are available. If acute portal thrombus is present, manual thrombectomy is performed at surgery (8). If chronic PV thrombosis is present or the PV diameter is less than 4 mm, the donor PV is anastomosed to the splenomesenteric confluence, the superior mesenteric vein, or a splenic varix (9).

If the graft PV is not long enough to reach the confluence, an iliac vein graft is obtained from the donor (9).

Inflammatory stranding of the perivenous fat may be seen with phlebitis. Higher recipient morbidity due to uncontrolled bleeding has been seen in patients with phlebitis that is present with thrombosis (9).

Varices

Perihepatic and pericaval varices can cause increased bleeding when the native liver is excised. Varices in other parts of the abdomen do not affect the surgical procedure and decrease in size spontaneously after transplantation (9).

Celiac Artery Stenosis

Celiac artery stenosis occurs with atherosclerotic disease and from compression by the median arcuate ligament. Recipients with celiac artery stenosis are at risk for compromised blood flow to the transplanted organ (10). The stenosis is therefore corrected at surgery.

Splenic Artery Aneurysm

Splenic artery aneurysms result from increased flow in the splenic artery in patients with cirrhosis and portal hypertension (11). Consideration can be given to ligation of the aneurysms, since they may rupture after transplantation due to increased flow.

EVALUATION OF LIVING TRANSPLANT DONORS

Hepatic Arterial Anatomy to the Graft Lobe

Adequate hepatic arterial flow is necessary for successful graft function and the avoidance of necrosis of biliary structures. Since extrahepatic collateral routes that are present in the native liver are no longer available once it is removed from the donor, all vessels supplying the liver need to be identified prior to its removal (12).

Even when normal arterial anatomy is found, a hepatic artery with sufficient length for reconstruction is sometimes difficult to obtain because only a part of the liver is harvested. Thus, it is important to recognize the proper hepatic artery bifurcation and to measure the length of the RHA (in cases of right lobe donation) or LHA (in cases of LLS donation) before the next bifurcation (13). Even so, findings such as filiform or redundant arteries may impede arterial reconstruction (14).

Some variants are suitable for the transplantation surgeon, whereas others are not. Up to one third of potential donors may be ineligible for transplantation because of unsuitable hepatic arterial anatomy (10).

The right hepatic artery is replaced and arises from the superior mesenteric artery in 11% of the general population. The left hepatic artery is replaced and arises from the left gastric artery in 10%. Accessory right or left hepatic arteries are present in approximately 8% of subjects (9). The presence of accessory vessels to a lobe requires at least two arterial anastomoses, and small-caliber arteries are more likely to be present in donors with multiple vessels that supply a single lobe (15). In some cases, the presence of multiple small vessels precludes donation. Atherosclerotic disease in the celiac artery of a donor precludes donation (9).

Venous and Biliary Anatomy

Accessory right hepatic veins are estimated to occur in 6% of people (16). An accessory hepatic vein can cause increased bleeding if not recognized before surgery and may be necessary for venous drainage of the transplanted right lobe. If there are multiple veins, venoplasty is performed or each vein is anastomosed separately to the IVC.

The main PV may also "trifurcate," with an early branching pattern in the right lobe. If there are two branches to the right lobe, two anastomoses are required when the lobe is transplanted into an adult recipient (9).

Evaluation of the biliary tree is routinely performed in potential donors by magnetic resonance cholangiopancreatography (MRCP) or endoscopic retrograde cholangiopancreatography (ERCP) as variations in anatomy are very common. It permits preoperative detection of abnormalities and anatomic variants of the biliary tract that may complicate resection of the right hepatic lobe. Although such variant anatomy may be delineated at intraoperative cholan-

giography, the preoperative detection of such may allow the surgical team the opportunity to plan their approach accordingly.

Liver Volumes

CT or MRI is used for volumetric assessment. A minimum of 40% of the normal liver volume is needed by the recipient (17). The donor volume is also used to ensure that a minimum of 35% of the liver is left in the donor (17). If the donor liver is too large, closure of the abdomen can be difficult and respiratory status may be compromised (18).

Liver Parenchyma

It is necessary to evaluate the donor liver for any undiagnosed diffuse or focal diseases. Even a common condition like moderate to severe fatty change in a potential donor generally precludes donation due to lowering of the corrected graft mass (9).

POSTOPERATIVE EVALUATION OF DONOR AND RECIPIENT

Normal Appearance After Transplantation

OLT requires grafting of one arterial anastomosis (hepatic artery), at least two venous anastomoses (PV and IVC), and a biliary anastomosis. *It is extremely important to know which surgical technique was used in each patient before planning the helical CT examination so that all of the anastomoses will be included in the study.*

The hepatic artery is typically reconstructed with a "fish-mouth" anastomosis between the donor and recipient arterial anastomotic sites.

The PV anastomosis is typically an end-to-end type between the two portal veins. Arterialization of the PV (i.e., creation of anastomoses between both the PV and hepatic artery of the donor and arterial vessels of the recipient) is occasionally used as a last resort when a portal-visceral (splenic vein, superior or inferior mesenteric vein) venous anastomosis cannot be performed because of extensive venous thrombosis.

During hepatectomy, the retrohepatic IVC of the recipient is usually resected and the IVCs of the recipient and donor are sutured twice, with end-to-end anastomoses. New techniques have recently appeared, with preservation of the recipient retrohepatic IVC and creation of anastomoses between the donor and recipient IVCs in an end-to-side or side-to-side configuration or an end-to-end anastomosis between the donor IVC and a common stump of the three hepatic veins (the piggyback technique) (19).

The biliary anastomosis is made between the donor common bile duct and the recipient common hepatic duct, usually after a cholecystectomy.

There can be small right pleural effusion and a small amount of free intraabdominal fluid or hematomas in the perihepatic region, especially in the hepatic hilum, adjacent to the IVC anastomoses, or in the fissure for the ligamentum teres (20, 21). These usually resolve within a few weeks, although infiltration of the hepatic hilum fat can sometimes persist for months.

A periportal area of low attenuation is often seen. This finding is attributed to dilatation of lymphatic channels due to lack of normal lymphatic drainage into the extrahepatic lymphatic system (20-22). The periportal halo resolves within weeks following transplantation (possibly due to development of alternative pathways), although it can persist for months (19). This periportal edema was once considered a sign of graft rejection, but later studies have ruled out this relationship (19).

Regeneration of Liver

The liver has a remarkable capacity for regeneration after major resection (23, 24), particularly normal livers. A report of 37 donors who underwent MR imaging after left lateral segmentectomy or left lobectomy shows that the volume of the remnant liver is restored to some extent within 4 weeks (24).

Complications and Postoperative Observations

The major complications in donors include abscess, bile leakage, and liver dysfunction because of ligation of a major bile duct branch, hepatic artery injury, and duodenal ulcer.

The major complications in recipients include vascular problems such as hepatic artery thrombosis, stenosis of the PV anastomosis, outflow obstruction of the hepatic vein anastomosis, PV thrombosis, biliary issues such as anastomotic stenosis, bile leakage, biloma, and abscess formation. Although acute rejection is one of the most serious complications affecting graft survival, it cannot always be reliably detected with available diagnostic tests or radiologic methods.

Ultrasonography is the initial imaging technique used for the detection of complications in the early post transplantation phase, since it can be performed at the bedside and is capable of demonstrating the hepatic parenchyma and bile ducts. Doppler ultrasound (US) allows detection of vascular abnormalities, but it is associated with a significant frequency of false-negative results (25, 26). In cases where US results are incon-

clusive, confirmation is required, or clinical suspicion of a complication persists despite normal US results, helical CT) should be performed (19).

VASCULAR COMPLICATIONS

Vascular compromise is a frequent cause of graft loss, estimated to occur in 9% of patients (27). Most transplantation centers perform routine postoperative Doppler US as the initial imaging study to evaluate the integrity of the graft vasculature.

The most important vascular complication, with a potential to cause graft failure, is thrombosis of the hepatic artery or PV. Vascular complications related to the IVC are much less frequent.

Hepatic Artery Thrombosis

Hepatic artery thrombosis is the most common vascular complication of OLT, with a prevalence of 4-12% in adult recipients and up to 40% in children. It has a mortality rate of 50-58% (28, 29). Unless thrombectomy can be promptly performed, most cases require retransplantation; even after retransplantation, the mortality rate is 27-30% (27, 30).

Risk factors for hepatic artery thrombosis include (a) significant differences in caliber between the donor and recipient hepatic arterial vessels or preexisting lesions such as celiac artery stenosis, (b) prolonged cold ischemia time of the donor liver, (c) ABO blood type incompatibility, and (d) rejection (19). Even in complete arterial thrombosis, small intrahepatic arterial vessels can sometimes be identified because of extensive collateralization to the liver. This situation can lead to false-negative results at Doppler US, although in most cases a tardus-parvus arterial waveform suggests the correct diagnosis (19). Hepatic artery thrombosis is often associated with bilomas, infarcts, abscesses, or bile duct dilatation (Figure 8.1).

Hepatic Artery Stenosis

The second most common vascular complication of orthotopic liver transplant (OLT), reported in about 5% of cases, is hepatic artery stenosis; which generally occurs at the anastomotic site within 3 months of OLT (19). If left untreated, it can eventually lead to hepatic artery thrombosis due to slow flow (31).

Risk factors are similar to those for hepatic artery thrombosis and include (but are not limited to) surgical issues, such as faulty technique, clamp injury, and/or intimal trauma caused by perfusion catheters (32, 33). Early identification and prompt reestablishment of ade-

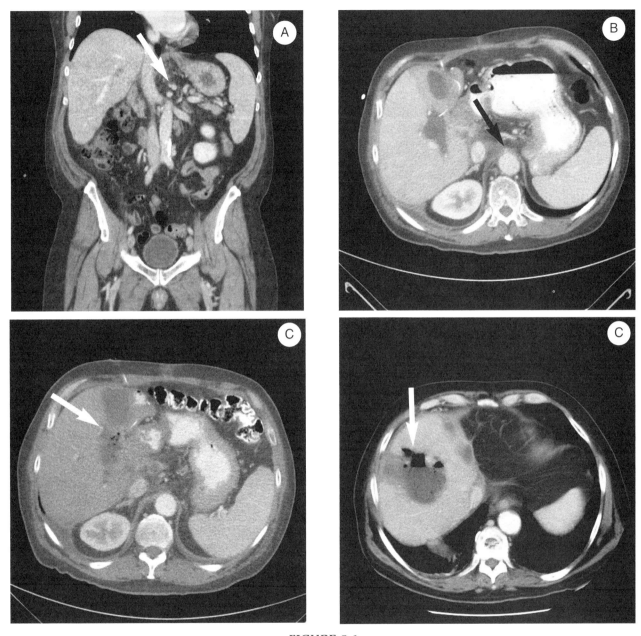

FIGURE 8.1

(A) Coronal reconstruction of contrast enhanced CT scan in a 55-year old post transplant patient (living donor) demonstrating thrombus in the native common hepatic artery (arrow) which developed as a consequence of dissection during the transplant. (B) Contrast CT in the same patient demonstrating thrombosis of the jump graft performed during transplant arising higher up from the aorta. The thrombosis was discovered a few weeks after transplant. (C) Contrast enhanced CT scans in the same patient at two levels demonstrating the air and bile containing collection (arrows) in the center of the liver, arising as a consequence of biliary necrosis secondary to hepatic artery thrombosis. Percutaneous CT guided drainage was performed.

quate blood flow (revascularization surgical procedures or arteriography and balloon angioplasty) usually resolve the stenosis resulting in long-term graft and patient survival (31), thus avoiding the need for retransplantation.

Hepatic Artery Pseudoaneurysm

This is an uncommon complication. Extrahepatic pseudoaneurysms usually develop at the vascular anastomosis or arise as a complication of angioplasty (19).

They can rupture intraperitoneally and lead to massive hemorrhage. Treatment for extrahepatic pseudoaneurysms includes surgical resection, embolization, or exclusion with stent placement. Intrahepatic pseudoaneurysms, which can occur after percutaneous needle biopsy or local infection (33), are often detected incidentally. A ruptured intrahepatic pseudoaneurysm may result in PV or biliary fistulas (34). Intrahepatic pseudoaneurysms can be treated with endovascular coil embolization.

Portal Vein Thrombosis or Stenosis

PV complications following OLT are relatively unusual, occurring in 1-3% of cases, and result from faulty surgical technique, vessel misalignment, differences in caliber of anastomosed vessels provoking turbulent flow, hypercoagulable states, previous PV surgery, or previous thrombosis in the recipient PV system (19). Helical CT can provide excellent visualization of filling defects within the PV or focal narrowing (usually at the anastomosis). However, such narrowing can occur naturally in patients in whom the discrepancy between donor and recipient PV sizes is significant. Percutaneous transhepatic direct portography allows measurement of the pressure gradient across the stenosis, with values higher than 5 mmHg being significant (32). Treatment includes percutaneous transluminal angioplasty with or without stent placement, surgical thrombectomy, placement of a venous jump graft, creation of a portosystemic shunt, or even retransplantation (19).

IVC Stenosis or Thrombosis

The prevalence of IVC complications is less than 1%. Stenosis of the IVC can occur at the anastomosis. IVC thrombosis can be caused by surgical problems and hypercoagulable states. Swelling of the graft can result in compression of the IVC, and sometimes a size discrepancy between the donor and recipient IVCs is misdiagnosed as stenosis (34). The functional significance is unclear until the pressure gradient across the stenosis is measured and found to be significant (32). Successful balloon angioplasty and stent placement has been reported in IVC stenosis (33).

Arterioportal Fistula

Intrahepatic arterio-portal fistula is a relatively frequent complication following surgical or percutaneous liver biopsy performed to rule out graft rejection. The helical CT findings of arterio-portal fistula include (a) early enhancement of peripheral PV branches during the

hepatic arterial phase and before the main PV is enhanced; (b) enhancement of peripheral PV branches and the main PV with nonenhanced superior mesenteric and splenic veins, signs that have been considered diagnostic on hepatic angiograms; and (c) transient, peripheral, wedge-shaped, usually straight-margined hepatic parenchymal enhancement during the hepatic arterial phase (35).

BILIARY COMPLICATIONS

Biliary complications following OLT occur in 6-34% of cases, most of them within 3 months of transplantation. They are the second most common cause of liver dysfunction in OLT patients, exceeded only by rejection (35). Biliary complications include leak, stricture, obstruction, and stone formation.

Bile leak is most often located at the T-tube site and rarely occurs at the anastomosis. A small bile leak may close spontaneously, or a stent can be placed across the site of leakage, but surgical revision of the anastomosis is often necessary. Formation of a bile collection can be treated with percutaneous drainage.

Most biliary strictures occur at the anastomotic site and may be secondary to scar formation that results in retraction and narrowing. Percutaneous dilation can be performed, although repeat surgery is occasionally required. Nonanastomotic strictures are probably caused by ischemia due to hepatic artery stenosis or thrombosis or preservation injury. Intrahepatic biliary strictures can also be due to recurrent sclerosing cholangitis. If a biliary stricture is suspected and CT shows no dilatation, endoscopic retrograde or percutaneous transhepatic cholangiography should be performed, since many liver transplants do not develop bile duct dilatation even in high-grade stenosis. (Figure 8.2)

Less common complications include sphincter of Oddi dysfunction and biliary obstruction due to kinking in a redundant common bile duct or to stones or sludge caused by alterations in bile composition. Mucocele of the cystic duct remnant is a rare complication resulting from ligation of the cystic duct both proximally and distally. It is seen as a round fluid collection that can compress the common bile duct, producing obstruction.

LIVER ISCHEMIA OR INFARCTION

Most cases of liver ischemia or infarction are due to vascular problems involving the hepatic artery (85% of cases) or, less frequently, the PV. These are seen at CT as wedge-shaped, low-attenuation peripheral lesions

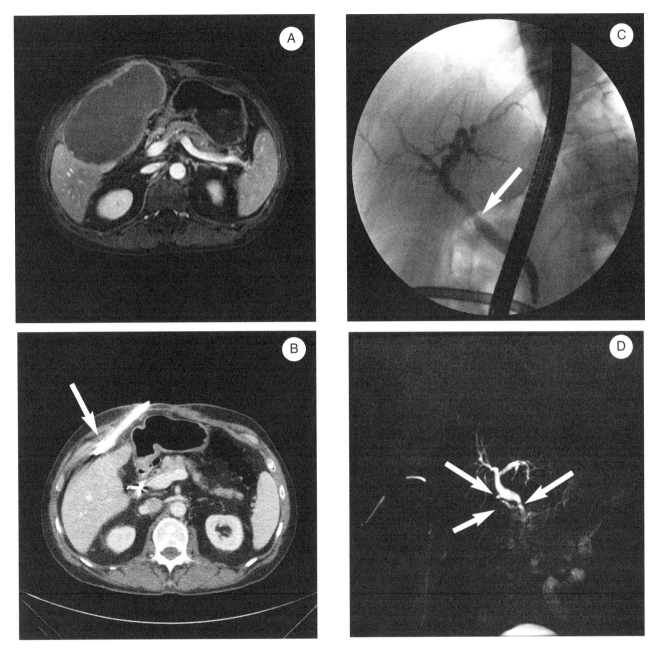

FIGURE 8.2

(A) Contrast enhanced T1 weighted axial LAVA image demonstrates a large fluid collection anterior and inferior to the transplanted liver in a 51-year-old man. The collection was suspected to be a bilomas and percutaneous drainage was performed. Chemical analysis showed the fluid to be biliary in origin.

(B) The percutaneous drainage catheter (arrow) was exchanged several times over a period of 10 weeks, until complete drainage was achieved. In the meanwhile, ERCP (Figure 8.2C) showed a mild anastomotic stricture that was stented (dashed arrow). Subsequently, the percutaneous drain was removed, and the collection did not recur. An actual bile leak was never demonstrated.

(C) ERCP demonstrating mild anastomotic narrowing (arrow) in this 51-year-old post transplant patient. No bile leak was demonstrated. A stent was placed.

(D) MRCP image demonstrating mild biliary stricture in a 53-year-old woman. There is mild dilation above the stricture (arrow). Incidental note is made of two cystic ducts (one each from the donor and recipient) (dashed arrows).

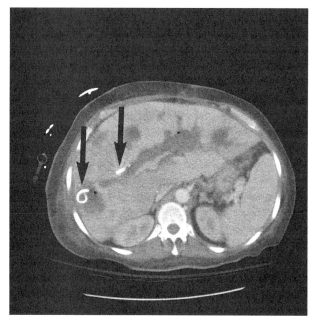

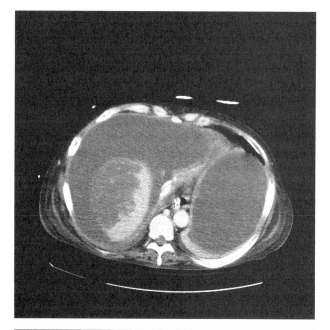

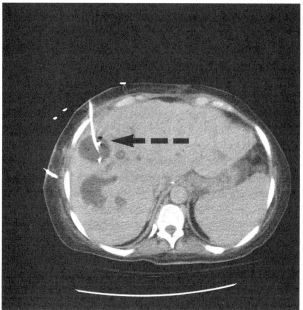

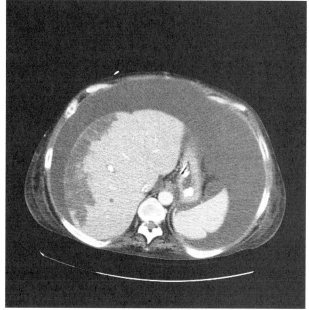

FIGURE 8.3

Contrast enhanced CT scan in a 52-year-old woman with biliary necrosis following liver transplant and hepatic arterial thrombosis. There is a biliary stent in place (solid arrow). Additionally, there are percutaneous drainage catheters in place (dashed arrows) draining the necrosed, infected pools of bile. Despite heroic measures, including a partial resection of the transplant liver, the patient eventually succumbed to sepsis.

(Figure 8.3). Extensive parenchymal and bile duct necrosis can lead to graft failure and require retransplantation (Figure 8.4).

FIGURE 8.4

Contrast enhanced CT scan images in a 55-year-old post transplant woman demonstrating extensive areas of necrosis in segment VII and VIII primarily. The necrosis was thought to be secondary to intraoperative hypotension, and was managed conservatively. However, the necrosed portion of the liver became infected, and had to be resected. Unfortunately, the patient died after prolonged hospitalization.

MALIGNANCY

These patients are at increased risk for developing malignancy, especially non-Hodgkin lymphoma and squamous cell skin cancer, because of the immunosuppressive therapy administered to avoid graft rejection (19). The primary tumor can recur in the graft or at any other location. The transplant recipients can also develop any type of neoplasm, as in the general population.

The diagnosis of acute rejection, one of the most serious complications of OLT, is established with graft biopsy and histologic study. The role of imaging methods consists of excluding the other complications described herein, which can have clinical signs and symptoms similar to those of acute rejection.

OLT patients are immunocompromised and prone to bacterial and opportunistic infections.

References

1. Jarnagin WR, Shoup M. Surgical management of cholangiocarcinoma. Semin Liver Dis 2004; 24:189-199.

2. Bismuth H, Nakache R, Diamond T. Management strategies in resection for hilar cholangiocarcinoma. Ann Surg 1992; 215:31-38.

3. Heimbach JK, Gores GJ, Nagorney DM, Rosen CB. Liver transplantation for perihilar cholangiocarcinoma after aggressive neoadjuvant therapy: a new paradigm for liver and biliary malignancies? Surgery 2006; 140:331-334.

4. Pandey D, Lee KH, Tan KC. The role of liver transplantation for hilar cholangiocarcinoma. Hepatobiliary Pancreat Dis Int 2007; 6:248-253.

5. Sudan DL. Transplantation for cholangiocarcinoma. Liver Transpl 2006; 12:S83-84.

6. Heimbach JK, Gores GJ, Haddock MG, Alberts SR, Nyberg SL, Ishitani MB, Rosen CB. Liver transplantation for unresectable perihilar cholangiocarcinoma. Semin Liver Dis 2004; 24:201-207.

7. Sudan D, DeRoover A, Chinnakotla S, Fox I, Shaw B, Jr., McCashland T, et al. Radiochemotherapy and transplantation allow long-term survival for nonresectable hilar cholangiocarcinoma. Am J Transplant 2002; 2:774-779,

8. Valls C, Guma A, Puig I, Sanchez A, Andia E, Serrano T, Figueras J. Intrahepatic peripheral cholangiocarcinoma: CT evaluation. Abdom Imaging 2000; 25:490-496.

9. Pannu HK, Maley WR, Fishman EK. Liver transplantation: preoperative CT evaluation. Radiographics 2001; 21 Spec No:S133-146.

10. Winter TC, 3rd, Freeny PC, Nghiem HV, Hommeyer SC, Barr D, Croghan AM, et al. Hepatic arterial anatomy in transplantation candidates: evaluation with three-dimensional CT arteriography. Radiology 1995; 195:363-370.

11. Nghiem HV, Dimas CT, McVicar JP, Perkins JD, Luna JA, Winter TC, 3rd, et al. Impact of double helical CT and three-dimensional CT arteriography on surgical planning for hepatic transplantation. Abdom Imaging 1999; 24:278-284.

12. Merion RM, Burtch GD, Ham JM, Turcotte JG, Campbell DA. The hepatic artery in liver transplantation. Transplantation 1989; 48:438-443.

13. Kruskal JB, Raptopoulos V. How I do it: pre-operative CT scanning for adult living right lobe liver transplantation. Eur Radiol 2002; 12:1423-1431.

14. Alonso-Torres A, Fernandez-Cuadrado J, Pinilla I, Parron M, de Vicente E, Lopez-Santamaria M. Multidetector CT in the evaluation of potential living donors for liver transplantation. Radiographics 2005; 25:1017-1030.

15. Inomoto T, Nishizawa F, Sasaki H, Terajima H, Shirakata Y, Miyamoto S, et al. Experiences of 120 microsurgical reconstructions of hepatic artery in living related liver transplantation. Surgery 1996; 119:20-26.

16. van Leeuwen MS, Fernandez MA, van Es HW, Stokking R, Dillon EH, Feldberg MA. Variations in venous and segmental anatomy of the liver: two- and three-dimensional MR imaging in healthy volunteers. AJR Am J Roentgenol 1994; 162:1337-1345.

17. Kamel IR, Raptopoulos V, Pomfret EA, Kruskal JB, Kane RA, Yam CS, Jenkins RL. Living adult right lobe liver transplantation: imaging before surgery with multidetector multiphase CT. AJR Am J Roentgenol 2000; 175:1141-1143.

18. Redvanly RD, Nelson RC, Stieber AC, Dodd GD, 3rd. Imaging in the preoperative evaluation of adult liver-transplant candidates: goals, merits of various procedures, and recommendations. AJR Am J Roentgenol 1995; 164:611-617.

19. Quiroga S, Sebastia MC, Margarit C, Castells L, Boye R, Alvarez-Castells A. Complications of orthotopic liver transplantation: spectrum of findings with helical CT. Radiographics 2001; 21:1085-1102.

20. Ito K, Siegelman ES, Stolpen AH, Mitchell DG. MR imaging of complications after liver transplantation. AJR Am J Roentgenol 2000; 175:1145-1149.

21. Shyn PB,Goldberg HI. Abdominal CT following liver transplantation. Gastrointest Radiol 1992; 17:231-236.

22. Dupuy DE, Costello P. Cross-sectional imaging of liver transplantation. Semin Ultrasound CT MR 1992; 13:399-409.

23. Chen MF, Hwang TL, Hung CF. Human liver regeneration after major hepatectomy. A study of liver volume by computed tomography. Ann Surg 1991; 213:227-229.

24. Nakagami M, Morimoto T, Itoh K, Arima Y, Yamamoto Y, Ikai I, Yamaoka Y. Patterns of restoration of remnant liver volume after graft harvesting in donors for living related liver transplantation. Transplant Proc 1998; 30:195-199.

25. Defrancq J, Trotteur G, Dondelinger RF. Duplex ultrasonographic evaluation of liver transplants. Acta Radiol 1993; 34:478-481.

26. Platt JF, Yutzy GG, Bude RO, Ellis JH, Rubin JM. Use of Doppler sonography for revealing hepatic artery stenosis in liver transplant recipients. AJR Am J Roentgenol 1997; 168:473-476.

27. Legmann P, Costes V, Tudoret L, Girardot C, Hazebroucq V, Uzan E, et al. Hepatic artery thrombosis after liver transplantation: diagnosis with spiral CT. AJR Am J Roentgenol 1995; 164:97-101.

28. Nolten A,Sproat IA. Hepatic artery thrombosis after liver transplantation: temporal accuracy of diagnosis with duplex US and the syndrome of impending thrombosis. Radiology 1996; 198:553-559.

29. Todo S, Makowka L, Tzakis AG, Marsh JW, Jr., Karrer FM, Armany M, et al. Hepatic artery in liver transplantation. Transplant Proc 1987; 19:2406-2411.

30. Wozney P, Zajko AB, Bron KM, Point S, Starzl TE. Vascular complications after liver transplantation: a 5-year experience. AJR Am J Roentgenol 1986; 147:657-663.

31. Abbasoglu O, Levy MF, Vodapally MS, Goldstein RM, Husberg BS, Gonwa TA, Klintmalm GB. Hepatic artery stenosis after liver transplantation-incidence, presentation, treatment, and long term outcome. Transplantation 1997; 63:250-255.

32. Glockner JF, Forauer AR. Vascular or ischemic complications after liver transplantation. AJR Am J Roentgenol 1999; 173:1055-1059.

33. Nghiem HV. Imaging of hepatic transplantation. Radiol Clin North Am 1998; 36:429-443.

34. Nghiem HV, Tran K, Winter TC, 3rd, Schmiedl UP, Althaus SJ, Patel NH, Freeny PC. Imaging of complications in liver transplantation. Radiographics 1996; 16:825-840.

35. Chen WP, Chen JH, Hwang JI, Tsai JW, Chen JS, Hung SW, et al. Spectrum of transient hepatic attenuation differences in biphasic helical CT. AJR Am J Roentgenol 1999; 172:419-424.

9 Magnetic Resonance Imaging

Alessandro Guarise
Giovanni Morana

Despite overall advances in the ability to diagnose and treat patients with cholangiocarcinoma, the prognosis for patients with this malignancy remains poor (1, 2). Further improvements in the survival of patients with cholangiocarcinoma will come with the early diagnosis of these lesions. New molecular techniques should improve the ability to screen high-risk patients, such as those with primary sclerosing cholangitis, hepatolithiasis, choledochal cysts, and ulcerative colitis (1). Improvements in magnetic resonance imaging (MRI) allow one to diagnose and stage patients with cholangiocarcinoma noninvasively.

The major clinical sign of cholangiocarcinomas is obstructive jaundice, which is persistent and progressive (3, 4). The first-line imaging investigation is ultrasonography (US), which always detects dilatation of the bile ducts, but more rarely the tumor itself (5, 6). Classically, endoscopic retrograde cholangiopancreatography (ERCP) or percutaneous transhepatic cholangiography (PTC), the "gold standard" investigations in case of obstructive jaundice, have been performed following US (7, 8). The actual recommendations, based on grade B and C evidence, are to start investigations with US and to continue with noninvasive methods-MRI/MR cholangiopancreatography (MRCP) or spiral computed tomography (CT)-whenever a malignant obstructive jaundice is suspected (9-11). The spread of MRI has drastically changed diagnostic management of obstructive jaundice as a result of the ability of MRCP sequences to provide a cholangiographic map of the bile ducts. Moreover, integration of the information provided by these sequences with that of T2- and T1-weighted (w) sequences obtained before and after contrast medium (c.m.) administration can suggest the nature of the obstruction with an accuracy that varies depending on the site (10, 12, 13). In addition, postcontrast dynamic acquisition obtained with three-dimensional (3D) T1w sequences makes possible angiographic evaluation of the hepatic vasculature (14-16). The "all-in-one" diagnostic role of MRI therefore allows one to limit the use of ERCP and PTC for tissue diagnosis or therapeutic decompression when cholangitis is present or for stent insertion in unresectable tumors (10, 17, 18).

The noninvasive nature and panoramic capabilities of MRCP and the fact that no contrast material is needed make it the examination of reference in the diagnosis of malignant stenosis of the distal bile duct thanks to its ability to visualize the entire biliary tree in the presence of critical strictures of the common bile duct (CBD). On the contrary, in the presence of obstructive stenosis ERCP is limited regarding the identification of distal bile ducts (7, 19). Technological advances, including new contrast agents and new sequences that are capable of improving spatial resolution, have shown promise for the increasing role of MR/MRCP as the initial modality in assessing postoperative hepato-biliary complications (20).

TECHNIQUE

MRCP is the newest modality for biliary and pancreatic duct imaging that combines the advantages of projectional and cross-sectional imaging techniques (10-12, 21). The aim of MRCP is to visualize selectively the fluid present in the biliary and pancreatic ducts as high signal intensity on heavy T2w sequences. Because it is a "fluid-based" imaging modality, we suggest giving patients, 10 minutes before the study, a superparamagnetic oral contrast agent to decrease the high signal intensity on T2w images of gastrointestinal (GI) fluid (10, 22). MRCP images can be obtained as a combination of multisection single-shot rapid acquisition with relaxation enhancement (RARE) images in the different spatial planes and "thick-slab" acquisitions (slice thickness: 50-70 mm) in oblique coronal angles using heavily T2w (TE: 1100 ms) RARE sequences (3, 20, 23-25). The "thick slab" is rotated with multiple acquisitions (six to eight) at progressive increments of about 15° angles. Acquisition time for thick slices is short (<2 seconds) limiting cardio-respiratory artefacts and eliminating the need for postprocessing. More recently a respiratory-triggered 3D turbo spin echo (TSE RT) sequence with a fairly isotropic 1-mm voxel was introduced, making possible high spatial resolution images in multiplanar views. Postprocessing maximum intensity projection (MIP) images and multiplanar reformations (MPR) give clinicians a 3D biliary map (26). Overall image quality of single-shot "thick-slab" MRCP can be superior, in particular in noncollaborating patients, compared to 3D sequences requiring longer acquisition time (27). In contrast, the original data from multisection thin partitions facilitate ductal visualization of different parts of the biliary system, periductal lesions, and adjacent structures. Therefore, a combination of both MRCP techniques is recommended for the diagnostic work-up and therapy planning of malignant hilar obstructions (28).

In addition, conventional T2w and T1w images and dynamic imaging after bolus injection of a gadolinium (Gd) chelate appear to be a fundamental component of an MRI examination of the liver for detection and characterization of biliary neoplasms (10). The combination of nonenhanced T1w and less heavily T2w images with MRCP images significantly improved the diagnostic accuracy of MR examinations of pancreaticobiliary disease (29).

Optimal dynamic scanning depends on the use of a multisection spoiled gradient-echo (GRE) technique that allows one to image the entire region of interest during a single suspended respiration. Images are obtained during four phases relative to the injection of the contrast agent: precontrast, arterial (presinusoidal), portal (sinusoidal), and delayed (equilibrium) phase (5-10 minutes after injection of c.m.). Liver-specific contrast agents, including hepatobiliary agents and reticoloendothelial system-targeted iron oxide particles, may offer advantages over gadolinium chelates in some clinical settings (30-32)

The following is the protocol adopted in our institution and diffusely accepted: single-shot T2w sequences in coronal and axial planes; precontrast acquisition of axial T1 GRE sequences with fat saturation (TR:140 ms, TE: 4.2 ms); axial T2 short tau inversion recovery (STIR) (TR: 6000 ms, TE: 66 ms) sequences; 3D T1w GRE sequences (i.e., volumetric interpolated breath-hold examination, VIBE; TR: 4.6 ms; TE: 1.8 ms); after administration of contrast material (Gd chelate): 0.2 ml/kg at flow rate of 2 ml/s. We acquire 3D T1w GRE sequences in arterial, venous, equilibrium, and delayed phases. Finally, a MRCP study is obtained.

MR FINDINGS OF CHOLANGIOCARCINOMA

Carcinoma of the biliary tree involves rare tumors of the GI tract with a rising incidence during the last years (1, 33). Cholangiocarcinoma arises from the bile ducts and is the most common primary malignancy of the biliary tree (34). Biliary neoplasms are classified into intra- and extrahepatic cholangiocarcinoma (Klatskin tumor, middle and distal extrahepatic tumors), gallbladder cancer, and ampullary carcinoma.

Intrahepatic cholangiocarcinoma (ICC) accounts for 10% of all cholangiocarcinomas, hilar cholangiocarcinoma for 25%, and extrahepatic cholangiocarcinoma for 65% (10, 35). Cholangiocarcinoma is classified according to its growth pattern as a mass-forming, periductal-infiltrating, or intraductal-growing type according to the recent classification of the Liver Cancer Study Group of Japan (36). Because the imaging findings and therapeutic options are different, we discuss those forms separately.

Intrahepatic Cholangiocarcinoma

Microscopically, cholangiocarcinoma represents an adenocarcinoma with a glandular appearance arising from the epithelium of the intrahepatic bile ducts (34).

Some underlying liver diseases may favor the development of intrahepatic cholangiocarcinoma, such as Caroli disease, sclerosing cholangitis, hepatolithiasis, and thorotrast deposition (1). Association between peripheral cholangiocarcinoma and clonorchiasis has also been reported (37, 38).

Mass-Forming Type

The usual gross appearance of mass-forming cholangiocarcinoma is a large, white, firm tumor that is solid and fibrous (Figure 9.1F,G), with a sclerotic appearance on

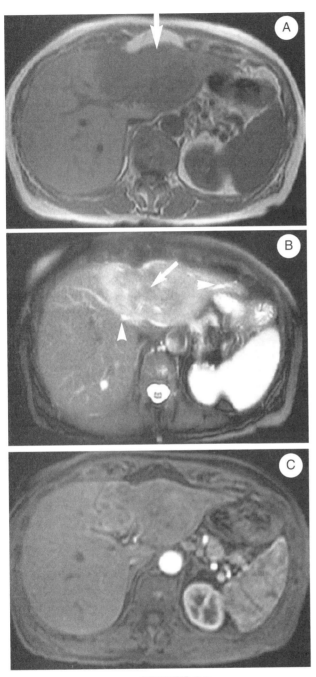

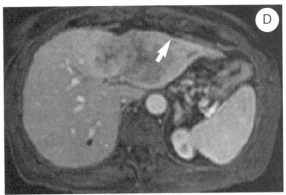

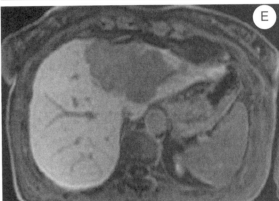

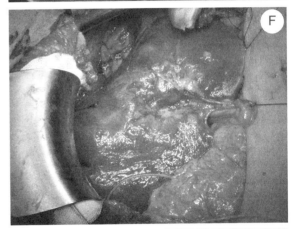

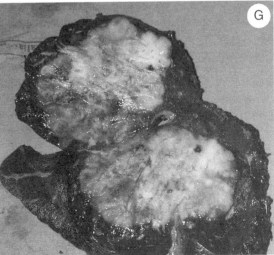

FIGURE 9.1

Mass-forming intrahepatic cholangiocarcinoma. (A) Unenhanced T1w GRE MR image shows a hypointense mass with an irregular margin (arrow) in the left lobe of the liver. (B) Unenhanced T2w TSE image demonstrates a mass hyperintense peripherically and hypointense in the central part (arrow) with initially dilated intra-hepatic bile ducts (arrowheads). (C) Arterial-phase dynamic MR sequence shows a low intense mass- with rim enhancement. (D) On a portal-phase sequence the central portion is now more enhanced. Capsular retraction is also seen (small arrow). (E) On delayed phase (2 hours) after e.v. Gd-BOPTA administration the mass is hypointense. The rim enhancement seen in the arterial phase is washed out. (F,G) Photograph of the pathologic specimen obtained at segmentectomy reveals a lobulated, yellow-white mass, due to fibrosis, with capsular retraction.

the cut surface of the specimen and frequently with dense fibrous stranding in the central portion (39). Mass-forming cholangiocarcinomas are usually large because they are rarely symptomatic early in their course, ranging from 6 to 10 cm of mean diameter; frequently (20-30% of cases) satellite nodules are present (39).

Cholangiocarcinoma appears as a homogeneous hypointense mass relative to the liver on T1w images and hyperintense on T2w sequences (Figure 9.1A,B)) (40-42). They are typically nonencapsulated with lobulated contours or smooth. On T2w images, the signal is usually heterogeneous because the amount of fibrosis, mucous secretion, and necrosis may vary in cholan-

giocarcinoma (Figure 9.1B) (12, 43). Central hypointensity corresponding to fibrosis may be seen on T2w images (Figure 9.1B) (43). Importantly, a central hypointensity can be a reliable feature for differentiating primary liver tumors from metastases on MRI evaluation (43). On the basis of signal intensity, MRI can differentiate two subtypes of cholangiocarcinomas: a scirrhous subtype with a large amount of fibrosis and a low content of mucous secretion and necrosis (Figure 9.1) and another subtype with a low or mild amount of fibrosis and a high content of mucous secretion and/or necrosis (Figure 9.2) (44).

On dynamic MR images, cholangiocarcinomas

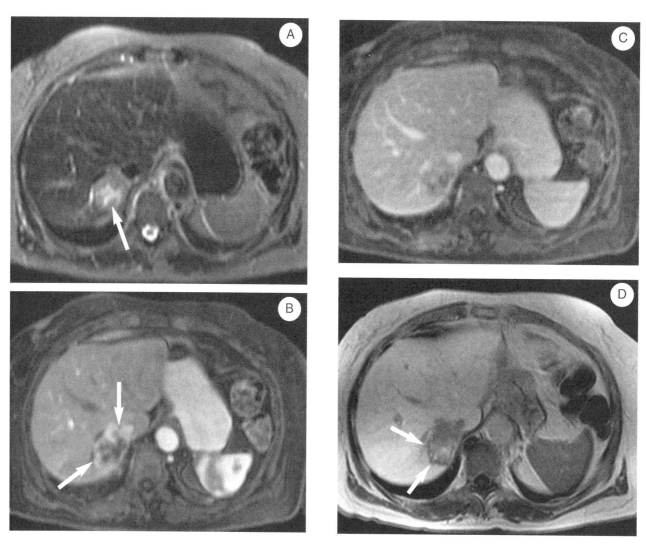

FIGURE 9.2

Dynamic MR findings of mass-forming type intrahepatic cholangiocarcinoma. (A) Unenhanced T2w STIR image shows a disomogeneous hyperintense mass (arrow) in the segment VII with lobulated margin. (B) On the arterial phase image, the mass shows a rim like enhancement along the periphery (arrows). (C) On the equilibrium phase image, the mass shows progressive and concentric filling of contrast material but the central part remains hypointense. (D) On the delayed-phase image obtained 2 hours after c.m. injection (Gd-BOPTA), the central portion of the mass is enhanced due to pooling phenomena of c.m. Peripheral washout is evident (arrows).

show moderate peripheral enhancement followed by progressive and concentric filling in the tumor with contrast material (Figures 9.1 and 9.2) (40). Pooling of contrast within the tumor on delayed MR images is suggestive of peripheral cholangiocarcinoma (Figure 9.2D). The entire mass may be enhanced only on delayed-phase images, many minutes after contrast administration (Figure 9.1D). Some cholangiocarcinomas are depicted only on delayed-phase images because of slow diffusion of contrast material into the interstitial spaces of the tumor (39, 45). The degree of enhancement on delayed-phase MR images is a useful indicator for predicting the prognosis of patients with mass-forming ICC (46). Asayama et al. (46) recently demonstrated that the degree of enhancement on the delayed-phase images is statistically significant correlated with the amount of fibrous stroma and the frequency of perineural invasion making the survival rate significantly worse. In this article multivariate analysis revealed that enhancement of more than two thirds of the ICC is a significant and independent prognostic factor (46).

This enhancing pattern differs from that of hypervascular tumors such as hepatocellular carcinomas, which most commonly show totally high intensity in the hepatic arterial phase and iso- or low intensity on the portal venous phase (47). Even if rarely, we found that small ICC can be hypervascular enhancing early in the arterial phase mimicking HCC (Figure 9.3) (48).

Mixed HCC-ICC frequently show the same MRI findings of classing ICC, making it impossible a differential diagnosis based only on imaging findings.

Hemangioma can cause a pitfall showing peripheral enhancement with central fill-in. In these cases the key findings are the homogeneous high T2 signal and the globular peripheral enhancement with complete fill-in characteristics of hemangioma.

Hypovascular metastases from fibrous tumors, especially colorectal, may show an enhancing pattern similar to that of peripheral cholangiocarcinomas (Figure 9.4) (49). Absence of the possible primary site, a relatively large tumor size, and other ancillary findings such as bile duct dilation (Figure 9.5) can be clues for differentiating mass-forming cholangiocarcinomas from metastases that also are usually multiple. Because of fibrosis fibrolamellar HCC can also show a similar pattern of enhancement (Figure 9.5).

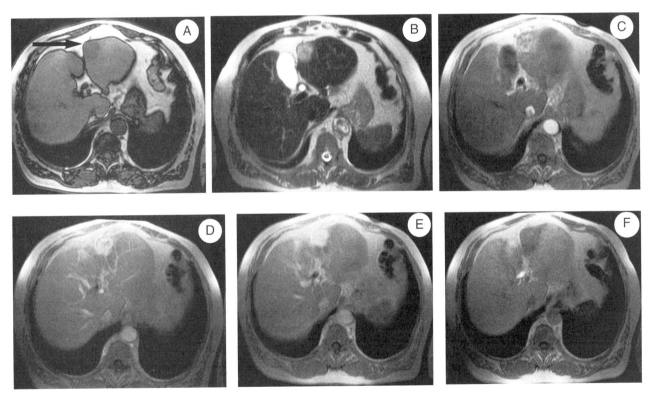

FIGURE 9.3

Dynamic MR findings of a small mass-forming type intrahepatic cholangiocarcinoma. (A) Unenhanced T1w GRE MR image shows a small hypointense mass with sharp margin (arrow) in the left lobe of the liver. (B) Unenhanced T2-weighted turbo spin-echo image demonstrates a hyperintense mass. (C) On the arterial phase image, the mass shows a disomogeneous enhancement. (D,E) On the equilibrium phase image, the mass shows more homogeneous enhancement. (F) On the delayed-phase image obtained 2 hours after c.m. (Gd-BOPTA) the lesion is hypointense.

The use of hepato-specific c.m. like Gd-EOB-DTPA and Gd-BOPTA that are selectively taken up by hepatocytes allow a selective enhancement of the liver parenchyma on T1w images. Liver parenchyma signal intensity is influenced by the extent to which liver function is compromised, in that residual hepatocytic functionality permits Gd-BOPTA uptake by certain lesions composed by normal hepatocytes; in contrast, metastases and neoplasms do not take up Gd BOPTA and EOB on delayed phase (Figures 9.1E,G, 9.3F, 9.4C) (50). The presence of desmoplastic tissue with large extracellular spaces allows a pooling effect of c.m (Fig-

ures 9.1E, 9.2D,). Therefore, most scirrhous-type ICC appear on delayed images hyperintense centrally with a peripheral hypointense rim (Figure 9.2D). These contrast agents may improve the MR imaging capability to detect focal liver lesions and to characterize them. Also, superparamagnetic c.m. (USPIO) was useful in characterizing ICC, which became markedly hyperintense 10 minutes after c.m. injection due to the absence of reticoloendotelial cells (Figure 9.6) (51).

The presence of ancillary signs such as intrahepatic bile duct dilatation (30%) may indicate cholangiocarcinoma (Figure 9.7) (52). The most common pattern of

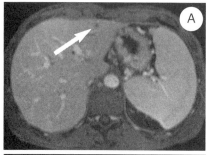
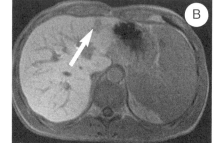
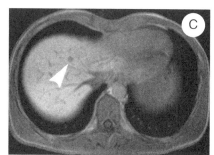
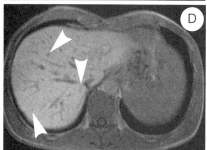

FIGURE 9.4

Dynamic MR findings of metastasis from colon cancer. (A) On the venous phase image, a small mass in the segment IV shows a disomogeneous enhancement at the periphery (arrow). (B) On the delayed-phase image (2 hours) after e.v. Gd-BOPTA administration, the lesions show a central enhancement due to the presence of fibrosis with rim washout (arrow). (C,D) Other lesions are seen in the liver (arrowheads).

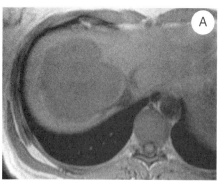
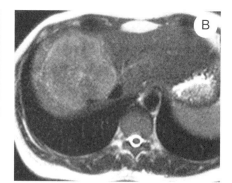
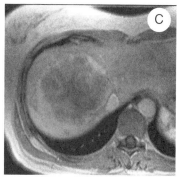
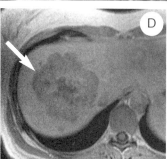
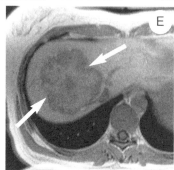

FIGURE 9.5

Fibrolamellar hepatocarcinoma mimicking ICC: MR imaging findings. (A) Unenhanced T1w GRE image shows a hypointense mass with an irregular margin in the right lobe of the liver. (B) Unenhanced T2w TSE image demonstrates disomogeneous high signal of the mass. (C) On the venous phase image, the mass shows progressive and concentric filling of contrast material. (D,E) On the delayed-phase image obtained 2 hours after c.m. administration (Gd-BOPTA), the central portion of the mass is enhanced with peripheral washout (arrows).

biliary duct dilation is diffuse, mild dilation with focally severe dilation around the tumor (15). Capsular retraction (20%) (Figure 9.1) and dilation with thickening of the peripheral intrahepatic ducts (especially when associated with clonorchiasis) (37) are corollary signs. The dense fibrotic nature of mass-forming cholangiocarcinoma may be the cause of retraction of the adjacent liver capsule. Capsular retraction adjacent to a hepatic tumor is an unusual finding, with a reported prevalence of 2% of HCC (53). This finding can be associated with a variety of tumors, including epithelioid hemangioendothelioma, metastasis from colorectal cancer, fibrolamellar hepatocellular carcinoma, carcinoid tumor, and lymphoma (Figure 9.8) (53). Although this sign is not specific for cholangiocarcinoma, it is suggestive of a malignant tumor with a relatively prominent desmoplastic reaction (53). Finally, useful associated findings are vascular invasion (50%), ipsilater lobar hypotrophy, and controlateral hypertrophy (20-40%). Narrowing or encasement of the portal vein is not an uncommon finding in mass-forming cholangiocarcinoma located centrally within the liver (Figure 9.9)

Parenchymal changes of the liver such as segmental or lobar atrophy (Figure 9.6) and increased transient degree of enhancement (THAD) of the liver parenchyma on postcontrast MR or CT images can be seen in hilar and intrahepatic cholangiocarcinoma (12). This area is generally hyperintense on T2w images.

Extrahepatic spread of mass forming cholangiocarcinoma is common, with an autopsy incidence of 50-67% (43). Lymph node metastasis with involvement of the celiac and left gastric areas or direct invasion of the omentum is frequently detected (1)

Periductal-Infiltrating Type

This form matches radiologically and pathologically infiltrating hilar cholangiocarcinoma but has a different location (i.e., peripheral to the secondary confluence). It grows along the bile ducts, and frequently

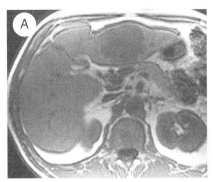
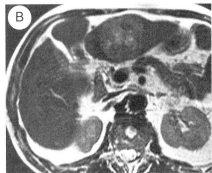
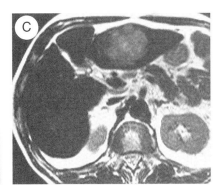

FIGURE 9.6

Mass-forming intrahepatic cholangiocarcinoma. (A,B) Axial T1w and T2w MR images of extrahepatic cholangiocarcinoma in the left lobe, respectively, hypo and hyperintense. (C) After the administration of superparamagnetic iron oxide (SPIO), the liver shows loss of signal because of the strong T2 shortening effect of SPIO. On the contrary, the mass is more hyperintense due to the absence of reticoloendothelial (RES) cells.

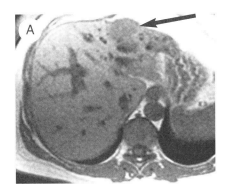
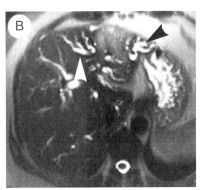
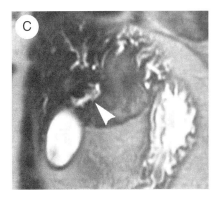

FIGURE 9.7

Mass-forming intrahepatic cholangiocarcinoma. (A) Unenhanced T1w GRE MR image shows a hypointense mass with well-defined margin (arrow) in the left lobe of the liver. (B,C) Unenhanced T2w turbo spin-echo images in the axial (B) and coronal (C) planes demonstrate hyperintense signal of the mass with dilated intrahepatic bile ducts (arrowheads).

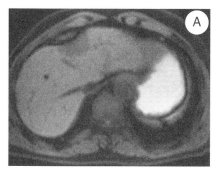
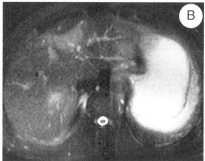
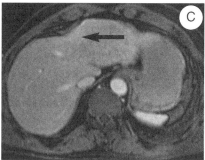
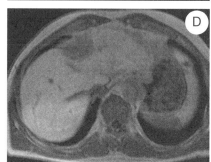

FIGURE 9.8

Non-Hodgkin lymphoma mimicking ICC: MR imaging findings. (A,B) Unenhanced T1w and T2w images show a subcapsular mass, respectively, hypointense and hyperintense with sharp margin located in segment IV. Slight dilation of the bilary tree is seen. (C) On the venous phase image the mass shows a progressive enhancement (small arrow). On the delayed-phase image obtained 2 hours after c.m. administration (Gd-BOPTA), the mass is hypointense. Capsular retraction is present in the area adjacent to the lesion.

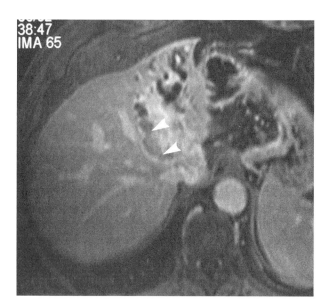

FIGURE 9.9

Intrahepatic cholangiocarcinoma. The infiltrating-type mass causes dilation of the biliary tree. The lesion is adjacent to a branch of the portal vein for segment IV without a defined surgical plane (arrowheads).

irregular narrowing of the involved bile duct or obstruction is present. In the early phase the tumor causes segmental dilatation of the bile ducts. In the advanced phase, the tumor may invade the hepatic parenchyma and hepatic hilum (40). On MR, ill-defined infiltrating tumor tissue can be detected as focal wall thickening (Figure 9.10), usually with a lower signal than the liver parenchyma, and the bile ducts proximal to the cholangiocarcinoma are dilated and hyperintense on T2w images unless secondary biliary stones or sludges are formed. Usually periductal-infiltrating cholangiocarcinoma results in obliteration of the bile ducts and proximal dilatation without an identifiable mass. MRCP shows focal stricture or complete obstruction of the bile ducts (Figure 9.10D). The correlation between the length of the stricture and the enhancement of the parietal bile duct after c.m. administration obtained by conventional and MRCP images determines the extent of disease with a good correlation with pathology (54, 55).

Primary sclerosing cholangitis (PSC) can show the same MR appearance as ICC, in particular the infiltrating type. In the absence of a clinical and laboratory setting typical of PSC, the differential diagnosis can be very difficult to achieve, in particular in the early stage. Patients with PSC are at increased risk for developing cholangiocarcinoma (1% for each year). The direct imaging finding useful for an early diagnosis is the presence of mass effect. The indirect signs are the presence of segmental biliary dilatation, lobar atrophy, and vascular involvement. The diagnosis of ICC on PSC remains challenging for Radiologists.

Intraductal-Growing Type

Intraductal intrahepatic cholangiocarcinoma is often limited to the mucosa invading the wall in the late phase.

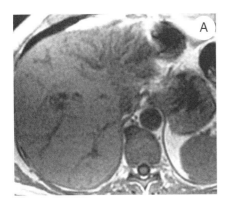
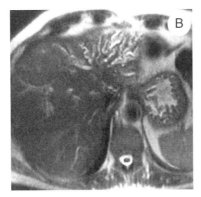
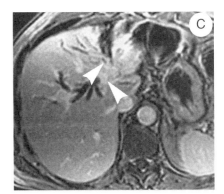
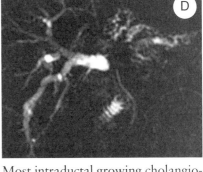

FIGURE 9.10

Infiltrating hilar cholangiocarcinoma with tumoral involvement of the right secondary confluence and common hepatic duct. (A,B) Unenhanced T1w and T2w images show dilation of the biliary tree but not evidence of mass causing the obstruction. (C) Postcontrast T1w image clearly shows circumferential thickening and infiltration of intrahepatic ducts (arrowheads). (D) MRCP shows dilation of the right and left hepatic biliary ducts. The common hepatic duct is not seen.

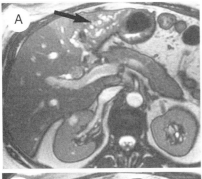
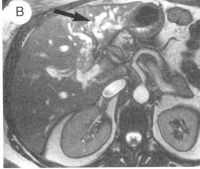
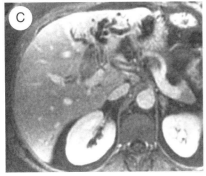
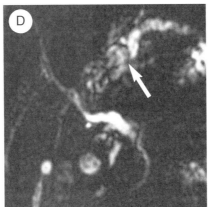

FIGURE 9.11

Intraductal papillary cholangiocarcinomas. (A,B) Axial balanced images (True-Fisp) show multiple polypoid tumors (arrows) involving the intrahepatic bile ducts. (C) Postcontrast T1w image shows tiny enhancement of the endoluminal masses. (D) MRCP demonstrates multiple intraductal papillary tumors (arrow) with upstream ductal dilatation.

Most intraductal growing cholangiocarcinomas are small, sessile, or polypoid; they often spread superficially along the mucosal surface and result in multiple tumors (papillomatosis) along different segments of the bile ducts (Figure 9.11) (56). They also can slough spontaneously, simulate bile duct stones, and occlude the bile ducts (56). Occasionally, the tumor produces a profuse amount of mucus, resulting in partial biliary obstruction (57). At MRCP intraductal-growing cholangiocarcinoma presents with focal or segmental bile duct dilatation with or without visible intraductal papillary tumors (Figure 9.11D) (56).

The mucin-producing form can be similar at MRCP to the intraductal papillary mucinous form of the pancreas. The biliary ducts can be segmental or diffusely dilated and filled by thick mucin. For this reason patients frequently present with symptoms. The cystic form of ICC is very rare. The differential diagnosis is with benign epithelial serous cyst or biliary cystadenoma, often being impossible only using imaging criteria.

Hilar Cholangiocarcinoma

Hilar cholangiocarcinomas account for more than 50% of bile duct malignancies

(43). At pathologic analysis, infiltrating hilar cholangiocarcinoma manifests as a sclerotic lesion with abundant fibrous tissue (34). Tumors originating from a large bile duct are in a critical location and are discovered early due to the presence of jaundice or cholangitis (58). Thus, these tumors are usually very small. The role of MR imaging in hilar cholangiocarcinoma is to confirm a diagnosis, suspected by ultrasound as a first-step imaging modality, and to assess resectability (10). Because of its intrinsic high tissue contrast and multiplanar capability, MR imaging and MRCP are able to detect and preoperatively assess patients with cholangiocarcinoma, investigating all involved structures such as bile ducts, vessels, and hepatic parenchyma (13, 17, 21).

Cholangiography through a retrograde endoscopic or percutaneous transhepatic approach may provide the most accurate anatomic information pertaining to which segmental branches are involved (Figure 9.12A). However, because direct cholangiography provides information only on the ductal system, any data on extraductal extension or the cause of the biliary obstruction cannot be obtained (59). In addition, cross-sectional MRI and MRCP can directly visualize hilar cholangiocarcinoma (Figure 9.12) (13, 17, 21). The morphology of bile duct stricture detectable on MRCP closely reflects the gross morphologic changes occurring along the biliary ductal walls (Figure 9.12D,E) (59).

Combined use of MRCP and dynamic MRI can display the overall extent of biliary tree involvement and the correct diagnosis of biliary malignancies (13, 17, 21).

Other diseases that can cause hilar obstruction indistinguishable from hilar cholangiocarcinoma are metastases to periportal lymph nodes, gallbladder cancer invading the hepato-duodenal ligament, lymphadenopathy due to other inflammation, and idiopathic benign focal stricture of the bile duct (60).

Periductal-Infiltrating Hilar Cholangiocarcinoma

Infiltrating hilar cholangiocarcinoma is the most common type of hilar cholangiocarcinoma (70% of cases) (43). Although the tumor can appear as a mural thickening or an encircling mass along the bile duct wall, a definite mass is rarely seen on US (6). On MRCP images, it appears as an irregular thickening of the bile duct wall (≥5 mm) with symmetric upstream dilation of the intrahepatic bile ducts (Figure 9.13) (13). The lumen may be completely obstructed or markedly narrowed. Nonunion of the right and left hepatic ducts with or without a visibly thickened wall is a typical finding of infiltrating hilar cholangiocarcinoma (Figure 9.13C) (43, 55). On cross-sectional MR images, the lesion appears hypointense to the liver on T1w images and moderately hyperintense until a high signal on T2w images (61).

On contrast-enhanced MR images, infiltrating tumors are better seen as a focally thickened ductal wall obliterating the lumen (Figure 9.13). About 80% of these tumors are hyperintense relative to the liver on arterial or portal phase or both. They usually are better seen at equilibrium phase due to fibrosis (Figure 9.13) (10).

One of the most challenging differential diagnoses is with inflammatory myofibroblastic tumor (IMT). On MR images IMT may manifest as either a mass-like lesion with heterogeneous signal intensity characteristics or as an area of periportal soft-tissue infiltration

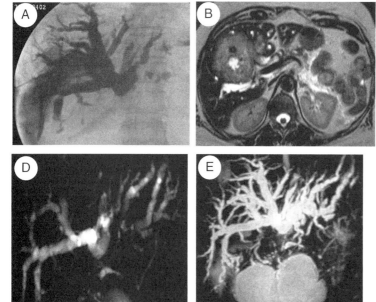

FIGURE 9.12

Hilar mass-like cholangiocarcinoma involving the perihilar and upper parts of the extrahepatic ducts. (A) PTC shows dilated intrahepatic bile duct with an obstructed common hepatic duct. (B) Axial conventional T2w MR image shows an expansive mass at the confluence of the common hepatic duct and the cystic duct. The lesion has a hypointense central component. (C) Postcontrast T1w image shows enhancement of the peripheral and central component. Most of the mass does not enhance because of the necrotic component. (D,E) A single thick slab (D) and 3D MRCP (E) demonstrate the intrahepatic bile ducts diffusely dilated with a stop at the level of the commun hepatic duct.

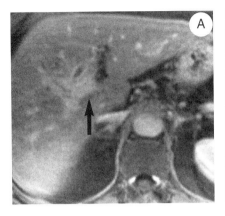
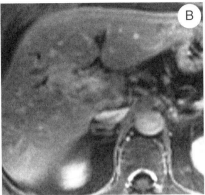
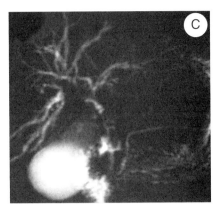

FIGURE 9.13

Hilar infiltrating cholangiocarcinoma. (A,B) Postcontrast T1w images clearly demonstrate circumferential neoplastic thickening of the common bile duct (CBD) with extension to main right duct (arrow). (C) At MRCP the intrahepatic bile ducts are slightly dilated and a right duct is obstructed.

with variable signal intensity at unenhanced T2w imaging and a variable enhancement pattern after the administration of c.m. (Figure 9.14) (62-64). The MRI findings can be explained by the varied composition of these lesions. Histologically, IMTs are composed of fibrous tissue associated with a mixed inflammatory infiltrate consisting of macrophages, lymphocytes, eosinophils, and neutrophils intermixed with areas of necrosis (Figure 9.14D,E) (62-64). The presence of fibrosis and granulation tissue can explain occlusive portal phlebitis visualized as periportal soft-tissue infiltration on MR images (Figure 9.14A,B). Both IMT and cholangiocarcinoma are more often seen in male patients and, when present as a focal mass, are more

common in the right lobe of the liver. Both tumors have moderately low signal intensity on T1w MR images and moderately high signal intensity on T2w MR images. Also, the pattern of enhancement after c.m. administration is similar and varies, with mild to moderate enhancement, in the early postcontrast phase and moderate to progressive enhancement on delayed postcontrast MR images (62-64).

Secondary involvement of the liver occurs commonly in stage IV Hodgkin and non-Hodgkin lymphoma (65). Histopathologically, liver involvement is heralded by tumor deposits within the portal tracts (65). This is typically seen at MR imaging as periportal soft-tissue infiltration. Periportal tumor infiltration

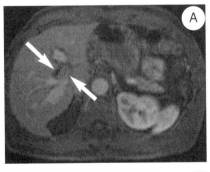
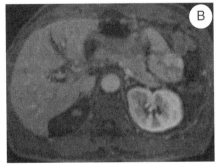
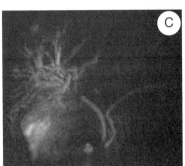

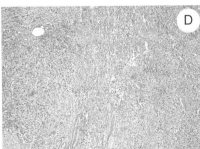

FIGURE 9.14

Inflammatory myofibroblastic tumor of the hilum. (A,B) Transverse T1w fat-suppressed spoiled GRE MR images obtained after gadolinium chelate administration show soft-tissue infiltration (arrows) along the intrahepatic ducts. (C) Biliary dilatation is visualized at MRCP. (D,E) Spindled myofibroblast and plasma cells set in a collagenized background (D) (hematoxylin-eosin). Immunohistochemical stain for smooth muscle actin (E), highlighting the myofibroblastic nature of the spindle cell proliferation.

is more common in lymphoma than in other forms of malignant disease (65). Lymphoma can also manifest as focal mass-like lesions (Figure 9.8). As reported by Kelekis et al. (65), lymphomatous hepatic lesions have two different appearances at MR. This variation in signal intensity was due to the differences in the relative amount of vascularity, the size of the extracellular space, and the presence of fibrosis and necrosis. The enhancement pattern after gadolinium chelate administration ranged from minimal to intense peripheral enhancement on the early images, to persistent enhancement, progression of enhancement, and washout with delayed peripheral enhancement on images obtained at equilibrium phase (65).

Considerable similarities between IMT and lymphoma and IMT and cholangiocarcinoma make the differentiation difficult, and, hence, histologic examination is necessary.

Mass-Forming Exophytic Hilar Cholangiocarcinoma

Hilar cholangiocarcinoma shows the same signal intensity pattern of peripheral tumors both on precontrast T1w and T2w images and after c.m. administration (Figure 9.15) (13, 17, 21). It can be difficult or even impossible to ascertain whether the carcinoma arises at the main hepatic juncture or represents a peripheral cholangiocarcinoma that secondarily obliterates the hilar area.

Intraductal Polypoid Hilar Cholangiocarcinoma

Polypoid hilar cholangiocarcinoma manifests as an intraductal soft tissue mass that has the same gross and histologic features as intraductal intrahepatic cholangiocarcinoma. The site of origin determines the presenting symptoms (jaundice in large duct lesions or incidentally found segmental ductal dilatation in intrahepatic lesions). On cross-sectional MR images, the lesion appears hypointense to the liver on T1w images and moderately hyperintense with a high signal on T2w images (Figure 9.16) (43). The tumors are frequently multiple or disseminated within the biliary system and involve both the intrahepatic and extrahepatic bile ducts.

Preoperative Evaluation

Before determining the best treatment method for a cholangiocarcinoma, its precise location must be known and the presence of intrahepatic metastases or other lesions and tumor thrombi must be confirmed or ruled out. MR imaging staging of biliary neoplasm has to define the following aspects: (a) the extent and location of intrahepatic disease, (b) the involvement of surgically critical areas such as the portal vein, inferior vena cava, and major bile ducts, and (c) the presence of extrahepatic disease (13). The principal question is whether an apparently free segment of the right and left lobes is uninvolved, thus permitting the obviously involved seg-

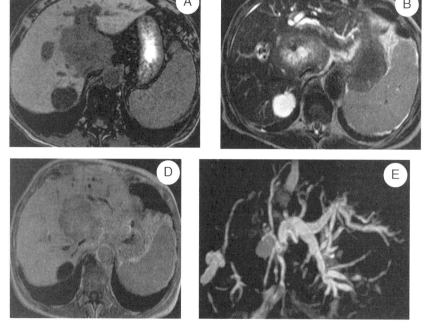

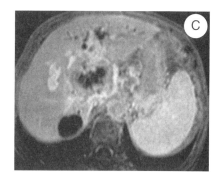

FIGURE 9.15

Mass-forming hilar cholangiocarcinoma. (A,B) Axial T1w and T2w images clearly depict a large mass, respectively, hypointense and disomogeneously hyperintense at the hilum. (C) Contrast-enhanced T1w axial section after administration of gadolinium chelate shows peripheral enhancement of the mass with a hypointense necrotic component. (D) On delayed (2h) contrast enhancement (Gd-BOPTA) the mass shows a central pooling of c.m. with peripheral washout. (E) 3D MRCP shows severe strictures at the hilum with dilation of the left biliary system.

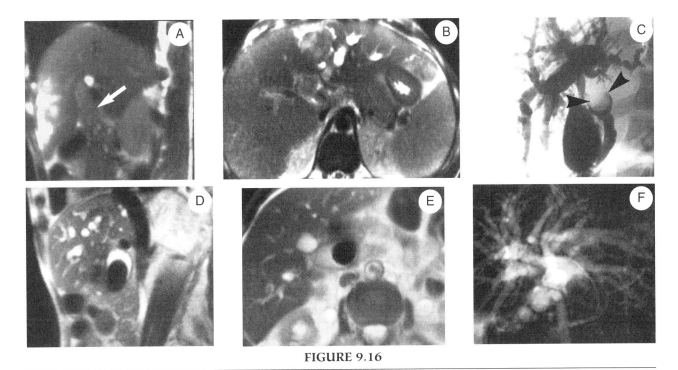

FIGURE 9.16

Intraductal-growing papillary cholangiocarcinoma of the hilum. (A,B) Coronal and axial half Fourier single shot TSE sequences depict a dilated common bile duct (arrow) filled by a mass isointense to the hepatic parenchyma. (C) Direct cholangiogram obtained by PTC demonstrates expansile growth of a spherical tumor (arrowheads) within the midportion of the extrahepatic bile duct. (D,E) Coronal and axial half Fourier single shot TSE sequences depict a dilated common bile duct filled by a marked hypointense ovoid structure (stone) (F) MRCP is similar to the previously described PTC (C) showing a marked dilated biliary tree and common hepatic duct with a meniscus sign due to the presence of a large stone.

ment to be excised (17). Delineation of tumor site and number relative to segment anatomy involved can be obtained from multidetector CT or MRI.

The biliary extension of the tumor is defined according to Bismuth's classification (Table 9.1). Most surgeons accept the nonresectability of hilar cholangiocarcinoma in the following cases: (a) cholangiographic evidence of severe bilateral involvement of the secondary confluence, (b) involvement of the main trunk of the portal vein, (c) involvement of both branches of the portal vein or bilateral involvement of the hepatic artery and portal vein, or (d) vascular involvement on one side of the liver and extensive bile duct involvement on the other side. Unilateral involvement of the hepatic artery, portal vein, or both vessels is compatible with resection (13). Precise preoperative evaluation of tumor extent often requires several imaging modality. MRI with a technique called "all in one" offers all the information needed. MRCP is competitive with cholangiography for detecting these neoplasms and determining the intraductal extent. The extent of tumor in the bile duct is one of the important factors that determine resectability. Therefore, identification of the proximal extent of the tumor is important in planning surgical treatment. MRI is also effective in detecting spreading tumor that extends above the level of bil-

iary obstruction showing enhancement of the inner wall of the bile duct with a preserved lumen: this appearance differentiates it from inflammation. The extent of intraductal tumor spread tends to be underestimated with MR. MR angiography and venography easily evaluate vascular involvement of the hepatic artery and portal vein as focal or segmental narrowing (encasement) of the involved vessel (66). In contrast, digital angiography cannot depict vascular invasion that does not change the diameter of the involved vessel. With MR as well as CT, obliteration of the fat plane between the biliary tumor and the hepatic artery or portal vein can be used as a criterion for vascular invasion (Figure 9.9). In addition, because the liver has a dual blood supply, obstruction or significant stricture of one vessel causes compensatory hyperperfusion of the other (67).

Gallbladder Malignant Neoplasms

Since the symptoms and signs of gallbladder carcinoma are vague, it is difficult to diagnose it clinically (68). Early-stage carcinoma is typically diagnosed incidentally because of inflammatory symptoms related to coexistent cholelithiasis or cholecystitis (68). Cholelithiasis is a well-established risk factor for the development of gallbladder carcinoma (68), and gallstones are pre-

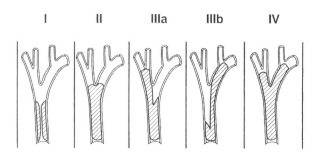

TABLE 9.1

*Bismuth's Classification of Hilar and Extrahepatic
Cholangiocarcinomas*

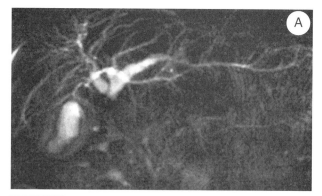

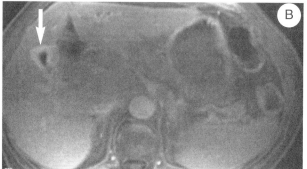

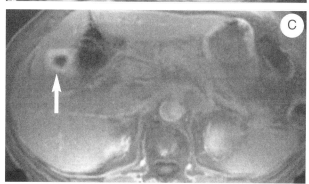

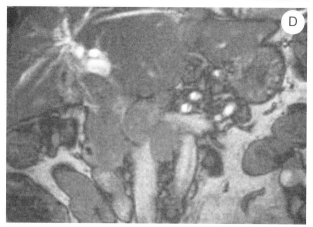

FIGURE 9.17

sent in 74-92% of affected patients (69). Porcelain gall-bladder is an uncommon condition in which there is diffuse calcification of the gallbladder wall, and 10-25% of patients with this condition have gallbladder carcinoma (69). Several pathologic and congenital anatomic anomalies are associated with a higher prevalence of gallbladder carcinoma. These conditions include congenital cystic dilatation of the biliary tree, choledochal cyst, anomalous junction of the pancreaticobiliary ducts (with or without a coexistent choledochal cyst), and low insertion of the cystic duct (69). Gallbladder abnormalities are frequently seen in patients with primary sclerosing cholangitis with the increased incidence of this tumor (68).

The majority (68%) of gallbladder carcinomas are diffusely infiltrating lesions, and the remainder exhibit intraluminal polypoid growth (32%) (69). Approximately 60% of tumors originate in the gallbladder fundus, 30% in the body, and 10% in the neck (69).

At MRCP neoplasms appear as filling defects that may represent tumor or stones, a mass displacing and invading the gallbladder (11). When the mass is huge or sludge fills the gallbladder, MRCP cannot display the lesion and the organ itself because of the absence of fluid. MRCP may demonstrate malignant strictures or obstruction involving the extrahepatic bile ducts, confluence of the right and left common ducts (70, 71) (Figure 9.17). Associated findings from MRCP include intraductal filling defects that may represent tumor or coexistent choledocholithiasis in the common hepatic ducts and/or intrahepatic ducts in the right lobe.

The cross-sectional imaging patterns of gallbladder carcinoma have been described as mass replacing the gallbladder, focal or diffuse gallbladder wall thickening, and an intraluminal polypoid mass (69, 70).

1. Mass replacing the gallbladder. This is the most common form of gallbladder cancer and represents 40-65% of all tumors (70). MR shows a hyperintense mass on T2w images in the gallbladder fossa, featuring dyshomogeneous

Gallbladder carcinoma: thickening of the wall. (A) MRCP shows dilated intrahepatic bile ducts obstructed at the hilum. (B,C) Postcontrast T1w MR image in the axial plan shows an irregular and diffuse thickening of the gallbladder wall markedly enhanced (arrows). (D) Coronal balanced image demonstrate multiple nodes.

enhancement after injection of gadolinium (Figure 9.18) (69, 70). The enhancement of the mass is better visualized on T1w images after fat saturation. Intraneoplastic stones or necrosis of the tumor are frequently observed. Areas of enhancement reflect viable tumor. Direct extension to the liver and biliary tree is a common associated finding with large, advanced carcinomas (11, 69, 70). In these cases, the tumor is inseparable from the adjacent liver. Biliary obstruction at the level of the porta hepatis and lymph node metastasis are frequent associated findings (Figure 9.17A,D).

2. Thickening of the gallbladder wall secondary to tumor infiltration and inflammatory changes is seen in 20-30% of cases of gallbladder carcinoma and can be diffuse (Figure 9.17) or focal (70). This is the most diagnostically challenging of the three patterns because it mimics the appearance of more common acute and chronic inflammatory conditions of the gallbladder. Pronounced wall thickening (i.e., more than 1 cm), demonstrated by MRCP or T1w images after c.m. administration, with associated mural irregularity or marked asymmetry, should raise concerns for malignancy or complicated cholecystitis (72). It is therefore particularly important to look for signs of local or metastatic involvement in such cases. Focal thickening of the wall may represent an early stage of cancer involvement.

3. Intraluminal mass within the gallbladder is the least common form of gallbladder carcinoma, representing 15-25% of tumors (70). These carcinomas tend to expand into the lumen of the gallbladder before invading the wall and seem to be associated with a less invasive, papillary-type carcinoma. MR imaging demonstrates a hypointense and hyperintense mass, respectively, on T1w and T2w images (11, 69, 70). Ill-defined early enhancement is a typical appearance of these tumors at dynamic gadolinium-enhanced MR imaging (72).

Whether T2w imaging and MRCP have high sensitivity to edema and fluid and are paramount in the evaluation of certain gallbladder diseases (cholelithiasis, cholecystitis, adenomyomatosis, and cystic duct abnormalities), dynamic gadolinium-enhanced MR imaging has the potential to differentiate among the many non-specific-appearing lesions involving the gallbladder (72). Dynamic MRI is useful for the differentiation of chronic cholecystitis from carcinoma and for the evaluation of its local extension (72).

MR imaging may not yet replace US as the workhorse of acute gallbladder imaging. Currently, MRCP is an ideal complementary study to inconclusive US studies and can help plan surgical intervention in the setting of acute cholecystitis. Unfortunately, the diagnosis of gallbladder carcinoma is not usually established until after the tumor has spread to the liver and other viscera (11, 69, 70).

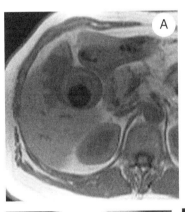
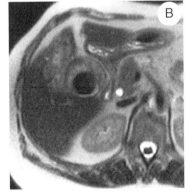
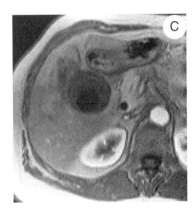
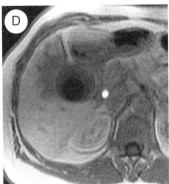
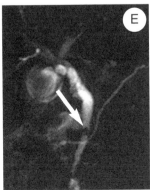

FIGURE 9.18

Gallbladder carcinoma: mass replacing the lumen. (A,B) Conventional T1w and T2w images show the gallbladder filled by a mass hypointense on T1w and hyperintense on T2w images. A big hypointense stone is present. (C) Gadolinium-enhanced axial T1w image shows irregular enhancement of the gallbladder carcinoma and of the adjacent infiltrated liver parenchyma. (D) On delayed-phase image (2 hours) after e.v. administrations of Gd-BOPTAthe infiltrated liver parenchyma is hypointense. (E) MRCP shows a small stone migrated into the distal CBD (arrow) and the presence of pancreas divisum.

The most common route of dissemination for gall-bladder carcinoma to adjacent organs is direct extension, followed by lymphatic and vascular extension. Contiguous spread of the tumor is facilitated by the thin gallbladder wall, narrow lamina propria, and only a single muscle layer. The liver is the organ most frequently involved by direct continuous spread. The incidence of liver involvement at the time of diagnosis varies from 34 to 89% according to the series, followed by involvement of the duodenum (15%), colon (15%), and pancreas (6%) (69). On MR images, tumor extension has the same signal intensity as the primary tumor (Figure 9.18), and biliary dilatation is a common associated finding (Figures 9.17 and 9.18). Infiltrative tumor growth alongside or within the cystic duct with spread to the extrahepatic bile duct causes biliary obstruction and dilatation (62%) (71).

Seeding of viable tumor cells into the peritoneal cavity can lead to peritoneal implants.

The prevalence of lymphatic spread is high in gallbladder carcinoma (76%) (71); positive lymph nodes are 1 cm in diameter or larger and show ring-like or heterogeneous enhancement at CT and MR. The pericholedochal lymph nodes are the primary nodes draining the gallbladder. Enlargement of these nodes provides another mechanism for obstruction of the extrahepatic biliary system from gallbladder carcinoma. Further lymphatic spread leads to involvement of the postero-superior pancreato-duodenal, retroportal, right celiac, hepatic, and superior mesenteric nodes. The inter-aorto-caval nodes represent the terminal nodes of the regional lymphatic drainage system of gallbladder. Spread to these lymph nodes is regarded as distant metastasis. Hematogenous metastases are most commonly seen in the liver.

Differential Diagnosis

Gallbladder carcinoma manifesting as diffuse gallbladder wall thickening has a differential diagnosis that includes the more common inflammatory and noninflammatory causes of wall thickening. These conditions include heart failure, cirrhosis, hepatitis, hypoalbuminemia, renal failure, and cholecystitis (69). Occasionally, a pericholecystic abscess, gallbladder necrosis, or fistula formation to adjacent bowel can complicate acute cholecystitis (Figure 9.19). The findings in these cases may simulate those of an aggressive neoplastic process. Gallbladder carcinoma should be suspected when there are features of a focal mass, lymphadenopathy, hepatic metastases, and biliary obstruction at the level of the porta hepatis (11, 69, 70).

Xanthogranulomatous cholecystitis is a pseudotumoral inflammatory condition of the gallbladder that radiologically simulates gallbladder carcinoma (73).

The MR features of xanthogranulomatous cholecystitis and gallbladder carcinoma overlap substantially; thus, these entities cannot be reliably differentiated (73). Both diseases may demonstrate gallbladder wall thickening, infiltration of the surrounding fat, hepatic involvement, and lymphadenopathy (73).

Adenomyomatosis is a common tumor-like lesion of the gallbladder with discussed malignant potential (69). It may involve the gallbladder in a focal, segmental, or diffuse form. Its histologic features include a proliferation of epithelial and mural elements, and Rokitansky-Aschoff sinuses are seen as prominent infoldings of the epithelium (69). Rokitansky-Aschoff sinuses are best visualized on T2w sequences; therefore, MR imaging can be useful for distinguishing this benign entity from gallbladder carcinoma (Figure 9.20) (74).

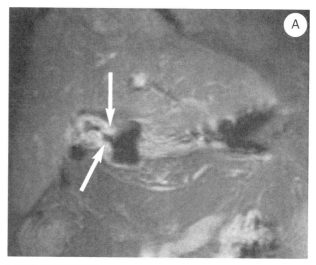

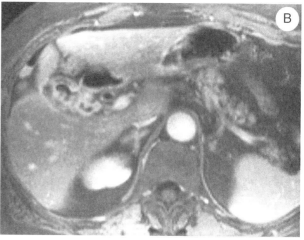

FIGURE 9.19

Complicated cholecystitis: thickening of the wall. Coronal (A) and axial (B) gadolinium-enhanced T1w images show irregular enhancement of the thickened gallbladder wall communicating with the duodenum (arrows)

The differential diagnosis for those tumors that manifest as an intraluminal polypoid mass includes adenomatous, hyperplastic, and cholesterol polyps; carcinoid tumor; metastatic melanoma; and hematoma within the gallbladder.

The differential diagnosis for a mass replacing the gallbladder fossa includes hepatocellular carcinoma, cholangiocarcinoma, and metastatic disease to the gallbladder fossa.

Extrahepatic Cholangiocarcinoma

Extrahepatic cholangiocarcinoma is an adenocarcinoma arising from the bile ducts below the bifurcation of the right and left hepatic ducts. Fifty to 75% of extrahepatic cholangiocarcinomas occur in the upper third, 10-30% in the middle third, and 10-20% in the

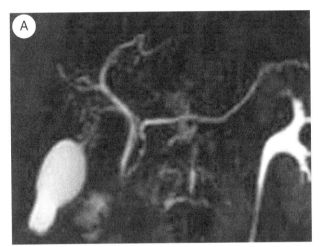

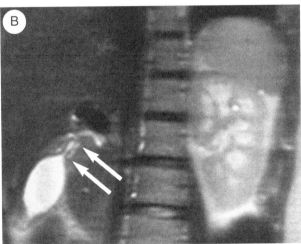

FIGURE 9.20

Gallbladder focal adenomyomatosis. MRCP (A) and coronal single shot T2w images (B) show focal thickening of the gallbladder neck with hyperintense small dots corresponding with Rokitansky-Aschoff sinuses (arrows).

lower third of the extrahepatic duct (75). Many extrahepatic cholangiocarcinomas, because the bile ducts are occluded during the early stage, are diagnosed when they are small (10, 75). Bile ducts proximal to the tumor are dilated, and the severity of this dilatation depends on the degree and duration of the obstruction. Like the previous forms, they are divided into mass-forming, periductal-infiltrating, and intraductal-growing types (75).

Mass-Forming Cholangiocarcinoma

This usually is a single nodule measuring 1-2 cm in diameter obstructing the bile duct. Because it is small, US may not identify the mass, which may be masked by adjacent structures or obscured by duodenal gas (6, 10). The bile ducts are usually completely obstructed, whereas the duct distal to the mass regains its normal diameter. MRCP shows dilated bile ducts proximally (Figure 9.21C). Like the previously described "mass-forming" type, the tumor is hypointense and hyperintense, respectively, on T1w and T2w images, demonstrating enhancement better visualized on delayed phase (5-10 minutes after injection of c.m.) (Figure 9.21B) (10, 42, 76).

Periductal-Infiltrating Cholangiocarcinoma

In periductal-infiltrating extrahepatic cholangiocarcinoma, the involved bile ducts show a concentric thickening of the bile duct wall that varies in length (10). On CT and MR images, this parietal thickening can be depicted better on enhanced images as a ring or spot (Figure 9.22). The tumor margin appears as an abrupt transition or as an asymmetrically thickened bile duct wall at the transition zone (Figure 9.22) (10, 24, 75). Adjacent periductal fat may be infiltrated by direct invasion, and lymph node metastasis is relatively frequent.

Because of bile duct obstruction, ERCP depicts only the distal normal segment of the bile duct, and PTC may depict only the dilated proximal ducts (10). However, MRI depicts the cancer involved segment as well as the proximal and distal normal bile ducts (77). In patients with a partial obstruction, the cancer-involved segment may be delineated as a string-like stenotic bile duct (10, 75, 77). Only MRI demonstrating the extraductal component of the tumor indicates the true extent of the lesion (10).

Intraductal-Growing Cholangiocarcinoma

Intraductal-growing cholangiocarcinoma of the extrahepatic duct accounts for about 10% of cholangiocarcinomas (75). It may be polypoid, sessile, or superfi-

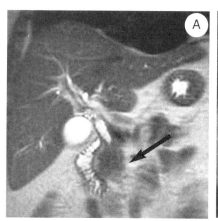
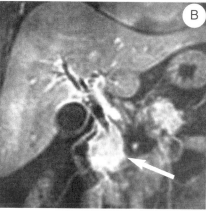
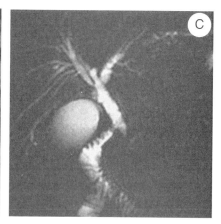

FIGURE 9.21

Mass-forming cholangiocarcinoma of the distal extrahepatic duct. Coronal image from thin-slices T2w single-shot TSE sequence (A) and contrast-enhanced T1w image (B) clearly depict a well defined mass (arrows) involving the wall of the distal bile duct, highly enhanced after c.m administration. (C) Single thick slab MRCP (coronal projection) shows severe strictures in the distal bile duct and the dilated upstream duct.

cially spreading along the bile duct lumen, single or ,more frequently, multiple (56). Most intraductal-growing cholangiocarcinomas are papillary cholangiocarcinomas. Sometimes the tumor can slough spontaneously and simulate a bile duct stone, which intermittently occludes the bile duct (57). On CT and MRI, the tumor usually appears as an intraluminally enhancing mass or as eccentric wall thickening (Figure 9.23) (40, 56). Precontrast T1w sequences are important in the differential diagnosis because a tumor attached to the wall of the bile duct will be enhanced (Figure 9.23C), whereas detached tumor fragments or stones will not. Rarely,

lymph nodes are enlarged. MRCP allows visualization of papillary intraductal tumors as a defect in the hyperintense duct (Figure 9.23A). Sometimes multiple papillary proliferations can involve intra- and extrahepatic ducts, resulting in floating masses mimicking bile duct stones. On MR, stones have a low signal intensity on T2w images; in contrast, a mass protruding into the bile duct lumen usually has the same signal intensity of the liver. At MRCP stones usually have a smooth, sometimes faceted surface, whereas papillary tumors are irregular or velvety (57).

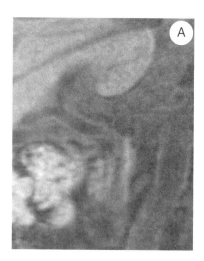
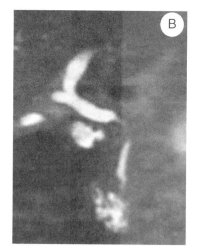
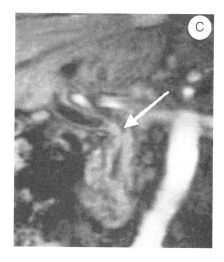

FIGURE 9.22

Periductal infiltrating extrahepatic cholangiocarcinoma. Coronal images from nonenhanced T1w (A) and thin-slice T2w (B) sequences show initial dilatation of the intrahepatic bile ducts with focal circumferential narrowing of the middle portion of CBD. (C) After administration of c.m., late-phase coronal image shows peripheral enhancement that envelops the wall of the CBD, which appears thickened (arrow).

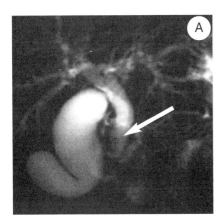 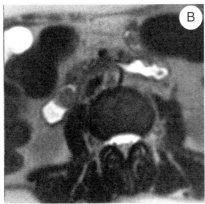 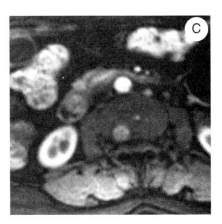

FIGURE 9.23

Intraductal-growing papillary cholangiocarcinoma of the distal common bile duct. (A) MRCP shows a small defect (arrow) in the mild dilated lower bile duct. T2w (B) and contrast-enhanced (C) MR images show a hypointense (B) well-defined mass protruding into the duodenal lumen. After c.m. administration the lesion is enhanced (C).

Differential Diagnosis

Most extrahepatic cholangiocarcinomas are of the infiltrative type and manifest as a focal stricture of the bile duct, whereas papillary carcinoma is occasionally found (78). Preoperative histologic diagnosis of extrahepatic cholangiocarcinoma depends solely on endoscopic tissue sampling and cytologic analysis. Endoscopic biopsy or brushing of the stricture requires a high degree of skill on the part of the endoscopist, and the lesions may not always be accessible; sensitivity of the test therefore ranges from 44 to 100% (79). Moreover, in the infiltrative type, endoscopic findings and tissue sampling frequently are unsatisfactory because intramural spread beneath the bile duct epithelium and abundant fibrosis interfere with adequate tissue sampling and lead to high false-negative rates (78, 79). MRCP has been reported to be highly sensitive (72-98%) for the diagnosis of biliary obstruction (24). The reported sensitivity of MRCP for differentiating benign from malignant biliary obstructions, however, ranges very widely, from 30 to 98% (4, 16, 24, 29, 79). An irregular and asymmetric stricture margin is more common in cholangiocarcinoma, and a smooth and symmetric stricture margin is more common in benign stricture (Figure 9.24). Irregular margins and asymmetric narrowing, however, were not specific to malignant strictures but were seen also in benign strictures. The involved segment of stricture is longer in cholangiocarcinoma than in benign stricture. The degree of bile duct dilatation and the frequency of depiction of the double-duct sign are not significantly specific to differentiate cholangiocarcinoma and benign stricture. In summary, a lengthy biliary stricture with asymmetric narrowing and an irregular margin may indicate cholangiocarcinoma (78). On the other hand, a short stricture with symmetric narrowing and a smooth mar-

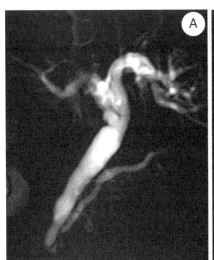 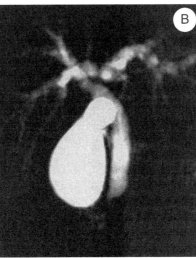

FIGURE 9.24

Benign versus malignant distal biliary stenosis: MRCP appearance. (A) MRCP shows mild dilation of the common bile duct, which presents as "mouse-tail" morphology in its distal tract with tapered margin (sclero-odditis). (B) MRCP shows irregular, asymmetric, and angled stenosis at the level of ampulla (ampulloma).

gin may indicate a benign lesion rather than cholangiocarcinoma (78). A malignant CBD stricture is characterized by strong enhancement during the hepatic arterial or portal venous phase, a thick wall (more than 1.5 mm), a longer involved segment and a more dilated duct proximal to the involved CBD than observed in cases of benign stricture (10, 78) .

As reported by Andersson et al. (80) MRI with MRCP was significantly more accurate than CT in differentiating between malignant and benign lesions in patients with suspected distal biliary tumors, mainly due to the information obtained on the MRCP images of the biliary and pancreatic duct anatomy.

The performance of MRCP in enabling differentiation of benign strictures from strictures caused by extrahepatic cholangiocarcinoma is comparable with that of ERCP, and the differential diagnosis may be similarly difficult with both tests (78).

References

1. Sherlock S. Disease of the Liver and Biliary System. 10th ed. London: Blackwell, 1997:642-649
2. Lygidakis NJ, et al. Long-term results following resectional surgery for Klatskin tumors. A twenty-year personal experience. Hepatogastroenterology 2001; 48(37):95-101.
3. Brink JA, Borrello JA. MR imaging of the biliary system. Magn Reson Imaging Clin N Am 1995; 3(1):143-160.
4. Low RN, et al. Evaluation of malignant biliary obstruction: efficacy of fast multiplanar spoiled gradient-recalled MR imaging vs spin-echo MR imaging, CT, and cholangiography. AJR Am J Roentgenol 1994; 162(2):315-323.
5. Bloom CM, Langer B, Wilson SR. Role of US in the detection, characterization, and staging of cholangiocarcinoma. Radiographics 1999; 19(5):1199-1218.
6. Hann LE, et al. Cholangiocarcinoma at the hepatic hilus: sonographic findings. AJR Am J Roentgenol 1997; 168(4):985-989.
7. Takehara Y. Can MRCP replace ERCP? J Magn Reson Imaging 1998; 8(3):517-534.
8. Nichols DA, MacCarty RL, Gaffey TA. Cholangiographic evaluation of bile duct carcinoma. AJR Am J Roentgenol 1983; 141(6):1291-1294.
9. Kim HJ, et al. Biliary ductal evaluation of hilar cholangiocarcinoma: three-dimensional direct multi-detector row CT cholangiographic findings versus surgical and pathologic results—feasibility study. Radiology 2006; 238(1):300-308.
10. Guarise A, et al. Role of magnetic resonance in characterising extrahepatic cholangiocarcinomas. Radiol Med (Torino) 2006; 111(4):526-538.
11. Heller SL, Lee VS. MR imaging of the gallbladder and biliary system. Magn Reson Imaging Clin N Am 2005; 13(2):295-311.
12. Manfredi R, et al. Magnetic resonance imaging of cholangiocarcinoma. Semin Liver Dis 2004; 24(2):155-164.
13. Vogl TJ, et al. Staging of Klatskin tumors (hilar cholangiocarcinomas): comparison of MR cholangiography, MR imaging, and endoscopic retrograde cholangiography. Eur Radiol 2006; 16(10):2317-2325.
14. Vahldiek G, Broemel T, Klapdo R. MR-cholangiopancreaticography (MRCP) and MR-angiography: morphologic changes with magnetic resonance imaging. Anticancer Res 1999; 19(4A):2451-2458.
15. Takehara Y. Fast MR imaging for evaluating the pancreaticobiliary system. Eur J Radiol 1999; 29(3):211-232.
16. Pavone P, Laghi A, Passariello R. MR cholangiopancreatography in malignant biliary obstruction. Semin Ultrasound CT MR 1999; 20(5):317-323.
17. Slattery JM, Sahani DV. What is the current state-of-the-art imaging for detection and staging of cholangiocarcinoma? Oncologist 2006; 11(8):913-922.
18. Wiedmann M, et al. (Current diagnostics and therapy for carcinomas of the biliary tree and gallbladder). Z Gastroenterol 2005; 43(3):305-315.
19. Adamek HE, et al. A prospective evaluation of magnetic resonance cholangiopancreatography in patients with suspected bile duct obstruction. Gut 1998; 43(5):680-683.
20. Zhong L, et al. Imaging diagnosis of pancreato-biliary diseases: a control study. World J Gastroenterol 2003; 9(12):2824-2827.
21. Hanninen EL, et al. Magnetic resonance imaging including magnetic resonance cholangiopancreatography for tumor localization and therapy planning in malignant hilar obstructions. Acta Radiol 2005; 46(5):462-470.
22. Lorenzen M, et al. [Quality rating of MR-cholangiopancreatography with oral application of iron oxide particles]. Rofo 2003; 175(7):936-941.
23. Reinhold C, Bret PM. Current status of MR cholangiopancreatography. AJR Am J Roentgenol 1996; 166(6):1285-1295.
24. Lee MG, et al. Extrahepatic biliary diseases: 3D MR cholangiopancreatography compared with endoscopic retrograde cholangiopancreatography. Radiology 1997; 202(3):663-669.
25. Mehta SN, Reinhold C, Barkun AN. Magnetic resonance cholangiopancreatography. Gastrointest Endosc Clin N Am 1997; 7(2):247-270.
26. Schaible R, et al. (Value of selective MIP reconstructions in respiratory triggered 3D TSE MR-cholangiography on a workstation in comparison with MIP standard projections and single-shot MRCP). Rofo 2001; 173(5):416-423.
27. Boraschi P, et al. MR cholangiopancreatography: value of axial and coronal fast Spin-Echo fat-suppressed T2-weighted sequences. Eur J Radiol 1999; 32(3):171-181.
28. Ito K, Koike S, Matsunaga N. MR imaging of pancreatic diseases. Eur J Radiol 2001; 38(2):78-93.
29. Kim MJ, et al. Biliary dilatation: differentiation of benign from malignant causes—value of adding conventional MR imaging to MR cholangiopancreatography. Radiology 2000; 214(1):173-181.
30. Patrizio G, et al. [A comparative study between Gd-BOPTA, a biliary excretion contrast medium, and Gd-DTPA in the magnetic resonance imaging of the rat liver]. Radiol Med (Torino) 1990; 79(5):458-462.
31. Ferrucci JT. Advances in abdominal MR imaging. Radiographics 1998; 18(6):1569-1586.
32. Schima W. [Organ specific MRI contrast media in general practice]. Wien Med Wochenschr Suppl 2002; (113):8-11.
33. Patel T. Increasing incidence and mortality of primary intrahepatic cholangiocarcinoma in the United States. Hepatology 2001; 33(6):1353-1357.
34. Nakajima T, et al. A histopathologic study of 102 cases of intrahepatic cholangiocarcinoma: histologic classification and modes of spreading. Hum Pathol 1988; 19(10):1228-1234.
35. Lim JH. Cholangiocarcinoma: morphologic classification according to growth pattern and imaging findings. AJR Am J Roentgenol 2003; 181(3):819-827.
36. Japan, L.C.S.G.o. The General Rules for the Clinical and Pathological Study of Primary Liver Cancer. 4th ed. Tokyo: Kanehara, 2000.
37. Choi BI, et al. Clonorchiasis and cholangiocarcinoma: etiologic relationship and imaging diagnosis. Clin Microbiol Rev 2004; 17(3):540-552, table of contents.
38. Watanapa P, Watanapa WB. Liver fluke-associated cholangiocarcinoma. Br J Surg 2002; 89(8):962-970.
39. Ros PR, et al. Intrahepatic cholangiocarcinoma: radiologic-pathologic correlation. Radiology 1988; 167(3):689-693.
40. Lee WJ, et al. Radiologic spectrum of cholangiocarcinoma: emphasis on unusual manifestations and differential diagnoses. Radiographics 2001; 21(Spec No):S97-S116.
41. Fan ZM, et al. Intrahepatic cholangiocarcinoma: spin-echo and contrast-enhanced dynamic MR imaging. AJR Am J Roentgenol 1993; 161(2):313-317.

42. Worawattanakul S, et al. Cholangiocarcinoma: spectrum of appearances on MR images using current techniques. Magn Reson Imaging 1998; 16(9):993-1003.
43. Choi BI, Lee JM, Han JK. Imaging of intrahepatic and hilar cholangiocarcinoma. Abdom Imaging 2004; 29(5):548-557.
44. Gabata T, et al. Delayed MR imaging of the liver: correlation of delayed enhancement of hepatic tumors and pathologic appearance. Abdom Imaging 1998; 23(3):309-313.
45. Han SL, et al. Diagnosis and surgical treatment of primary hepatic cholangiocarcinoma. Hepatogastroenterology 2005; 52(62):348-351.
46. Asayama Y, et al. Delayed-phase dynamic CT enhancement as a prognostic factor for mass-forming intrahepatic cholangio-carcinoma. Radiology 2006; 238(1):150-155.
47. Awaya H, et al. Differential diagnosis of hepatic tumors with delayed enhancement at gadolinium-enhanced MRI: a pictorial essay. Clin Imaging 1998; 22(3):180-187.
48. Yoshida Y, et al. Intrahepatic cholangiocarcinoma with marked hypervascularity. Abdom Imaging 1999; 24(1):66-68.
49. Choi BI, et al. Characterization of focal hepatic tumors. Value of two-phase scanning with spiral computed tomography. Cancer 1995; 76(12):2434-2442.
50. Giovagnoni A, Paci E. Liver. III: Gadolinium-based hepatobiliary contrast agents (Gd-EOB-DTPA and Gd-BOPTA/Dimeg). Magn Reson Imaging Clin N Am 1996; 4(1):61-72.
51. Braga HJ, Imam K, Bluemke DA. MR imaging of intrahepatic cholangiocarcinoma: use of ferumoxides for lesion localization and extension. AJR Am J Roentgenol 2001; 177(1):111-114.
52. Maetani Y, et al. MR imaging of intrahepatic cholangiocarcinoma with pathologic correlation. AJR Am J Roentgenol 2001; 176(6):1499-1507.
53. Soyer P, et al. CT of hepatic tumors: prevalence and specificity of retraction of the adjacent liver capsule. AJR Am J Roentgenol 1994; 162(5):1119-1122.
54. Soto JA, et al. Biliary obstruction: findings at MR cholangiography and cross-sectional MR imaging. Radiographics 2000; 20(2):353-366.
55. Yeh TS, et al. Malignant perihilar biliary obstruction: magnetic resonance cholangiopancreatographic findings. Am J Gastroenterol 2000; 95(2):432-440.
56. Han JK, Lee JM. Intrahepatic intraductal cholangiocarcinoma. Abdom Imaging 2004; 29(5):558-564.
57. Lim JH, et al. Radiological spectrum of intraductal papillary tumors of the bile ducts. Korean J Radiol 2002; 3(1):57-63.
58. Jarnagin WR, et al. Staging, resectability, and outcome in 225 patients with hilar cholangiocarcinoma. Ann Surg 2001; 234(4):507-17; discussion 517-59.
59. Lopera JE, Soto JA, Munera F. Malignant hilar and perihilar biliary obstruction: use of MR cholangiography to define the extent of biliary ductal involvement and plan percutaneous interventions. Radiology 2001; 220(1):90-96.
60. Koea J, et al. Differential diagnosis of stenosing lesions at the hepatic hilus. World J Surg 2004; 28(5):466-470.
61. Manfredi R, et al. (Malignant biliary hilar stenosis: MR cholangiography compared with direct cholangiography). Radiol Med (Torino) 2001; 102(1-2):48-54.

62. Venkataraman S, et al. Inflammatory myofibroblastic tumor of the hepatobiliary system: report of MR imaging appearance in four patients. Radiology 2003; 227(3):758-763.
63. Choi BY, et al. Inflammatory myofibroblastic tumor of the liver in a child: CT and MR findings. Pediatr Radiol 2003; 33(1):30-33.
64. Tublin ME, et al. Biliary inflammatory pseudotumor: imaging features in seven patients. AJR Am J Roentgenol 2007; 188(1):W44-48.
65. Kelekis NL, et al. Focal hepatic lymphoma: magnetic resonance demonstration using current techniques including gadolinium enhancement. Magn Reson Imaging 1997; 15(6):625-636.
66. Zhong L, Li L, Yao QY. Preoperative evaluation of pancreaticobiliary tumor using MR multi-imaging techniques. World J Gastroenterol 2005; 11(24):3756-3761.
67. Lee MG, et al. Preoperative evaluation of hilar cholangiocarcinoma with contrast-enhanced three-dimensional fast imaging with steady-state precession magnetic resonance angiography: comparison with intraarterial digital subtraction angiography. World J Surg 2003; 27(3):278-283.
68. Misra S, et al. Carcinoma of the gallbladder. Lancet Oncol 2003; 4(3):167-176.
69. Levy AD, Murakata LA, Rohrmann, Jr., CA. Gallbladder carcinoma: radiologic-pathologic correlation. Radiographics 2001; 21(2):295-314; questionnaire, 549-555.
70. Adusumilli S, Siegelman ES. MR imaging of the gallbladder. Magn Reson Imaging Clin N Am 2002; 10(1):165-184.
71. Schwartz LH, et al. Gallbladder carcinoma: findings at MR imaging with MR cholangiopancreatography. J Comput Assist Tomogr 2002; 26(3):405-10.
72. Demachi H, et al. Dynamic MRI using a surface coil in chronic cholecystitis and gallbladder carcinoma: radiologic and histopathologic correlation. J Comput Assist Tomogr 1997; 21(4):643-651.
73. Gore RM, et al. Imaging benign and malignant disease of the gallbladder. Radiol Clin North Am 2002; 40(6):1307-1323, vi.
74. Yoshimitsu K, et al. MR diagnosis of adenomyomatosis of the gallbladder and differentiation from gallbladder carcinoma: importance of showing Rokitansky-Aschoff sinuses. AJR Am J Roentgenol 1999; 172(6):1535-1540.
75. Lim JH, et al. Imaging of extrahepatic cholangiocarcinoma. Abdom Imaging 2004; 29(5):565-571.
76. Di Cesare E, et al. Malignant obstructive jaundice: comparison of MRCP and ERCP in the evaluation of distal lesions. Radiol Med (Torino) 2003; 105(5-6):445-453.
77. Takehara Y. Preoperative assessment of extrahepatic cholangiocarcinoma with imaging. Abdom Imaging 2004; 29(5):572-580.
78. Park MS, et al. Differentiation of extrahepatic bile duct cholangiocarcinoma from benign stricture: findings at MRCP versus ERCP. Radiology 2004; 233(1):234-240.
79. Cohen MB, et al. Brush cytology of the extrahepatic biliary tract: comparison of cytologic features of adenocarcinoma and benign biliary strictures. Mod Pathol 1995; 8(5):498-502.
80. Andersson M, et al. MRI combined with MR cholangiopancreatography versus helical CT in the evaluation of patients with suspected periampullary tumors: a prospective comparative study. Acta Radiol 2005; 46(1):16-27.

10 Functional Imaging

Antonio Rodríguez-Fernández
Manuel Gómez-Río
José Manuel Llamas-Elvira

In gallbladder cancer (GBC), the challenge for any diagnostic imaging procedure is to be early and specific. The nonspecific clinical manifestations of this disease hamper an early diagnosis, and this situation is complicated by the fact that surgery remains the only available curative treatment. Because GBC is therefore usually only detected in advanced stages, there is a need for accurate presurgical staging to avoid unnecessary surgery in patients with metastatic disease.

As in conventional radiology, GBC diagnosis by nuclear medicine (NM) procedures is based on the detection of indirect signs produced by the growth and invasion of the tumor. These signs are often only detected in advanced stages and are also commonly produced by benign diseases of the gallbladder (1). Although conventional NM techniques can contribute valuable functional data on the hepato-biliary system, they are less useful for direct examination of GBC. This information is frequently related to tumor-induced obstruction or hepatic invasion and can assist treatment planning and interpretation of the local and systemic repercussions of the disease. We recommend the reviews by Zeismman et al. on the use of these procedures in acute cholecystitis, biliary obstruction, and biliary leakage (2) and on the examination of chronic acalculous gallbladder or biliary disease (3).

The relatively recent inclusion of positron emission tomography (PET) tracers may be useful for the specific study of GBC. This chapter describes the contribution of biochemical imaging with PET procedures to the study of GBC.

POSITRON EMISSION TOMOGRAPHY: THE PHYSICS

PET is the volumetric imaging registration of the biodistribution of biomolecules labeled with radionuclides decaying by positron emission. These radionuclides are produced in a cyclotron and usually have a relatively short physical half-life, which means that the cyclotron must be in close physical proximity to the detection devices, designated positron cameras, scanners, or tomographs. From its beginnings, the development of PET instrumentation has been based on advances in multiple scientific fields, e.g., atomic physics, electronics, and computing. Since the introduction by Phelps and Hoffman (1974-1976) of the first PET devices (4), major technological improvements have been made, especially in the labeling of metabolic substrates with radiotracers that use biologically ubiquitous atoms (e.g., carbon, oxygen, nitrogen) and can offer direct physiologic information.

Positrons are antiparticles of electrons, having the same properties but an opposite electric charge. They derive from the disintegration of an unstable nucleus with a neutron:proton ratio of <1. The positron (β^+) emitted by the nucleus loses its kinetic energy in the tissue through which it moves. When most of its kinetic energy has been lost, the positron collides with a resident electron in an annihilation reaction, resulting in two 511 keV gamma photons emitted in a straight line of coincidence (also called formally the "line of response" or LOR) but opposite direction (Figure 10.1).

Since PET radionuclides have a short half-life, they must be rapidly added to the radiopharmaceuticals at a laboratory situated alongside the cyclotron. The most widely used PET radionuclides are C-11, N-13, O-15, and F-18, and their key physical characteristics are summarized in Table 10.1 (5). F-18 is the most interesting radionuclide for diagnostic use because of its chemistry and physics (half-life: 109.6 minutes), allowing it to be used in centers at some distance from the cyclotron (6).

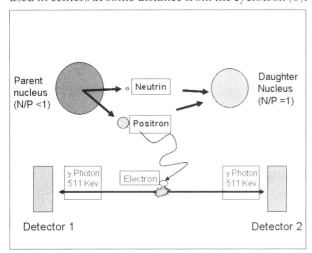

FIGURE 10.1

Annihilation diagram.

TABLE 10.1
Mean Physical Characteristics of PET Radionuclides for Clinical Use

		POSITRONS			PHOTONS		
ISOTOPE	T1/2 (min)	n°	%	$E_{\beta+}$ (KeV)	n°	%	$E_{\beta+}$ (KeV)
C-11	20.4	1	99.7	960	2	193.46	511
N-13	9.9	1	99.8	1198	2	199.61	511
O-15	2.0	1	99.9	1732	2	199.80	511
F-18	109.6	1	96.73	634	2	193.46	511

Source: Ref. 5.

PHARMACOLOGIC AND BIOCHEMICAL BASES

The most important phase of the process is the recording of temporal changes in the radioactivity proceeding from the distribution of the radiopharmaceutical after its administration (usually intravenous) to the patient. Several characteristics have been proposed for the ideal radiopharmaceutical for PET, e.g., an easy uptake by target tissue, low unspecific absorption, elevated affinity for the binding site, and an appropriate time period related to clearance, nonspecific vascular activity, and low or no catabolism to facilitate mathematic modeling (7).

PET permits the study and quantification of various biochemical pathways and parameters, e.g., energetic metabolism, protein synthesis rate, cell proliferation, intracellular pH, blood flow, signal transmission, or gene expression and regulation. Some of these aspects are summarized in Table 10.2.

FDG: 2-Deoxy-2-(18F)Fluoro-D-Glucose

The most widely used radiopharmaceutical in PET is 2-deoxy-2-(18F)fluoro-D-glucose (FDG) (8), due to its relatively long half-life (110 minutes), easy synthesis, and metabolic characteristics, allowing its use in a wide range of clinical situations.

FDG is a structural analog of D-glucose (missing an OH group in position 2) and can therefore be introduced into the cell by two types of specific cell membrane receptors: (a) Na+/glucose transporters (SGLT1 and SGLT2), with expression of both subtypes even in low molar concentrations of glucose and allowing introduction of glucose against the concentration gradient; and (b) passive diffusion transporters, designated Glut 1-5 , with the passage of glucose into the cell related to the number and activity of these receptors and to blood insulin levels (8).

Once within the cell, FDG is phosphorylated by hexokinase to 18F-2-DG-6P, an intermediary compound that has a higher polarity than glucose and does not freely cross the membrane, remaining trapped within tumor cells. This molecule could convert to fructose-6P and enter the Krebs cycle or (theoretically) undergo gluconeogenesis as glucose-6P due to an isomerase, although this enzyme does not act on 18F-2-DG-6P. 18F-2-DG-6P may be dephosphorylated by glucose-6-Pase, allowing it to pass through the cell membrane to interstitial space. This pathway is relatively slow in tumor cells, which usually lack this enzyme, resulting in a selective metabolic trapping of 18F-2-DG-6P in the cells. This allows external detection of the decay of 18F and

TABLE 10.2
Biochemical Use of PET Radiopharmaceuticals

Metabolic pathways	Glycolysis	2-Deoxy-2-(18F)fluoro-D-glucose (FDG)
	ß-Oxidation	(^{11}C)Palmitate (^{11}C)Acetate
	DNA synthesis	(^{11}C)Thymidine (^{18}F)Fluorothymidine
	Protein synthesis	(^{11}C)Methionine (^{18}F)Tyrosine (^{18}F)Fluoro-L-DOPA
Regional blood flow	By diffusion	(^{15}O)Water Rubidium-82
	By extraction	(^{13}N)Ammonia

study of its in vivo distribution in the patient (8, 9) (Figure 10.2).

The metabolic behavior of the FDG is different in tumor cells than in normal cells, which is especially useful for the study of oncologic processes. The underlying mechanisms proposed for this differentiation are (9):

1. Higher expression of glucose transporters (Glut receptors) on the cell surface. Intake of glucose (and therefore FDG) is accelerated due to a higher need for nutrients and a decreased metabolic rate (oxygen/glucose consumption), implying a predominantly anaerobic metabolism of the glucose.

2. Higher hexokinase activity.

3. Lower glucose-6-phosphatase level compared with most normal tissues (tumor dedifferentiation?).

As a general rule, images are acquired 45-60 minutes after intravenous injection of the radiopharmaceutical, an adequate time for all of the metabolic processes described above (10).

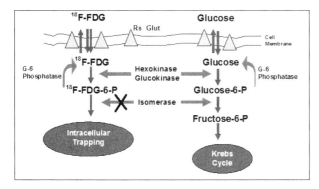

FIGURE 10.2

Metabolism of glucose and FDG.

IMAGE ANALYSIS

After the image is acquired and processed, it is can be analyzed by visual or semiquantitative analysis. **Visual interpretation** is the most common method. Tumors are identified as an area with higher FDG activity in comparison with surrounding healthy tissue. Grading can be carried out with respect to neighboring tissue, usually the liver in GBC cases (10).

Semiquantitative methods use an imaging matrix in which the value of the pixel is proportional to the concentration (measured as activity) of the radiopharmaceutical in the studied area. Quantitation can be based on a semiquantitative index that relates lesion activity to the administered dose and body weight (standardized uptake value, SUV) or to activity in a reference area (tumor-to-background ratio). The most common semiquantitative index is the SUV, defined by the ratio between tumor FDG activity (mCi/g) and injected dose (mCi) divided by the body weight in grams. The resulting parameter is adimensional.

SUV measurements can be influenced by the following factors (7, 11): the **spatial resolution** of the PET camera, which determines the capacity to detect or miss small (<10-15 mm) lesions; the **body weight** of the patient, which affects the SUV because the body fat compartment is not part of the volume of FDG distribution; **blood glucose levels**, which affect the biodistribution of FDG, with high levels reducing tumor FDG uptake (which does not occur in inflammatory disease). Finally (10, 12, 13), the FDG **injection-image acquisition** interval has important effects. With a longer interval, FDG uptake is higher in tumor tissue but lower in benign lesions, providing the "differential clearance."

SUV measurements can be used to characterize a lesion. A value above 2.5 should raise the possibility of a malignancy (14), although this is not always the case. FDG accumulation can also be observed in benign conditions or lesions, since inflammation or infection (e.g., granulomatous diseases) can produce focal infiltration of metabolically active host cells. Consequently, numerous groups have considered SUV to be complementary to visual analysis (14, 15). In order to obtain a high specificity, it is necessary to know the patterns of normal and pathologic FDG distribution and to use semiquantitative algorithms.

CLINICAL APPLICATIONS

Study of the diagnostic accuracy of FDG-PET in GBC is limited by the low prevalence of GBC (0.5-7.4% of autopsies, 1% of cholecystectomies) (16) and by the poor prognosis of the disease in advanced stages, leading to a reluctance to use invasive procedures to confirm the diagnosis. Therefore, most of the information on the clinical use of FDG-PET in GBC derives from relatively small case series in reports on positive findings for GBC and on the potential shortcomings and pitfalls of this diagnostic method. No studies have been conducted in large series of patients covering the full spectrum of disease, and ethical considerations impede the performance of examinations under independent and blinded conditions. Nevertheless, although high-quality evidence is not available, published studies offer some valuable information with immediate repercussions for the clinical management of patients.

In routine clinical practice, the diagnostic accuracy in GBC is related to the algorithm applied in different local settings, i.e., the order in which structural imaging, notably ultrasonography (US), and functional imaging is applied (17). FDG-PET has been used in the diagnostic workup for malignancy in gallbladder lesion and after the incidental finding of GBC after cholecystectomy, when posttreatment FDG-PET has been applied for residual tumor detection and staging.

Diagnostic Workup for Malignancy in Gallbladder Lesion

Despite unfavorable outcomes, surgery usually represents the only therapeutic option in GBC. Hence, a reliable staging algorithm is required to distinguish between patients who can and cannot benefit from surgery.

As already mentioned, FDG-PET is generally performed after structural procedures. In GBC cases, these procedures include conventional or helical computed tomography (CT) and magnetic resonance (MR) or MR cholangiopancreatography, etc., whose results are influenced by the skill of the ultrasonographer and use of contrast media, among others (17). These factors can affect the sensitivity for diagnosing GBC and lead to potential pitfalls in both directions, i.e., false-negative or false-positive results. This may produce a bias in the selection for FDG-PET that might in part explain why the diagnostic accuracy of FDG-PET has proven superior to that of CT (usually helical CT) in all published series. In general, radiology is expected to be more specific with respect to unspecific clinical findings and FDG-PET more specific with respect to unspecific radiologic signs. The most common findings by structural imaging techniques are (a) complete occupation or replacement of gallbladder lumen by the mass (in 40-65% of published series), (b) focal or diffuse parietal thickening (20-30% of series), and (c) intraluminal polyp (15-25%) (18).

In most FDG-PET reports, GBC is described as a "hot" lesion that results from active incorporation of FDG into tumor cells and occupies the gallbladder layer or is found near the hepatic hilum, with a higher uptake than observed in the surrounding liver tissue (17) (Figures 10.3, 10.4). This uptake of the radiotracer can be quantified on a subjective visual analysis scale (establishing relationship with surrounding tissue) (10) or by objective determination of the SUV, which usually shows a value of >2.5 in GBC.

Koh et al. (19) studied the differential diagnosis of GBC with FDG-PET in 16 candidates for surgery with only protuberant lesions of the gallbladder. A global diagnostic accuracy of 81% (sensitivity, 75%; specificity, 87.5%) was obtained by this approach compared with an accuracy of 68.8% obtained with CT (sensitivity, 62.5%; specificity, 75%), in a series with a GBC prevalence of 50%. Two false negatives were produced in a patient with diabetes and in another with a small lesion (13 mm) and one false negative in a patient with xanthogranulomatous cholecystitis.

When only the finding of parietal thickening was considered (20), the global accuracy for GBC diagnosis was 93% (sensitivity, 75%; specificity, 100%; tumor prevalence, 3/12), with one false positive in a patient with chronic cholecystitis. FDG-PET findings that rule out GBC and therefore avoid surgical management are of value.

Similar results to the above were obtained by our group (21) using FDG-PET in the presurgical workup of 16 patients with suspected GBC lesions (sensitivity, 80%; specificity, 82%; tumor prevalence, 31.2%). There was one false negative in a mucinous adenocarcinoma with low metabolic rate and two false positives, one in a tuberculous granuloma (22) with caseous necrosis and the other in a polyp with adenomy-

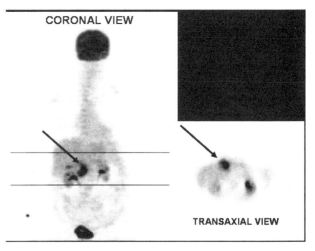

FIGURE 10.3

Gallbladder carcinoma. FDG-PET coronal and transaxial images showing high uptake at the gallbladder (arrows).

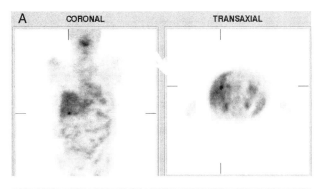

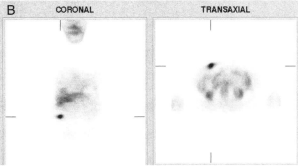

FIGURE 10.4

Gallbladder carcinoma. (A) FDG-PET coronal and transaxial images showing high uptake in liver at gallbladder bed. (B) Unexpected peritoneal implants.

omatosis. A more recent study (23) of a wider sample (24 patients) showed comparable results (sensitivity, 88%; specificity, 80%; tumor prevalence, 37.5%), with a false positive in an acute gangrenous cholecystitis and two cases of unsuspected dissemination (22.2% of patients with GBC, 8.3% of series). No significant difference in global diagnostic accuracy was found between the examination of protuberant lesions and lesions with parietal thickening.

In a similar group of patients (with suspicion of GBC by conventional radiologic studies), Nishiyama et al. (10) reported a significant increase in sensitivity (from 82.6 to 91.3%) by visually analyzing early (62 ± 8 min) and delayed imaging (146 ± 14 min), with no change in the specificity. This improvement is based on an increase in the contrast resolution, which gives a better lesion-to-background ratio. They also reported a greater accuracy for early and delayed SUV and retention index in patients with normal versus high C-reactive protein (CRP) levels. The prevalence of GBC in their series was 72%, and the specificity was relatively low (44.4%), especially in patients with severe inflammation (estimated by CRP levels). These authors suggest that only delayed imaging may be adequate for clinical diagnostic purposes.

No clear relationship has been established (20) between FDG-PET findings and CRP levels (10) or biochemical changes that indicate the severity of inflammatory disease (24). Nevertheless, our group shares the view that FDG-PET results should be interpreted with caution in patients with elevated inflammation, especially in the acute phase, given the possibility of false positive studies due to glucose uptake in activated inflammatory cells (10).

Incidental Finding of GBC after Cholecystectomy: Posttreatment FDG-PET for Residual Tumor Detection and Staging

GBC is often an incidental finding during cholecystectomy. In this situation, FDG-PET may be useful for initial staging or for restaging when recurrence is suspected.

After the first description by Lomis et al. (16) of recurrent GBC at laparoscopy port sites, there have been further reports of changes in the staging of GBC when FDG-PET examination has revealed unexpected presence (26) or spread (27) of the disease. Anderson et al. (28) used FDG-PET to examine 14 GBC patients with suspicion of residual carcinoma (defined as primary tumor, local gallbladder fossa invasion, or hepatic metastases) or distant metastases. Using these definitions, they found a sensitivity of 78% and specificity of 80% for FDG-PET in the diagnosis of residual carcinoma and a sensitivity of 0.56 in the detection of distant metastases or carcinomatosis, detecting peritoneal carcinomatosis in three out of six affected patients. This relatively low sensitivity in the case of carcinomatosis was attributed to the small size of the lesions (below the limits of detection of the equipment). There was one false-positive examination in a patient studied at one month after cholecystectomy, and this possibility must be kept in mind when the GBC diagnosis is incidental and postsurgical staging is performed. The prevalence of tumor activity was 64.3% in patients studied for the first time. Based on their results in this small sample of patients, Anderson et al. questioned the value of FDG-PET in the routine follow-up of these patients.

Possible regional lymph node involvement cannot usually be accurately established by the use of PET devices alone due to their low spatial resolution and the absence of anatomic reference structures. One case report has been published in this respect (26), but most groups have not adopted a specific approach for lymph node staging. Initial expectations about the contribution of new hybrid devices have been not endorsed by the only published study on this issue (29), which reported a detection rate of regional lymph node metastases by PET-CT of only 12% of affected cases, similar to that obtained with conventional systems (30). Although the impact on patient survival of regional lymph node spread in primary biliary cancer is controversial (31, 32), regional nodal involvement does not appear to alter the surgical approach and does not clearly contraindicate surgery (33).

Unlike N staging, the detection of distant metastases has immediate negative repercussions for survival, ruling out surgery with curative intent. FDG-PET has been described as a useful tool in this respect, not only to assess the prognosis but also to select patients for surgical resection. Although no specific approach has been proposed, detection of unsuspected distant metastases has been reported in 17% (29) to 30% (30) of patients with primary biliary tumors. In the former study, the majority of cases with unsuspected metastases (7/12) were in patients with GBC (29). In our experience with FDG-PET, unsuspected dissemination has been discovered in 22.2% of GBC patients, ruling out surgery (Figure 10.4). Evidently, this proportion could be lower in patients with suspicion of malignancy due to a space-occupying lesion than in patients evaluated for residual carcinoma. Moreover, account should be taken of the possibility of missing diffused carcinomatosis by this method.

HYBRID IMAGING TOOLS: PET-CT

Hybrid PET (functional imaging) and CT (structural imaging) equipment has recently been developed. Initial expectations were raised by the possibility of obtaining invaluable complementary information in a single examination for assessing possible tumor participation in nonspecific structural changes and determining the precise topographic limits of this involvement (19) (Figure 10.5). Another potential use of this equipment is in the difficult evaluation of patients after biliary stent placement (28).

Petrowsky et al. (29) contributed important data on this issue in their study of biliary tumors (GBC and cholangiocarcinoma). In the 14 patients with GBC, they compared the diagnostic accuracy and clinical relevance of PET-CT with those of enhanced-contrast CT (CTec). PET-CT showed a sensitivity of 100% versus 71% for CTec in the detection of primary or recurrent GBC. CTec failed to differentiate between local recurrence and scarring in one out of the four patients with recurrent GBC after previous surgery. Both CTec and PET-CT gave a false-positive result for a patient with Mirizzi's syndrome. As already stated, PET-CT was not superior to a single FDG-PET examination for the detection of regional lymph node involvement. PET-CT influenced the therapeutic management of 17% of the whole group of patients with primary biliary tumor,

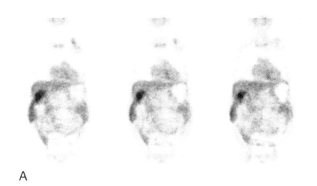

A

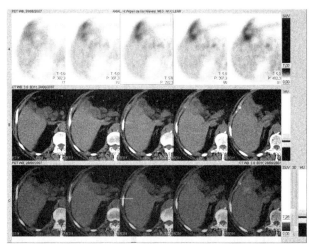

B

FIGURE 10.5

PET-CT imaging of gallbladder carcinoma. (A) FDG-PET coronal view showing high uptake in gallbladder wall. (B) FDG-PET (top row), CT (middle row), and fusion imaging (bottom row) showing hypermetabolism at gallbladder with spread to liver.

largely due to its better detection (versus CTec) of unsuspected distant metastases, especially in GBC. Therefore, initial results of the use of PET-CT in GBC are encouraging, and the study of larger populations is required to establish its role.

OTHER RADIOPHARMACEUTICALS

Although any PET tracer used in oncology could theoretically be of interest, there are no definitive data to guide us. Thus, (18F)·FDOPA-PET may be considered a suitable alternative to (18F)·FDG-PET, based on the metabolism of amino acids by the tumor, although the physiologic excretion pathway of FDOPA may include the gallbladder, and nonspecific retention in the hepatic hilum may mimic a GBC (34).

FDG-PET: LIMITATIONS AND PITFALLS

The main limitations of FDG-PET are that it is not yet widely available for routine clinical use and is often wrongly considered an expensive examination (19, 35) for use in only a few clinical situations. In addition, the low prevalence of GBC (0.5-7.4% of autopsies) (16) has meant that little information is yet available on the possible contribution of these procedures in the functional imaging diagnosis of this disease or on their cost-effectiveness.

The potential pitfalls of this technique are independent of the clinical context of the diagnosis (e.g., workup of gallbladder lesion or tumor persistence) and must be taken into account. Although errors can be explained on a case-by case basis, general conclusions cannot be drawn. Table 10.3 summarizes published reports of diagnostic errors. The possibility of a false positive is of special interest in the postsurgical staging of patients with an incidental diagnosis of GBC after cholecystectomy (28) and in patients with biliary stents or known granulomatous disease (21, 28).

The marked biochemical-metabolic character of the information offered by FDG-PET is counterbalanced by its relative limited spatial resolution, resulting in the failure to detect lesions smaller than double the equipment resolution, which is usually 4-5 mm (partial volume effect). At any rate, this minimum detection size should be corrected as a function of the density and metabolic rate (marked avidity for glucose) of the cells that form the tumor (36, 37).

There is a general consensus (10, 28, 29) that FDG-PET has a low sensitivity for small lesions, probably due to the partial-volume effect, the respiratory

TABLE 10.3
Pitfalls of FDG-PET in Gallbladder Cancer

Ref.	Clinical Context	Pitfall	Explanation
Koh 2003 (19)	(2)	FN	Diabetes mellitus Small 13-mm lesion
		FP	Xanthogranulomatous cholecystitis
Anderson 2004 (28)	Gallbladder cancer (2)	FP	Postsurgical (1 mo) tissue repair
		FN	Bulky intra-abdominal metastases Carcinomatosis
	Cholangiocarcinoma	FP	Sclerosing cholangitis Carcinomatosis
		FN	Carcinomatosis Carcinomatosis
Rodríguez 2004 (21)	(1)	FN	Mucinous adenocarcinoma
		FP	Tuberculosis Adenomyomatosis
Oe 2004 (20)	(1)	FP	Chronic cholecystitis
Nishiyama 2006 (10)	(1)	FN	10-mm tubular adenocarcinoma 10-mm tubular adenocarcinoma
Petrowsky 2006 (29)	(1)	FP	Mirizzi´s syndrome
Serradilla 2007 (23)	(1)	FP	Acute gangrenous cholecystitis

Reference and clinical context of studies are shown, describing the type of error (FN = false-negative; FP = false-positive) and proposed explanation.
(1) = Diagnostic workup for malignancy in a gallbladder lesion.
(2) = Incidental gallbladder cancer: posttreatment FDG-PET for residual tumor and staging; type of error, and its possible explanation (see text).

movements of the upper abdomen, and the presence of background activity in the liver parenchyma (10). Although 10 mm could be considered a reasonable limit of detection, some authors (19) have reported false-negative results in 13-mm lesions. As already mentioned, the size limitation could be modified by the cell metabolic activity.

However, the relationship between tumor type and FDG metabolic behavior has yet to be fully clarified, and false-negative findings have been reported for different forms of GBC. It can reasonably be considered that infiltrative and highly aggressive patterns of growth may not reach the minimal critical tumor cell mass required to produce a sufficiently intense positron emission signal (29). Anderson et al. (28) found a lower diagnostic accuracy for FDG-PET in the whole series of biliary cancers than in those showing a nodular pattern. They also described three false-negative examinations in lesions >3 cm, which they attributed to a change in the tumor biology due to the advanced stage of the disease. This proposition is supported by reports of false-negative findings in infiltrative cholangiocarcinoma (tumor mass diameter < 8-10 mm). It may also explain false-negative findings in patients with carcinomatosis.

SUMMARY

Despite the methodologic limitations of the different studies, some conclusions can be drawn that are of value to clinicians and surgeons in the management of patients under suspicion of GBC. The resectability of the tumor is usually the main issue, and it is especially important to rule out the presence of distant metastases. Functional imaging (and specifically metabolic imaging) used in the appropriate clinical situation appears able to optimize the use of costly and invasive procedures for the diagnosis and staging in patients with suspicious lesions (e.g., endoscopic retrograde cholangiopancreatography or percutaneous transhepatic cholangiography) in the standard workup of these patients (29). It can also offer reliable information for appropriate treatment planning, avoiding unnecessary surgery.

In general, FDG-PET shows a higher sensitivity versus structural imaging for GBC detection, with a sensitivity of 75-85% for the initial diagnosis and for staging. This sensitivity can be increased by using hybrid equipment (PET-CT) (29) and/or by acquiring delayed images (10).

Our group agrees with comments made by Petrowsky et al. (29) on the repercussions of positive examinations. It should be kept in mind that diagnostic doubts usually arise in patients with a surgical indication due to their symptoms and clinical status rather than in patients with a tumor diagnosis. Thus, in the case of a cholecystitis, a negative FDG-PET does not preclude surgery and a false-positive FDG-PET due to inflammatory activity has no repercussions for the surgical management of the patient. In this context, the key objective is to avoid unnecessary surgery with curative intent in patients with metastatic disease, for whom surgical management should be ruled out and who could be expected to represent as many as 17-30% of cases.

Regardless of the theoretical and practical advantages of functional imaging and especially hybrid systems, its use requires a consensual diagnostic algorithm according to the procedures available at each center, and the information from functional imaging must form a complementary part of the complete set of data on each individual patient (e.g., clinical signs, biochemical inflammation markers, tumor markers, structural appearance). In our view, functional imaging procedures should be considered immediately after first-line structural procedures (usually US-CT) if GBC is suspected before applying invasive procedures for staging or treatment. Studies of long series are warranted to offer definitive information on the role of FDG-PET in GBC, especially in terms of its cost-effectiveness.

References

1. Kokudo N, Makuuchi M, Natori T, Sakamoto Y, Yamamoto J, Seki M, et al. Strategies for surgical treatment of gallbladder carcinoma based on information available before resection. Arch Surg 2003; 138:741-750.
2. Ziessman HA. Acute cholecystitis, biliary obstruction, and biliary leakage. Sem Nucl Med 2003; 33:279-296.
3. Ziessman HA. Functional hepatobiliary disease: chronic acalculous gallbladder and chronic acalculous biliary disease. Sem Nucl Med 2006; 36:119-132.
4. Phelps ME, Hoffman EJ, Mullani NA, Ter-Pogossian MM. Application of annihilation coincidence detection to transaxial reconstruction tomography. J Nucl Med 1975; 16:210-224.
5. Ruiz JA, Carreras JL. Bases de la tomografía por emisión de positrones. In: Carreras JL, Lapeña L, Asensio C (eds.). PET en Oncología. Madrid: Nova Sidonia Oncología-Hematología, 2002:7-31.
6. Bailey DL, Kart JS, Surti S. Physics and instrumentation in PET. In: Valk PE, Bailey DL, Townsend DW, Maisey MN (eds.). Positron Emisión Tomography. Basic Science and Clinical Practice. London: Springer, 2003:41-67.
7. Newiger H, Hämisch Y, Oehr P, et al. Physical principles. In: Ruhlmann J, Oehr P, Biersack H-J (eds.). PET in Oncology. Basis and Clinical Applications. Berlin: Springer, 1999:3-34.
8. Oehr P. Metabolism and transport of glucose and FDG. In: Ruhlmann J, Oehr P, Biersack H-J (eds.). PET in Oncology. Basis and Clinical Applications. Berlin: Springer, 1999:44-57.
9. Coleman RE. Single photon emission computed tomography and positron emission tomography in cancer imaging. Cancer 1991; 67:1261-1270.
10. Nishiyama Y, Yamamoto Y, Fukunaga K, Kimura N, Miki A, Sasakawa Y, et al. Dual-time-point 18F-FDG PET for the evaluation of gallbladder carcinoma. J Nucl Med 2006; 47:633-638.
11. Zhuang HM, Cortés-Blanco A, Pourdehnad M, Adam LE,

Yamamoto AJ, Martínez-Lázaro R, et al. Do high glucose levels have differential effect on FDG uptake in inflammatory and malignant disorders? Nucl Med Commun 2001; 21:1123-1128.

12. Kubota K, Itoh M, Ozaki K, Ono S, Tashiro M, Yamaguchi K, et al. Advantage of delayed whole-body FDG-PET imaging tumour detection. Eur J Nucl Med 2001; 28:696-703.

13. Hustinx R, Smith RJ, Bernard F, Rosenthal DI, Machtay M, Farber LA, et al. Dual time point 18fluorine fluorodeoxyglucose positron emission tomography: a potential method to differentiate malignancy from inflammation and normal tissue in the head and neck. Eur J Nucl Med 1999; 26:1345-1348.

14. Duhaylongsod FG, Lowe VJ, Patz EF Jr, Vaughn AL, Coleman RE, Wolf WG. Detection of primary and recurrent lung cancer by means of F-18 fluorodeoxyglucose positron emission tomography (FDG-PET). J Thorac Cardiovasc Surg 1995; 110:130-140.

15. Graeter TP, Hellwig D, Hoffmann K, Ukena D, Kirsch CM, Schäfers HJ. Mediastinal lymph node staging in suspected lung cancer: comparison of positron emission tomography with F-18 fluorodeoxyglucose and mediastinoscopy. Ann Thorac Surg 2003; 75:231-236.

16. Lomis KD, Vitola JV, Delbeke D, Snodgrass SL, Chapman WC, Wright JK, et al. Recurrent gallbladder carcinoma at laparoscopy port sites diagnosed by positron emission tomography: implications for primary and radical second operations. Am Surg 1997; 63:341-345.

17. Rodríguez-Fernández A, Gómez-Río M, Medina-Benítez A, Moral JV, Ramos-Font C, Ramia-Angel JM, et al. Application of modern imaging methods in diagnosis of gallbladder cancer. J Surg Oncol 2006; 93(8):650-664.

18. Levy AD, Murakata LA, Rohrmann CA. Gallbladder carcinoma: radiologic-pathologic correlation. Radiographics 2001; 21:295-314.

19. Koh T, Taniguchi H, Yamaguchi A, Kunishima S, Yamagishi H. Differential diagnosis of gallbladder cancer using positron emission tomography with fluorine-18 labeled fluoro-deoxyglucose (FDG-PET). Surg Oncol 2003; 84:74-81.

20. Oe A, Kawabe J, Torii K, Kawamura E, Higashiyama S, Kotani J, et al. Distinguishing benign from malignant gallbladder wall thickening using FDG-PET. Ann Nucl Med 2006; 20:699-703.

21. Rodríguez-Ferníndez A, Gómez-Río M, Llamas-Elvira JM, Ortega-Lozano S, Ferrón-Orihuela JA, Ramia-Angel JM, et al. Positron-emission tomography with fluorine l8-2-deoxy-d-glucose for gallbladder cancer diagnosis. Am J Surg 2004; 188:171-175.

22. Ramia JM, Muffak K, Fernández A, Villar J, Garrote D, Ferrón A. Gallbladder tuberculosis: false-positive PET diagnosis of gallbladder cancer. World J Gastroenterol. 2006; 12:6559-65650.

23. Serradilla M, Villegas T, Muñoz N, Villar JM, Rodríguez A, Gómez M, et al. Aportación de la Tomografía por Emisión de Positrones en el diagnóstico preoperatorio del Cáncer de Vesícula. (Abst.) Cirugía Española. 2007, 82 (supl 1): 26.

24. Fritscher-Ravens A, Bohuslavizki KH, Broering DC, Jenicke L, Schaefer H, Buchert R, et al. FDG PET in the diagnosis of hilar Cholangiocarcinoma. Nucl Med Commun 2001; 22:1277-1285.

25. Koh T, Taniguchi H, Kunishima S, Yamagishi H. Possibility of differential diagnosis of small polypoid lesions in the gallbladder using FDG-PET. Clin Positron Imaging 2000; 3:213-218.

26. Cózar MP, Ortega F, Fuster C, Vázquez-Albadalejo C, Santos J, Almenar S. Detección por PET de una tumoración primaria de vesícula biliar y adenopatía metastásica pericística. Rev Esp Med Nucl 2006; 25:113-114.

27. Chander S, Lee P, Zingas AP, Joyrich RN, Zak IT, Bloom DA. PET imaging of gallbladder carcinoma. Clin Nucl Med 2005; 30:804-805.

28. Anderson CD, Rice MH, Pinson CW, Chapman WC, Chari RS, Delbeke D. Fluorodeoxyglucose PET imaging in the evaluation of gallbladder carcinoma and cholangiocarcinoma. J Gastrointest Surg 2004; 8:90-97.

29. Petrowsky H, Wildbrett P, Husarik DB, Hany T, Tam S, Jochum W, et al. Impact of integrated positron emission tomography and computed tomography on staging and management of gallbladder cancer and cholangiocarcinoma. J Hepatol 2006; 45:43-50.

30. Kluge R, Schmidt F, Caca K, Barthel H, Hesse S, Georgi P, et al. Positron emission tomography with FDG for diagnosis and staging of bile duct cancer. Hepatology 2001; 33:1029-1035.

31. Jarnaging WR, Fong Y, DeMatteo RP, Gonen M, Burke Ec, Bodniewicz BJ, et al. Staging, resectability, and outcome in 225 patient with hilar cholangiocarcinoma. Ann Surg 2001:507-517, discussion 517-519.

32. Rea DJ, Muñoz-Juarez M, Farnell MB, Donohue JH, Que FG, Crownhart B, et al. Major hepatic resection for hilar cholangiocarcinoma: analysis of 46 patients. Arch Surg 2004; 139:514-523, discussion 523-525.

33. Henning AW, Reed AI, Fujita S, Foley DP, Howard RJ. Surgical management of hilar cholangiocarcinoma. Ann Surg. 2005; 241:693-699, discussion 699-702.

34. Balan KK. Visualization of the gall bladder on F-18 FDOPA PET imaging: a potential pitfall. Clin Nucl Med. 2005; 30:23-24.

35. Miles KA, Connelly LB. Cost-effectiveness studies of PET in oncology. In: Oehr P, Biersack HJ, Coleman RE (eds.). PET and PET-CT in Oncology. Berlin: Springer-Verlag, 2004:321-329.

36. Rota Kops E, Krause HJ. Partial volume effects/corrections. In: Wieler HJ, Coleman RE (eds.). PET in Clinical Oncology. Darmstadt: Springer, 2000:33-42.

37. Bockisch A, Freudenberg L, Antoch G, Muller St. PET/CT: clinical considerations. In: Oehr P, Biersack HI, Coleman RE (eds.). PET and PET-CT in Oncology. Berlin: Springer-Verlag, 2004:101-112.

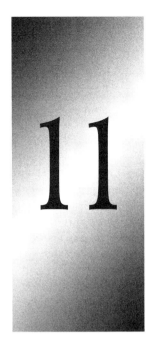

11 Computed Tomography

Leonardo Marcal
Chitra Viswanathan
Janio Szklaruk

Imaging of primary gallbladder and biliary tract tumors is challenging due to the anatomic complexity of the biliary tree and the large number and frequency of anatomic variations. The different morphologic subtypes of cholangiocarcinomas and their patterns of spread in the liver and along the biliary tree add to the complexity of imaging gallbladder and biliary cancers, placing additional demands on radiology to precisely demonstrate the extent of disease.

Computed tomography (CT) is a method of acquiring and reconstructing the image of a thin cross section on the basis of measurement of its attenuation. Since its inception in 1972, CT has rapidly become an essential imaging modality with numerous clinical applications in a wide variety of diseases. Dramatic improvements in CT technology have resulted in unparalleled advancements in image quality, acquisition speed, and patient throughput. The development of helical or spiral CT around 1990 represented a revolutionary advancement in CT technology, allowing a three-dimensional volume of tissue to be imaged within a single breathhold. The advent of thin section imaging with multislice computed tomography (MSCT) in 1998 was a major technological breakthrough. MSCT resulted in unprecedented advances in the clinical practice of CT, with important contributions to imaging of the gallbladder and biliary tree. One of the most promising advantages of multidetector row technology is its ability to obtain true "isotropic" voxels. Isotropic voxels are essential for a variety of different postprocessing techniques, translating into high-quality multiplanar and three-dimensional reconstructions. In our institution, MSCT has solidified its role as the prime imaging modality for the initial diagnostic evaluation, staging workup, and oncologic surveillance of patients with gallbladder and biliary tract cancer.

GALLBLADDER CANCER

Epidemiology

Gallbladder carcinoma is the most common malignancy of the biliary tree and the fifth most common gastrointestinal cancer following cancers of the colon, pancreas, stomach, liver, and esophagus. The estimated incidence of gallbladder cancer is 3 cases per 100,000 persons and approximately 6500 new diagnoses per year in the United States alone (1). Women are two to six times more commonly affected than men, and the incidence increases with age. Obesity, high-carbohydrate diet, alcohol use, and smoking have also been implicated with a higher incidence of gallbladder cancer (2).

Although the exact etiology is unclear, chronic irritation of the gallbladder mucosa by stones is believed to play a major role. The proposed pathophysiology consists of chronic inflammation and repetitive epithelial repair, which result in epithelial dysplasia with eventual progression to carcinoma in situ and then to invasive carcinoma. Most tumors are adenocarcinomas. Squamous cell carcinoma, adenosquamous carcinoma, and small cell carcinoma also occur. Other tumors are sarcomas, lymphomas, carcinoids, and other unusual malignancies.

Clinical Presentation

The clinical presentation is usually insidious, and early-stage gallbladder cancer is typically diagnosed incidentally on pathologic review of cholecystectomy specimens. Some patients may present with right upper quadrant pain and symptoms indistinguishable from those of cholecystitis. Presenting symptoms include chronic abdominal pain, unintentional weight loss, jaundice, and hepatomegaly. These are poor prognostic signs and usually indicate advanced disease.

Laboratory studies rarely show any abnormalities in patients with early disease. Elevated levels of serum bilirubin, transaminase, and γ-glutamyl transpeptidase may be seen in advanced cases, which present with obstructive jaundice (3). The prognosis is generally poor at the time of diagnosis. The mean survival rate is 6 months and the 5-year survival rate is approximately 5% for nonresected gallbladder cancer (4).

Imaging

The main role of imaging in gallbladder cancer is to provide accurate information regarding the extent of disease. The size and location of the primary tumor, the depth of hepatic parenchymal invasion, nodal disease, vascular anatomy, and presence of distant metastases constitute the key elements to be addressed by imaging. Radical surgical resection (usually including excision of segments V and IVb) has been shown to improve survival in patients whose tumors are locally confined to the cystic fossa and adjacent hepatic parenchyma (5, 6).

Protocol and Technique

The preoperative imaging of gallbladder cancer is performed in a selected population. In many cases, gallbladder cancer is detected after laparoscopic cholecystectomy for benign indications (7). In a patient with clinical suspicion of gallbladder carcinoma, we initially perform a nonenhanced scan through the liver and kidneys with a 5-mm collimation acquisition reconstructed at 2.5-mm intervals. Images are routinely reconstructed at 2.5-mm intervals for better spatial resolution. Nonenhanced images are useful for detecting fatty infiltration of the liver, parenchymal calcifications, and calcified gallstones. Following intravenous injection of 125–150 cc of nonionic iodinated contrast at a rate of 3 cc/sec, a multidetector (MDCT) imaging acquisition is performed from the diaphragm to the ischial tuberosities after a 60-second delay. This routine protocol results in imaging of the liver during the portal-venous phase of contrast enhancement and the kidneys in the early nephrographic phase, ensuring a comprehensive evaluation of the entire abdomen.

In the setting of preoperative evaluation of gallbladder cancer, a multiphasic liver protocol is performed. One hundrred and fifty cc of intravenous iodinated contrast is injected at 5 cc/sec over 33 seconds. SmartPrep® (GE Healthcare, Milwaukee) is used for contrast tracking, monitoring the aorta at the level of the celiac artery until 100 Hounsfield units is obtained. This takes roughly 20 seconds. Dynamic imaging through the liver in the late arterial phase is then obtained over approximately 5 seconds. Portal venous phase imaging is then obtained after 90 seconds, and delayed images through the liver are obtained at 180 seconds.

Imaging Findings

The imaging analysis of gallbladder cancer should focus on the parameters used to judge the chances of achieving a complete surgical resection. Familiarity with the normal appearance of gallbladder, cystic fossa, and adjacent structures on CT is essential for the accurate interpretation of CT findings.

Normal Gallbladder

The gallbladder lies within the cystic fossa along with the inferior vena cava (IVC). On contrast-enhanced CT the normal gallbladder appears as an elongated tubular structure of homogeneous low attenuation with a thin wall, not exceeding 3 mm when adequately distended. Thin homogeneous mucosal enhancement may be observed during the early arterial or portal venous phases of enhancement and constitutes a normal finding (Figure 11.1). When contracted, the gallbladder wall appears thickened (more than 3 mm) and may show more significant enhancement. The size and shape of the normal gallbladder are highly variable and depend on the fasting state of the patient.

Primary Tumor

When detected de novo, the appearance of gallbladder cancer on CT depends upon the morphology of the tumor and extent of disease at the time of imaging. Carcinomas of the gallbladder can be divided into five sub-

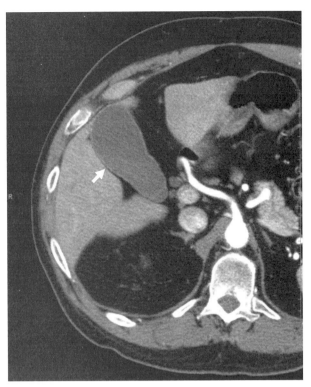

FIGURE 11.1

Normal gallbladder. Axial contrast-enhanced image obtained during the arterial phase shows a normal gallbladder. Its walls are sharply demarcated from the adjacent liver parenchyma and peritoneal fat. Thin homogeneous wall enhancement (arrow) during the arterial or portal venous phase is a normal finding.

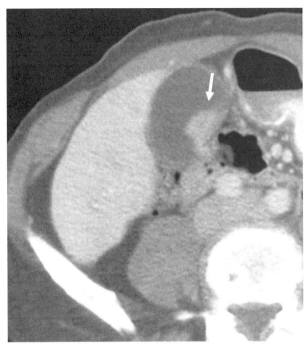

FIGURE 11.2

Papillary gallbladder cancer: 55-year-old female with gallbladder cancer incidentally found on cholecystectomy specimen. Axial contrast-enhanced image shows a soft tissue mass protruding into the homogeneous low attenuation lumen of the gallbladder (arrow).

types, according to their gross morphologic appearance, as papillary, nodular, flat, filling, and massive (8). Papillary, nodular, and filling tumors usually present on imaging as an enhancing soft tissue mass protruding into the normally low-density fluid attenuation lumen of the gallbladder (Figure 11.2). Flat tumors may present as irregular thickening of the gallbladder wall without a discrete soft tissue mass or nodule. Massive tumors are more commonly identified on imaging and appear as a large mass that completely replaces the gallbladder and adjacent hepatic parenchyma (Figure 11.3).

According to the AJCC staging criteria, T1 tumor invades the lamina propria or muscle layer. T2 tumor invades the perimuscular connective tissue but does not extend beyond the serosa. T3 tumor perforates the serosa and directly invades the liver (less than 2 cm) or one other adjacent organ or structure, such as the bile duct, colon, duodenum, or pancreas. T4 tumor invades the liver (greater than 2 cm), the main portal vein or hepatic artery, or multiple (two or more) adjacent organs and structures. CT is not useful for T-staging except to discriminate between T3 and T4 tumors.

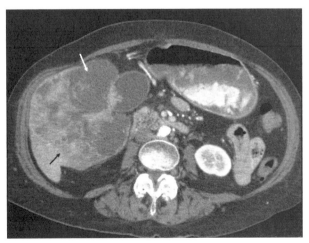

FIGURE 11.3

Sixty-six-year-old female with advanced gallbladder cancer. A large heterogeneous mass replaces most of the right liver. There is irregular peripheral enhancement (black arrow) and central areas of low attenuation indicative of necrosis (white arrow).

Radial Tumor Growth and Adjacent Organ Invasion

The liver is the organ most commonly involved by direct extension (65% of cases), and tumors of the fundus and body of the gallbladder have a propensity to invade segments IVb and V at an early stage (6, 9). Direct hepatic invasion is demonstrated on contrast-enhanced CT as an irregular soft tissue mass disrupting the adjacent liver parenchyma, usually in segments IVb and V (Figures 11.4–11.6).

Anatomic structures in the hepatic hilum and in close proximity to the gallbladder can also be involved by direct tumor extension. The bile duct and the portal vein are the structures more commonly involved by direct local extension of gallbladder cancer (9, 10). The colon and duodenum are also frequently involved, comprising 15% of cases each, followed by the pancreas with 6% (10, 11). Disruption of the fat planes between the tumor and adjacent structures is used as a criterion for diagnosis of infiltration by tumor (11). Extension into the hepatic flexure of the colon is shown on CT as infiltration of the normal low-density pericolonic fat by soft tissue with obliteration of vessels (Figure 11.7A and Figure 11.7B). Wall thickening with possible luminal narrowing and eventual obstruction may also occur.

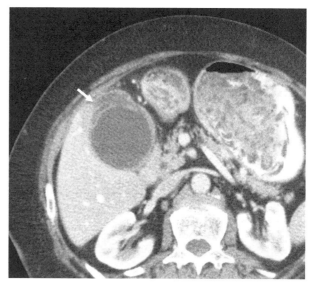

FIGURE 11.5

Fifty-five-year-old female with gallbladder carcinoma. Contrast-enhanced MSCT image shows a low density mass in the fundus of the gallbladder (arrow). Indistinct margins with segment V are indicative of invasion. The depth of invasion is less than 2 cm (T3 tumor).

Nodal Disease

The presence or absence of nodal disease is important for accurate staging. The prevalence of lymphatic metastases is high in gallbladder carcinoma and surpasses 70% in some series (3, 6). Lymphatic spread in gallbladder cancer occurs first to the hepatoduodenal nodes (N1 nodes). Disease can then spread to the celiac, superior mesenteric, and peripancreatic nodes, which comprise the N2 nodes (Figures 11.8 and 11.9). Left paraaortic and interaoartocaval adenopathy in the retroperitoneum are regarded as distant nodal metastases. Detection of nodal involvement on CT is based on size and internal imaging features of the nodes. Nodes greater than 1 cm in short axis are likely malignant (12). Nodes with a low attenuation center indicating central necrosis are also likely to harbor metastatic disease (12). The sensitivity of CT in the detection of positive nodes in gallbladder cancer is 36 and 47% for N1 and N2 nodes, respectively (13).

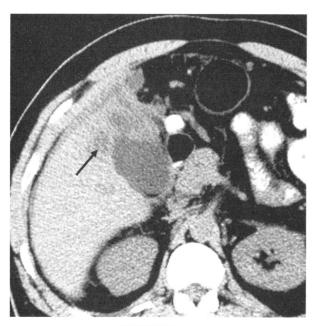

FIGURE 11.4

Locally invasive gallbladder cancer. Noncontrast axial MSCT image shows a soft tissue mass in the fundus of the gallbladder. There is greater than 2 cm invasion into segment V of the liver (arrow) and also in segment IV (T4 tumor). Tumor of the fundus of the gallbladder has a propensity for early invasion of segments V and IVb.

Metastatic Disease

Hematogenous metastases occur most commonly to the liver. Hepatic metastases appear as multifocal areas of low attenuation in relation to the adjacent hepatic parenchyma, usually with a peripheral rim of contrast enhancement, and are identified on routine contrast-enhanced CT (Figure 11.10). Lung, cerebral, and osseous metastases occur less frequently. Gallbladder cancer has

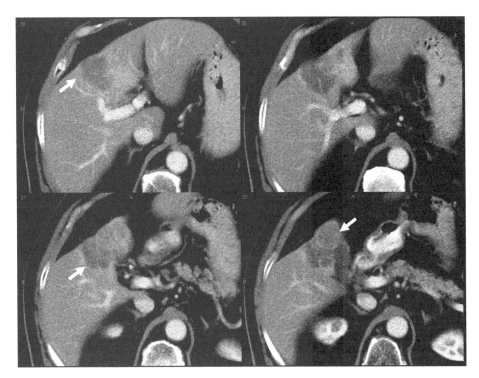

FIGURE 11.6

Sixty-two-year-old female with locally invasive gallbladder carcinoma. Contiguous contrast-enhanced axial MSCT images show an enhancing mass (arrows) of heterogeneous attenuation involving segments IVb and V, consistent with locally invasive gallbladder carcinoma.

a remarkable propensity to seed and grow in the peritoneal cavity (10, 14). Peritoneal deposits appear on imaging as nodularity or fat stranding of the normal low-density peritoneal fat (Figure 11.11). Peritoneal metastases may be difficult to diagnose and are easily overlooked. The sensitivity of CT for detection of peritoneal metastases is in the range of 63–79% (15).

Overall, MSCT has been found to be an accurate technique to determine resectability of gallbladder car-

cinoma when factors such as vascular invasion, adjacent organ invasion, and metastases are considered, with a sensitivity of 72.7%, specificity of 100%, and accuracy of 85% (16)

Differential Diagnosis

A variety of clinical conditions may mimic gallbladder carcinoma on imaging studies, for example, inflamma-

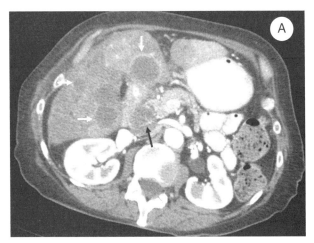
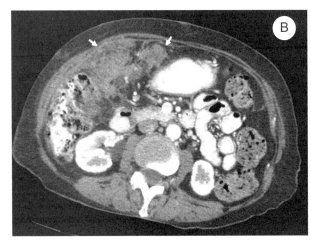

FIGURE 11.7

(A) Seventy-one-year-old female with advanced gallbladder carcinoma. Contrast-enhanced axial MSCT shows multiple low-density masses with a peripheral rim of contrast enhancement in segments IVb, V, and VI (white arrows). An enlarged centrally necrotic portocaval node is also identified (black arrow). (B) Contrast-enhanced axial MSCT in the same patient shows soft tissue nodules infiltrating the transverse mesocolon and involving the hepatic flexure of the colon. Note infiltration of the pericolonic fat, which should display homogeneous fat attenuation (arrows).

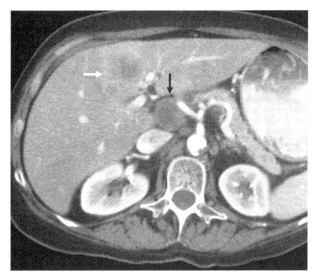

FIGURE 11.8

Lymphangitic spread in gallbladder carcinoma. Contrast-enhanced MSCT shows a large lobulated enhancing mass in segment IV, consistent with gallbladder carcinoma (white arrow). An enlarged low-density node is noted in the hepatoduodenal ligament (black arrow), consistent with a N1 node. Nodes larger than 1 cm in short axis or nodes of central low attenuation are likely metastatic.

tory conditions such as acute cholecystitis. The imaging features of acute cholecystitis on CT are gallbladder wall thickening, cholelithiasis, pericholecystic fluid, and infiltration of the pericholecystic fat (Figure 11.12). CT can readily identify calcified gallstones, but detec-

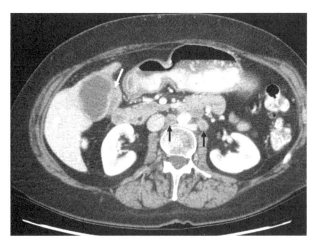

FIGURE 11.9

Lymphangitic spread in gallbladder carcinoma. Contrast-enhanced axial MSCT image shows an enhancing soft tissue mass in the medial wall of the gallbladder, consistent with gallbladder cancer (white arrow). Prominent intera-ortocaval and left para-aortic nodes are identified indicative of distant nodal metastases (black arrows).

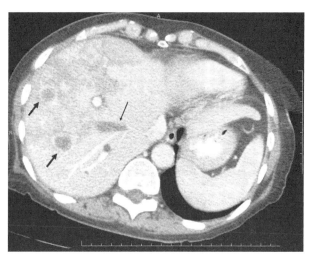

FIGURE 11.10

Hematogenous metastases in gallbladder cancer: 71 year-old female with advanced gallbladder carcinoma. Multiple contrast-enhanced axial MSCT images obtained during the portal venous phase show multiple ring-enhancing nodules, compatible with hematogenous metastases (arrows). There is a filling defect in segment VIII portal vein (thin long arrow), consistent with thrombus.

tion of cholesterol stones is difficult due to the similar attenuation of the bile. Gallstones are a well-known risk factor for gallbladder cancer, and the two condi-

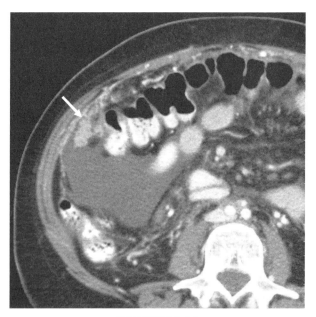

FIGURE 11.11

Peritoneal metastases. Contrast-enhanced MSCT image shows nodular soft tissue thickening in the omentum consistent with peritoneal deposits (arrow). Nodularity and stranding of the peritoneal fat are signs indicative of peritoneal carcinomatose

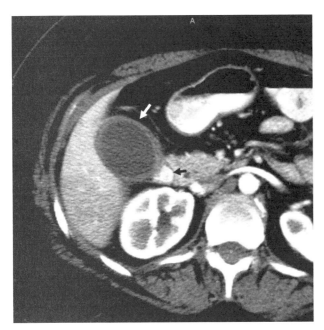

FIGURE 11.12

Acute cholecystitis. Axial contrast-enhanced MSCT image shows a distended gallbladder with a thick enhancing wall (white arrow), consistent with acute cholecystitis. Note a calcified gallstone impacted at the gallbladder neck (black arrow). Wall thickening in acute cholecystitis is usually symmetric along the entire wall of the gallbladder and cholelithiasis is almost always present.

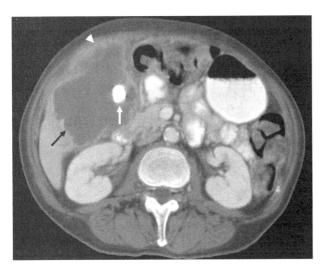

FIGURE 11.13

Cholelithiasis and gallbladder carcinoma. Contrast-enhanced axial CT image shows a large necrotic mass replacing the cystic fossa and invading segments IVb and V (black arrow). A large calcified gallstone is present (white arrow). Note direct tumor invasion into the anterior abdominal wall (arrowhead).

tions may coexist, making differentiation more difficult (Figure 11.13). Enhancement of the liver parenchyma adjacent to the cystic fossa has been reported in acute cholecystitis and should not be misinterpreted as a focal hepatic lesion (Figure 11.14). Also, tumors arising in the neck of the gallbladder not infrequently may cause obstruction of the cystic duct and present clinically as acute cholecystitis.

Adenomyomatosis, a benign, nonneoplastic condition of the gallbladder, may mimic malignancy on imaging studies. Adenomyomatosis is an acquired hyperplastic lesion of benign etiology, characterized by proliferation of the surface epithelium, thickening of the muscle layer, and multiple enlarged and deepened invaginations of the mucosa into the thickened muscle layer (17). Imaging features of adenomyomatosis on CT include focal or diffuse cystic-appearing gallbladder wall thickening (18) (Figure 11.15). Although it is not possible to reliably differentiate gallbladder carcinoma from this condition in all cases, the presence of cystic-appearing spaces in the thickened gallbladder wall allows the diagnosis of adenomyomatosis to be made with reasonable confidence (18).

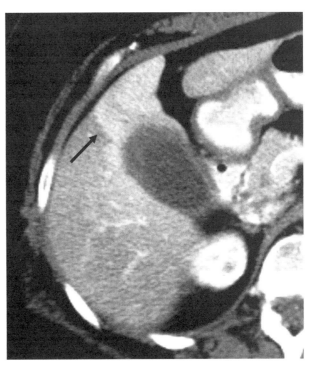

FIGURE 11.14

Hyperemia of the hepatic parenchyma in a 56-year-old female with acute cholecystitis. Contrast-enhanced axial MSCT image shows hyperemia of the hepatic parenchyma adjacent to the gallbladder (arrow). Hyperemia of the hepatic parenchyma adjacent to the gallbladder fossa is commonly seen in patients with acute cholecystitis and should not be confused with a hepatic lesion.

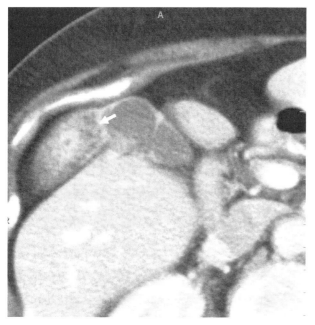

FIGURE 11.15

Adenomyomatosis of the gallbladder. Axial contrast-enhanced MSCT image shows a focal area of significant wall thickening involving the fundus of the gallbladder. Small cystic-appearing spaces are noted in the focal area of segmental wall thickening (arrow). When cystic-appearing spaces are identified within the area of gallbladder wall thickening, the diagnosis of adenomyomatosis can be made with reasonable accuracy.

Cholesterol polyps represent approximately 50% of all polypoid lesions in the gallbladder and have no malignant potential. Cholesterol polyps may be single or multiple and are usually less than 1 cm in diameter (19). On unenhanced CT, cholesterol polyps are difficult to see, but are readily apparent on contrast-enhanced scans due to vascularity within the polyp.

There are other benign tumors of epithelial and nonepithelial origin that may involve the gallbladder and biliary tract. Adenoma of the gallbladder is a rare benign epithelial tumor found in approximately 0.5% of cholecystectomy specimens. Patients with familial adenomatous polyposis and Peutz-Jeghers syndrome have a reported higher prevalence of adenomas of the gallbladder and biliary tract. A small proportion of gallbladder adenomas progress to carcinomas. At contrast-enhanced CT, gallbladder adenoma presents as an enhancing intraluminal soft tissue mass or nodule that may be iso- or hypo-attenuating relative to the liver (19).

Treatment Response and Recurrence

CT is used to monitor patients following treatment for gallbladder carcinoma. Following surgery, a nonenhancing fluid collection may be seen at the resection margin. This fluid collection usually decreases in size after 3–6 months but may never completely disappear. If a catheter is left in the surgical bed, small pockets of air may be present and not necessarily imply infection.

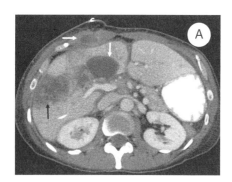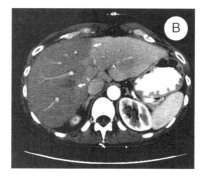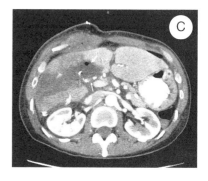

FIGURE 11.16

(A) Postoperative abscess following surgery for gallbladder cancer. Contrast-enhanced follow-up CT examination obtained a month following surgery reveals a low-density collection in the surgical bed with peripheral rim enhancement compatible with an abscess (vertical white arrow). An additional collection with similar imaging features is noted in the right rectus abdominis, representing a smaller abscess (horizontal white arrow). Note evolving infarct in segment V (black arrow). (B) Lobar hepatic infarction following radical resection of gallbladder cancer: 60-year-old female status post resection of gallbladder carcinoma, with abnormal liver function tests in the postoperative. Axial contrast-enhanced MSCT obtained in the late arterial phase shows a sharp demarcation between the right and left liver (arrow). The entire right liver is homogeneously lower attenuation when compared with the left liver. (C) Lobar hepatic infarction following surgery for gallbladder cancer. Contrast-enhanced axial MSCT image at a lower level shows a filling defect within the right hepatic artery (thin white arrow), consistent with a thrombus. A geographic area of low density is noted in segments V and VI, compatible with hepatic infarction (black arrow). The fluid collection in the resection bed with a small pocket of air does not necessary imply an abscess in the early postoperative period (thick white arrow). Close continual follow-up is required to document involution of the collection and to exclude abscess formation.

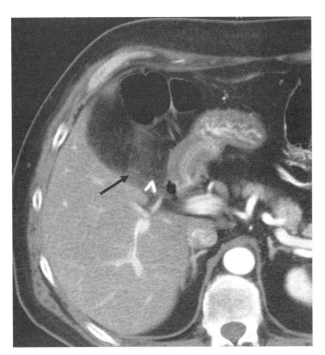

FIGURE 11.17

Normal postoperative CT appearance after radical chole-cystectomy for gallbladder cancer. Infiltration of peritoneal fat following surgery is a normal finding and does not imply peritoneal seeding or metastases (arrow). The degree of soft infiltration and stranding decreases with time.

Increasing amounts of fluid and gas, development of a thick rim of peripheral enhancement, and progressive infiltration of the adjacent fat are signs of abscess formation (Figure 11.16A). Differentiating an abscess from a postoperative seroma or hematoma can be extremely difficult in the early postoperative period.

Hepatic segmental infarction due to portal vein or hepatic artery thrombosis may be seen in the early postoperative period. Segmental hepatic infarction is demonstrated on CT as a sharply marginated area of decreased enhancement in the anatomic distribution of the thrombosed or occluded vessel (Figure 11.16B,C).

Infiltration of the peritoneal fat in the operative bed and focal areas of fat necrosis are normal postsurgical findings and should not be misinterpreted as recurrent disease (Figure 11.17). The degree of soft tissue infiltration regresses gradually and may never completely disappear. A discrete nodule of soft tissue attenuation that increases in size 3–6 months following surgery is concerning for peritoneal metastasis and needs to be followed closely on subsequent imaging studies (Figure 11.18A). Recurrent disease may also occur at the resection margin in the liver or along the tract of previous drainage catheters in the abdominal wall (Figure 11.18B).

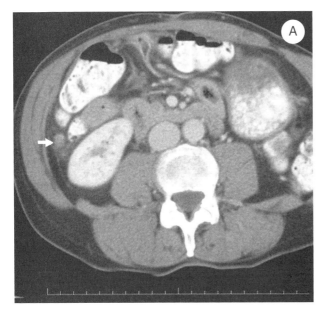

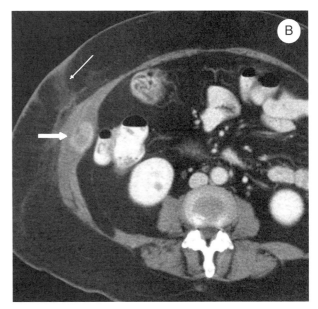

FIGURE 11.18

(A) Recurrent disease after surgery for gallbladder. Axial contrast-enhanced image shows a soft tissue nodule in the right paracolic gutter that increased in size 4 months after surgery for gallbladder cancer, consistent with a metastatic peritoneal deposit. (B) Recurrent disease 6 months following surgery for gallbladder cancer. An enhancing lobulated nodule is identified in the right transversalis, internal oblique muscles, consistent with metastases (thick arrow). The subcutaneous tract of prior drains should be carefully evaluated in routine oncologic surveillance CT examination (thin arrow). Not infrequently, metastatic deposits will be discovered in close proximity to these tracts.

INTRAHEPATIC CHOLANGIOCARCINOMA

Epidemiology

Intrahepatic cholangiocarcinoma (ICC), also called peripheral cholangiocellular carcinoma, is a malignant tumor arising from intrahepatic bile duct epithelium. It is thought to arise from the secondary bile duct or proximal branches of the intrahepatic bile ducts. Intrahepatic cholangiocarcinomas account for 8% of all cholangiocarcinomas, with extrahepatic perihilar tumors representing 50%, and extrahepatic distal tumors 42% (19). The estimated annual incidence in the United States is 1 per 100,000 persons. ICC accounts for approximately 7% of all malignant liver tumors, with hepatocellular carcinoma (HCC) being the most common primary liver malignancy (20). Approximately 2–6% of primary malignant liver tumors exhibit hepatocellular and bile duct differentiation, and these are called combined HCC-ICC (cHCC-ICC) (21). Risk factors for developing ICC include primary sclerosing cholangitis, choledochal cysts, inflammatory bowel disease, biliary cirrhosis, cholelithiasis, alcoholic liver disease, thyrotoxicosis, chronic pancreatitis, familial polyposis, congenital hepatic fibrosis, parasitic infestation of *Opisthorchis senensis*, and thorotrast exposure (22).

Clinical Presentation

Patients present with nonspecific symptoms, such as malaise, weight loss, abdominal pain, or nausea (23). In contrast to patients with extrahepatic cholangiocarcinoma (ECC), patients with ICC do not present with jaundice due to biliary obstruction. In contrast to patients with HCC, patients do not have ascites or symptoms associated with portal hypertension or cirrhosis.

Laboratory abnormalities include elevation of CA 19-9 and carcinoembryonic antigen (CEA); this is also seen in ECC. α-Fetoprotein (AFP), frequently elevated in patients with HCC, is usually normal in ICC. In combined tumors of HCC-ICC pathology, there will be elevated α-fetoprotein and modestly elevated CA19-9, versus elevation of AFP alone for HCC and CA19-9 for ICC (24).

Imaging: Protocol and Technique

The clinical presentation for imaging in our institution is a patient with an incidentally found liver mass with abdominal pain. The differential diagnosis for a liver mass in this setting includes ICC, HCC, or metastatic disease. For diagnosis and staging, a liver MSCT protocol as described in the section for gallbladder carcinoma is utilized.

Imaging Findings

There are three macroscopic presentations of intrahepatic cholangiocarcinoma described by the Liver Cancer Study Group: mass-forming (MF), periductal-infiltrating (PD), and intraductal (ID) types (25). A fourth group has been created to combine tumors that exhibit mixed characteristics, for example, MF + PD.

Mass-Forming Type

The mass-forming and the combination types are the most common, accounting for over 70% of cases. On noncontrast images, there is a large hypoattenuating mass with lobular or irregular margins (Figure 11.19A). On late arterial phase images (Figure 11.19B) there is minimal to no peripheral enhancement of the tumor. On portal venous phase images, continued centripetal enhancement can be seen in the tumor (Figure 11.19C). On the delayed images, there is continued, homogeneous enhancement (Figure 11.19D). The delayed enhancement in ICC is due to the presence of a fibrous stroma, which retains contrast over time. Associated

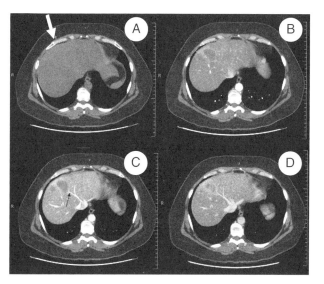

FIGURE 11.19

Enhancement pattern of ICC: 43-year-old female with intrahepatic cholangiocarcinoma presenting with right upper quadrant abdominal pain. (A) MSCT noncontrast image shows low-attenuation mass in segment IV with extension into segment VIII (thick white arrow). (B) MSCT late arterial phase image shows mass to be hypointense to adjacent hepatic parenchyma. Minimal peripheral enhancement is seen. Enhancement of the surrounding liver is due to transient hepatic attenuation. (C) MSCT portal venous phase image shows continued peripheral enhancement of the mass. The mass involves the middle hepatic vein (black arrow). (D) MSCT delayed image shows continued peripheral enhancement, with near-complete enhancement of the mass.

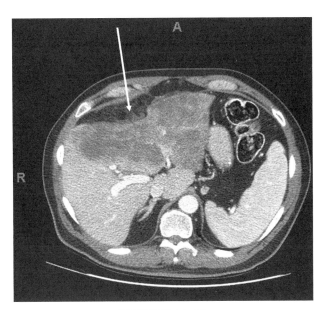

FIGURE 11.20

Capsular retraction: 65-year-old male with intrahepatic cholangiocarcinoma presenting with weight loss, fatigue and weakness. MSCT portal venous phase image shows capsular retraction (arrow) due to desmoplastic reaction. Adjacent stranding of the fat represents metastatic spread to peritoneum.

findings include peripheral ill-defined calcification due to mucin production in 18% and capsular retraction due to desmoplastic response (Figure 11.20) (26–28).

The differential diagnosis of this type is metastasis from colorectal carcinoma, which has a similar enhancement pattern. This enhancement pattern helps exclude HCC or hypervascular metastases (for example, neuroendocrine carcinoma), which are intensely enhancing on arterial phase, wash out quickly in the portal venous phase, and are hypoattenuating on delayed images.

Periductal-Infiltrating

The periductal-infiltrating type accounts for approximately 15–20% of cases (25, 29). On noncontrast CT, this tumor pattern presents as proximal ductal dilation without a discrete mass or as periductal soft tissue. On the arterial phase, there is minimal ductal wall enhancement or periductal soft-tissue enhancement (30). In the portal venous phase, more intense enhancement is seen in the ductal wall and periductal soft tissues (25).

The differential diagnosis of this type includes benign stricture due to hepatolithiasis or cholangitis. The presence of portal vein obliteration and lymph node involvement is more suggestive of a malignant etiology.

Intraductal Type

The intraductal type of ICC accounts for approximately 5% of cases (25, 29). This pattern of ICC is considered similar to the intraductal papillary mucinous neoplasm of the pancreas and has the best prognosis (31). On noncontrast CT, a dilated duct with or without a mass greater than 1 cm can be seen. On the arterial and portal venous phases, a hypoattenuating mass or a hyperattenuating duct may be seen (32) (Figure 11.21A,B). The differential diagnosis of a high-attenuation intraductal mass includes stone, tumor such as HCC or metastatic disease, or stricture with debris. Intraductal HCC will usually have the typical pattern of HCC enhancement, being slightly less hypoattenuating on the noncontrast images and showing marked enhancement on arterial phase images and washout on the portal venous images (33).

Combined HCC-ICC

The rare tumors of mixed HCC and ICC (cHCC-CC) present as large, solitary tumors with irregular margins (24). The contrast enhancement pattern is dependent on the percentage of each tumor. An HCC pattern with intense arterial enhancement is most common occurring in over 50%, followed by an ICC pattern representing 33%, and the remainder represents a combination of the two. It can be very difficult to predict prospectively whether the mass represents HCC or ICC. On noncontrast CT there is a large hypoattenuating tumor. During the arterial phase, the HCC portion will enhance avidly, while the ICC portion may stay

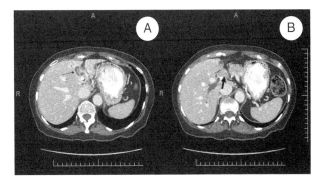

FIGURE 11.21

Imaging appearance of intraductal type of ICC: 83-year-old female with ICC intraductal type presenting with right upper quadrant pain, jaundice, and dark urine. A stent has been placed to reduce jaundice. (A) MSCT delayed image shows dilated duct with enhancing material (thin arrow) in segment IV of liver. Note adjacent atrophy of the remainder of the left lobe. (B) MSCT delayed image inferior to (A) shows enhancing mass (thick arrow) contained within the left intrahepatic duct.

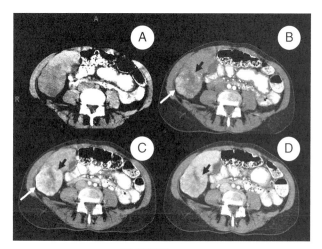

FIGURE 11.22

Enhancement pattern: 55-year-old female with cHCC-ICC presenting with metastatic skull mass. (A) MSCT noncontrast image shows low-attenuation mass in right lobe of liver with central calcification. (B) MSCT late arterial phase image shows lateral aspect of mass has intense nodular enhancement (arrow). More medial portion of tumor (short arrow) remains hypoattenuating to liver. (C) MSCT portal venous phase image shows slight washout in the previously enhancing lateral portion (arrow). There is peripheral enhancement of the medial portion of the mass (short arrow). (D) MSCT delayed image shows continued peripheral enhancement of the medial portion (short arrow), with near-complete enhancement of the mass.

hypointense. At the portal venous phase, the enhancing portion representing HCC will wash out and the portion representing ICC continues to enhance. On the delayed phase, the HCC component is hypoattenuating, and the ICC portion is homogeneously enhancing (Figure 11.22).

STAGING

Primary Tumor

Mass-forming ICC and cHCC-ICC are staged according to the AJCC hepatocellular carcinoma system. The discriminating factors for T-staging are tumor size, satellite nodules, vascular invasion, and extracapsular extension. MSCT is a good initial study for identifying the presence of the mass and assessing local organ involvement. Thin-section imaging with 1.25-mm reconstructed images is very useful for evaluating arterial and venous involvement; however, MSCT tends to underestimate the extent of biliary ductal involvement. ICC has a propensity to encase and even invade small branches of portal veins through direct extension (34).

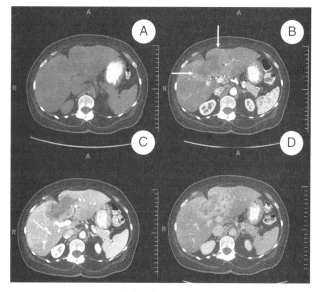

FIGURE 11.23

Transient hepatic attenuation due to obstruction of portal flow: 65-year-old female with ICC presenting with pain in the right flank. (A) MSCT noncontrast image shows a large mass involving the left lobe with extension into the right lobe. (B) MSCT late arterial phase image shows an area of hyperattenuation (arrow), which corresponds to altered blood supply due to encasement of portal vein. (C) MSCT portal venous phase image shows a large mass involving the left lobe with extension into the right lobe. (D) MSCT delayed image shows a large mass involving the left lobe with extension into the right lobe and inferior extension to involve the gallbladder.

There can be wedge-shaped enhancement of the liver surrounding the tumor due to arterial supply as a result of portal vein encasement (Figure 11.23) (35). Biliary ductal dilation and gallbladder involvement due to direct extension of the tumor into the gallbladder fossa can also be seen (Figure 11.24).

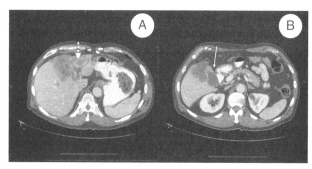

FIGURE 11.24

Ductal dilation and gallbladder involvement: 68-year-old male with ICC presenting with abnormal liver function tests. (A) Mass involves the left lobe of the liver and causes ductal dilation (fat arrow). (B) More inferiorly, the mass is seen to involve the gallbladder wall (long arrow) by direct extension.

Nodal Disease

Lymph node status is one of the most important prognostic indicators. Helpful clues for metastatic lymph nodes include size greater than 1 cm, low-density center due to necrosis, or delayed enhancement. CT has a high negative predictive value but a low positive predictive value for lymph node involvement (36).

ICC typically spreads into the hepatoduodenal ligament first, and then into the para-aortic nodes, retropancreatic nodes, and common hepatic artery nodes, in that order. Involvement is also seen along the left gastric nodes along the lesser curvature as well as the paracardiac nodes for tumors in the left lobe (37). Classification is divided into N0, with no regional lymph node metastasis, and N1, with spread to regional lymph nodes such as perihepatic, periportal, portocaval, and periceliac nodes (Figure 11.25). Peripancreatic and para-aortic/retroperitoneal nodes are rare.

Metastatic Disease

The most common site of metastatic spread is to the hepatic parenchyma via the portal venous system (38). CT has high sensitivity for assessing distal metastatic disease but underestimates the extent of peritoneal disease, spread along Glisson's capsule, and metastatic liver disease(39).

In the portal venous phase images, enhancing nodules with peripheral enhancement are seen in the noncontiguous lobe (Figure 11.26). Distal metastastic disease affects the lung, bone, adrenal gland, peritoneum, and brain. Lung metastasis can be present as single or multiple nodules (Figure 11.27). Bony involvement can be seen as lytic lesions. Adrenal metastases present as

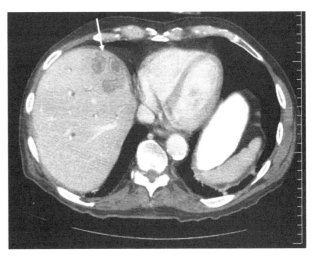

FIGURE 11.26

Hepatic metastases in the right liver: 68-year-old male with ICC in the left lobe presenting with abnormal liver function tests. MSCT portal venous image shows hypoattenuating hepatic metastases in the right lobe of the liver. Peripheral enhancement (arrow) is seen.

large, irregular masses (Figure 11.28). Spread to the peritoneum results in peritoneal carcinomatosis and thickening of the omentum (Figure 11.29).

Treatment Response and Recurrence

Curative treatment of intrahepatic cholangiocarcinoma is primarily surgical (19, 40). Factors that preclude sur-

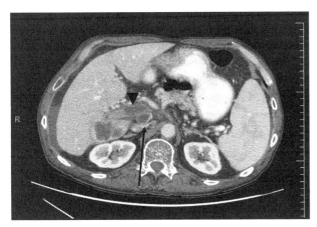

FIGURE 11.25

Portocaval lymph node: 54 year old male with ICC presenting with right upper quadrant pain. MSCT portal venous image shows portocaval lymph node (arrow). There is also portal vein bland thrombosis (arrowhead).

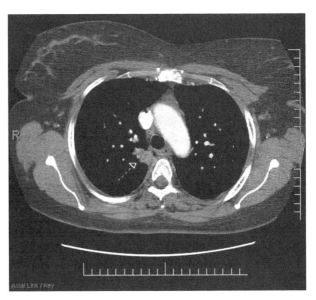

FIGURE 11.27

Lung metastasis: 49-year-old female with ICC resected 3 years prior. MSCT contrast image shows lobulated mass in the lung (dashed arrow), biopsy-proven metastasis.

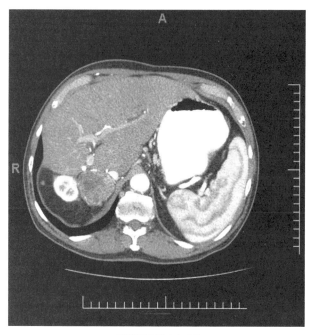

FIGURE 11.28

Adrenal metastasis: 79-year-old male with cHCC-ICC 2 years s/p extended right hepatectomy. MSCT contrast image shows a heterogeneous mass in the right adrenal gland, presumed metastatic disease. Patient was treated with radiofrequency ablation.

gical resection are bilobar involvement, main portal vein involvement, involvement of two or more hepatic veins, and metastatic spread. Other factors that can impact surgery are degree of cirrhosis, degree of steatosis, and comorbid factors.

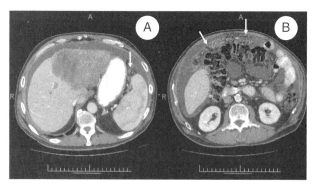

FIGURE 11.29

Peritoneal disease: 65-year-old male with ICC presenting with weight loss, fatigue, and weakness. (A) MSCT portal venous phase image shows the primary tumor in the left lobe of the liver. Arrow shows peritoneal disease between stomach and spleen. (B) Inferiorly, there is ascites and nodularity of the transverse mesocolon and omentum (white arrows), consistent with peritoneal dissemination of tumor.

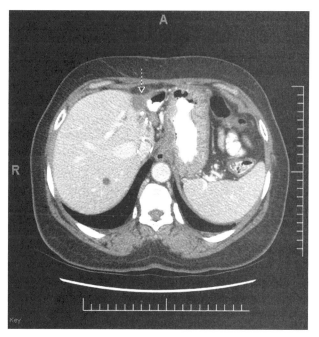

FIGURE 11.30

Volume calculation: 35-year-old female with ICC of the right lobe. Multiple volume-rendered images of the whole liver and expected residual liver segments (I, II, and III), whole liver volume of 1923.1 cc, segment I 27.2 cc, segment II 151 cc, segment III 168.2 cc.

Prior to surgery, CT volumetric analysis of the liver is usually performed to assess residual liver volume (Figure 11.30). The liver is marked into individual segments by the radiologist, and then 3D volumetric reconstructions are performed using 1.25-mm collimation images. Calculations of the future liver volume (FLV)/total expected liver volume (TELV) ratio are made. If this ratio is less than 20% in noncirrhotic livers or less than 40% in cirrhotic livers, then portal vein embolization is utilized to increase liver volume to avoid liver failure after surgery (41).

Postoperative changes include stranding of the peritoneal fat and seroma, which appears as low-density fluid collection at the surgical site and resolves within 3–6 months (Figure 11.31). The most common site of recurrence is local, with patients presenting with elevation of CA19-9 or jaundice. On MSCT, there is a nodular mass underneath the hemidiaphragm or contiguous to the surgical site (Figure 11.32).

Chemotherapy can be used alone or combined with radiotherapy for preoperative debulking of the tumor or for palliation. Imaging findings after chemotherapy include decrease in the size of the mass, decrease in enhancement of solid components, and decrease in the adjacent perfusion abnormalities (Figure 11.33). Findings after radiotherapy include

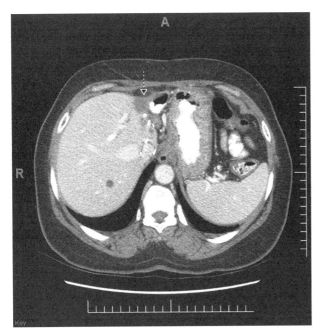

FIGURE 11.31

Seroma: 49-year-old female with ICC status post–left hepatectomy. MSCT contrast-enhanced image shows a low-density fluid collection (arrow) at the surgical site (clips shown by fat arrow).

low attenuation in the liver parenchyma adjacent to the radiation port (Figure 11.34). This is due to peritumoral edema, which appears as a lower attenuation area compared to adjacent liver.

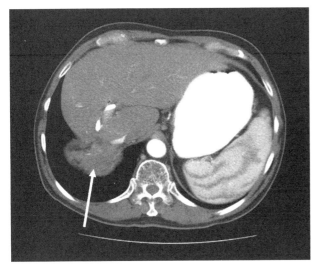

FIGURE 11.32

Recurrent tumor at the surgical site: 79-year-old male with cHCC-ICC 2 years s/p extended right hepatectomy. MSCT contrast-enhanced image shows nodularity in the infradiaphragmatic region (arrow).

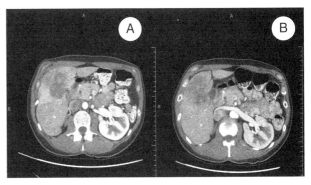

FIGURE 11.33

Changes of chemotherapy: 35-year-old female with ICC with tumoral reponse status post–3 months of chemotherapy. MSCT contrast-enhanced images show decrease in peripheral enhancement and the size of the tumor.

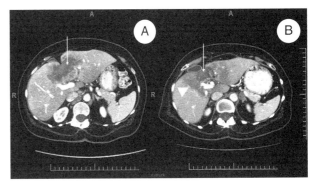

FIGURE 11.34

Changes of chemoradiation: 65-year-old male with ICC after 11 months of chemoradiation. MSCT contrast-enhanced images show a decrease in the size of the tumor (white arrows) involving segment IV extending into segment V. Adjacent low-density changes in the liver are edema due to radiation therapy (arrowhead).

EXTRAHEPATIC CHOLANGIOCARCINOMA

Extrahepatic cholangiocarcinomas are adenocarcinomas of the bile ducts that arise proximal in the right or left hepatic ducts, at the confluence of the ducts, or in the common hepatic or common bile ducts. They are usually subdivided into hilar or distal cholangiocarcinomas if they arise at the confluence of the ducts or in the distal bile duct near the ampulla, respectively. Hilar cholangiocarcinomas are the most prevalent, with a reported incidence ranging from 40 to 60% in large series (49). Tumors of the distal bile duct are less common, accounting for approximately 20–30% (49).

A classification system has been proposed by The Liver Cancer Study Group of Japan that provides information on the gross appearance, tumor growth, and biologic behavior and is useful for radiologic interpretation. According to this classification, cholangiocarcinoma can be divided into three subtypes: (a) mass forming, (b) periductal-infiltrating, and (c) intraductal-growing (37).

Epidemiology

Extrahepatic cholangiocarcinoma is a disease of the elderly, and the majority of patients are over 65 years of age. The prognosis is poor, and, if untreated, it usually leads to death in approximately 12 months.

Risk factors for the development of extrahepatic cholangiocarcinoma are similar to those for intrahepatic cholangiocarcinoma. Primary sclerosing cholangitis is probably the most widely recognized risk factor (2). The reported incidence of cholangiocarcinoma in patients with primary sclerosing cholangitis varies from 8 to 40%, and, unlike sporadic cholangiocarcinoma, these patients are at risk for multifocal disease. An increased incidence has also been reported in patients with choledochal cysts and Caroli's disease (2). Oriental cholangiohepatitis has shown an association with a higher incidence of cholangiocarcinoma, particularly in Japan and parts of Southeast Asia, where the disease is more prevalent.

Clinical Presentation

Most patients with extrahepatic cholangiocarcinoma present with obstructive jaundice. Jaundice may not occur if biliary obstruction is not complete, such as when only the right or left hepatic ducts are involved or with segmental ductal obstruction. Abdominal pain, pruritus, weight loss, and anorexia are present in about one third of patients. The alkaline phosphatase level is usually elevated. Tumor markers such as CEA and CA 19-9 are elevated after the mass has become very large

Imaging

The imaging approach for ECC should focus on providing a comprehensive noninvasive resectability evaluation in order to assist the surgeon in correctly stratifying patients preoperatively into operable and nonoperable categories. The CT imaging protocol must be tailored to provide accurate information on the following factors: location and extent of the primary tumor within the biliary tree, vascular anatomy and involvement by the tumor, nodal disease, and the presence of metastases.

Protocol and Imaging Technique

In our institution, CT has become the primary imaging modality for workup of biliary tract malignancy. Recent developments in multidetector CT have made possible imaging the entire abdomen at 0.7-mm slice thickness in one breathhold. These capabilities decrease volume averaging artifacts and significantly lower the chance of motion artifacts that may hinder the detection of small tumors and their true extent along the biliary tree.

In order to increase tumor conspicuity, rapid intravenous injection (4–8 cc/sec) of 120–150 cc of iodinated contrast is required (50). Dual-phase imaging of the entire abdomen during the hepatic arterial dominant phase and during the peak of portal venous enhancement optimizes detection of the primary tumor, visualization of arterial and venous structures for staging, and identification of hepatic metastasis (50).

Our dual-phase protocol for imaging on a 64-detector row scanner results in a 5-second image acquisition for the entire abdomen. Images are then reconstructed for both phases to 0.625 mm for problem solving and multiplanar 3D reconstructions. We inject at 5 cc/sec for a 30-second injection duration. Smart-Prep® (GE Healthcare, Milwaukee) is used for bolus tracking, monitoring the aorta at the level of the celiac artery until a trigger value of 100 Hounsfield units is reached. After a diagnostic delay of 20 seconds, we begin imaging at the level of the diaphragm at 40 seconds postinjection and complete scanning the abdomen at 45 seconds. After another 15-second delay, the abdomen is imaged again for portal venous imaging.

Imaging Findings: Tumor Location and Extension into the Biliary Tree

A thorough understanding of the normal anatomy of the hilar fissure of the liver is essential for the correct interpretation of CT images. In the hilar fissure, the left hepatic duct (which drains segments II, III, and IV) joins the right hepatic duct (which drains segments V, VIII, VII, and VI) to form the common bile duct. The confluence of the hepatic ducts is located anterior to the bifurcation of the portal vein or just anterior to the origin of the left portal vein. The intrahepatic biliary ducts are not visible on contrast-enhanced CT unless dilated. The normal right and left hepatic ducts and the common hepatic duct may be seen as thin tubular structures of water attenuation and imperceptible walls anteriorly to the portal vein (Figure 11.35). The left hepatic duct is usually longer than the right duct, measuring approximately 2–5 cm, while the right duct measures around 1 cm.

The Bismuth and Corlette Classification System is used to stage patients with hilar cholangiocarcinoma. This system takes into account the location of the primary tumor in relation to the confluence of the right and left ducts and the extent of ductal involvement (51, 52) According to this system, hilar cholangiocarcinomas are classified into four types: Type I lesions involve only the common hepatic or common bile duct but do not extend

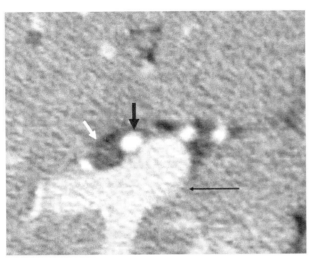

FIGURE 11.35

Normal anatomy of the hepatic hilum on MSCT. In the hilar fissure the hepatic artery (thick black arrow) and the bile duct (thick white arrow) are anterior to the portal vein (long thin black arrow). The bile duct is lateral to the hepatic artery. Note the homogeneous water attenuation of the bile duct. Its walls are thin and imperceptible.

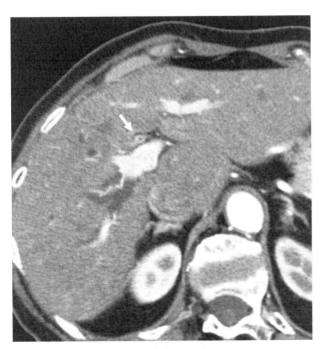

FIGURE 11.36

Bile duct enhancement in cholangiocarcinoma. Axial contrast-enhanced MSCT image shows enhancement and irregular thickening of the right bile duct in the hilar fissure (arrow). Bile duct thickening and enhancement is always an abnormal finding and should raise concerns for tumor involvement in the absence of recent instrumentation or infection.This tumor involves the confluence of the ducts and extends in the right duct consistent with a bismuth Type IIIa hilar cholangiocarcinoma.

to the bifurcation of the hepatic duct . Type II lesions involve the confluence of the right and left hepatic ducts. Type IIIa lesions involve the right secondary confluence, and type IIIb, the left secondary confluence. Type IV lesions involve both secondary confluences.

The CT imaging features we use to determine tumor location and extension are: enhancement of the bile duct wall (Figures 11.36 and 11.37), changes of attenuation from water to soft tissue within the bile ducts (Figure 11.38), abrupt caliber changes, and presence of a mass within the bile duct with proximal dilatation of the biliary tree (Figures 11.39 and 11.40).

Most extrahepatic cholangiocarcinomas are of the periductal infiltrating type, and these tumors present on contrast-enhanced CT as areas of irregular circumferential thickening and luminal narrowing of the bile duct associated with proximal biliary dilatation (Figures 11.41 and 11.42). Bile duct wall enhancement or thickening is always an abnormal finding and is an indication of tumor involvement in the absence of inflammatory disease or recent instrumentation. Mass-forming and intraductal-growing types of extrahepatic cholangiocarcinoma present as an enhancing soft tissue mass filling and expanding the lumen of the bile duct (Figure 11.43).

The periductal-infiltrating cholangiocarcinoma shows a tendency to disseminate submucosally, which underestimates the extent of disease on imaging studies. In a study by Tillich et al., CT was able to detect the primary tumor, but the exact proximal tumor

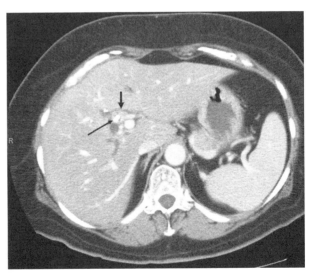

FIGURE 11.37

Circumferential thickening and enhancement of the bile duct in Type IIIa hilar cholangiocarcinoma. Contrast-enhanced axial MSCT image shows prominent circumferential thickening of the right bile duct with bile duct wall and enhancement (arrow), consistent with a hilar cholangiocarcinoma. There is a stent in the bile duct extending into segment VIII bile duct (long arrow).

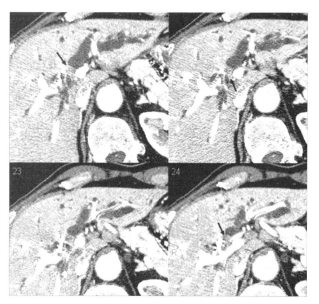

FIGURE 11.38

Transition from water to soft tissue attenuation within bile duct in cholangiocarcinoma. Multiple axial contrast-enhanced MSCT images show dilatation of the segment III bile duct and of the left bile duct. Note transition from water to soft tissue attenuation within the left bile duct in the left hilar fissure extending into the confluence of the ducts, consistent with a Type IIIb hilar cholangiocarcinoma (arrows).

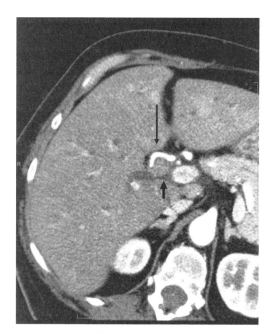

FIGURE 11.39

Mass-forming hilar cholangiocarcinoma. Axial contrast-enhanced MSCT image shows a soft tissue mass in the common hepatic duct involving the confluence of the ducts, consistent with a type II hilar cholangiocarcinoma (arrow). Note the hepatic artery (long arrow) is anterior to the duct, an anatomic variation that occurs in approximately 13% of cases.

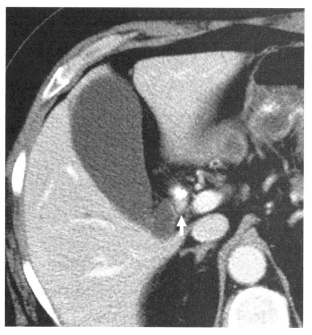

FIGURE 11.40

Type I hilar cholangiocarcinoma. Axial contrast-enhanced MSCT image shows a focal area of mural soft tissue thickening in the common bile duct, at the level of the insertion of the cystic duct, consistent with a type I cholangiocarcinoma (arrow). In cases when there is a low insertion of the cystic duct just above the pancreatic head or the tumor is located more than 2 cm from the confluence of the ducts, it should be classified as distal or suprapancreatic cholangiocarcinoma.

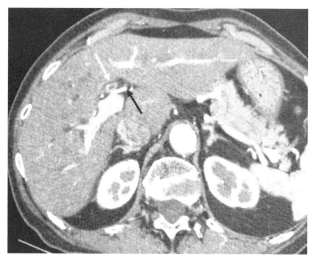

FIGURE 11.41

Periductal-infiltrating cholangiocarcinoma. Axial contrast-enhanced image shows circumferential thickening and enhancement of the right bile duct, just proximal to the confluence (white arrow). There is a clear fat plane surrounding the hepatic artery, which is not narrowed (black arrow). Enhancement and irregular soft tissue thickening are features of periductal-infiltrating type of cholangiocarcinoma.

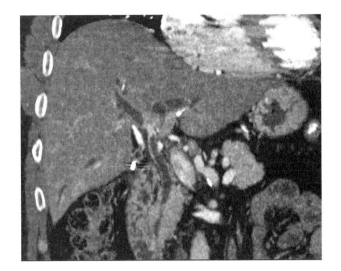

FIGURE 11.42

Periductal-infiltrating type of hilar cholangiocarcinoma. Coronal reformation shows a focal area of narrowing, irregular thickening, and enhancement of the common hepatic duct, at the level of the confluence (arrow), consistent with a periductal-infiltrating type of cholangiocarcinoma. There is prominent proximal biliary dilatation. This type of tumor infiltrates the periductal soft tissues and causes a desmoplastic response that results in significant enhancement.

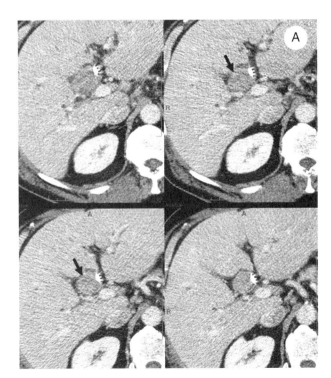

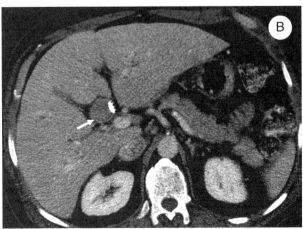

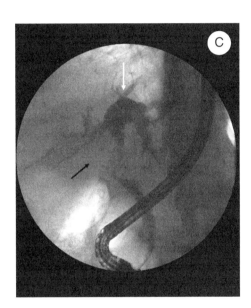

FIGURE 11.43

(A) Intraductal-growing hilar cholangiocarcinoma. Multiple axial contrast-enhanced MSCT images show a soft tissue mass expanding the right duct and extending into the common hepatic duct, consisting with an intraductal-growing type of cholangiocarcinoma (arrow). A plastic stent is displaced medially with the duct by the large polypoid tumor. (B) Intraductal-growing hilar cholangiocarcinoma. Axial contrast-enhanced image shows with better detail the large mass filling the lumen of the bile duct. Note the thin wall of the expanded bile duct (arrow). This is a distinct feature of this type of cholangiocarcinoma. There is no infiltration of the periductal soft tissues or desmoplastic response with narrowing of the lumen of the bile, as commonly seen in periductal-infiltrating tumors. (C) Intraductal-growing hilar cholangiocarcinoma. Fluoroscopic image obtained during ERCP shows a polypoid mass arising in the right duct (black arrow), which is not opacified with contrast. The mass fills the lumen of the common hepatic duct and obstructs the left ducts, which are markedly dilated (white arrow).

extent was underestimated by CT, accounting for an overall accuracy of resectability of only 60% (53). In a recent study by Aloia et al. utilizing thin section MSCT, CT was proven accurate in predicting resectability of hilar cholangiocarcinoma when factors such as tumor location within the biliary tree, vascular invasion, and metastatic disease were taken into consideration. MSCT shows a sensitivity of 94%, specificity of 79%, and negative and positive predictive values of 92 and 85%, respectively, with an overall accuracy of 74.5% (54).

After the anatomic site of the primary tumor has been determined by imaging, attention needs to be paid to the extent of radial growth and adjacent organ invasion. The periductal-infiltrating type of cholangiocarcinoma commonly invades the surrounding periductal fat and has a propensity to spread along the peribiliary nerve plexus and arteries (53). Soft tissue attenuation with obliteration of the fat surrounding the vessels in the hepatic hilum is a feature of periarterial and perineural spread of cholangiocarcinoma (Figures 11.44–11.47). It is important to carefully evaluate the ducts and vessels in the hilar fissure for signs of invasion. Similar to gallbladder carcinoma, extrahepatic cholangiocarcinoma can invade adjacent structures. Adjacent organ invasion is usually readily apparent on CT as direct tumor extension into the hepatic parenchyma, gallbladder, or bowel.

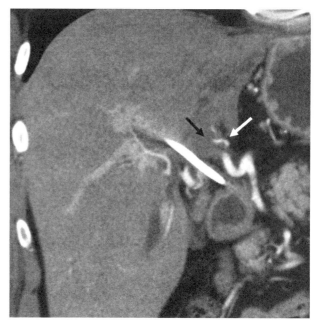

FIGURE 11.45

Periarterial perineural spread in cholangiocarcinoma. Oblique coronal volume rendered image shows infiltrating soft tissue (black arrow) encasing the left hepatic artery (white arrow), consistent with periarterial perineural spread of a hilar cholangiocarcinoma. Note atrophy of the left lobe of the liver.

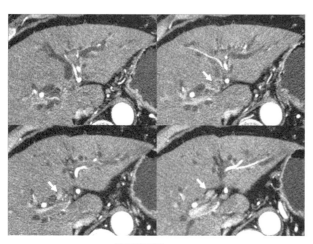

FIGURE 11.44

Type IV periductal-infiltrating cholangiocarcinoma. Multiple contiguous contrast-enhanced axial MSCT images show dilatation of BIII, BIV, and BVIII ducts. There is an infiltrative enhancing mass growing in the left and right hilar fissure (arrow). The left portal vein is occluded, and there is and there is soft tissue infiltration surrounding the left hepatic artery branches in the left hilar fissure. Periarterial and perineural spread is a feature commonly seen with periductal-infiltrating cholangiocarcinoma.

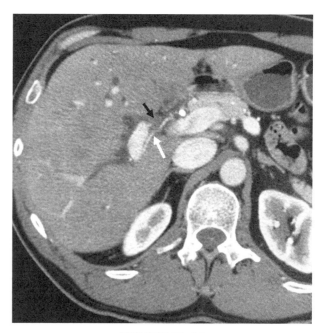

FIGURE 11.46

Periarterial perineural spread of cholangiocarcinoma. Axial contrast-enhanced MSCT image shows infiltrative soft tissue (black arrow) encasing the right hepatic artery (white arrow) in the hilar fissure, compatible with periarterial spread of tumor.

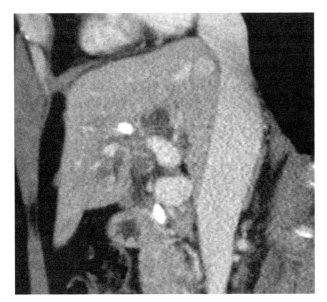

FIGURE 11.47

Perineural periarterial spread of cholangiocarcinoma. Sagittal oblique reformation shows infiltrative soft tissue in the hepatic hilum (short black arrow) encasing the right hepatic artery (long black arrow). A stent is noted in the right duct (white arrow). Perineural periarterial spread of tumor is seen on imaging as soft tissue infiltration along the course of the artery. The vessel may be narrowed, angulated, or occluded depending upon the degree of invasion into the adventitia.

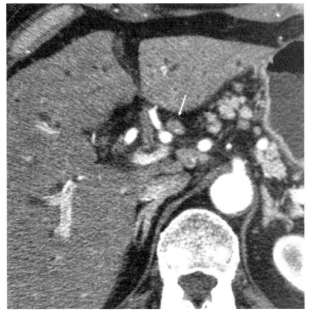

FIGURE 11.48

Axial contrast-enhanced image shows a common hepatic artery node (arrow). Although this not does not exceed 1 cm in short axis diameter, because it is larger than the adjacent nodes and is located along the lymphangitic path of spread of cholangiocarcinoma, it was considered suspicious for malignancy.

Nodal Disease

Lymphatic spread represents crucial information with direct impact in patient management and prognosis. Five-year survival of 39% has been reported for patients with N0 disease as opposed to only 3% in patients with N2 disease (51, 55). The cystic and pericholedochal nodes (N1 disease) are usually resected with the primary tumor and do not represent a contraindication to surgery. These need to be differentiated from the celiac, periduodenal, and superior mesenteric nodes (N2 nodal station), since they usually represent a contraindication to surgical resection (9, 10) (Figures 11.48 and 11.49). Imaging features that indicate metastatic involvement of lymph nodes are nodal enlargement (short axis greater than 1 cm) and its internal attenuation. Nodes with lower attenuation are generally necrotic, and necrotic nodes are more likely to harbor metastatic disease, even if not enlarged by CT criteria (12). Enlarged nodes distant to the primary such as retroperitoneal, para-aortic, and mesenteric nodes should be biopsied prior to surgical planning to exclude the possibility of lymphoproliferative disorders or reactive lymphadenopathy. MSCT has been proven accurate in predicting nodal metastasis in patients with hilar cholangiocarcinoma with a positive predictive value of

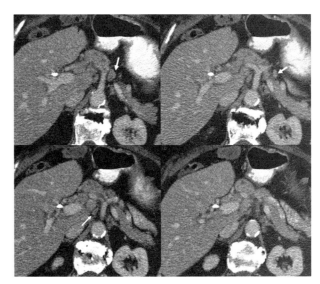

FIGURE 11.49

Lymphangitic spread in cholangiocarcinoma. Multiple contiguous axial contrast-enhanced images of a patient with hilar cholangiocarcinoma show multiple enlarged nodes along the common hepatic artery and celiac axis, consistent with N2 nodes.

80%, negative predictive value of 84.4%, and sensitivity and specificity of 53.3 and 95%, respectively, yielding an overall accuracy of 83.6% (56)

Distant Metastases

Common sites of distant metastases are the liver, peritoneal implants, and distant nodal metastases. Small hepatic and peritoneal metastases are a well-recognized cause of nonresectability. Lesions larger than 1 cm are readily identified on thin slice MSCT and can generally be confidently differentiated from benign lesions such as cysts or hemangiomata. Hepatic metastases generally present as hypoattenuating lesions in relation to the contrast-enhanced hepatic parenchyma and are best appreciated during the portal-venous phase of contrast enhancement. Subcentimeter hepatic metastases remain a diagnostic dilemma since even state-of-the-art MSCT may not be able to accurately characterize these lesions. Peritoneal implants usually present as soft tissue infiltration or discrete nodularity against the normal low attenuation intraperitoneal fat (Figures 11.50–11.52). Again, subcentimeter peritoneal implants are a common source of error in the imaging analysis of resectability. In a recent study involving 32 patients who underwent laparotomy for hilar cholangiocarcinoma, MSCT predicted resectability in three patients who were deemed inoperable at surgery (54). Subcentimeter peritoneal disease and subcentimeter hepatic metastases were responsible factors.

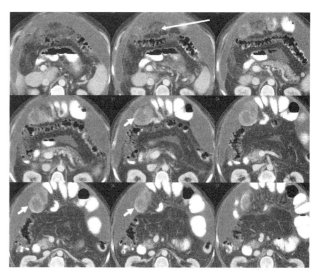

FIGURE 11.51

Peritoneal carcinomatose from hilar cholangiocarcinoma. Multiple axial contiguous contrast-enhanced images show ascites and infiltration and stranding of the omental fat, consistent with peritoneal carcinomatose (long arrow). Note a large enhancing implant in the omentum (short arrows).

Differential Diagnosis

Several nonneoplastic and neoplastic conditions may mimic extrahepatic cholangiocarcinoma on imaging studies. In our opinion, inflammatory conditions of the biliary tree can pose a significant diagnostic challenge.

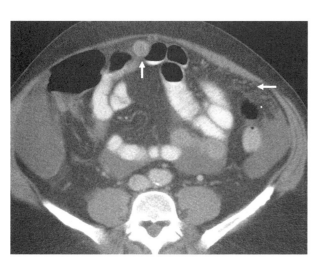

FIGURE 11.50

Peritoneal carcinomatose. Axial contrast-enhanced image in a patient with metastatic hilar cholangiocarcinoma shows infiltration and stranding of the omental fat in the left lower quadrant, consistent with peritoneal carcinomatose (horizontal arrow). Note a large enhancing soft tissue nodule in the omentum along the midline (vertical arrow).

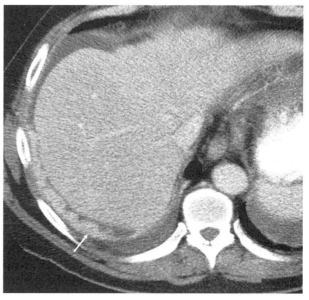

FIGURE 11.52

Pleural and diafragmatic metastases in a patient with extensive peritoneal carcinomatose from hilar cholangiocarcinoma. Note nodular thickening of the undersurface of right hemidiaphragm and of the right pleura in the posterior sulcus (arrow).

Mirizzi's syndrome is defined as compression of the common hepatic duct due to inflammation associated with an impacted stone in the cystic duct or neck of the gallbladder. Figures 11.53 and 11.54 show the imaging features of Mirizzi's syndrome. In the setting of inflammation, thickening and enhancement of the bile duct wall is commonly seen and can be virtually indistinguishable from biliary cancer. Careful attention to clinical history and presentation, the presence of cholelithiasis, and adjacent inflammatory changes may help the radiologist make the appropriate distinction.

Likewise, neoplastic processes such as lymphoma and plasmocytoma may occasionally involve the biliary tree and need to be included in the differential diagnosis in the appropriate clinical setting. Diffuse homogeneous soft tissue thickening and infiltration may be seen in patients with lymphoproliferative disorders in the biliary tree.

Treatment Response and Recurrence

Similar to gallbladder cancer, CT is the imaging modality of choice to monitor patients with extrahepatic cholangiocarcinoma after curative surgical resection. Familiarity of the normal postoperative CT appearance following partial hepatectomy with bilioenteric anastomosis is essential for adequate interpretation of the images. A nonenhancing fluid collection at the hepatic resection margin is a normal finding following surgery.

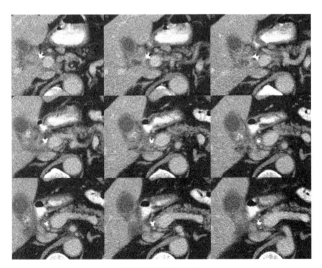

FIGURE 11.53

Mirizzi's symdrome. Multiple axial contrast-enhanced images show an ill-defined enhancing mass in the neck of the gallbladder (arrows). The common hepatic duct obstruction has been relieved by a plastic stent (long black arrow). There is gallbladder wall thickening and cholelithiasis. These findings should alert the radiologist to the possibility of an inflammatory condition mimicking cholangiocarcinoma.

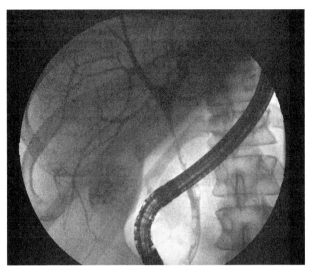

FIGURE 11.54

Spot fluoroscopic image obtained during ERCP shows a long smooth stricture of the common hepatic and common bile duct. Multiple filling defects are seen within the gallbladder, compatible with gallstones.

This collection should progressively decrease in size on serial follow-up examinations. No soft tissue nodule or solid components should be present. Soft tissue infiltration and blurring is commonly noted at the site of choledochojejunostomy or hepaticojejunostomy and does not necessarily indicate recurrent disease. It usually becomes less prominent on serial examinations. In our experience, postradiation fibrosis can be very difficult to differentiate from recurrent disease. The importance of serial imaging with similar technique (collimation, reconstruction interval, field of view, etc.) cannot be overemphasized, since posttreatment changes such as scarring and postradiation fibrosis can masquerade underlying disease and decrease sensitivity of CT for recurrence. Despite state-of-the-art CT technique, early diagnosis of recurrence in the setting of prominent radiation fibrosis remains a diagnostic dilemma. Findings that indicate recurrent disease on imaging are progressive enhancement and irregular thickening of the remaining bile duct wall, development of a soft tissue mass within the residual ducts, and obstruction of the choledochal jejunostomy or hepaticojejunostomy with development of biliary obstruction.

Vascular Information

Information regarding variant vascular anatomy and involvement of the portal vein and hepatic artery is extremely important for proper staging and surgical planning of hepatobiliary malignancies. The presence of variations of the vascular anatomy or vascular invasion plays a major role in determining resectability. Common vascular variants include replaced right hepatic artery from the superior mesenteric artery (SMA) (Figure 11.55), accessory right hepatic artery and common hepatic artery replaced from the SMA, and replaced left hepatic artery from the left gastric artery (Figures 11.56 and 11.57). The overall incidence of hepatic branches from the SMA is approximately 20%. Careful evaluation of the hepatic artery is critical. The presence of an accessory or replaced right hepatic artery may change management of a patient with unresectable biliary cancer due to encasement of the common hepatic artery by tumor. Variation of the portal venous anatomy is also equally important. In patients with trifurcation of the main portal vein, the right anterior portal vein arises from the left portal vein (Figure 11.58). Resection of the left portal vein proximal to the origin of the right anterior portal vein in such cases would compromise perfusion to the right liver. MSCT is accurate for the preoperative vascular evaluation of patients with hepatobiliary neoplasms. It depicts hepatic arterial and venous anatomy with an overall accuracy of 97%, sensitivity of 94%, and specificity of 100% (57), obviating the need for catheter angiography before oncologic liver surgery.

The presence of vascular invasion has a major impact on surgical planning. Encasement or occlusion of the main portal vein or hepatic artery, or involvement of the portal vein contralateral to the primary tumor, constitutes criteria for irresectability in most institutions. A cholangiocarcinoma in the left duct may extend inferiorly along the hilar fissure and occlude the main or the contralateral portal vein (Figure 11.59). The imaging criteria commonly used in CT to determine vascular invasion include occlusion, irregular luminal narrowing, and loss of the fat plane between the tumor and the vessel wall with tumor encasing more

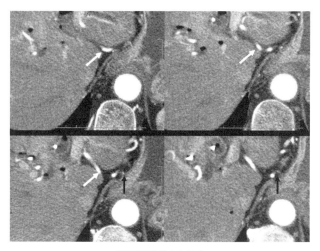

FIGURE 11.56

Replaced left hepatic artery (LHA) from the left gastric artery (LGA). Multiple axial contrast-enhanced images show the LHA (white arrow) arising from the LGA (black arrow) within the gastrohepatic ligament.

than 180 degrees of vessel circumference (58). MSCT has proven to be a reliable technique to predict vascular invasion in patients with hepatobiliary cancer with reported sensitivity, specificity, positive predictive value, negative predictive value, and overall accuracy of 92.3, 100, 100, 94.1, and 96.6% , respectively (56).

CONCLUSION

Gallbladder and biliary tract cancers are highly lethal diseases. The prognosis is dismal and surgical resection remains the only chance for a cure. Cross-sectional imaging with MSCT is a valuable technique in the preoperative evaluation of gallbladder and intra- and

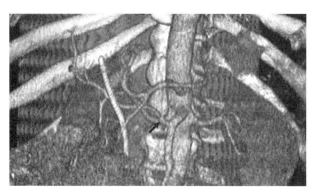

FIGURE 11.55

Replaced right hepatic artery (RHA) from the superior mesenteric artery (SMA). Three-dimensional volumetric reconstruction shows the RHA arising from the SMA (arrow).

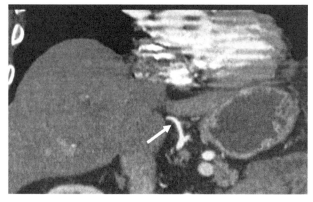

FIGURE 11.57

Replaced LHA from the LGA. Coronal reformation illustrates the LHA (arrow) arising from the LGA and coursing throgu the gastrohepatic ligament into the left liver.

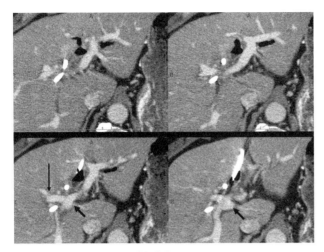

FIGURE 11.58

Trifurcation of the portal vein. Multiple axial contrast-enhanced images show a common origin of the left portal vein and right anterior and posterior portal veins (short black arrows). Injury to the right anterior portal vein supplying segments VIII and V can occur during surgery for a left hepatectomy if this anatomic variation is overlooked.

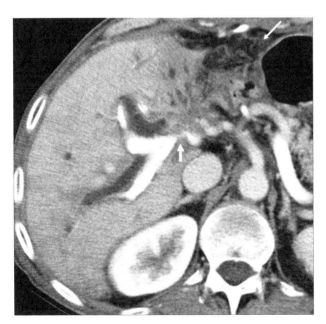

FIGURE 11.59

Vascular invasion in advanced hilar cholangiocarcinoma. Axial contrast-enhanced image shows an infiltrative tumor growing in the left hilar fissure, which has occluded the left portal vein and caused atrophy of the left lobe of the liver. Stranding and infiltration of the omental fat in the left sub-hepatic space is noted, consistent with peritoneal seeding (thin arrow). The tumor grows into the right fissure, obstructs the right anterior and posterior ducts, and encases and virtually occludes the right portal vein (arrow). Periarterial spread is noted along the common hepatic artery, which is surrounded by soft tissue attenuation (white arrow).

extrahepatic cholangiocarcinoma. MSCT is capable of providing, in a single study, information on tumor location and depth of hepatic invasion, extent into the biliary tree, adjacent organ invasion, regional lymphadenopathy, and distant metastases. This information constitutes the basis for proper staging and effectively predicting resectability preoperatively. In our institution, state-of-the-art MSCT is the imaging modality of choice for the staging workup and in monitoring treatment response in patients with gallbladder and biliary tract cancers.

References

1. Greenlee RT, et al. Cancer statistics, 2000; CA Cancer J Clin 2000; 50(1):7–33.
2. Khan ZR, et al. Risk factors for biliary tract cancers. Am J Gastroenterol 1999; 94(1):149–152.
3. Bartlett DL. Gallbladder cancer. Semin Surg Oncol 2000; 19(2):145–55.
4. Barr LH, Wright FH. Carcinoma of the gallbladder. Am Surg 1984; 50(5):275–276.
5. Matsumoto Y, et al. Surgical treatment of primary carcinoma of the gallbladder based on the histologic analysis of 48 surgical specimens. Am J Surg 1992; 163(2):239–245.
6. Bartlett DL, et al. Long-term results after resection for gallbladder cancer. Implications for staging and management. Ann Surg 1996; 224(5):639–646.
7. Yoshikawa T, et al. (The study for the surgical treatment on distal bile duct carcinoma). Nippon Geka Gakkai Zasshi 1997; 98(5):501–504.
8. Fong Y, Jarnagin W, Blumgart LH. Gallbladder cancer: comparison of patients presenting initially for definitive operation with those presenting after prior noncurative intervention. Ann Surg 2000; 232(4):557–569.
9. Blumgart LH, Fong Y. Hepatobiliary cancer. Semin Surg Oncol, 2000; 19(2):83.
10. Sussman SK, et al. Gastric adenocarcinoma: CT versus surgical staging. Radiology 1988; 167(2):335–340.
11. Noji,T, et al. Computed tomography evaluation of regional lymph node metastases in patients with biliary cancer. Br J Surg 2008; 95:92–96.
12. Ohtani T, et al. Spread of gallbladder carcinoma: CT evaluation with pathologic correlation. Abdom Imaging 1996; 21(3):195–201.
13. Levin B. Gallbladder carcinoma. Ann Oncol 1999; 10(suppl 4):129–130.
14. Coakley FV, et al. Peritoneal metastases: detection with spiral CT in patients with ovarian cancer. Radiology 2002; 223(2):495–499.
15. Kalra N, et al. MDCT in the staging of gallbladder carcinoma. AJR Am J Roentgenol 2006; 186(3):758–762.
16. Owen CC, Bilhartz LE. Gallbladder polyps, cholesterolosis, adenomyomatosis, and acute acalculous cholecystitis. Semin Gastrointest Dis 2003; 14(4):178–188.
17. Ching BH, et al. CT differentiation of adenomyomatosis and gallbladder cancer. AJR Am J Roentgenol 2007; 189(1):62–66.
18. Levy AD, et al. From the archives of the AFIP. Benign tumors and tumorlike lesions of the gallbladder and extrahepatic bile ducts: radiologic-pathologic correlation. Armed Forces Institute of Pathology. Radiographics 2002; 22(2):387–413.
19. DeOliveira ML, et al. Cholangiocarcinoma: thirty-one-year experience with 564 patients at a single institution. Ann Surg 2007; 245(5):755–762.
20. Martin R, Jarnagin W. Intrahepatic cholangiocarcinoma. Current management. Minerva Chi 2003; 58(4):469–478.
21. Liu CL, et al. Hepatic resection for combined hepatocellular and cholangiocarcinoma. Arch Surg 2003; 138(1):86–90.

22. Welzel TM, et al. Risk factors for intrahepatic and extrahepatic cholangiocarcinoma in the United States: a population-based case-control study. Clin Gastroenterol Hepatol 2007; 5(10): 1221–1228.

23. Fu XH, et al. Clinicopathologic features, diagnosis and surgical treatment of intrahepatic cholangiocarcinoma in 104 patients. Hepatobiliary Pancreat Dis Int 2004; 3(2):279–283.

24. Lin G, et al. Combined hepatocellular cholangiocarcinoma: prognostic factors investigated by computed tomography/magnetic resonance imaging. Int J Clin Pract 2007; 62(8): 1199–1205.

25. Yamasaki S. Intrahepatic cholangiocarcinoma: macroscopic type and stage classification. J Hepatobiliary Pancreat Surg 2003; 10(4):288–291.

26. Ros PR, et al. Intrahepatic cholangiocarcinoma: radiologic-pathologic correlation. Radiology 1988; 167(3):689–693.

27. Asayama Y, et al. Delayed-phase dynamic CT enhancement as a prognostic factor for mass-forming intrahepatic cholangiocarcinoma. Radiology 2006; 238(1):150–155.

28. Blachar A, Federle MP, Brancatelli G. Hepatic capsular retraction: spectrum of benign and malignant etiologies. Abdom Imaging 2002; 27(6):690–699.

29. Hirohashi K., et al. Macroscopic types of intrahepatic cholangiocarcinoma: clinicopathologic features and surgical outcomes. Hepatogastroenterology 2002; 49(44):326–329.

30. Park HS, et al. CT Differentiation of cholangiocarcinoma from periductal fibrosis in patients with hepatolithiasis. AJR Am J Roentgenol 2006; 187(2):445–453.

31. Gulluoglu MG, et al. Intraductal growth-type mucin-producing peripheral cholangiocarcinoma associated with biliary papillomatosis. Ann Diagn Pathol 2007; 11(1):34–38.

32. Lee JW, et al. CT features of intraductal intrahepatic cholangiocarcinoma. AJR Am J Roentgenol 2000; 175(3):721–725.

33. Jung AY, et al. CT features of an intraductal polypoid mass: Differentiation between hepatocellular carcinoma with bile duct tumor invasion and intraductal papillary cholangiocarcinoma. J Comput Assist Tomogr 2006; 30(2):173–181.

34. Lim JH. Cholangiocarcinoma: morphologic classification according to growth pattern and imaging findings. AJR Am J Roentgenol 2003; 181(3):819–27.

35. Zhang Y, et al. Intrahepatic peripheral cholangiocarcinoma: comparison of dynamic CT and dynamic MRI. J Comput Assist Tomogr 1999; 23(5):670–677.

36. Grobmyer SR, et al. Perihepatic lymph node assessment in patients undergoing partial hepatectomy for malignancy. Ann Surg 2006; 244(2):260–264.

37. Tsuji T, et al. Lymphatic spreading pattern of intrahepatic cholangiocarcinoma. Surgery 2001; 129(4):401–407.

38. Shimoda M, Kubota K. Multi-disciplinary treatment for cholangiocellular carcinoma. World J Gastroenterol 2007; 13(10):1500–1504.

39. Ohtsuka M, et al. Results of surgical treatment for intrahepatic cholangiocarcinoma and clinicopathological factors influencing survival. Br J Surg 2002; 89(12):1525–1531.

40. Nakeeb A, et al. Cholangiocarcinoma. A spectrum of intrahepatic, perihilar, and distal tumors. Ann Surg 1996; 224(4):463–473; discussion 473–475.

41. Madoff DC, Abdalla EK, Vauthey JN. Portal vein embolization in preparation for major hepatic resection: evolution of a new standard of care. J Vasc Interv Radiol 2005; 16(6):779–790.

42. Parker SL, et al. Cancer statistics, 1996. CA Cancer J Clin 1996; 46(1):5–27.

43. Slattery JM, Sahani DV. What is the current state-of-the-art imaging for detection and staging of cholangiocarcinoma? Oncologist 2006; 11(8):913–922.

44. Jarnagin WR, et al. Staging, resectability, and outcome in 225 patients with hilar cholangiocarcinoma. Ann Surg 2001; 234(4):507–517; discussion 517–519.

45. D'Angelica M, et al. The role of staging laparoscopy in hepatobiliary malignancy: prospective analysis of 401 cases. Ann Surg Oncol 2003; 10(2):183–189.

46. Tillich M, et al. Multiphasic helical CT in diagnosis and staging of hilar cholangiocarcinoma. AJR Am J Roentgenol 1998; 171(3):651–658.

47. Aloia TA, et al. High-resolution computed tomography accurately predicts resectability in hilar cholangiocarcinoma. Am J Surg 2007; 193(6):702–706.

48. Otto G, et al. Hilar cholangiocarcinoma: resectability and radicality after routine diagnostic imaging. J Hepatobiliary Pancreat Surg 2004; 11(5):310–318.

49. Lee HY, et al. Preoperative assessment of resectability of hepatic hilar cholangiocarcinoma: combined CT and cholangiography with revised criteria. Radiology 2006; 239(1):113–121.

50. Sahani D, et al. Using multidetector CT for preoperative vascular evaluation of liver neoplasms: technique and results. AJR Am J Roentgenol 2002; 179(1):53–59.

51. Cha JH, et al. Preoperative evaluation of Klatskin tumor: accuracy of spiral CT in determining vascular invasion as a sign of unresectability. Abdom Imaging 2000; 25(5):500–507.

III

THERAPEUTIC APPROACHES

12 Radiofrequency Ablation

Ronald S. Arellano

Among the treatment options available to patients with intrahepatic cholangiocarcinoma, hepatic resection or liver transplantation offer the only chances for cure (1, 2). Even so, the 5-year survival rates for surgical resection range from 33.5 to 63% (3–5) compared to 5-year survival rates for untreated tumors of less than 5%. However, not all patients are suitable surgical candidates due to size, location, and/or medical comorbidities that render patients inoperable. Image-guided percutaneous radiofrequency ablation (also referred to as thermoablation) offers a newer and minimally invasive therapeutic option for the management of intrahepatic cholangiocarcinoma. A growing body of clinical and laboratory evidence supports the use of thermal ablative therapies, including radiofrequency ablation, to treat a variety of hepatic tumors. While the largest body of evidence is in the use of radiofrequency ablation to treat hepatocellular carcinoma, the guiding principles that govern the clinical application of radiofrequency ablation can be applied to the treatment of peripheral cholangiocarcinoma.

RADIOFREQUENCY ABLATION TECHNIQUE

Liver tumor ablation is accomplished with radiofrequency by using radio waves to generate heat within tissues. Most currently available radiofrequency generator systems have incorporated circuitry that allows measurement of generator output (measured in milliamperage and wattage) as well as local tissue impedance and temperature measurements. Any one of these variables can be used to monitor the effects of active radiofrequency ablation, and most commercially available radiofrequency systems employ one or more of these variables to guide treatment. Radiofrequency energy is deposited within a tumor by means of radiofrequency electrodes that are available in a variety of configurations and are typically 14–16 gauge in size. Electrode designs include expandable thermally active tines that are incrementally deployed throughout the tumor during treatment or straight electrodes that can be configured as a single electrode embedded on one handle or as a clustered arrangement spaced 5 mm apart, on a single handle. All electrode designs share the common feature of electrical insulation along all but the distal 1–3 cm of the electrode or variable lengths of the active tines for the expandable systems. Placement of the radiofrequency electrodes is accomplished using imaging guidance, typically with ultrasound or computed tomography. Magnetic resonance–compatible radiofrequency equipment is not widely available (6). Following verification that satisfactory placement of the electrode within the tumor has occurred, the electrode is connected to the appropriate generator and radiofrequency energy is emitted through the distal noninsulated portion of the electrode or tines (Figures 12.1 and 12.2). As radiofrequency energy passes

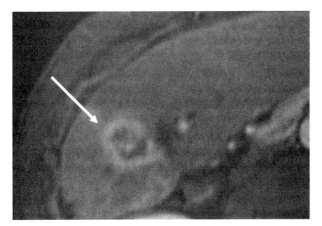

FIGURE 12.1

T1WI gadolinium-enhanced MRI obtained during the arterial phase demonstrates an enhancing lesion within segment IV of the liver (white arrow). The patient had a previous right hepatectomy for intrahepatic cholangiocarcinoma. Subsequent biopsy of the segment IV lesion confirmed the diagnosis of intrahepatic cholangiocarcinoma.

through tissue and attempts to reach electrical ground, the oscillating radiowaves induce ionic agitation within the tissues adjacent to the electrode that is converted to heat, resulting in coagulative necrosis (7). Via this mechanism, temperatures of up to 90°C can be achieved within a matter of minutes, and experimental studies have shown that irreversible coagulative necrosis of tissue can be achieved in as little as 6 minutes when tissue temperatures are at least 55–60°C. Increasing tissue temperatures to greater than 100°C does not necessarily result in larger volumes of ablated tissue. Instead, tissue charring and vaporization that result at these temperatures often result in increased local tissue impedance that acts to limit radiofrequency deposition, diffusion of heat, and ultimately coagulative necrosis (8). An early limitation of percutaneous radiofrequency ablation was the limitation in size of the coagulated tissue to approximately 1.6 cm with a single, straight electrode. Currently available electrode designs and generator systems, however, can now generate diameters of coagulated tissue of up to 5–7 cm. The availability of electrodes capable of generating large volumes of necrosis, coupled with treatment protocols that include serial and overlapping ablations to be performed, may facilitate treatment of tumors up to 5 cm diameter.

Image-guided percutaneous radiofrequency ablation is typically performed with ultrasound or computed tomography (CT) guidance and with the use of local anesthesia and intravenous procedural sedation. Intravenous procedural sedation is achieved with a combination of midazolam and short-acting narcotic such as fentanyl. General anesthesia may be required for patients with significant comorbidities in whom

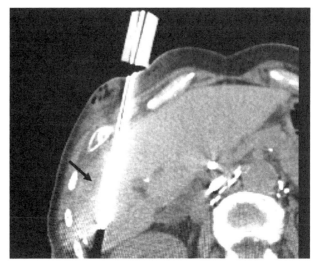

FIGURE 12.2

Axial CT image demonstrating radiofrequency electrode within the tumor (black arrow).

local anesthesia with intravenous sedatives and narcotic analgesia may be insufficient to maintain the comfort levels necessary to perform the ablation. Continuous cardiovascular and hemodynamic monitoring is required for all radiofrequency ablations. Dispersive grounding pads placed on the patient's thigh are an essential component of radiofrequency ablation equipment, and these act to disperse the electrical energy deposited within the body. It is essential that adhesive contact with the skin be maintained throughout the ablation in order to prevent skin burns.

Successful treatment requires that all identifiable tumor as well as a margin of adjacent hepatic parenchyma be included within the ablated tissue. Ideally, a zone of ablation with a margin of 0.5–1.0 cm around the tumor should be included with treatment as a means to prevent local tumor recurrence. Lack of an adequate ablative margin can result in peripheral tumor growth, necessitating additional treatments. In order to achieve adequate treatment with a sufficient size ablative margin, overlapping ablations following electrode repositioning within and around the tumor are often necessary for most lesions 3–4 cm in size, even with currently available electrode designs that can larger volumes of coagulated tissues.

FOLLOW-UP IMAGING

Computed Tomography

Follow-up imaging after radiofrequency ablation can be performed using dynamic contrast-enhanced CT or magnetic resonance imaging (MRI). The timing of post-procedure imaging varies by institution, but follow-up imaging with CT or MRI at 1- to 3-month intervals is useful for assessing treatment results as well as for the detection of residual tumor (9–11). The follow-up imaging schedule employed at our institution includes imaging 1 month after the ablation to evaluate the results of treatment and then repeat imaging at 3-month intervals thereafter for continued surveillance imaging. Accurate assessment of residual disease requires that high-quality imaging be obtained before and after radiofrequency ablation. An important imaging characteristic of cholangiocarcinoma is the tendency of this tumor to demonstrate delayed enhancement following administration of intravenous contrast material, so it is imperative to include delayed imaging when assessing treatment results. When no residual tumor is identified on the 1-month scan, repeat imaging is obtained at 3-month intervals, relative to the time of treatment, for 1 year.

The postablation CT protocol used at the Massachusetts General Hospital is a contrast-enhanced dynamic scan of the abdomen and pelvis using a 16-slice CT (Lightspeed, GE Healthcare, Madison, WI). Contrast material–enhanced images of the liver and abdomen are obtained following 30- and 70-second delays after the administration of contrast material. A total of 110 cc of contrast material is injected through an 18 gauge peripheral intravenous cannula at a rate of 5 cc/sec. Images are acquired at 5-mm slice thickness using a pitch of 1.375 and table speed of 27.5. Coronal reconstructions are also performed and may be helpful to evaluate lesions treated near the hepatic dome.

Completely treated tumor should manifest as a well-demarcated volume of low attenuation tissue that lacks enhancement following the administration of intravenous contrast. The CT findings of residual disease often appear as irregular, thickened soft tissue enhancement at the periphery or possibly within the zone of coagulated tissue. This is not to be confused with a thin rim of benign enhancement frequently identified at the margin of the coagulated tissue that is often seen immediately after an ablation when contrast is used to assess the immediate results of ablation. This can persist for several months after an ablation and is believed to represent inflammatory or reactive tissue. When residual disease is suspected, additional treatments are necessary to extend the zone of ablation to incorporate the residual disease within an adequate volume of ablated tissue. When follow-up imaging shows lack of irregular or thickened enhancement by 6 months, this suggests that tumor regrowth is unlikely to occur.

Magnetic Resonance Imaging

Magnetic resonance imaging is also useful to assess treatment results following radiofrequency ablation of peripheral cholangiocarcinoma (Figures 12.3 and 12.4). The MR signal of treated tumors can manifest as areas of high, low, or heterogeneous T1- and T2-weighted signal in the acute setting. The signal characteristics of the treated tissue evolve over time, but typically show decreased T2 signal characteristics following treatment and lack of enhancement following administration of Gd-DTPA. The changes in signal intensity likely reflect areas of altered protein within coagulated tissue.

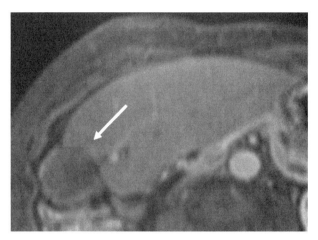

FIGURE 12.3

T1WI gadolinium-enhanced MRI obtained during the arterial phase, 2 years after radiofrequency ablation of intrahepatic cholangiocarcinoma. The examination shows absence peripheral or intratumoral enhancement on delayed imaging, consistent with successfully treated tumor (white arrow).

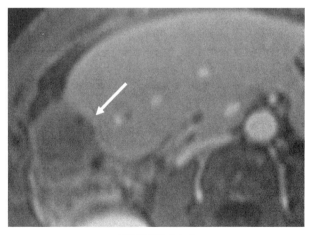

FIGURE 12.4

T1WI gadolinium-enhanced MRI obtained 120 seconds following the administration of intravenous contrast, 2 years after radiofrequency ablation of intrahepatic cholangiocarcinoma. The examination shows no delayed peripheral or intratumoral enhancement on delayed imaging, consistent with successfully treated tumor (white arrow).

Untreated tumors show irregular, thickened enhancement following intravenous administration of Gd-DTPA, similar to the findings observed on contrast-enhanced CT. The benign peripheral rim of enhancement along the margin of the ablative zone that is observed on CT can also be detected on MR imaging. This has been shown to represent inflammatory changes secondary to coagulative necrosis (12). As with follow-up CT imaging, this is not to be confused with bulky or irregular enhancement, which likely indicates residual disease.

Ultrasound

Gray-scale ultrasound is usually insufficiently sensitive to evaluate the extent of coagulative necrosis on follow-up imaging (9). Ultrasonographic blood pool agents may have a role in the future to assess treatment results, but these agents are not yet widely available.

COMPLICATIONS OF RADIOFREQUENCY ABLATION

Hepatic abscess is a potential major complication associated with radiofrequency ablation liver tumors and has a reported prevalence of 0.3–2% (13–17). Air within the zone of ablation from tissue vaporization is frequently observed immediately after treatment and should not be confused with an infectious process. This usually resolves within 1 week. Persistent air within the zone of ablation in the setting of leukocytosis and clinical findings of infection should raise the suspicion of an evolving hepatic abscess. When present, abscess can be treated with percutaneous aspiration or drainage. Surgical debridement is seldom necessary. The role of intravenous antibiotics for treatment of liver tumors is controversial, but should be considered in patients with previous bilioenteric anastamoses.

Mild dilation of the bile ducts around the zone of ablation can be detected on follow-up CT imaging in up to 87% of treated tumors (18). Hemobilia has also been described with radiofrequency ablation (19). This finding, however, is usually inconsequential and seldom results in cholangitis. Symptomatic bilomas can be treated with percutaneous drainage or aspiration.

Vascular injury associated with percutaneous radiofrequency ablation is a rare complication. Hepatic infarction is a rare occurrence following radiofrequency ablation of hepatic tumor, due primarily to the dual blood supply to the liver from the hepatic artery and portal vein. However, when a Pringle maneuver is performed with intraoperative radiofrequency, prolonged ischemic changes to the liver can be observed.

A variety of other complications following radiofrequency of hepatic tumors have been described, including bowel perforation, diaphragmatic and cardiac injury, and bleeding(20). Fortunately, these are all rare occurrences.

RESULTS

The largest clinical series specifically aimed at the use of percutaneous radiofrequency ablation for the treatment of peripheral cholangiocarcinoma is reported by Chiou et al. (21), who used ultrasound guidance to perform radiofrequency ablation as the primary treatment of 10 patients with 10 peripheral cholangiocarcinomas. Using contrast-enhanced CT to assess treatment results, the authors reported complete necrosis in all tumors with diameters of 3.0 cm or less and 67% complete necrosis of tumor 3.1–5.0 cm diameter (21). These results are similar to those reported for hepatocellular carcinoma of similar size treated with radiofrequency ablation (22). In additional to the series reported by Chiou et al., several case reports have documented the utility for treatment of primary intrahepatic (23) as well as recurrent cholangiocarcinoma (24, 25) with local control of tumor following radiofrequency ablation of up to 24 months.

FUTURE DIRECTIONS

Minimally invasive thermal ablative therapies, including radiofrequency ablation, are likely to become an integral tool in the multidisciplinary management of patients with hepatic tumors. The role of radiofrequency ablation in the management of peripheral cholangiocarcinoma shows promise and in time may emerge as a primary treatment modality for this disease. Its role in the management of recurrent peripheral cholangiocarcinoma requires further study, and the use of radiofrequency ablation as a bridge to transplantation has yet to be determined.

References

1. Pandey D, Lee KH, Tan KC. The role of liver transplantation for hilar cholangiocarcinoma. Hepatobiliary Pancreat Dis Int 2007; 6:248–253.
2. Giuliante F, Gauzolino R, Vellone M, Ardito F, Murazio M, Nuzzo G. Liver resection for intrahepatic cholangiocarcinoma. Tumori 2005; 91:487–492.
3. Maeno H, Ono T, Yamanoi A, Nagasue N. Our experiences in surgical treatment for hilar cholangiocarcinoma. Hepatogastroenterology 2007; 54:669–673.
4. Seyama Y, Makuuchi M. Current surgical treatment for bile duct cancer. World J Gastroenterol 2007; 13:1505–1515.
5. DeOliveira ML, Cunningham SC, Cameron JL, et al. Cholangiocarcinoma: thirty-one-year experience with 564 patients at a single institution. Ann Surg 2007; 245:755–762.
6. Bathe OF, Mahallati H. MR-guided ablation of hepatocellular carcinoma aided by gadoxetic acid. J Surg Oncol 2007; 95:670–673.

7. Cosman ER, Nashold BS, Ovelman-Levitt J. Theoretical aspects of radiofrequency lesions in the dorsal root entry zone. Neurosurgery 1984; 15:945–950.

8. Goldberg SN, Gazelle GS, Halpern EF, Rittman WJ, Mueller PR, Rosenthal DI. Radiofrequency tissue ablation: importance of local temperature along the electrode tip exposure in determining lesion shape and size. Acad Radiol 1996; 3:212–218.

9. Solbiati L, Ierace T, Goldberg SN, et al. Percutaneous US-guided radio-frequency tissue ablation of liver metastases: treatment and follow-up in 16 patients. Radiology 1997; 202:195–203.

10. Kim SK, Lim HK, Kim YH, et al. Hepatocellular carcinoma treated with radio-frequency ablation: spectrum of imaging findings. Radiographics 2003; 23:107–121.

11. Sironi S, Livraghi T, Meloni F, De Cobelli F, Ferrero C, Del Maschio A. Small hepatocellular carcinoma treated with percutaneous RF ablation: MR imaging follow-up. AJR Am J Roentgenol 1999; 173:1225–1229.

12. Lim HK, Choi D, Lee WJ, et al. Hepatocellular carcinoma treated with percutaneous radio-frequency ablation: evaluation with follow-up multiphase helical CT. Radiology 2001; 221:447–454.

13. Choi D, Lim HK, Kim MJ, et al. Liver abscess after percutaneous radiofrequency ablation for hepatocellular carcinoma: frequency and risk factors. AJR Am J Roentgenol 2005; 184:1860–1867.

14. Akahane M, Koga H, Kato N, et al. Complications of percutaneous radiofrequency ablation for hepato-cellular carcinoma: imaging spectrum and management. Radiographics 2005; 25(suppl 1):S57–68.

15. Rhim H, Dodd GD, 3rd, Chintapalli KN, et al. Radiofrequency thermal ablation of abdominal tumors: lessons learned from complications. Radiographics 2004; 24:41–52.

16. Rhim H. Complications of radiofrequency ablation in hepatocellular carcinoma. Abdom Imaging 2005; 30:409–418.

17. Livraghi T, Solbiati L, Meloni MF, Gazelle GS, Halpern EF, Goldberg SN. Treatment of focal liver tumors with percutaneous radio-frequency ablation: complications encountered in a multicenter study. Radiology 2003; 226:441–451.

18. Kim SH, Lim HK, Choi D, et al. Changes in bile ducts after radiofrequency ablation of hepatocellular carcinoma: frequency and clinical significance. AJR Am J Roentgenol 2004; 183:1611–1617.

19. Francica G, Marone G, Solbiati L, D'Angelo V, Siani A. Hemobilia, intrahepatic hematoma and acute thrombosis with cavernomatous transformation of the portal vein after percutaneous thermoablation of a liver metastasis. Eur Radiol 2000; 10:926–929.

20. Rhim H, Yoon KH, Lee JM, et al. Major complications after radio-frequency thermal ablation of hepatic tumors: spectrum of imaging findings. Radiographics 2003; 23:123–134; discussion 134–136.

21. Chiou YY, Hwang JI, Chou YH, Wang HK, Chiang JH, Chang CY. Percutaneous ultrasound-guided radiofrequency ablation of intrahepatic cholangiocarcinoma. Kaohsiung J Med Sci 2005; 21:304–309.

22. Lu DS, Yu NC, Raman SS, et al. Radiofrequency ablation of hepatocellular carcinoma: treatment success as defined by histologic examination of the explanted liver. Radiology 2005; 234:954–960.

23. Zgodzinski W, Espat NJ. Radiofrequency ablation for incidentally identified primary intrahepatic cholangiocarcinoma. World J Gastroenterol 2005; 11:5239–5240.

24. Rai R, Manas D, Rose J. Radiofrequency ablation of recurrent cholangiocarcinoma after orthotopic liver transplantation—a case report. World J Gastroenterol 2005; 11:612–613.

25. Slakey DP. Radiofrequency ablation of recurrent cholangiocarcinoma. Am Surg 2002; 68:395–397.

13 Chemoembolization

Kenneth J. Kolbeck
John Kaufman

As described throughout this book, cholangiocarcinoma and gallbladder cancer can present with a multitude of imaging properties. From an interventional radiology point of view, biliary malignancy can be subdivided into two categories: lesions primarily contained within the biliary tree or lesions with a focal, mass-like, intrahepatic component. The lesions that tend to spread superficially throughout the biliary tree have a diffuse arterial supply and are generally not treated with chemoembolization techniques; however, the lesions with a mass-like intrahepatic component frequently have a dominant arterial supply and can be treated with intraarterial techniques. The overall goal of chemoembolization is to place a high concentration of chemotherapeutic agent directly into the arterial supply of the malignancy with reduced/minimal toxicity to adjacent normal hepatic parenchyma. Using current catheter technology and fluoroscopic techniques, the hepatic arterial supply to specific liver segments can be successfully cannulated. Accessing the arterial supply of a lesion and introducing pharmaceuticals from this proximity can result in significantly higher concentrations of agent within the tumor and potentially reduced systemic side effects when compared to similar intravenous therapies (1–3). Hence, there exists the potential to increase the therapeutic ratio.

The blood supply to the liver is from a combination of the portal vein and the hepatic artery. Normal liver parenchyma is frequently perfused with a 3:1 ratio of portal venous to hepatic arterial supply. Studies evaluating the perfusion to hepatocellular carcinoma indicate a significantly higher proportion of hepatic arterial supply over the portal venous supply (3). Although comparative studies have not been performed with cholangiocarcinoma, it is well known that the bile ducts are an "end-organ" vascular supply of the hepatic arterial system. Therefore, an arterial approach to treat bile duct malignancy is within reason.

Chemoembolization is a technique designed to help gain "local control" of the malignancy. In general, chemoembolization slows or stops growth of a focal liver lesion. In some cases, the lesion will decrease in size over the initial months of therapy. In rare cases, the lesion can shrink enough to allow surgical resection. Obviously, the majority of cases do not result in a "cure," and the patient should be prepared for and advised as such. A successful chemoembolization would include a procedure that slows the radiographic growth of the tumor, reduces current clinical symptoms associated with the offending lesion, or delays the onset of disease-related liver failure. Chemoembolization has been shown to increase survival in prospective randomized studies in hepatocellular carcinoma and shown to be of benefit in other intrahepatic malignancies (neuroendocrine, colorectal, ocular melanoma, and other hepatic metastases) (4–7).

TECHNIQUES OF CHEMOEMBOLIZATION

Chemoembolization is a technique designed to deliver a chemotherapeutic or cytotoxic agent to a malignant lesion. The embolic component of the procedure ideally reduces the perfusion to the lesion with the intent of both decreasing washout of the chemotherapeutic agent and limiting the overall metabolic activity of the treated tissue. There are several chemotherapeutic agents available to be delivered via the arterial route. In general, cisplatin, adriamycin, and mitomycin C represent a three-drug combination frequently used to treat malignancies within the liver. Additional medications that have been infused arterially include fluorouracil, irinotecan, and ibuprofen. Other agents have been developed that carry a β-emitting isotope (yttrium-90) directly to the tumor in order to selectively irradiate intrahepatic malignancies. Embolic agents include an iodinated oil emulsion, gel foam particles, and a variety of polymer compounds (polyvinyl alcohol, polyacrylamide copolymers, gelatin, and hydrogels). Newer embolic agents have recently been under development that allow a "sustained release" of the chemotherapeutic agent (1, 3).

The procedure is relatively straightforward for those experienced in the techniques (2, 3, 8). In short, arterial access is generally obtained via the common femoral artery. Seldinger technique is used to exchange the arterial access needle for a 4-5 Fr steerable catheter. The catheter is used to select both the superior mesenteric artery and the celiac axis. Digital subtraction arteriograms are obtained of both vessels to evaluate the visceral vascular supply and the patency of the portal vein.

Figure 13.1 demonstrates an arterial phase of a diagnostic visceral arteriogram. In this patient, the left hepatic artery originates from a separate origin and the right lobe of the liver is supplied via a branch of the celiac axis. A metallic stent maintains patency of the common bile duct in this patient. The mass-like tumor is identified by the blush of contrast present within the liver. For a more selective treatment, a microcatheter (Figure 13.2) can be advanced into the distal branches of the right hepatic artery to deliver the chemoembolic agents.

The vascular supply to the liver is extremely variable, and care must be taken to avoid delivery of the chemoembolic agent to adjacent stomach, small, or large bowel. Once an adequate map of the visceral vasculature has been obtained, segmental and subsegmental evaluation of the hepatic arterial supply to the malignant lesion can be obtained. Frequently, cholangiocarcinoma is located within the hilum of the liver, and there is hepatic arterial supply from both left and right hepatic arterial branches. In rare cases a single hepatic arterial supply to the lesion can be identified. In cases with multiple sources of hepatic arterial supply, the treatment is

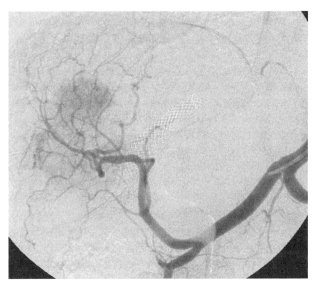

FIGURE 13.1

Digital subtraction arteriogram of a patient with a biopsy-proven mass-like cholangiocarcinoma in the right lobe of the liver. The catheter is positioned just distal to the origin of the splenic artery in the common hepatic artery from the celiac axis. The right hepatic artery supplies the tumor (enhancing blush). The tumor is located lateral to the existing metallic biliary stent. Subtraction artifact outlines the right renal pelvis and collecting system.

frequently divided into multiple settings. For instance, with a hilar tumor with several arterial feeding vessels, the right lobe hepatic artery may supply the majority of the lesion. In that case, the right lobe would be chemoembolized, with a majority of the chemoembolic material going to the tumor. However, as "collateral damage" the normal right lobe hepatic parenchyma is also somewhat affected. The left lobe has been left untreated and will continue to provide standard hepatic function. Four to 6 weeks later, the left half of the liver will be treated; allowing the right to function as the normal hepatic reserve.

The indication for regional therapy of malignant disease is predicated upon liver-dominant disease. In patients with extrahepatic disease, chemoembolization of liver lesions can be performed assuming the hepatic component of the malignancy is the dominant source of clinical symptoms. Chemoembolization is frequently performed in patients with hepatocellular carcinoma, metastases from neuroendocrine tumors, and ocular melanoma. Additional hepatic metastases that have been treated include primary cancers from the pancreas, colon, lung, breast, bladder, and other soft tissue sarcomas. The goal of regional therapy is to control the clinical symptoms and slow the progression of disease. Rarely is regional therapy performed in an attempt to cure a malignant disease.

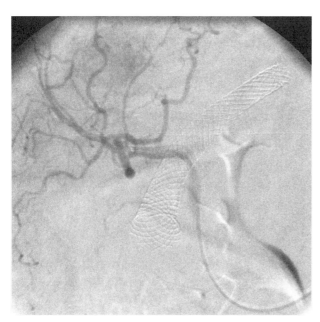

FIGURE 13.2

A microcatheter has been advanced into a distal branch of the right hepatic artery supplying the tumor. The chemoembolic mixture was delivered from this point with low risk of nontarget embolization to adjacent unaffected liver, stomach, and small bowel.

The contraindications to chemoembolization can be divided into categories. First, contraindications to the chemotherapeutic agent must be considered. Cisplatin therapy includes a risk of renal failure, and adriamycin includes a risk of cardiac toxicity. Contraindications to the visceral arteriogram include iodinated contrast reactions, uncorrectable coagulopathy, inability to lie flat for the interventional procedure and recovery period for the arterial puncture. Contraindications for the delivery of chemotherapy to the liver (at risk for going into liver failure) include significantly elevated bilirubin, hepatic tumor burden greater than 50%, hepatic encephalopathy or jaundice, portal vein occlusion without hepatopedal collateral flow, or focal obstruction of intrahepatic biliary tree (risk of abscess/sepsis).

The complications associated with chemoembolization include access site complications (>5%, infection, bleeding, hematoma, arteriovenous fistula, pseudoaneurysm), catheterization complications (>1%, vascular intimal injury-dissection, disruption, thrombosis, distal emboli), and complications related to hepatic artery embolization (>5%, liver failure, abscess, liver infarction). A common side effect following the procedure is postembolization syndrome: a self-limited constellation of symptoms (low-grade fever, elevated white count, abdominal pain, nausea, and occasionally vomiting). Rarely, contrast-induced nephropathy, life-

threatening liver failure, and hepatic abscess formation can result in hospital readmissions following the procedure. The most common reason for hospital readmission following chemoembolization appears to be dehydration (secondary to nausea and vomiting) or pain control. There is a reported 1–4% 30-day mortality rate associated with the procedure, most evident in the populations with decreased liver function at the beginning of therapy (2, 3).

SPECIFIC OUTCOMES OF CHEMOEMBOLIZATION FOR CHOLANGIOCARCINOMA

Clinical outcomes of chemoembolization techniques in cholangiocarcinoma are limited. In reviewing the published English literature, only one peer-reviewed article and a few conference abstracts specifically evaluate chemoembolization in patients with cholangiocarcinoma. Most articles and abstracts describe using chemoembolization in patients that have already progressed following standard chemotherapeutic and surgical options. In evaluating the chemoembolization data, one must keep in mind that the median survival of this group of patients with standard therapeutic treatment options is only 6–12 months (9–11).

Burger et al. reviewed 17 individual cases of unresectable intrahepatic cholangiocarcinoma treated with chemoembolization (12). The median survival following chemoembolization was 23 months. Two of the 17 patients were able to undergo successful resection of the tumor following the chemoembolization procedure. They reported two minor and one major complication associated with the procedure (including one death attributed to progression of disease). They concluded that chemoembolization "was effective at prolonging survival of patients with unresectable cholangiocarcinoma."

Similarly, Graf et al. reviewed another institution's experience with chemoembolization of cholangiocarcinoma (13). They reviewed the case history of 19 patients with biopsy-proven cholangiocarcinoma ($n = 13$) or poorly differentiated adenocarcinoma ($n = 6$, presumed cholangiocarcinoma). These patients were treated with 42 chemoembolization procedures with three-drug chemotherapy (cisplatin, adriamycin, and mitomycin C) and embolization with iodinated oil emulsion and polyvinyl alcohol polymer. They reported 1- and 2-year survival of 53 and 35%, respectively. By imaging criteria, they reported stabilization or regression in 60% of patients. One third of patients remain free from progression at 1 year. They reported two complications (pulmonary edema and hepatic lobe infarct) during their study. They concluded that "chemoembolization provided stabilization or regression of intrahepatic cholangiocarcinoma in 9/15 (60%) with 1/3 remaining free of progression at 1 year."

A third institution reviewed results of yttrium-90 therapy applied to eight patients with advanced cholangiocarcinoma (14). A total of 11 doses of the radioactive treatment were utilized in the treatment course. They reported median survivals of 616 and 204 days for patients with Eastern Cooperative Oncology Group (ECOG) performance status scores of 0 and 1, respectively. They also reported regression or stable disease (based upon 90-day cross-sectional imaging) in 81.8% of the treated liver segments. The most common side effects were fatigue (63%) and transient abdominal pain (50%). They also concluded that yttrium-90 brachytherapy is a viable therapeutic option in patients who are "not candidates for resection or have failed chemotherapy."

Similarly, Amesur et al. reviewed the use of chemoembolization with a specific embolic agent in patients with several types of hepatic malignancies (15). Eleven of the 43 patients treated carried the diagnosis of cholangiocarcinoma. They reported a 20–41% reduction in the size of an index lesion in 9 of the 11 patients with cholangiocarcinoma (depending upon the size of the embolic agent and frequency of the procedure). This group also concluded that chemoembolization can be safely performed.

Finally, Rilling et al. reviewed the clinical course of 10 patients with unresectable intrahepatic cholangiocarcinoma (16). A total of 28 treatments were deemed technically successful. Of 5 patients with an elevated tumor marker (CA19-9), 4 showed clinical response with decreasing serum tumor markers. Mean survival time from the initial chemoembolization treatment was 15.7 months. They also concluded that chemoembolization is "feasible and safe" in patients with intrahepatic cholangiocarcinoma.

Three cases of biopsy-proven cholangiocarcinoma have been treated with chemoembolization at the Dotter Interventional Institute. One patient survived 4 weeks following the treatment and had succumbed to overall progression of disease. The two other patients are still alive after the chemoembolization procedure. One has magnetic resonance evidence of progression of disease 3–4 months after treatment. The other patient has undergone a multidisciplinary treatment involving both chemoembolization and radiation therapy. This patient is alive 16 months after chemoembolization (and several rounds of radiation therapy) with cross-sectional imaging indicating stable disease.

CONCLUSIONS

From the limited data available for review, one can conclude that chemoembolization is a safe procedure to perform in patients with mass-like intrahepatic cholangiocarcinoma when the standard guidelines of chemoembolization for hepatocellular carcinoma are followed. There are small studies that show some benefit of chemoembolization in cholangiocarcinoma, including stable or decreasing tumor burden (based upon imaging criteria or serum tumor markers) as well as increased median survival (15–23 months). When compared to median survivals of 6–12 months in patients with standard therapeutic options, the chemoembolization techniques show promise. However, small sample size and variability in treatment parameters make generalizations to broader populations difficult. Chemoembolization with or without additional combined therapies remains a viable alternative treatment in patients who are not resection/transplant candidates and have failed first-line chemotherapy.

References

1. Liapi E, Geschwind JFH. Transcatheter and ablative therapeutic approaches for solid malignancies. J Clin Oncol 2007; 25:9787–986.
2. Soulen MC. Chemoembolization of hepatic malignancies. In: Kandarpa K, Aruny JE (eds.). Handboook of Interventional Radiologic Procedures. 3rd ed. Philadelphia: Lippincott Williams & Wilkins, 2002:227–231.
3. Hanjan T, De Sanctis J. Hepatic arterial interventions. In: Ray CE, Hicks ME, Patel NH (eds.). Interventions in Oncology: Society of Interventional Radiology; 2003:103–118.
4. Bruix J, Llovet JM. Prognostic prediction and treatment strategy in hepatocellular carcinoma. Hepatology 2002; 35(3):519–524.
5. Llovet JM, Real MI, Montana X, Planas R, Coll S, Aponte J, et al. Arterial embolisation or chemoembolisation versus symptomatic treatment in patients with unresectable hepatocellular carcinoma: a radomised controlled trial. Lancet 2002; 359:1734–1739.
6. Llovet JM, Bruix J. Systematic review of randomized trials for unresectable hepatocellular carcinoma: chemoembolization improves survival. Hepatology 2003; 37:429–442.
7. Camma C, Schepis F, Orlando A, Albanese M, Shahied L, Trevisani F, et al. Transarterial chemoembolization for unresectable hepatocellular carcinoma: meta-analysis of randomized controlled trials. Radiology 2002; 224:47–54.
8. Kernagis LY, Soulen MC. Multimodality therapy for hepatic malignancies. In: Ray CE, Hicks ME, Patel NH (eds.). Interventions in Oncology. Fairfax, VA: Society of Interventional Radiology; 2003:137–142.
9. Singh P, Patel T. Advances in the Diagnosis, Evaluation and Management of Cholangiocarcinoma. Curr Opin Gastroenterol 2006; 22:294–299.
10. Eckel F, Schmid RM. Chemotherapy in advanced biliary tract carcinoma: a pooled analysis of clinical trials. Br J Cancer 2007; 96:896–902.
11. de Groen PC, Gores GJ, LaRusso NF, Gunderson LL, Nagorney DM. Biliary tract cancers. NEJM 1999; 341(18):1368–1378.
12. Burger I, Hong K, Schulick R, Georgiades C, Thulavath P, Choti M, et al. Transcatheter arterial chemoembolization in unresectable cholangiocarcinoma: initial experience in a single institution. J Vasc Interv Radiol 2005; 16:353–361.
13. Graf WR, Soulen MC, Tuite CM. CAM/Ethiodol/PVA chemoembolization of intrahepatic cholangiocarcinoma. J Vasc Interv Radiol 2007; 18(1, Part 2):S142.
14. Lewandowski R, Atassi B, Ryu R, Sato K, Omary R, Salem R. Y-90 radioembolization of cholangiocarcinoma: preliminary results. Society of Interventional Radiology Annual Meeting, 2007, 18:S82.

15. Amesur NB, Patel SS, Zajko AB, Federle MP, Pealer KM, Carr BI. Transcatheter treatment of malignant liver tumors with intra-arterial chemotherapy and embolization with microspheres. J Vasc Interv Radiol 2003; 14(2, Part 2):S93.

16. Rilling WS, Pinchot JW, Quebbeman EJ, Pitt HA, Ritch PS. Segmental transcatheter arterial chemoembolization for treatment of intrahepatic cholangiocarcinoma. J Vasc Interv Radiol 2004; 15(2):S227.

14 Surgical Management of Intrahepatic Biliary Tract Cancer

Richard R. Smith
John F. Gibbs

holangiocarcinoma (CCA) is a cancer arising from the bile duct epithelium. CCA can be divided into extrahepatic and intrahepatic types based on the site of origin. Extrahepatic cholangiocarcinoma (EHC) arises from the left or right hepatic duct or more distally. Intrahepatic cholangiocarcinoma (IHC) or peripheral cholangiocarcinoma is variably defined as arising from the second or more distal branches of the intrahepatic bile ducts or involving the intrahepatic bile ducts not extending into the hepatic hilum (1–3). Although IHC and EHC are often indistinguishable histologically, they are distinct from one another in presentation, prognostic factors, and growth characteristics (4, 5). IHC typically presents with pain and an intrahepatic mass lesion, whereas EHC presents with jaundice (6). This review will focus on the surgical treatment of IHC. We will briefly discuss diagnosis and staging as it pertains to surgical management. We will then discuss emerging surgical considerations for treatment with a focus on technical aspects unique to surgical management of IHC.

IHC is the second most common primary hepatic malignancy representing 5–15% of all tumors (4, 7). There is marked geographic variability in incidence, being highest in areas of the Far East (8). This is most likely related to a high incidence of known predisposing conditions in these areas. These conditions include parasitic infestation (e.g., *Clonorchis sinensis* and

Opisthorchis viverrini), hepatolithiasis, and choledochal cyst (1, 9). Other predisposing conditions include primary sclerosing cholangitis (PSC), Caroli's disease, and exposure to the contrast medium thorotrast (1, 6, 10). Chronic inflammation and/or injury to the bile duct epithelium are common to all these conditions. The most common predisposing condition associated with CCA in the Western Hemisphere is PSC, with a reported incidence of 6–11% in cohort studies and as high as 36% in patients undergoing liver transplantation (6, 11). The incidence of IHC in the United States and the United Kingdom has been rising more recently (8, 12). The incidence of IHC in the United States increased from 0.13 per 100,000 in 1973 to 0.67 per 100,000 in 1997, an annual percentage change of 9% (8). This may be related to improved awareness and diagnosis using immunohistochemistry. Another factor may be related to increased immigration from high prevalence regions of the world (8, 13).

Patients with IHC typically present with abdominal pain, fever/chills, jaundice, or a mass lesion in the liver on imaging studies performed for other reasons (4). The differential would include benign liver lesions, hepatocellular carcinoma (HCC), and metastatic disease. A history of cirrhosis or hepatitis is less likely in IHC than in the typical patient with HCC. There are no specific blood tests or tumor markers diagnostic for CCA. However, a CA 19-9 level greater than 100 U/ml has been used to predict malignancy in patients with

PSC with a sensitivity of 75–89% and a specificity of 80–86% (14). When applied to patients without a history of PSC the sensitivity is 53–68% and specificity up to 87% (15, 16).

Typical imaging includes ultrasound (US), computed tomography (CT), and or magnetic resonance imaging (MRI). There are no specific imaging features on US to differentiate IHC from other solid benign or malignant lesions. Triphasic CT scan can show some features suggestive of IHC. The tumors typically show hyperattenuation on delayed intravenous contrast images because of interstitial uptake of contrast medium in the tumor (17, 18). The percentage of tumor volume showing delayed uptake has been shown to correlate with increased fibrous stroma, perineural invasion, and worse prognosis (19). Other features that may suggest IHC include capsular retraction, dilation, and thickening of intrahepatic ducts. Capsular retraction is not specific to IHC and can be seen in a variety of malignant liver tumors (20).

CT and MRI are generally complimentary to one another. IHC is hypointense relative to the normal liver on T1-weighted MRI images and hyperintense on T2-weighted images. The T2 hyperintensity is frequently seen centrally and corresponds to fibrosis (18, 21). Similarly to CT scan, peripheral enhancement of the tumor is seen frequently on delayed images.

Positron emission tomography (PET) scans have shown improved sensitivity in identifying disease for a variety of malignancies. A recent study by Petrowsky and associates found that integrated PET/CT and CT were comparable in identifying primary disease in 61 patients with biliary cancer. PET/CT was significantly more accurate in identifying distant metastatic disease. Unfortunately, neither PET/CT nor CT was accurate in identifying locoregional nodal disease with sensitivity of 12 and 24%, respectively (22). The benefit of PET scan in detecting distant disease has been limited in the preoperative assessment of IHC, which tends to progress locoregionally.

Several staging and classification systems are currently used for IHC. The American Joint Committee on Cancer (AJCC/ International Union Against Cancer (UICC) TNM classification (Table 14.1) system is widely used (23). The system was developed primarily for hepatocellular cancer (HCC) but is applied to IHC as well.

The Liver Cancer Study Group of Japan (LCSGJ) has developed a classification system for IHC specifically based on macroscopic appearance (Figure 14.1): mass forming (MF), periductal infiltrating (PI), and intraductal growth (IG) (7). Tumors can show more than one macroscopic appearance and are then described with the predominant type followed by the lesser type separated by a "+" (i.e., mass forming + periductal infiltrating). The macroscopic appearance of the disease reflects tumor cells with different biologic behaviors. This biologic difference can be seen in the 1-year overall survival (OS) of patients with IHC. MF lesions have an 80% 1-year OS, PI tumors a 69% 1-year OS, and MF + PI a 39% 1-year OS (p = 0.0072) (24).

MF tumors are the most common, particularly in Western series. They are localized rounded tumors with distinct borders in noncirrhotic liver parenchyma. PI tumors are diffusely infiltrating along the bile duct and can involve the periductal connective tissue or adjacent liver parenchyma. On imaging they typically show peripheral biliary ductal dilatation with a small more central mass. PI tumors can present similarly to a Klatskin's tumor, but the former is usually found at a higher stage and is associated with a larger mass as the tumor grows from the liver parenchyma into the hilum of the liver. IG tumors show intraductal papillary

FIGURE 14.1

Macroscopic types of intrahepatic cholangiocarcinoma. (a) Mass-forming tumors are localized rounded tumors with distinct borders in noncirrhotic liver parenchyma. (b) Periductal infiltrating tumors along the bile duct can involve the periductal connective tissue or adjacent liver parenchyma. (c) Intraductal growth tumors associated with superficial mucosal spread and or tumor thrombus. (d) Mass-forming and periductal infiltrating tumors. (From Ref. 29.)

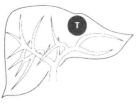

a Mass forming

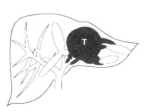

b Periductal infiltrating

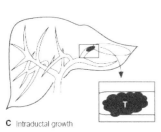

c Intraductal growth

d Mass forming and periductal infiltrating

TABLE 14.1
AJCC/UICC TNM Classification for Liver Cancer

PRIMARY TUMOR (T)

TX	Primary tumor cannot be assessed
T0	No evidence of primary tumor
T1	Solitary tumor without vascular invasion
T2	Solitary tumor with vascular invasion or multiple tumors none <5 cm
T3	Multiple tumors <5 cm or involving a major branch of the portal or hepatic vein
T4	Tumor with direct invasion of adjacent organ other than gallbladder or perforation of visceral peritoneum

REGIONAL LYMPH NODES (N)

NX	Regional lymph nodes cannot be assessed
N0	No regional lymph node metastasis
N1	Regional lymph node metastasis

DISTANT METASTASIS (M)

MX	Distant metastasis cannot be assessed
M0	No distant metastasis
M1	Distant metastasis

STAGE GROUPING

Stage I	T1	N0	M0
Stage II	T2	N0	M0
Stage IIIA	T3	N0	M0
Stage IIIB	T4	N0	M0
Stage IIIC	Any T	N1	M0
Stage IV	Any T	any N	M1

TABLE 14.2
Liver Cancer Study Group of Japan Staging Classification Factors

1. Solitary tumor
2. Tumor 2 cm or less
3. No invasion of portal vein, hepatic vein, or serous membrane

TUMOR STAGE (T)

T1 Meets all three factors
T2 Meets two of three factors
T3 Meets one of three factors
T4 Meets none of the three factors

LYMPH NODES (N)

N0	No regional lymph node metastasis
N1	Regional lymph node metastasis

METASTASIS (M)

M0	No distant metastasis
M1	Distant metastasis

STAGING SYSTEM

Stage I	T1	N0	M0
Stage II	T2	N0	M0
Stage III	T3	N0	M0
Stage IVA	T4	N0	M0
	or any T	N1	M0
Stage IVB	Any T	Any N	M1

in 136 patients with MF type IHC is shown in Figure 14.2 (26).

TREATMENT

General Surgical Considerations

In the following section we will discuss emerging surgical considerations for IHC. These will include the role of staging laparoscopy, portal vein embolization (PVE), and lymphadenectomy in surgical resection. In addition, extended hepatic resection with or without vascular resection and the role of orthotopic liver resection (OLT) will be addressed. Finally, we will discuss surgical and nonsurgical palliation.

Curative resection offers the best chance at long-term survival. Whereas palliation with surgical bypass was once the preferred surgical procedure even for resectable disease, aggressive surgical resection is now the standard. In addition, the surgical bypass for palliation in unresectable cases has now largely been replaced

growth associated with superficial mucosal spread and or tumor thrombus. On imaging typically marked biliary dilatation is seen. Precise delineation of the area of involvement is often difficult secondary to mucin production obscuring the primary tumor and the superficial mucosal spread that cannot be visualized. IG tumors are pathologically seen as papillary adenocarcinoma or well-differentiated tubular carcinomas. These tumors have less frequent vascular, lymphatic, or perineural invasion and hence better overall prognosis than the MF or PI types. In addition, PI tumors are associated with hepatolithiasis and thus more commonly found in Eastern series (25).

As mentioned previously, the AJCC TNM stage system is based on data from HCC. The criteria also include microscopic findings that cannot be applied preoperatively to staging. With these issues in mind, the LCSGJ developed a TNM staging specifically for IHC (Table 14.2). The survival curve based on this system

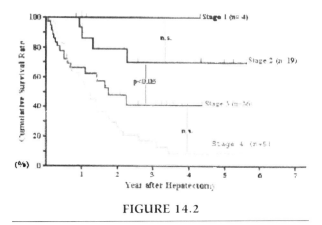

FIGURE 14.2

Survival by LCSGJ staging system. (From Ref. 26.)

by biliary endoprosthesis. Table 14.3 shows the largest reported series in the literature examining outcome with hepatectomy for IHC. The 5-year OS is 23–40% for resected patients (1–3, 27–36). The OS for an R0 resection is 36–63% at 5 years (2, 3, 34). The postoperative mortality rate is 0–8% in large series (2, 3, 27, 29, 30, 32, 35–37). The resection rate for patients explored for curative intent is 50–87% (5, 29, 30, 33, 35).

The series described in the literature are all relatively small, making conclusions difficult regarding prognostic factors. In series with multivariate analysis, the most frequently sited significant negative prognostic factors are the following: positive margin, satellite lesions, lymph node metastasis, lymphatic invasion, and vascular invasion (1–3, 27, 29–33, 35, 36, 38). Of these prognostic factors, lymphatic and microvascular inva-

sion cannot be readily determined preoperatively and do not improve patient selection for resection. Lymph node metastasis can also be difficult to determine preoperatively and will be discussed in a separate section.

Morimoto et al. found a positive surgical margin had a relative risk (RR) of death of 2.7 on multivariate analysis ($p = 0.02$) and a 3-year OS of 12% versus 56% when the margin was negative (2). Casavilla et al. found a median OS of 7 months when the resection margin was positive versus 38 months with a negative margin ($p = >0.0001$) and resection margin was a significant negative factor on multivariate analysis (39). Lang et al. found a median OS of 46 months for a microscopically negative margin versus 5 months for a microscopically positive (R1) margin ($p = <0.004$) (40).

Satellite lesions are identifiable preoperatively and appear to be a particularly poor prognostic factor. Ohtsuka et al. performed multivariate analysis on 36 patients with MF tumors undergoing resection and found that satellite lesions increased the relative risk of dying by a factor of 3.9 ($p = 0.03$). This risk was exceeded only by a CA 19-9 level greater than 10,000 units/L in predicting death following resection (29). Suzuki et al. examined 19 patients with MF tumor type undergoing resection and found that satellite lesions had the greatest impact on survival with a RR of dying 11.3 times greater than without satellite lesions with no 3-year survivors in this group (33). Uenishi et al. examined 28 patients with IHC undergoing resection and found a 1-year OS of 14% when satellite lesions were present (38). Shimada et al. examined 49 patients with IHC undergoing resection and found the presence of

TABLE 14.3

Outcomes After Resection for Intrahepatic Cholangiocarcinoma

Study	Year	Patients	Postoperative Mortality (%)	Median Survival (mos)	Median Survival R0 (mos)	1-yr OS (%)	3-yr OS (%)	5-yr OS (%)	5-yr OS R0(%)
Jan et al.	1996	41	0	12	22	54	37	26	44
Casavilla et al.	1997	34			38	60	37	31	45
Chu et al.	1999	48		16		60	30	22	
Valverde et al.	1999	30	3	28		86	22		
Weimann et al.	2000	95	5	18		64	31	21	
Inoue et al.	2000	52		18		63	36	36	55
Shimada et al.	2001	49	4	26		66			
Okabayashi et al.	2001	60	5	20	21	68	35	29	39
Ohtsuka et al.	2002	48	8	26		62	38	23	
Weber et al.	2001	33	3		46	83	55	31	
Morimoto et al.	2003	49	4			68	44	32	41
Nakagawa	2005	46	6			66	38	26	
Miwa et al.	2006	41	0			79	36	29	36
DeOliveira et al.	2007	44	4	28	80			4	63

R0, microscopically negative resection; OS, overall survival.

satellite lesions a significant factor with a RR 3.7 times greater of dying and no survival beyond 3 years in this group (31). Okabayashi et al. reported on 60 patients with MF IHC undergoing hepatic resection. Satellite lesions were a significant predictor of decreased survival with a RR of 4.6 for death and no 3-year survivors in the group identified preoperatively (32). Nakagawa et al. examined 28 patients undergoing resection for IHC and found a RR of dying 2.2 times for satellite lesions and no 3-year survivors (35). Given the existing literature we believe that the presence of multiple tumors (satellite lesions) would seem at least a relative contraindication to surgery.

The resection of IHC follows the basic principles of anatomic liver resection for malignant neoplasm and is described in detail elsewhere (41). The understanding of hepatic anatomy started in 1654 with Glisson's description of the liver capsule. This was followed by Cantilie's description of the division of the liver into functional halves in 1897. Finally, Couinaud defined the segmental anatomy of the liver in 1957 (42) (Figure 14.3). The anatomic division of the liver into right and left halves is based on Cantilie's line, which is an imaginary line that extends from the gallbladder fossa to the left of the vena cava. Anatomically this is defined by the middle hepatic vein. Each half of the liver is then divided into four other segments based on the venous drainage, portal venous inflow, and arterial inflow, for a total of eight segments. A thorough understanding of the hepatic segmental anatomy increases the safety of liver resection, and anatomic resection has been shown to result in increased survival (43). The remainder of this section will deal with several issues of resection specific to IHC and its clinicopathologic characteristics.

Staging Laparoscopy

Despite negative radiologic evaluation preoperatively, the rate of patients found to be unresectable at laparotomy remains high at 14–38% in several recent series (29, 30, 35, 37). Because of the relatively high rate of unresectability and the fact that survival of patients with incomplete resection is the same as for patients palliated conservatively, diagnostic laparoscopy has been used by several institutions as part of the staging of IHC. Washburn and associates performed diagnostic laparoscopy on 46 patients with potentially respectable biliary cancer. Five of 46 (11%) were found to have unresectable disease on laparoscopy. Another six patients were found on laparotomy to have unresectable disease for an overall sensitivity of 45% for laparoscopy (44). Weber and associates have adopted a policy of diagnostic laparoscopy as a routine assessment for IHC based on identifying that 27% of their patients deemed potentially respectable were found

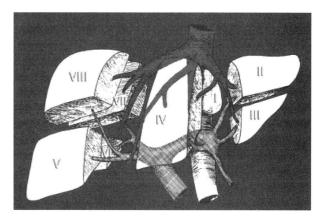

FIGURE 14.3

Segmental liver anatomy as described by Couinaud and Bismuth. Renz, J.F. et al. *Am J Transplant* 2003, 3:1323-1335

unresectable at laparoscopy for a sensitivity of 55% (30). Goere and associates found that 36% of their patients with IHC had unresectable disease on laparoscopy, with a sensitivity of 67% (45). The patients with unresectable disease that laparoscopy missed were patients with vascular invasion and metastasis to distant lymph nodes. Intraoperative ultrasound could increase the sensitivity in some of these patients by identifying vascular invasion.

Portal Vein Embolization

Postoperative liver failure is a known complication of extended hepatectomy. Portal vein embolization (PVE) is designed to increase the proposed functional liver remnant (FLR) prior to hepatectomy, thereby decreasing the risk of postoperative liver failure. PVE was first described by Makuuchi et al. in 1982 for the treatment of hilar cholangiocarcinoma (46). Subsequently the technique has been applied to a variety of malignancies primary and metastatic (47).

The indication for PVE varies from Eastern and Western reported series. The indication also varies with the patients underlying liver function. Many Far Eastern series consider PVE when the expected FLR is less than 40% for healthy liver tissue (47–49). Many Western authors believe that 25–30% FLR is the minimum for safe hepatic resection (50–52). For patients with mild liver dysfunction and a FLR of less than 50%, PVE should be considered (47) . The liver dysfunction can be related to cirrhosis, steatosis, or heavy chemotherapy pretreatment. Because of the risk for liver failure, patients with obstructive jaundice should undergo biliary decompression prior to PVE. The presence of cholestatic liver dysfunction may retard the degree of expected liver regeneration following resection. Ideally

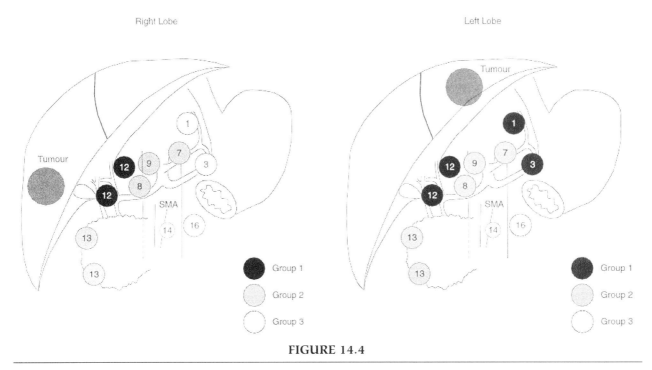

FIGURE 14.4

"Right" and "left" nodal drainage pathways. Nozaki, Y et al. *Cancer* 1998, 83:1923-1929

PVE is performed when the bilirubin is less than 5 mg/dL. Radical surgery would typically be performed 3–4 weeks later when the FLR has hypertrophied and the bilirubin is less than 2 mg/dl (53).

Nagino and associates described 240 consecutive patients with biliary tract cancer undergoing PVE prior to extended hepatectomy. Twenty percent of patients had progressive disease following PVE and were not offered resection. The perioperative mortality in the patients with CCA was 4.5%, and this was similar to a contemporary cohort undergoing hepatectomy for CCA without PVE at 3.7%. The FLR increased significantly from 33 to 43%. The 3- and 5-year OS rates in the patients with CCA were 41.7 and 26.8%, respectively (49). Abdalla et al. examined 42 patients undergoing extended hepatectomy for hepatobiliary malignancies. PVE was performed at the discretion of the surgeon when the FLR was determined to be les than 25%. The patients who did not undergo PVE were predominantly in the early study period and were younger with excellent performance status. Eighteen patients underwent PVE, and 24 did not. Median increase in FLR was 8%, increasing the median FLR from 18 to 26% in patients undergoing PVE. The median OS was similar in the PVE group and the non-PVE group at 40 and 52 months (*p* = 0.70) (50). PVE has shown efficacy in increasing FLR in patients with hepatobiliary malignancies. With the addition of PVE, the median OS after resection in patients with a preoperatively determined postresection FLR of less than 25% are comparable to patients on

adequate preoperative FLR. The use of PVE can offer resection to those patients with a FLR that might preclude resection and facilitate aggressive resection.

Lymph Node Dissection

The traditional nodal drainage pathway via the hepatoduodenal ligament for IHC has been described (54). More recent studies have shown that the drainage pathway can include transit via the lesser omentum to the lesser curve of the stomach and even up to the pericardial region of the stomach, particularly when the lesion is located within the left lobe of the liver (31, 54).

The LCSGJ has defined the nodal drainage for primary liver cancer and is shown in Figure 14.4 (7). The nodes are grouped as primary, secondary, and tertiary drainage and differ for right and left lesions. Okami et al. performed systematic lymphadenectomy to include the hepatoduodenal ligament (right pathway) and the cardiac portion of the stomach and along the lesser curve of the stomach (left pathway) in 13 consecutive patients with left lobe IHC. The "right" and "left" nodal drainage pathways are shown in Figure 14.4. Lymph nodes were examined by standard H&E as well as molecular-based analysis by RT-PCR. Eight of 13 patients were node positive by H&E or RT-PCR. An additional two patients who were initially identified as negative by H&E were subsequently found to be positive by RT-PCR. Positive nodes were identified in the right pathway in 38% of patients with H&E and 50%

with RT-PCR. Positive nodes were found in the left pathway in 31% of patients by H&E and 58% by RT-PCR. Two of the eight patients with positive nodes had disease only in the left-side pathway (55). Thus, in this study the distribution of positive lymph nodes was equally distributed between the traditional right-side pathway via the hepatoduodenal ligament and the left-side pathway via the lesser omentum.

The rate of positive lymph nodes found when routine radical lymphadenectomy is performed is 31–59% (2, 29, 31, 35, 38, 56, 57). Most series that include multivariate analysis show positive lymph nodes as a significant poor predictor of survival (2, 3, 5, 31, 32, 34, 36, 37). A few long-term survivors following curative resection with positive lymph nodes have been reported (2, 29, 32, 33, 35). However, many studies have shown no long-term survival with positive lymph nodes despite curative resection and systematic lymph node dissection (31, 32, 37, 54, 58). Nakagawa et al. performed extensive lymphadenectomies including hepatoduodenal ligament, posterior pancreatic, celiac nodes and lesser curve of stomach, gastric and cardia nodes for left-sided lesions in 28 patients with IHC. Positive lymph nodes in this series were not significant on multivariate analysis, and the 3-year OS for patients with no positive nodes, one to two positive nodes, and three or more nodes was 62, 50, and 0%, respectively (35). However, Okabayashi et al. found no 5-year survivors with positive lymph nodes in their series of 60 patients undergoing curative resection (32). Morimoto et al. reported that among 51 patients undergoing curative resection, only one of 16 patients with positive lymph nodes was alive at 5 years, and this patient had an IG tumor with favorable prognosis (2). Shimada et al. compared the survival of 41 patients undergoing systematic lymph node dissection with 8 patients who did not and found

no difference in survival. Specifically, no patient with positive lymph nodes survived to 3 years (31).

Given the frequency of nodal metastasis and the poor survival of these patients, it would be advantageous to identify those patients before subjecting them to extensive resections. Sentinel lymph node biopsy has been studied in an animal model and appears to be safe and effective when injected into the liver parenchyma (59). Lymphatic mapping of the liver has also been shown to safe and effective in patients with colorectal metastasis (60). Sentinel lymph node mapping may be more efficacious in IHC than colorectal metastasis because of the greater incidence of nodal metastasis in IHC.

There is no consensus on the need for or extent of lymph node dissection in IHC. Given the overall poor outcome for patients with lymph node–positive disease, the appropriateness of extensive surgery in node-positive patients or the need for lymph node dissection as a standard treatment for IHC is questionable at the present time.

Extended Resection

Because of their intrahepatic location, IHCs typically reach a large size prior to presentation and as such often invade contiguous structures or require extended hepatectomy (40). Roayaie et al. performed hepatic resection on 16 patients with IHC, and 88% had tumors within 1.5 cm of the vena cava (61). Extended hepatectomy is defined as resection of greater than 4 Couinaud segments and is required for curative resection in 7–54% of IHCs in large series (1, 2, 29, 30, 32, 37). Extended resection of contiguous vascular structures and or extrahepatic ducts in conjunction with hepatectomy is not uncommon. Extrahepatic bile duct resec-

TABLE 14.4
Incidence of Extended Resection in Hepatectomy for Intrahepatic Cholangiocarcinoma

Author	Year	Total resections	Extended resections N (%)	1-yr OS (%)	3-yr OS (%)	5-yr OS (%)	Median OS (mos)	Postoperative mortality (%)
Casavilla et al.	1997	34	15 (44)	60	37	31		6
Chu et al.	1997	39	8 (21)	57	24	16	12	
Roayaie et al.	1998	16	11 (69)	86	64	21	43	12
Yamamoto	1999	83	27 (33)			23		2
Valverde et al.	1999	30	16 (53)	86	22		28	3
Inoue et al.	2000	52	23 (44)	63	36	36	18	
Weber	2001	33	15 (45)	83	55	31	37	3
Ohtsuka et al.	2002	48	26 (54)	62	38	23	25	8
Morimoto et al.	2003	51	15 (29)	68	44	32		4
Lang et al.	2005	27	27 (100)	69	55			6

OS, overall survival.

TABLE 14.5

Incidence of Vascular Resection Combined with Hepatectomy in Intrahepatic Cholangiocarcinoma

Author	Year	Total Resections	Vascular Resections N (%)	1-YR OS (%)	3-YR OS (%)	5-YR OS (%)	Median OS (mos)	Postoperative Mortality (%)
Nakagawa et al.	2005	46	4 (9)	66	38	26	21	6
Chu et al.	1997	39		57	24	16	12	
Roayaie et al.	1998	16	2 (13)	86	64	21	43	12
Yamamoto	1999	83	21 (25)			23		2
Valverde et al.	1999	30	2 (7)	86	22		28	3
Inoue et al.	2000	52		63	36	36	18	
Ohtsuka et al.	2002	48	12 (25)	62	38	23	25	8
Morimoto et al.	2003	51	2 (4)	68	44	32		4
Lang et al.	2005	27	11 (41)	69	55			6

OS, overall survival.

tion was combined with hepatic resection in 27–74% of some large series (2, 29, 30, 33, 35, 37, 40). Vascular resection of the portal vein or IVC was included in 4–37% of these same series. Table 14.4 shows the incidence of extended resection reported in several large series and Table 14.5 the incidence of combined vascular resection and hepatectomy.

Lang et al. examined 50 patients with locally advanced IHC undergoing surgical exploration. These patients were determined by preoperative evaluation to require extended hepatectomy. A total of 27 (54%) patients underwent attempted curative resection; 16 (59%) of these resections required hepatectomy combined with vascular resection, diaphragmatic resection, o, extrahepatic biliary tract resection. The perioperative mortality of the entire group was 6%. The postoperative morbidity was 45% in the standard resection group and 56% in the combined resection group. A R0 resection was accomplished in 56% of the extended resection group and 64% of the standard resection group. The median OS after an R0 resection was 46 months for the entire group with a 3-year OS of 82%. The median survival in the R1 group was 5 months compared to 7 months in the explored only group (40).

Yamamoto and associates examined 83 patients with IHC undergoing resection. Fifty-six patients underwent a standard hepatectomy with or without extrahepatic bile duct resection. These were compared to 27 patients undergoing extended hepatectomy or standard hepatectomy combined with vascular resection and/or pancreatectomy. Perioperative mortality in the extended surgery group was significantly higher at 7% compared to the standard resection with 0% mortality ($p = 0.04$). The 1-year OS was also significantly lower in the extended resection group at 22% compared to 61% in the standard group ($p = 0.001$). The difference in survival may be related to a significantly higher rate of local recurrence and disseminated peritoneal recurrence. However, long-term survival was seen in patients undergoing extended surgery, with 3 of 27 patients surviving greater than 5 years. Two of the three patients had MF tumors and 1 an IG tumor. No patient with PI or MF + PI tumors had long-term survival (57). Weber and associates performed hepatic resection in 33 patients with IHC. Forty-six percent of patients required extended hepatectomy, and an equal number required resection of the extrahepatic biliary tree. In the total patient group vascular invasion was the only factor significantly associated with poor outcome ($p = 0.0007$). The median OS with vascular invasion was 15 months compared to 61 months when vascular invasion was absent (30).

Many series examining combined vascular resection and hepatectomy combine hilar and intrahepatic cholangiocarcinoma. Despite this limitation, these series provide the best available evaluation of the role of extended resections in IHC. Hemming et al. described 22 patients who underwent combined hepatic resection and resection of the inferior vena cava (IVC). The patients had a variety of primary and metastatic

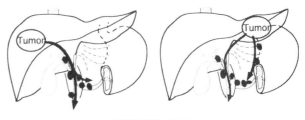

FIGURE 14.5

LCSGJ lymph node groups for right and left lobe tumors. Group 1: first order of lymph node drainage; Group 2: second order of lymph node drainage; Group 3: tertiary order of lymph node drainage. (From Ref. 31.)

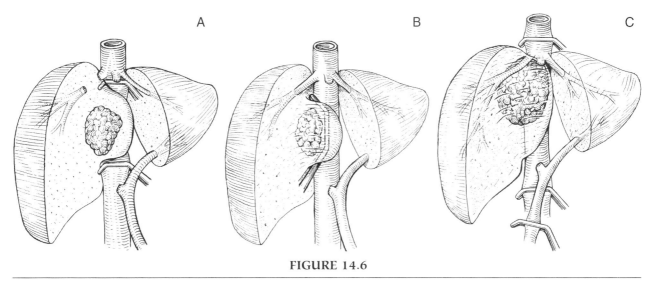

FIGURE 14.6

(a) Infrahepatic IVC occlusion. (b) Partial IVC occlusion. (c) Total vascular isolation of the liver. (From Ref. 62.)

liver tumors, of which five were CCA. The majority of patients were able to be approached in the standard lateral to medial approach to mobilizing the liver and exposing the IVC. In seven patients an anterior approach to the IVC was used. A variety of caval clamping techniques were utilized depending on the portion of the IVC involved with tumor (Figure 14.6). Perioperative mortality was 9%. An R0 resection was performed in 91% of cases. Actuarial 1-, 3-, and 5-year OS was 85, 60, and 33%, respectively (62). Madariaga et al. have published a series of combined hepatectomy with IVC resection in nine patients. Three of the nine patients had CCA. There was one perioperative death; the second patient survived for 10 months and the third was still alive at 43 months. They concluded that selected patients with advanced tumor stages can potentially benefit from aggressive surgical resection including cava resection. Warm ischemia time should be kept within 60–90 minutes, and veno-venous bypass should be available for patients that do not tolerate complete hepatic vascular exclusion (63).

Several series have described the outcome after combined vascular resection and hepatectomy for patients with hilar CCA. Centrally located IHCs can often present in a very similar manner to hilar CCA. Nimura et al. examined 142 patients undergoing resection for hilar CCA. Ninety-nine patients had a standard resection, and 43 patients had a standard resection combined with a vascular resection. The survival at 3 and 5 years was significantly worse for the patients with a portal vein resection at 18 and 6% compared to standard resection at 37 and 27% respectively (p = <0.0001). The survival of the patients with portal vein resection was still significantly better than patients with no resection (p < 0.003) (64). Miyazaki et al. examined 161 patients

who underwent resection for hilar CCA. Forty-three patients underwent combined hepatectomy and vascular resection. In this study, patients undergoing portal vein resection had similar operative morbidity and mortality to patients not undergoing vascular resection. However, patients undergoing hepatic artery resection had a significantly higher postoperative mortality rate than patients not undergoing vascular resection (p < 0.01). OS at 1, 3, and 5 years was significantly worse for patients undergoing portal vein resection than those with no vascular resection (p < 0.001). Five-year OS for portal vein resection was 16% compared to 30% in patients not undergoing vascular resection. Survival for hepatic artery resection was particularly bad, with no 3-year survivors and only 11% alive at 1 year (65).

The above studies are all relatively small and so specific conclusions about the appropriateness of extended resections in IHC are difficult. What seems to be most important to any resection is the need to obtain a microscopically negative margin (R0 resection). Patients with IHC and an incomplete resection seem to fare as poorly as patients without resection. Extended hepatectomy can be completed with acceptable morbidity and mortality, and survival appears comparable to standard hepatectomy if an R0 resection is obtained. Regarding combining extrahepatic resection with hepatectomy, long-term survival appears possible in a small number of patients, but overall survival of this population is significantly worse than for patients with less extensive disease.

Orthotopic Liver Transplantation

Because of the large size and central location of most IHCs, many patients are locally advanced and unresectable at presentation. OLT has been proposed as a potential option for curative resection. Many of the transplantation series combine IHC and hilar CCA as a single entity. Because these initial attempts were made in patients with advanced disease the rates of recurrent malignancy were high. The Cincinnati Transplant Tumor Registry collected data from transplant centers worldwide and identified 207 patients with CCA who received liver transplant. Twenty-one percent were found incidentally. There was a postoperative mortality rate of 10%. Median time to recurrence was 9.7 months. Interestingly, 47% of recurrences occurred in the transplanted liver. There was also no difference in recurrence rates between patients with known CCA and those found incidentally. The OS at 1, 2, and 5 years were 72, 48, and 23%, respectively. They conclude that long-term survival was possible in a small number of patients but there were no identifiable variables to predict these patients preoperatively (66). Similarly, Ghali and colleagues identified 10 patients in Canada who were found to have CCA incidentally. No patient had greater than stage II disease, and none had nodal metastasis. CCA recurred in 8 of 10 patients, with a median time to recurrence of 26 months and a 3-year OS of 30% (67). Based on these findings CCA has been considered a contraindication to liver transplantation in Canada. The authors also noted that the median time to recurrence was longer than most studies but probably reflected a lead time bias of the early stage, and the overall survival at 3 years was still poor. The Spanish experience with transplantation for both hilar and IHC was reviewed. A total of 59 patients (36 hilar and 23 peripheral) underwent OLT. The 1-, 3-, and 5-year OS in the IHC patients were 77, 65, and 42%, respectively. This survival was better than most previous reports, but the authors recognized that the survival was still below OLT survival rates for nonmalignant indications, and with a limited amount of organs the indication could be questioned (68).

Based on the high recurrence rate after transplantation, treatment programs incorporating neoadjuvant chemoradiation prior to transplantation for hilar CCA were developed. These studies have been limited to hilar CCA because of the ability to deliver brachytherapy directly to the tumor in the bile duct. The Mayo Clinic transplant division developed a protocol utilizing external beam radiation therapy (EBRT) plus bolus 5-FU, followed by brachytherapy plus infusional 5-FU and subsequent OLT in patients with hilar CCA. Inclusion criteria required no evidence of nodal metastasis, intrahepatic metastasis or distant disease. Two to 6 weeks following the transcatheter brachytherapy, patients underwent an exploratory laparotomy to evaluate for extrahepatic disease. The patients staged on laparotomy had to be stage II or less to be placed on the United Network for Organ Sharing (UNOS) list and subsequently transplanted. Seventy-one patients presenting with CCA were eligible for the study and underwent radiation. Thirty-eight patients were able to undergo transplant (54%). No residual tumor was seen in 16 of 38 patients in the explanted livers. One-, 3-, and 5-year recurrence rates were 0, 5, and 12%, respectively, with a mean time to recurrence of 40 months. OS at 1, 3, and 5 years were 92, 82, and 82%, respectively. The author's conclude that neoadjuvant therapy followed by OLT appears to have greater efficacy than resection for selected patients (69, 70). The University of Nebraska utilized a similar protocol with a higher dose of brachytherapy eliminating EBRT. Continuous 5-FU is started at the time of brachytherapy and continued until transplant. Seventeen patients were enrolled in the trial, 11 of whom completed the brachytherapy and went on to transplantation without progressive disease. The median OS of the transplanted patients was 25 months. Five patients (45%) were alive and without recurrence at 2.8–14.5 years posttransplant (10).

These studies have shown that despite removing the liver completely and performing OLT, a large number of patients will recur, with half of this recurrence within the new liver. There appears to be an improvement in recurrence prevention with the addition of neoadjuvant chemoradiation in early-stage hilar CCA. The survival in the Mayo Clinic series approaches that seen with OLT for nonmalignant indications. Even with these improvements, the majority of patients presenting with IHC will have advanced disease and not be considered a candidate for current protocols. Perhaps a better understanding of risk factors for recurrence could lead to broader applicability and the use of living related transplant could temper the ethical decision of using the limited resource of cadaveric livers in this population. The protocols from the Mayo Clinic and University of Nebraska have also raised the question of applying neoadjuvant chemoradiation to standard hepatic resection. However, because of previous poor results, transplantation for hilar CCA remains contraindicated outside a research protocol.

Palliative Procedures

The role of surgical palliation for biliary obstruction has decreased with the improvement in endobiliary prosthesis. Many centers question the need for decompression in asymptomatic patients. Because surgical bypass has not been demonstrated superior to stenting, palliation is accomplished conservatively when possible. Biliary obstruction is much less common with IHC when compared to hilar CCA and typically occurs as a late event as the tumor encroaches on the hilum from the

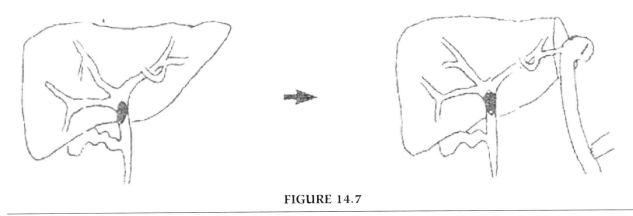

FIGURE 14.7

Longmire bypass to segment III. Lau, WY *Journal of the Hong Kong medical association* 1987, 39(1):11-17.

liver parenchyma or by extrinsic compression from bulky adenopathy. In addition, the survival after palliative surgery for IHC has been dismal, with 2- to 6-month median survival in surgical series (5, 28, 29, 36). Jan et al. examined 373 patients with IHC undergoing surgical procedures; 186 of these patients underwent nonresectional surgical procedures with a postoperative mortality of 11% and a median OS of 4 months (1).

When surgical bypass is necessary, the most common procedures employ a segment III or a right sectoral (segment IV) hepatic duct bypass. In most instances, a unilateral bypass may be performed as results appear to be satisfactory even when there is no communication between right and left biliary systems (71). Therefore the segment III bypass is typically employed, as it is technically easier and the location of the duct more consistent (72).

There are two main techniques for bypassing to segment III. The first was described by Longmire in 1948 and is shown in Figure 14.7 (73). This has been since modified to include preoperative placement of a catheter in the distal left bile duct to facilitate identification and isolation of the duct as described by Cameron et al. (74). The second technique was first described by Soupault and Couinaud, where the duct is accessed at the umbilical ligament in order to preserve the hepatic parenchyma and is depicted in Figure 14.8 (75). The umbilical ligament exposure of the segment III duct is most common and is exposed by making a hepatotomy to the left of the umbilical fissure at its base. A 3-cm section of duct is exposed and a 1- to 2-cm incision is made in the duct and a Roux-en-Y loop hepaticojejunostomy is performed (72, 76).

The right sectoral hepatic bypass is begun by exposing the right portal pedicle by performing hepatotomies at the base of the gallbladder fossa and the caudate process. The overlying hepatic parenchyma is divided with exposure of the sectoral branches. The anterior sectoral branch is typically used. A Roux-en-Y hepaticoje-

junostomy is then performed to the anterior sectoral branch (72, 76). Suzuki et al. reported on 15 patients undergoing intrahepatic cholangiojejunostomy for unresectable biliary tumors; two of these had IHC (72). There were no postoperative deaths, and the morbidity rate was 13%. The median OS was 9 months; 13.5 months in the IHC group. The rate of recurrent cholangitis was 44% in patients surviving more than 6 months, and these were treated with percutaneous transhepatic biliary drainage. Jarnagin et al. examined 55 patients undergoing intrahepatic biliary-enteric bypass; 20 patients with IHC (76). The postoperative mortality was 11% and morbidity 45%. The median OS of the patients with CCA was 52 weeks. Readmission was required in 47% of patients; 35% for recurrent cholangitis.

Biliary obstruction can often be palliated by percutaneous transhepatic cholangiography (PTHC) or endoscopic placement of an endobiliary prosthesis.

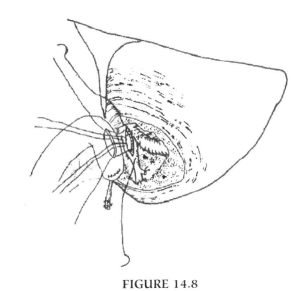

FIGURE 14.8

Exposure of segment III bile duct at base of umbilical ligament for anastomosis. (From Ref. 72.)

When this fails or is not possible, surgical bypass can be considered. This can have durable patency and effective palliation, but not without significant morbidity and mortality associated. In addition, recurrent biliary sepsis can be seen in 35–44% of patients.

ADJUVANT THERAPY

There are no trials comparing adjuvant chemotherapy, radiation, or chemoradiation versus resection only. The surgical series that include patients receiving adjuvant therapy do not delineate the indications, and the regimens are variable. The University of Pittsburgh group found no difference in survival between patients receiving adjuvant therapy with a median OS of 7.2 months versus 18.3 months median survival for those not receiving adjuvant therapy (39). The John Hopkins University group found no significant difference in survival between patients receiving adjuvant therapy and those who did not. There was no difference in the overall group undergoing resection or when the subgroups of patients who had R0 or R1/R2 resections were analyzed separately (3).

Jan et al. examined 373 patients with IHC who underwent a variety of both curative and palliative procedures in which chemotherapy with 5-FU–based regimens and external beam radiation therapy (EBRT) were given for positive margin or recurrence. They showed a significant improvement in OS with a median survival of 11 months in patients receiving chemotherapy and 5 months in the group not receiving chemotherapy ($p = 0.0001$). The lack of chemotherapy remained a significant factor on multivariate analysis (1). The OS of the patients not receiving chemotherapy in this study is not representative of patients undergoing curative resection in other studies, and so the applicability of these findings to the adjuvant setting is questionable. Roayaie et al. reported on 26 patients with IHC undergoing exploration, 16 of whom underwent attempted curative resection. Patients with positive margins received 5-FU–based chemotherapy and EBRT. The five patients with positive margins all recurred intrahepatically, but the median DFS in this group was 18 months compared to 31 months in the negative margin group. The median OS of the margin positive group was 43 months compared to 7 months for the unresected group. There was no difference in OS for patients receiving chemotherapy and radiation compared to those who did not (61). The authors suggested that the lack of difference in survival between those receiving chemotherapy and radiation and those who did not implied a benefit to adjuvant therapy.

Currently there is no level 1 evidence to support postsurgical adjuvant therapy (77–79). More recently combination therapy, including addition of cisplatin, epirubicin, and or gemcitabine to standard 5-FU regimens, has been used in unresectable cases, and response rates up to 40% have been achieved (80–82). Unfortunately, median survival is still approximately 9 months with chemotherapy (83). This has been increased in some series up to 13.3 months when radiation is combined with hepatic intra-arterial chemotherapy, with the suggestion that improved survival is directly correlated to increasing doses of EBRT (83, 84). The improved response of combination chemotherapy and possibly the use of intensity-modulated radiation therapy, allowing increased dose tolerance, will offer opportunities for further trials.

CONCLUSIONS

The surgical management of IHC remains complex. Resection often requires extended surgery to include extended hepatectomy, resection of the bile duct, and/or vascular resection. The morbidity and mortality is significantly increased with extended resection. However, long-term survival is possible if a microscopically negative resection can be performed. Currently the role of lymphadenectomy in resection of IHC is of questionable benefit. There have been intriguing results in using neoadjuvant chemoradiation in patients with cholangiocarcinoma undergoing transplantation. The role of neoadjuvant chemoradiation in resection of IHC would be an area for future exploration.

References

1. Jan YY, et al. Prognostic analysis of surgical treatment of peripheral cholangiocarcinoma: two decades of experience at Chang Gung Memorial Hospital. World J Gastroenterol 2005; 11(12):1779–1784.
2. Morimoto Y, et al. Long-term survival and prognostic factors in the surgical treatment for intrahepatic cholangiocarcinoma. J Hepatobiliary Pancreat Surg 2003; 10(6):432–440.
3. DeOliveira ML, et al. Cholangiocarcinoma: thirty-one-year experience with 564 patients at a single institution. Ann Surg 2007. 245(5):755–762.
4. Chen MF, Peripheral cholangiocarcinoma (cholangiocellular carcinoma): clinical features, diagnosis and treatment. J Gastroenterol Hepatol 1999; 14(12):1144–1149.
5. Hanazak, K, et al. Prognostic factors of intrahepatic cholangiocarcinoma after hepatic resection: univariate and multivariate analysis. Hepatogastroenterology 2002; 49(44):311–316.
6. Yoon JH, Gores GJ. diagnosis, staging, and treatment of cholangiocarcinoma. Curr Treat Options Gastroenterol 2003; 6(2):105–112.
7. Liver Cancer Study Group of Japan. The General Rules for the Clinical and Pathological Study of Primary Liver Cancer (English ed.). 4th ed. Tokyo: Kanehara, 2000.
8. Patel T. Increasing incidence and mortality of primary intrahepatic cholangiocarcinoma in the United States. Hepatology 2001; 33(6):1353–1357.
9. Franko J, Nussbaum ML, Morris JB. Choledochal cyst cholangiocarcinoma arising from adenoma: case report and a review of the literature. Curr Surg 2006; 63(4):281–284.

10. Sudan D, et al. Radiochemotherapy and transplantation allow long-term survival for nonresectable hilar cholangiocarcinoma. Am J Transplant 2002; 2(8):774–779.

11. Miros M, et al. Predicting cholangiocarcinoma in patients with primary sclerosing cholangitis before transplantation. Gut 1991; 32(11):1369–1373.

12. Taylor-Robinson SD, et al. Increase in mortality rates from intrahepatic cholangiocarcinoma in England and Wales 1968–1998. Gut 2001; 48(6):816–820.

13. Monson JR, et al. Intraoperative radiotherapy for unresectable cholangiocarcinoma—the Mayo Clinic experience. Surg Oncol 1992; 1(4):283–290.

14. Chalasani N, et al. Cholangiocarcinoma in patients with primary sclerosing cholangitis: a multicenter case-control study. Hepatology 2000; 31(1):7–11.

15. John AR, et al. Is a raised CA 19-9 level diagnostic for a cholangiocarcinoma in patients with no history of sclerosing cholangitis ? Dig Surg 2006; 23(5–6):319–324.

16. Patel AH, et al. The utility of CA 19-9 in the diagnoses of cholangiocarcinoma in patients without primary sclerosing cholangitis. Am J Gastroenterol 2000; 95(1):204–207.

17. Lacomis JM, et al. Cholangiocarcinoma: delayed CT contrast enhancement patterns. Radiology 1997; 203(1):98–104.

18. Slattery JM, Sahani DV. What is the current state-of-the-art imaging for detection and staging of cholangiocarcinoma? Oncologist 2006; 11(8):913–922.

19. Asayama Y, et al. Delayed-phase dynamic CT enhancement as a prognostic factor for mass-forming intrahepatic cholangiocarcinoma. Radiology 2006; 238(1):150–155.

20. Soyer P, Capsular retraction of the liver in malignant tumor of the biliary tract MRI findings. Clin Imaging 1994; 18(4):255–257.

21. Manfredi R, et al. Magnetic resonance imaging of cholangiocarcinoma. Semin Liver Dis 2004; 24(2):155–164.

22. Petrowsky H, et al. Impact of integrated positron emission tomography and computed tomography on staging and management of gallbladder cancer and cholangiocarcinoma. J Hepatol 2006; 45(1):43–50.

23. Greene FL. American Joint Committee on Cancer and American Cancer Society. AJCC Cancer Staging Manual. 6th ed. New York: Springer, 2002.

24. Hirohashi, K, et al. Macroscopic types of intrahepatic cholangiocarcinoma: clinicopathologic features and surgical outcomes. Hepatogastroenterology 2002; 49(44):326–369.

25. Sano T, et al. Macroscopic classification and preoperative diagnosis of intrahepatic cholangiocarcinoma in Japan. J Hepatobiliary Pancreat Surg 1999; 6(2):101–107.

26. Yamasaki S. Intrahepatic cholangiocarcinoma: macroscopic type and stage classification. J Hepatobiliary Pancreat Surg 2003; 10(4):288–291.

27. Jan YY, et al. Factors influencing survival after hepatectomy for peripheral cholangiocarcinoma. Hepatogastroenterology 1996; 43(9):614–619.

28. Berdah SV, et al. A western surgical experience of peripheral cholangiocarcinoma. Br J Surg 1996. 83(11):1517–1521.

29. Ohtsuka M, et al. Results of surgical treatment for intrahepatic cholangiocarcinoma and clinicopathological factors influencing survival. Br J Surg 2002; 89(12):1525–1531.

30. Weber SM, et al. Intrahepatic cholangiocarcinoma: resectability, recurrence pattern, and outcomes. J Am Coll Surg 2001; 193(4):384–391.

31. Shimada M, et al. Value of lymph node dissection during resection of intrahepatic cholangiocarcinoma. Br J Surg 2001; 88(11):1463–1466.

32. Okabayashi T, et al. A new staging system for mass-forming intrahepatic cholangiocarcinoma: analysis of preoperative and postoperative variables. Cancer 2001; 92(9):2374–2383.

33. Suzuki S, et al. Clinicopathological prognostic factors and impact of surgical treatment of mass-forming intrahepatic cholangiocarcinoma. World J Surg 2002; 26(6):687–693.

34. Miwa S, et al. Predictive factors for intrahepatic cholangiocarcinoma recurrence in the liver following surgery. J Gastroenterol 2006; 41(9):893–900.

35. Nakagawa T, et al. Number of lymph node metastases is a significant prognostic factor in intrahepatic cholangiocarcinoma. World J Surg 2005; 29(6):728–733.

36. Weimann A, et al. Retrospective analysis of prognostic factors after liver resection and transplantation for cholangiocellular carcinoma. Br J Surg 2000; 87(9):1182–1187.

37. Valverde A, et al. Resection of intrahepatic cholangiocarcinoma: a Western experience. J Hepatobiliary Pancreat Surg 1999; 6(2):122–127.

38. Uenishi T, et al. Histologic factors affecting prognosis following hepatectomy for intrahepatic cholangiocarcinoma. World J Surg 2001; 25(7):865–869.

39. Casavilla FA, et al. Hepatic resection and transplantation for peripheral cholangiocarcinoma. J Am Coll Surg 1997; 185(5): 429–436.

40. Lang H, et al. Extended hepatectomy for intrahepatic cholangiocellular carcinoma (ICC): when is it worthwhile? Single center experience with 27 resections in 50 patients over a 5-year period. Ann Surg 2005; 241(1):134–143.

41. Blumgart LH, Fong Y (eds.). Surgery of the Liver and Biliary Tract. 3rd ed. New York: W.B. Saunders, 2000.

42. Couinaud C. Le Foie: Etudes Anatomiques et Chirurgicales. Paris: Masson, 1957.

43. Wakai T, et al. Anatomic resection independently improves long-term survival in patients with T1–T2 hepatocellular carcinoma. Ann Surg Oncol 2007; 14:1356–1365.

44. Washburn WK, Lewis WD, Jenkins RL. Aggressive surgical resection for cholangiocarcinoma. Arch Surg 1995;. 130(3):270–276.

45. Goere D, et al. Utility of staging laparoscopy in subsets of biliary cancers : laparoscopy is a powerful diagnostic tool in patients with intrahepatic and gallbladder carcinoma. Surg Endosc 2006; 20(5):721–725.

46. Makuuchi M, et al. Percutaneous transcatheter embolization of the portal venous branch for patients receiving extended lobectomy due to the bile duct carcinoma (in Japanese). J Jpn Soc Clin Surg 1984; 45:14–20.

47. Kokudo N, Makuuchi M. Current role of portal vein embolization/hepatic artery chemoembolization. Surg Clin North Am 2004; 84(2):643–657.

48. Kubota K, et al. Measurement of liver volume and hepatic functional reserve as a guide to decision-making in resectional surgery for hepatic tumors. Hepatology 1997; 26(5): 1176–1181.

49. Nagino M, et al. Two hundred forty consecutive portal vein embolizations before extended hepatectomy for biliary cancer: surgical outcome and long-term follow-up. Ann Surg 2006; 243(3):364–372.

50. Abdalla EK, et al. Extended hepatectomy in patients with hepatobiliary malignancies with and without preoperative portal vein embolization. Arch Surg 2002; 137(6):675–680; discussion 680–681.

51. Hemming AW, et al. Preoperative portal vein embolization for extended hepatectomy. Ann Surg 2003; 237(5):686–691; discussion 691–693.

52. Vauthey JN, et al. Standardized measurement of the future liver remnant prior to extended liver resection: methodology and clinical associations. Surgery 2000; 127(5):512–519.

53. Shimada K, et al. Safety and effectiveness of left hepatic trisegmentectomy for hilar cholangiocarcinoma. World J Surg 2005; 29(6):723–727.

54. Shirabe K, et al. Intrahepatic cholangiocarcinoma: its mode of spreading and therapeutic modalities. Surgery 2002; 131(1 suppl):S159–164.

55. Okami J, et al. Patterns of regional lymph node involvement in intrahepatic cholangiocarcinoma of the left lobe. J Gastrointest Surg 2003; 7(7):850–856.

56. Yamamoto M, et al. Recurrence after surgical resection of intrahepatic cholangiocarcinoma. J Hepatobiliary Pancreat Surg 2001; 8(2):154–157.

57. Yamamoto M, Takasaki K, Yoshikawa T. Extended resection for intrahepatic cholangiocarcinoma in Japan. J Hepatobiliary Pancreat Surg 1999; 6(2):117–121.

58. Uenishi T, et al. Clinicopathologic features in patients with long-term survival following resection for intrahepatic cholangiocarcinoma. Hepatogastroenterology 2003; 50(52):1069–1072.

59. Kahlenberg MS, et al. Hepatic lymphatic mapping: a pilot study for porta hepatis lymph node identification. Cancer Invest 2001; 19(3):256–260.

60. Kane JM, 3rd, et al. Intraoperative hepatic lymphatic mapping in patients with liver metastases from colorectal carcinoma. Am Surg 2002; 68(9):745–750.

61. Roayaie S, et al. Aggressive surgical treatment of intrahepatic cholangiocarcinoma: predictors of outcomes. J Am Coll Surg 1998; 187(4):365–372.

62. Hemming AW, et al. Combined resection of the liver and inferior vena cava for hepatic malignancy. Ann Surg 2004; 239(5):712–719; discussion 719–721.

63. Madariaga JR, et al. Liver resection combined with excision of vena cava. J Am Coll Surg 2000; 191(3):244–250.

64. Nimura Y, et al. Aggressive preoperative management and extended surgery for hilar cholangiocarcinoma: Nagoya experience. J Hepatobiliary Pancreat Surg 2000; 7(2):155–162.

65. Miyazaki M, et al. Combined vascular resection in operative resection for hilar cholangiocarcinoma: does it work or not? Surgery 2007; 141(5):581–588.

66. Meyer CG, Penn I, James L. Liver transplantation for cholangiocarcinoma: results in 207 patients. Transplantation 2000; 69(8):1633–1637.

67. Ghali P, et al. Liver transplantation for incidental cholangiocarcinoma: analysis of the Canadian experience. Liver Transpl 2005; 11(11):1412–1416.

68. Robles R, et al. Spanish experience in liver transplantation for hilar and peripheral cholangiocarcinoma. Ann Surg 2004; 239(2):265–271.

69. Heimbach JK, et al. Liver transplantation for unresectable perihilar cholangiocarcinoma. Semin Liver Dis 2004; 24(2):201–207.

70. Rea DJ, et al. Liver transplantation with neoadjuvant chemoradiation is more effective than resection for hilar cholangiocarcinoma. Ann Surg 2005; 242(3):451–458; discussion 458–461.

71. Baer HU, et al. The effect of communication between the right and left liver on the outcome of surgical drainage for jaundice due to malignant obstruction at the hilus of the liver. HPB Surg 1994; 8(1):27–31.

72. Suzuki S, et al. Intrahepatic cholangiojejunostomy for unresectable malignant biliary tumors with obstructive jaundice. J Hepatobiliary Pancreat Surg 2001; 8(2):124–129.

73. Longmire WP Jr. Intrahepatic cholangiojejunostomy with partial hepatectomy for biliary obstruction. Surgery 1948; 24:264–276.

74. Cameron JL, Gayler BW, Harrington DP. Modification of the Longmire procedure. Ann Surg 1978; 187(4):379–382.

75. Soupault R, Couinaud C. [New procedure for intrahepatic biliary shunt: left cholangiojejunostomy without hepatic sacrifice]. Presse Med 1957; 65(50):1157–1159.

76. Jarnagin WR, et al. Intrahepatic biliary enteric bypass provides effective palliation in selected patients with malignant obstruction at the hepatic duct confluence. Am J Surg 1998; 175(6): 453–460.

77. Yamamoto M, Ariizumi S. Intrahepatic recurrence after surgery in patients with intrahepatic cholangiocarcinoma. J Gastroenterol 2006; 41(9):925–926.

78. Khan SA, et al. Guidelines for the diagnosis and treatment of cholangiocarcinoma: consensus document. Gut 2002; 51(suppl 6):VI1-9.

79. Benson AB, 3rd, et al. Hepatobiliary cancers. Clinical practice guidelines in oncology. J Natl Compr Canc Netw 2006; 4(8):728–750.

80. Thongprasert S, et al. Phase II study of gemcitabine and cisplatin as first-line chemotherapy in inoperable biliary tract carcinoma. Ann Oncol 2005; 16(2):279–281.

81. Park SH, et al. Phase II study of epirubicin, cisplatin, and capecitabine for advanced biliary tract adenocarcinoma. Cancer 2006; 106(2):361–365.

82. Knox JJ, et al. Combining gemcitabine and capecitabine in patients with advanced biliary cancer: a phase II trial. J Clin Oncol 2005; 23(10):2332–2338.

83. Ben-Josef E, et al. Phase II trial of high-dose conformal radiation therapy with concurrent hepatic artery floxuridine for unresectable intrahepatic malignancies. J Clin Oncol 2005; 23(34):8739–8747.

84. Cantore M, et al. Phase II study of hepatic intraarterial epirubicin and cisplatin, with systemic 5-fluorouracil in patients with unresectable biliary tract tumors. Cancer 2005; 103(7): 1402–1407.

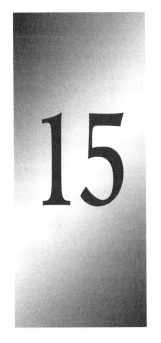

15 Surgical Management of Extrahepatic Biliary Tract Cancer

Swee H. Teh
Susan L. Orloff

Bile duct cancer is a rare clinical entity with an incidence of 2000–3000 new cases per year (1). The most common type of bile duct cancer is cholangiocarcinoma which arises from the epithelial lining of the biliary tree. In general, it can be subdivided into 4 subcategories according to the origin of the tumor in the billiary tree (2). These are intrahepatic cholangiocarcinoma, gallbladder carcinoma, hilar cholangiocarcinoma, and periampullary (distal) cholangiocarcinoma. In this chapter we will focus on the surgical technique for the treatment of hilar cholangiocarcinoma.

Prognosis of untreated hilar cholangiocarcinoma (HC) is poor, with the median survival of 6–12 months, with a 1- and 2-year survival rate of 15 and 0%, respectively (3–5). Aggressive surgical resection remains the only chance for long-term survival (6–9). Resectability of HC depends, in part, on the tumor's anatomic location, extent of involvement, and stage. However, HC often presents with advanced disease, precluding curative surgical intervention. Less than 30% of patients with HC are suitable candidates for surgical resection (8, 10, 11). Surgical resection for HC, however, is highly complex and often involves major biliary tract reconstruction with or without hepatic resection (more than two segments). Perioperative complications are not uncommon; therefore, an understanding of the pathologic and anatomic characteristics of the tumor preoperatively is paramount. Treating HC with chemother-apy or radiation therapy alone has had limited success in prolonging survival (12, 13). In combination, these treatment modalities may palliate pain and improve biliary decompression (14, 15). Multimodality therapy following a curative resection may improve local control (16). The role of combination chemoradiatherapy followed by liver transplantation (Mayo Clinic protocol) for a highly selected group of patients with HC has shown some promising results and should be validated prospectively (17).

PATHOLOGIC CHARACTERISTICS

Subtype of HC and Mode of Spread

Sclerosing HC (70%) is the most common subtype (18). These tumors spread both longitudinally and radially. Cholangiography usually underestimates the longitudinal extent of tumor spread both proximally and distally (Figure 15.1). Sclerosing HC also spreads directly through the wall of the bile duct into adjacent structures (19).

Desmoplastic reaction, a characteristic of sclerosing HC, frequently causes adherence of the primary tumor to adjacent hilar structures. The hepatic artery and portal veins are at risk of tumor encasement and invasion (Figure 15.2A). Therefore, any fibrosis near the hilus must be treated as malignancy, unless histopatho-

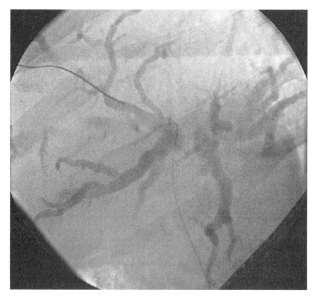

FIGURE 15.1

This patient's endoscopic retrograde cholangiopancreatography (ERCP) showed what appeared to be a potentially resectable cholangiocarcinoma with findings consistent with a stricture in the common hepatic duct at the hilum near the bifurcation of the left and right ducts. On exploration of this patient the tumor extended both proximally into the right duct and distally toward the pancreas. The tumor was of the sclerosing type and was much more extensive than the ERCP had portrayed. The patient had a gastrohepatic node positive for tumor in addition to a separate lesion in the left intrahepatic ductal system, rendering him unresectable.

logic examination confirms otherwise. Hepatic parenchyma involvement can occur either by direct tumor invasion into hepatic segment IVb or by longitudinal spread along the bile ducts directly into the caudate lobe biliary pedicle (Figure 15.3). The nodular and papillary HC subtype tends to growth intraluminally with late radial extension (20). Current imaging modalities including ultrasound, helical computed tomography (CT) scan, magnetic resonance cholangiopancreatography (MRCP), or endoscopic ultrasound (EUS) can underestimate the extensiveness of local disease.

Staging (TNM)

It is imperative to perform a complete staging by imaging studies to rule out distance or regional disease that may preclude patients from a major resection. The current TNM staging system (Table 15.1) for HC is suboptimal (21). This is based on histopathologic criteria, which can only be used accurately following resection, and its application preoperatively is limited.

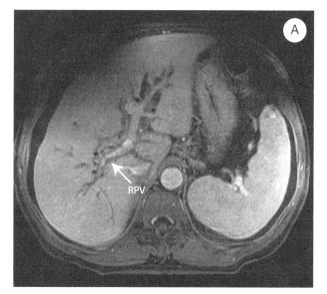

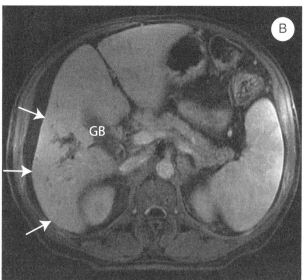

FIGURE 15.2

(A) This patient's MRI/MRA shows encasement and narrowing of the right portal vein (long arrow); left and main portal veins are patent. RPV, right portal vein. (B) Atrophy of the right lobe of the liver (arrows) secondary to central cholangiocarcinoma involving the central right hepatic duct and extending to the ductal confluence. There is relative hypertrophy of the left lobe of the liver due to the long-standing right-sided biliary and vascular obstruction. GB, gallbladder.

Atrophy–Hypertrophy Complex

Hepatic lobar atrophy can be the result of reduced lobar inflow secondary to ipsilateral lobar portal vein occlusion or thrombosis and less commonly the involvement of the hepatic artery. This often results in the contralateral hepatic lobar hypertrophy (Figures

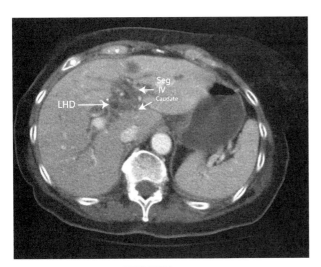

FIGURE 15.3

Patient with unresectable cholangiocarcinoma. Contrast-enhanced CT scan demonstrates diffuse ductal dilatation involving the intrahepatic ducts. In this specific image, there is thickening of the left hepatic duct (LHD, long arrow) due to tumor which extends from the common hepatic duct into the hilum and extends into the left hepatic duct greater than the right. There is extension of the tumor into segment IV and to a small degree into the caudate lobe (short arrow).

15.2B and 15.4). This may be an indication of a more advanced disease and may therefore translate into unresectability or need for major vascular reconstruction during the resection. Chronic lobar biliary obstruction can also result in lobar atrophy but typically with less contralateral hepatic lobar hypertrophy. This atrophy–hypertrophy complex can be seen on CT or magnetic resonance imaging (MRI).

ANATOMIC CHARACTERISTICS

Cholangiographic Extension

The Bismuth-Corlette classification (Table 15.2) allows cholangiographic assessment of the longitudinal extension of tumor along the bile duct and provides vital information of the status of proximal bile duct involvement (2). Any involvement of bile duct proximal to lobar biliary pedicle dictates the need for hepatic resection. This extension is best visualized via percutaneous transhepatic cholangiography (PTC) (Figure 15.5). Endoscopic retrograde cholangiography (ERC) may not provide adequate visualization in the patient with a more proximal tumor. In order to best delineate the extent of biliary tract involvement with tumor, it is often most helpful to perform both a PTC and and ERC.

TABLE 15.1
TNM Staging for Hilar Cholangiocarcinoma

TNM DEFINITION

Primary tumor (T)
TX: Primary tumor cannot be assessed
T0: No evidence of primary tumor
Tis: Carcinoma in situ
T1: Tumor confined to the bile duct histologically
T2: Tumor invades beyond the wall of the bile duct
T3: Tumor invades the liver, gallbladder, pancreas, and/or unilateral branches of the portal vein (right or left) or hepatic artery (right or left)
T4: Tumor invades any of the following: main portal vein or its branches bilaterally, common hepatic artery, or other adjacent structures, such as the colon, stomach, duodenum, or abdominal wall

Regional lymph nodes (N)
NX: Regional lymph nodes cannot be assessed
N0: No regional lymph node metastasis
N1: Regional lymph node metastasis (hilar, cholecystic, pericholedochal nodes)
N2: Regional lymph node metastasis (peripancreatic, periduodenal, periportal, celiac, and superior mesenteric nodes)

Distant metastasis (M)
MX: Distant metastasis cannot be assessed
M0: No distant metastasis
M1: Distant metastasis

AJCC STAGE GROUPINGS

Stage 0
Tis, N0, M0
Stage IA
T1, N0, M0
Stage IB
T2, N0, M0
Stage IIA
T3, N0, M0
Stage IIB
T1, N1, M0
T2, N1, M0
T3, N1, M0
Stage III
T4, any N, M0
Stage IV
Any T, any N, M1

Source: Ref. 21.

Vascular Involvement

Prior to the sophisticated current imaging techniques, such as CT angiogram with dual phase liver or MRI/magnetic resonance angiography (MRA), the gold standard for assessing vascular involvement by the

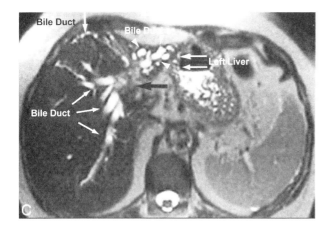

FIGURE 15.4

Axial magnetic resonance cholangiopancreatography images of a patient with hilar cholangiocarcinoma. The bile ducts appear white. The left liver is shrunken; its medial extent is indicated by the white arrows. The bile ducts in the left liver are dilated and crowded (white arrowheads), with little interposed liver tissue. The tumor is indicated by the black arrow. (From Ref. 8.)

tumor, which would include encasement and/or thrombosis, was a visceral angiogram. The CT angiogram allows better spatial resolution, as well as smaller-caliber vessel visualization, than does the MRI/MRA. In addition, CT imaging is less sensitive to small movements from the patient (requires less breath holding), hence it is easier to obtain a clear and optimal exam. The choice of CT angiogram versus MRI/MRA depends somewhat upon the individual center's sophistication with each of these imaging techniques as well as the staff radiologists' ability to accurately interpret the studies.

SURGERY

The goal of the operation is to achieve an R0 resection while preserving an adequate hepatic remnant with intact inflow (hepatic artery and portal vein) and outflow (hepatic vein) and restoration of enterohepatic circulation. The current contraindications for biliary and hepatic resection for HC are as shown in Table 15.3.

Essential Components of Resection for HC

1. Cholecystectomy
2. Resection of extrahepatic bile duct from the hilus to the pancreas
3. Regional lymphadenectomy (hilar, cystic, pericoledochal, portal, hepatic artery, and posterior pancreaticoduodenal lymph nodes)

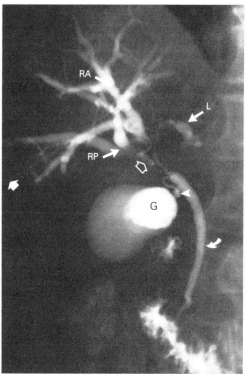

FIGURE 15.5

Cholangiogram of a patient with cholangiocarcinoma. RA denotes the right anterior ductal system, RP the right posterior ductal system, L the left ductal system, and G the gallbladder. The broad, open arrow points to part of the duct that is narrowed by the tumor; the broad solid arrow to the track of the percutaneous needle used to inject contrast material; the arrowhead to the cystic duct; the curved arrow to the common hepatic duct.

4. Hepatic lobar resection (only Bismuth-Corlette Type I, and potentially Type II, do not require hepatic resection)
5. Caudate lobe resection (required in Bismuth-Corlette Type III and if grossly involved in Type I and II)
6. Roux-en-Y hepaticojejunostomy
7. ±Vascular resection/reconstruction

Preoperative Planning

Disease Factors

Once the diagnosis is made and regional and distant metastasis has been ruled out, the surgeon needs to conceptualize the extent of the disease and therefore the extent of the resection. This is based on preoperative pathologic and anatomic characteristics of the tumor mentioned above. If extended hepatic resection is required to achieve an R0 resection, one may consider

TABLE 15.2
The Bismuth-Corlette Classification

Type I: Tumors below the confluence of left and right hepatic duct
Type II: Tumors at the confluence of the hepatic ducts
Type IIIa: Tumors at the confluence and extends into the right hepatic duct
Type IIIb: Tumors at the confluence and extends into the left hepatic duct
Type IV: Tumors at the confluence and extends to the right and left hepatic ducts or multicentric

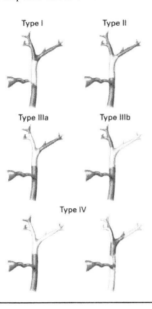

TABLE 15.3
Contraindications for Resection for Hilar Cholangiocarcinoma

A. Advanced hilar disease
 1. Bile duct
    a. Bilateral extension of tumor into segmental bile ducts (cannot get R0 resection)
    b. Unilateral lobar hepatic bile duct tumor extension with contralateral lobar hepatic artery or lobar portal vein invasion.
    c. Unilateral lobar hepatic bile duct tumor extension with contralateral lobar atrophy
 2. Portal vein
    a. Tumor invasions proximal to PV bifurcation
    b. Tumor extension to bilateral secondary portal vein branches
 3. Hepatic artery
    a. Tumor extension to bilateral secondary hepatic artery branches
B. Inadequate remnant liver volume
 1. Less than 30% of the whole liver volume (despite PV embolization)
 2. Hepatic cirrhosis
C. Metastasis
 1. Regional lymph node disease (N2)
 2. Peritoneal disease
 3. Distance metastasis

preoperative portal vein embolization if the planned hepatic remnant is deemed to be less than 25–30% of the total liver volume (29).

Patient Factors

Resection with curative intent for HC often means a major operation with significant perioperative mortality rate ranging from 5 to 17% and morbidity rate of 30–76% (6–11). Therefore, only patients with The Eastern Cooperative Oncology Group (ECOG) performance status of 0, 1, or 2 are candidates for surgery. Many people would say only 0 and 1 patients are candidates for major hepatectomy. Patients with performance status less than 50% of normal and who have significant medical comorbidities should not be considered for resection.

Billiary Stenting

Almost all HC patients present with obstructive jaundice. Patients with a bilirubin level of 10–20 mg/dl or above inevitably have underlying hepatic dysfunc-

tion and are at significant risk of infection either directly related to the biliary tract or from distant sources. The coagulation profile is often abnormally elevated. We advocate preoperative decompression of the biliary tree to improve the cholestatic environment (22–24). This may reverse the hepatic dysfunction and improve postoperative hepatic regeneration and function. If portal vein embolization is considered, the planned hepatic remnant may be further augmented when the cholestasis is decreased by drainage with a biliary stent. Preoperative biliary stenting has been shown to increase the risk of postoperative infection, and therefore, preoperative broad-spectrum antibiotics are indicated (25).Overall, preoperative drainage may reduce the incidence of postoperative hyperbilirubinemia and hepatic insufficiency in patients who require extended hepatic resection. The use of a Wall stent for decompression is not advised, as this type of metal stent is indicated only in patients who are deemed unresectable. Of note, preoperative biliary instrumentation may cause enlarged reactive periportal lymph nodes that mimic metastatic disease. Therefore, complete cross-sectional imaging is recommended to evaluate the potential resectability before any biliary instrumentation.

OPERATIVE TECHNIQUE

Laparoscopy

The first goal of the operation conduct is to assess resectability. Despite modern imaging modalities, only about 30–50% of patients submitted to surgery for curative intent have tumor that is resectable with negative margins (8). Fifteen to 25% of patients may have unrecognized peritoneal and regional (N2) disease. The remainder may have advanced hilar disease that precludes resection. Routine and systemic diagnostic laparoscopic exploration for peritoneal and regional lymph nodes (N2) may avoid unnecessary laparotomy. However, advanced hepatic hilar disease cannot be accurately accessed via laparoscopy.

Laparotomy

Exposure, Mobilization, and Assessment

A bilateral subcostal incision (chevron) allows wide exposure. If liver resection is included in the operation,

a midline extension should be performed in most cases to facilitate control of the inferior vena cava–hepatic vein junction. All the congenital perihepatic adhesions, which include flaciform ligament, ligamentum teres, coronary ligament, triangular ligaments, and the gastrohepatic ligament, are divided (if liver resection is not planned, the coronary ligament and triangular ligaments do not have to be taken down.) This is followed by assessment of the hepatic hilus (m). The goals are to assess the ductal extension into the contralateral bile duct pedicle and vascular involvement. This is achieved by having full control of the portal hepatis by incising the pars flaccida and gaining access into the foramen of Winslow. The primary HC is then palpated at the confluence of the bile ducts and traced toward the left and right hepatic ducts. This tactile information will provide the surgeon with a sense of tumor extension. The hilar plate is lowered by incising the fibrofatty tissue at the base of segment 4. This allows access to the left bile duct and is a critical move for assessment of tumor extension (8). Sclerosing HC is often associated with periportal fibrosis and ductal thickening; therefore, in

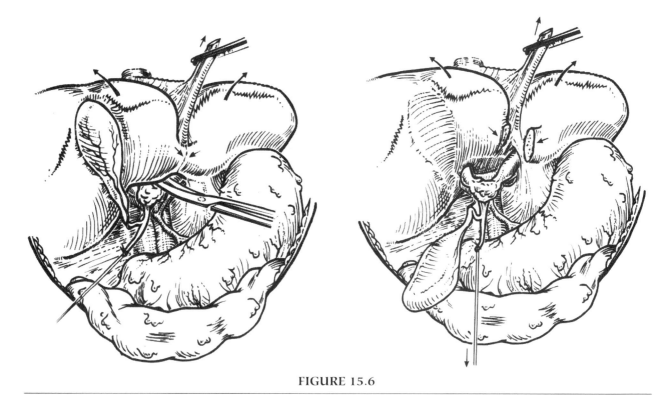

FIGURE 15.6

(A) Dissection to expose structures at the hilus of the liver. The ligamentum teres is elevated, and the liver is turned upward. Dissection at the base of the quadrate lobe (scissors) lowers the hilar plate. The bridge of the liver tissue connecting segments III and IV is still intact (arrows). The common bile duct is divided immediately above the duodenum, and its lower end has been separated from the underlying portal vein and hepatic artery and elevated together with associated connective tissue and lymph nodes. (B) The bridge of liver tissue at the base of the umbilical fissure has been divided (arrows). This is readily accomplished by dividing it with diathermy. The gallbladder has been mobilized together with the common bile duct. The biliary confluence and left hepatic duct together with the tumor have been lowered from beneath the quadrate lobe, which is facilitated by lowering the hilar plate.

this type of tumor, one may underestimate the actual proximal extent of tumor. However, if the patient has had longstanding obstruction and or cholangitis, the hilum can be very fibrotic due to the inflammatory reaction, rather than tumor involvement. It is therefore critical to perform intraoperative biopsies of the suspicious tissue for histologic evaluation in order to appropriately assess resectability. In addition, the left hepatic duct is longer, more extrahepatic, and has more angulation compared to the right hepatic duct, leading to a more challenging assessment of the right ductal extension. The hilar plate is lowered to assess the ductal extension (Figure 15.6A). Excising the bridge of liver tissue between segments III and IVa will allow better exposure of the base of the umbilical fissure and, therefore, the left hepatic pedicles (Figure 15.6B). The gallbladder is taken down, still allowing the cystic duct to remain attached to the common hepatic duct. Mobilization of the ductal system allows identification of the hepatic artery and portal vein, which then allows assessment of tumor involvement (Figure 15.7). Lack of vascular involvement by the tumor allows biliary and hepatic resection to proceed as appropriate.

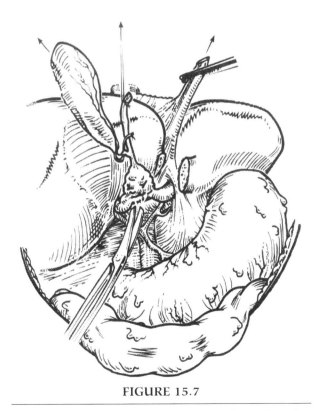

FIGURE 15.7

The entire extrahepatic biliary apparatus is elevated together with associated portal connective tissue and nodes to allow dissection anterior to the bifurcation of the portal vein and elevation of the tumor, which is now completely mobilized. The hepatic artery and portal vein are skeletonized.

In selected cases, vascular reconstruction may be indicated only if there is no regional disease (N2), because proven nodal involvement may preclude potentially curative resection. Reconstruction of portal vein almost always requires autologous venous graft despite full mobilization of the main portal vein. Reconstruction of the left portal vein can sometimes be done with primary end-to-end anastomosis due to the angulation and the extrahepatic length of the left portal vein. Once the tumor is deemed resectable, the retrohepatic inferior vena cava is mobilized off of the posterior aspect of the liver to the degree that is needed to obtain adequate resection margins of the tumor, and the respective hepatic veins are dissected and controlled (this is not needed unless parenchymal resection is required to encompass the tumor).

Dissection of Bile Duct, Hepatic Artery, and Portal Vein

Kocherization of the duodenum is performed in order to obtain the posterior pancreaticoduodenal lymph node as part of the regional lymphadenectomy. The most distal bile duct is then transected, and negative distal bile margin is confirmed on frozen section. The dissection of porta hepatis lymph nodes should be left intact with the bile duct. Therefore, dissection is performed close to the adventitia of the hepatic artery and portal vein. Ideally, one starts on the anterior wall of these vascular structures and works circumferentially. If vascular encasement of tumor is suspected, frozen sections of the fibrous tissue surrounding the vasculature should be sent to for histologic evaluation to determine the degree (or not) of tumor involvement. The lobar bile duct above the tumor draining the planned hepatic remnant is then transected, leaving behind adequate length for hepaticojejunostomy. A negative proximal bile duct margin must be confirmed by frozen section histology. The vascular inflow and outflow to and from the hepatic lobe to be removed is then divided. The respective hepatic artery should be doubly ligated with suture. The respective portal vein and hepatic vein(s) can be ligated and divided and then oversewn with prolene-type vascular suture. Use of the endo-GI vascular load stapler is another very effective way to ligate and divide the appropriate portal vein and hepatic vein branch(es) (tributary(ies)).

Hepatic Parenchyma Transection

The hepatic parenchyma is then transected by the preferred method of the surgeon. Each method has its advantages and disadvantages. Regardless, bile ducts or blood vessels more than 2–3 mm in size should be ligated with suture, clips, staple device, or suture. Of note, en bloc hepatic lobar and caudate resection should be performed in many HCs to achieve adequate tumor clearance. This form of hepatic resection addresses the longitudinal extension of HC along the intrahepatic ducts and radially into the hepatic parenchyma and, therefore, increases the ability to achieve a tumor-free margin (3, 5, 6, 11, 20). If intra-operatively there is a suspicion for gross tumor involvement at the hepatic transection margin, the transection plan should be extended to achieve an R0 resection. The margin of resection should never risk damage to the major hepatic vasculature. In addtion, the inflow and outflow vascular structures to the remnant liver must be carefully protected.

Reconstruction

A 60-cm (±20 cm) Roux-en-Y limb is then brought up to the portal hepatis to allow a tension-free hepatico-jejunostomy to restore enterohepatic circulation (Figure 15.8).

OUTCOMES

The overall perioperative morbidity rate ranges from 30 to 60%, and the mortality rate ranges from 5 to 17% (6–11, 26–28). Major morbidities include hyper-bilirubinemia, bleeding, bile leaks, anastomosis break-down, infection, and hepatic insufficiency. As the operative technique has evolved, incorporating vascular resection into the surgical management of HC is becoming more prevalent. Overall, approximately 50% of patients who are deemed intraoperatively to have tumor infiltration into the vasculature have histologic evidence of tumor invasion beyond the adventitia. In selected patients and centers, portal vein resection alone seems to offer a survival benefit when the tumor involves the portal vein, without increasing operative risk (9). In contrast, there is no survival benefit in patients who have undergone hepatic artery resection (26). In the face of a significantly higher adverse peri-operative outcome, the practice of hepatic artery resection in the management of HC is, therefore, currently unjustified.

The independent prognostic factors for long-term survival include resection with negative margins (R0) and an early pathologic stage by histologic evaluation (6–11). The recent trend of advocating a more aggressive surgical intervention that incorporates partial hepatic resection has increased the number of patients with negative surgical margins. This has been translated into a parallel increase in the 5-year survival rate to approximately 25–50% (7, 11, 26). Adjuvant chemora-diatherapy may improve local control. However, the

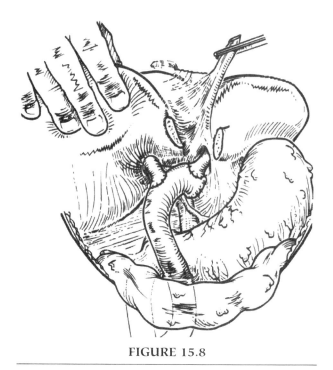

FIGURE 15.8

The exposed right and left hepatic ducts are anastomosed using a single layer of 3-0 absorbable suture to a 70-cm retrocolic Roux-en-Y loop of jejunum. If there are multiple ducts exposed at the hilus, these may be approximated one to another, if possible. All exposed ducts must be included in the anastomosis.

disease recurrence is not uncommon despite an R0 resection. Approximately, one third of patients will have the local tumor recurrence and two thirds will have distance recurrence. The next major improvement in survival in patients with HC is not likely to be derived from advancements through more aggressive and sophisticated surgical techniques. Rather, research in this area should be focused on chemoprevention and early disease detection in patients who are at risk. The development of next-generation adjuvant chemoradio-therapy will be paramount in improving the outcomes of patients with hilar cholangiocarcinoma.

References

1. Landis SH, Murray T, Bolden S, Wingo PA. Cancer statistics, 1999. CA Cancer J Clin 1999: 49(1):8–31.
2. Bismuth H, Nakache R, Diamond T. Management strategies in resection for hilar cholangiocarcinoma. Ann Surg 1992: 215(1):31–38.
3. Jarnagin WR, Burke E, Powers C, Fong Y, Blumgart LH. Intra-hepatic biliary enteric bypass provides effective palliation in selected patients with malignant obstruction at the hepatic duct confluence. Am J Surg 1998; 175(6):453–460.
4. Nordback IH, Pitt HA, Coleman J, et al. Unresectable hilar cholangiocarcinoma: percutaneous versus operative palliation. Surgery 1994; 115(5):597–603.
5. Stain SC, Baer HU, Dennison AR, Blumgart LH. Current management of hilar cholangiocarcinoma. Surg Gynecol Obstet 1992; 175(6):579–588.

6. Washburn WK, Lewis WD, Jenkins RL.Aggressive surgical resection for cholangiocarcinoma. Arch Surg 1995: 130(3):270–276.

7. Hidalgo E, Asthana S, Nishio H, et al. Surgery for hilar cholangiocarcinoma: The Leeds experience. Eur J Surg Oncol 2007; Nov 22; epub.

8. Jarnagin WR, Fong Y, DeMatteo RP, et al. Staging, resectability, and outcome in 225 patients with hilar cholangiocarcinoma. Ann Surg 2001; 234(4):507–517; discussion 517–519.

9. Hemming AW, Kim RD, Mekeel KL, et al. Portal vein resection for hilar cholangiocarcinoma. Am Surg 2006; 72 (7):599–604; discussion 604–605.

10. Nakeeb A, Pitt HA, Sohn TA, et al. Cholangiocarcinoma. A spectrum of intrahepatic, perihilar, and distal tumors. Ann Surg 1996; 224(4):463–473; discussion 473–475.

11. Kosuge T, Yamamoto J, Shimada K, Yamasaki S, Makuuchi M. Improved surgical results for hilar cholangiocarcinoma with procedures including major hepatic resection. Ann Surg 1999; 230(5):663–671.

12. Witzigmann H, Berr F, Ringel U, et al. Surgical and palliative management and outcome in 184 patients with hilar cholangiocarcinoma: palliative photodynamic therapy plus stenting is comparable to r1/r2 resection. Ann Surg 2006; 244(2):230–239.

13. Simmons DT, Baron TH, Petersen BT, et al. A novel endoscopic approach to brachytherapy in the management of hilar cholangiocarcinoma. Am J Gastroenterol 2006; 101(8):1792–1796.

14. Kuvshinoff BW, Armstrong JG, Fong Y, et al. Palliation of irresectable hilar cholangiocarcinoma with biliary drainage and radiotherapy.Br J Surg 1995; 82(11):1522–1525.

15. Benjamin IS, McPherson GA, Blumgart LH. Iridium-192 wire for hilar cholangiocarcinoma. Lancet 1981; 2(8246):582–583

16. Gerhards MF, van Gulik TM, González González D, Rauws EA, Gouma DJ. Results of postoperative radiotherapy for resectable hilar cholangiocarcinoma. World J Surg 2003; 27(2):173–179.

17. Rea DJ, Heimbach JK, Rosen CB, et al. Liver transplantation with neoadjuvant chemoradiation is more effective than resection for hilar cholangiocarcinoma. Ann Surg 2005; 242(3): 451–458; discussion 458–461.

18. de Groen PC, Gores GJ, LaRusso NF, Gunderson LL, Nagorney DM. Biliary tract cancers.N Engl J Med 1999; 341(18): 1368–1378.

19. Sakamoto E, Nimura Y, Hayakawa N, et al. The pattern of infiltration at the proximal border of hilar bile duct carcinoma: a histologic analysis of 62 resected cases. Ann Surg 1998; 227(3):405–411.

20. Burke EC, Jarnagin WR, Hochwald SN, Pisters PW, Fong Y, Blumgart LH. Hilar cholangiocarcinoma: patterns of spread, the importance of hepatic resection for curative operation, and a presurgical clinical staging system. Ann Surg 1998; 228(3): 385–394.

21. Fleming ID, Copper JS, Henson DE. AJCC Cancer Staging Manual. 6th ed. New York: Springer-Verlag, 2002.

22. Maguchi H, Takahashi K, Katanuma A, et al. Preoperative biliary drainage for hilar cholangiocarcinoma. J Hepatobiliary Pancreat Surg 2007; 14(5):441–446.

23. Nimura Y, Kamiya J, Kondo S, Nagino M, Uesaka K, Oda K, Sano T, Yamamoto H, Hayakawa N. Aggressive preoperative management and extended surgery for hilar cholangiocarcinoma: Nagoya experience. J Hepatobiliary Pancreat Surg 2000; 7(2):155–162.

24. Takada T. Is preoperative biliary drainage necessary according to evidence-based medicine? J Hepatobiliary Pancreat Surg 2001; 8(1):58–64.

25. Hochwald SN, Burke EC, Jarnagin WR, Fong Y, Blumgart LH. Association of preoperative biliary stenting with increased postoperative infectious complications in proximal cholangiocarcinoma. Arch Surg 1999; 134(3):261–266.

26. Klempnauer J, Ridder GJ, von Wasielewski R, Werner M, Weimann A, Pichlmayr R. Resectional surgery of hilar cholangiocarcinoma: a multivariate analysis of prognostic factors. J Clin Oncol 1997; 15(3):947–954

27. Gazzaniga GM, Filauro M, Bagarolo C, Mori L. Surgery for hilar cholangiocarcinoma: an Italian experience. J Hepatobiliary Pancreat Surg 2000; 7 (2):122–127.

28. Nishio H, Kamiya J, Nagino M, Kanai M, Uesaka K, Sakamoto E, Fukatsu T, Nimura Y. Value of percutaneous transhepatic portography before hepatectomy for hilar cholangiocarcinoma. Br J Surg 1999; 86(11):1415–1421.

29. Nagino M, Kamiya J, Nishio H, Ebata T, Arai T, Nimura Y. Two hundred forty consecutive portal vein embolizations before extended hepatectomy for biliary cancer: surgical outcome and long-term follow-up.Ann Surg 2006; 243(3):364–372.

16 Surgical Management of Gallbladder Cancer

Rebecca J. McClaine
Syed A. Ahmad
Andrew M. Lowy

In the United States, gallbladder cancer is a relatively rare disease, with an incidence of 1.2 cases per 100,000, and 2418 new cases reported to the National Cancer Data Base in 2004 (1). It is estimated that approximately 4600 new cases will be diagnosed in 2007, with over 1600 deaths (2). However, it is the most common of the biliary tract cancers, and the sixth most common gastrointestinal tumor. Approximately 1–2% of all gallbladder specimens contain carcinoma (3). Within the U.S. population, Hispanics, Native Americans, and Asian-Pacific Islanders experience significantly higher rates of gallbladder cancer compared to Caucasians (3). Worldwide, the highest rates of gallbladder cancer occur in the Native American populations of North, Central, and South America. The next highest rates are found in Eastern European countries, northern India, and Japan (4). Incidence peaks at age 50–60 years. Unlike other biliary cancers, women are affected two to three times more often than men (3).

ETIOLOGY

Personal history of gallstone disease is the most common risk factor for development of gallbladder cancer and is present in 75–92% of cases (4). The epidemiologic patterns described for gallbladder cancer directly mirror the incidence of cholelithiasis worldwide.

Patients with large stones (>3 cm) are at 10 times the risk of cancer development than those with small stones (<1 cm). Obesity and multiparity, known risk factors for cholelithiasis, are also strongly associated with gallbladder cancer. In Japan, where males and females are affected at similar rates, many cases of gallbladder cancer are associated with anomalous pancreaticobiliary junction, which leads to reflux of pancreatic enzymes into the biliary tree and gallbladder with subsequent inflammation (4). Gallbladder cancer is also associated with chronic cholecystitis, porcelain gallbladder, as diagnosed by plain film (cancer rates of 10–25%), and chronic infection with *Salmonella typhi* and *Helicobacter pylori* (4). Other associated conditions may include cholecystoenteric fistulas, exposure to chemical carcinogens, inflammatory bowel disease, and Mirrizi syndrome (4).

PATHOLOGY

The gallbladder wall is composed of five histologic layers: (a) mucosa composed of tall columnar epithelium, (b) lamina propria, (c) muscle layer with loosely organized longitudinal and circular fibers, (d) subserosa containing connective tissue, nerves, and lymphatics, and (e) serosa, except where the gallbladder is embedded in the liver. Mucus is normally secreted only by tubuloalveolar glands in the infundibulum and neck of the gland. Adenocarcinoma represents 90% of all gall-bladder malignancies. Histologically, these are divided into papillary and tubular subtypes, based upon the pattern of growth. Papillary tumors tend to grow intra-luminally and spread intraductally, with a somewhat more favorable prognosis. Both types contain mucin-producing, signet-ring cells (5). Most cases of gall-bladder cancer arise from areas of metaplasia, which is seen in about 50% of chronic cholecystitis specimens. Pathologic specimens of cancer typically contain areas of metaplasia in an intestinal or gastric pattern, dys-plasia, and carcinoma-in-situ in addition to invasive carcinoma, suggesting a stepwise progression to malig-nancy, which is estimated to occur over 10 years after the development of dysplasia. Approximately 3% of gallbladder adenocarcinomas arise from large adeno-mas that undergo malignant transformation (6). Muta-tions and abnormal expression of multiple genes, including tumor suppressor gene p53, cell cycle regu-lator cyclin E, apoptosis regulator Bcl-2, and ras onco-genes, have all been associated with the development of gallbladder cancer (5).

In general, gallbladder cancers are aggressive and tend to spread locally and via the lymphatics early in the disease process. Invasion of liver segments IVb and V occurs by direct extension; metastases to all liver lobes can occur via draining veins. In the lymphatic sys-tem, tumor cells typically spread first via the hepato-duodenal ligament to the cystic, pericholedochal, and hilar nodes (7). Second echelon nodes include retropan-creatic nodes (right-sided drainage), celiac nodes (left-sided drainage), and superior mesenteric nodes (central drainage via the mesentery) (8).Tumor cells often metastasize first to peritoneal surfaces; the most com-mon site of extra-abdominal metastasis is the lung.

Adenosquamous/squamous cell carcinoma of the gallbladder accounts for 1–10% of cases of gallbladder cancer. Compared to adenocarcinoma, this tumor is associated with more direct liver invasion and less lymph node metastasis, but is similar in terms of prog-nosis and treatment (9). Primary gallbladder carcinoid is very rare, representing 1% of carcinoid tumors, and can be difficult to distinguish from adenocarcinoma his-tologically (10). The most common metastatic lesion to the gallbladder (50–60% of cases) is malignant melanoma. While less than 5% of malignant melanoma patients present with symptomatic gallbladder disease, 15% have gallbladder involvement at autopsy (11).

STAGING

The AJCC staging system is utilized for gallbladder car-cinoma. The T stage is based upon depth of invasion. The staging system was last updated in 2002 and

TABLE 16.1

American Joint Commission on Cancer Staging System for Gallbladder Carcinoma

PRIMARY TUMOR (T)

TX	Primary tumor cannot be assessed
T0	No evidence of primary tumor
Tis	Carcinoma in situ
T1a	Tumor invades lamina propria
T1b	Tumor invades muscle layer
T2	Tumor invades perimuscular connective tissue
T3	Tumor perforates serosa and/or directly invades the liver and/or one other adjacent organ or structure
T4	Tumor invades main portal vein or hepatic artery or invades multiple extrahepatic organs or structures

REGIONAL LYMPH NODES (N)

NX	Lymph nodes cannot be assessed
N0	No regional lymph node metastasis
N1	Regional lymph node metastasis

DISTANT METASTASIS (M)

MX	Distant metastasis cannot be assessed
M0	No distant metastasis
M1	Distant metastasis

STAGES

Stage 0	Tis	N0	M0
Stage IA	T1	N0	M0
Stage IB	T2	N0	M0
Stage IIA	T3	N0	M0
Stage IIB	T1–T3	N1	M0
Stage III	T4	Any N	M0
Stage IV	Any T	Any N	M1

Source: Adapted from Ref. 16.

reflected changes based upon disease resectability, omit-ting depth of liver invasion to distinguish T3 from T4 tumors (Table 16.1).

CLINICAL PRESENTATION AND EVALUATION

Gallbladder cancer is typically diagnosed in one of two scenarios, as demonstrated by a bimodal pattern of pre-senting stage (Table 16.2). Most cancers are diagnosed either incidentally, during routine pathologic examina-tion of gallbladders removed for benign indications, or in advanced stages, after more troubling symptoms

TABLE 16.2
Gallbladder Cancer Stage at Diagnosis

STAGE	% OF TOTAL DIAGNOSES
0	4.5
I	20.2
II	24.2
III	3.8
IV	31.1
Unknown	16.1

Source: Adapted from Ref. 1.

have appeared. Less than 10% of gallbladder cancers are diagnosed prior to an operative intervention. In the early stages of gallbladder cancer, symptoms mimic those of cholecystitis and include right upper quadrant pain, nausea, vomiting, and anorexia. In advanced stages, jaundice and weight loss may also occur, and physical exam may reveal a palpable distended gallbladder with hepatomegaly.

To date, no laboratory studies have been found to consistently correlate with the presence of gallbladder carcinoma. Liver function tests may reveal an obstructive pattern (elevated bilirubin and alkaline phosphatase) when the tumor mass interferes with normal biliary drainage. In one study analyzing blood samples from patients with known gallbladder cancer, carbohydrate antigen 19-9 (CA 19-9) >20 units/ml was found to have a sensitivity and specificity of 79% in distinguishing carcinoma from benign gallbladder disease. Carcinoembryonic antigen (CEA) >4 ng/ml yielded a sensitivity of 50% and specificity of 93% in the same study. Utilization of CA 19-9 and CEA in combination did not improve diagnostic accuracy (12). Recently, a similar study demonstrated cancer antigen 125 (CA 125) >11 units/ml to differentiate gallbladder cancer from both benign disease and normal controls with 64% sensitivity and 90% specificity (13).

Routine radiographic studies have proven to be largely unreliable in the diagnosis of early gallbladder cancer. The most common imaging modality to evaluate cholelithiasis symptoms continues to be right upper quadrant ultrasound. While this modality provides accurate diagnoses of acute cholecystitis and cholelithiasis, it is difficult to differentiate these benign processes from early malignant disease. Early cancers are associated with some characteristic ultrasound findings: irregularly shaped hypo- or isoechogenic intraluminal masses with or without entrapped gallstones (40–65% of tumors), irregular wall thickening >1 cm diameter, less echogenic than that seen with chronic cholecystitis (20–30% of tumors), or intraluminal polyps >10 mm in diameter (15–25% of tumors). Polyps can represent both malig-

nant and benign disease processes (cholesterol polyp, adenomyomatosis) and are therefore nondiagnostic for cancer. In all, routine right upper quadrant ultrasound has a sensitivity of only about 30% in diagnosing early gallbladder cancer. Routine abdominal computed topography (CT) and magnetic resonance imaging (MRI) reveal similar findings and provide similar sensitivities to ultrasound in the diagnosis of early disease. Ultrasound with color Doppler capabilities, which demonstrates high blood flow in malignant lesions, may help to improve the diagnostic sensitivity of ultrasound, but is not yet widely used. Likewise, fluorodeoxyglucose positron emission tomography (FDG-PET) demonstrates increased uptake in malignant versus benign lesions. However, false-negative results are generated by lesions <0.5–1 cm in diameter, and benign processes such as adenomyomatosis and xanthogranulomatous cholecystitis may generate false positives. More studies are needed to validate the utility of these modalities in diagnosing early gallbladder cancer (14).

Advanced gallbladder cancer is diagnosed easily by standard imaging modalities, and radiographic staging is paramount in determining the appropriate treatment course. Right upper quadrant ultrasound has a sensitivity of 85% in diagnosing locally invasive cancer, which appears as an irregular hypo- to isoechogenic mass obscuring the gallbladder–liver border. Ultrasound may also reveal lymphadenopathy, invasion of the hepatic pedicle, invasion of extrahepatic structures, and peritoneal metastases, but with sensitivity of only 30–40%, necessitating further radiographic evaluation when these findings are not visualized. Helical (thin-cut) CT with contrast is superior to ultrasonography at determining depth of hepatic invasion and involvement of the hepatic portal structures, with sensitivities of 86 and 93%, respectively. Finally, a few limited studies evaluating FDG-PET suggest that this modality may be helpful in assessing peritoneal and distant metastases; its role in determining lymph node involvement has not been assessed (14).

SURGICAL THERAPY

The goal of surgical therapy in gallbladder cancer is complete, microscopic margin-negative resection (R0) of the tumor mass. This point bears emphasis as in a 20-year series at one North American medical center, no patient survived 5 years after R1 resection, and incomplete (R2) resection confers no survival advantage as documented in multiple studies (7). Selection of the appropriate operation is dictated by the stage of disease and timing of diagnosis.

A large proportion of gallbladder cancers are diagnosed incidentally at pathologic examination following a cholecystectomy that has been performed for benign indications. In this situation, a large number of tumors (81% in one recent series) are Stage I or II (15). For tumors confined to the mucosa (Tis, T1a), if the cystic duct margin is free of tumor, no further surgical intervention is required and 5-year survival approaches 100%. In a Japanese retrospective review, no survival advantage was conferred to patients undergoing more radical resection following the initial cholecystectomy for this stage of cancer (7). In this group, survival is significantly decreased in patients who demonstrate recurrence of disease at the incision site and in whom bile spillage occurs. Incision site recurrence likely occurs both by spillage of cancer cells during removal of the specimen through the wound and because of the predilection of cancer cells for healing wounds, rich in growth factors (7, 8). In patients with unsuspected gallbladder cancer, port site recurrence has been reported in 10–29% of cases of laparoscopic cholecystectomy; wound recurrence has been reported in 0–31% of cases of open cholecystectomy. Several retrospective reviews have compared laparoscopic and open approaches, with mixed results in terms of both incision-site recurrence and survival (8). However, a single prospective trial demonstrated no difference in incision-site recurrence or survival between the two approaches (7). Bile spillage, which occurs in 14–44% of routine laparoscopic cholecystectomies, has been associated with poorer survival in early-stage gallbladder cancer in multiple trials and likely contributes to incision-site recurrences in both types of procedures (7, 8). In all patients undergoing laparoscopic cholecystectomy, the potential presence of gallbladder cancer, though remote, should be considered. Several surgical techniques could be employed to reduce the intraperitoneal or incision-site spread of any potential malignancy: securing trocars to the abdominal wall, preventing gas and fluid leakage through the incision sites, careful handling of the specimen to avoid bile spillage, placing the specimen in an isolating bag prior to removal, minimizing trauma to the abdominal wall, and closing the peritoneum (7).

In some situations, gallbladder cancer is diagnosed intraoperatively, either by frozen section examination or by gross appearance of tumor, even when it was not suspected preoperatively. In such instances, precautions to limit intraperitoneal spread of cancer cells should be undertaken and conversion to open cholecystectomy strongly considered. Furthermore, R0 resection of the tumor should be attempted at the initial operation. In circumstances where the operating surgeon has limited experience with oncologic resection of the gallbladder, the operation should be terminated. Two recent retrospective reviews found that patients experience no worse outcomes when the initial operation is termi-

nated and complete resection performed during a second (staged) procedure. In one study, 39 patients underwent surgery with curative intention—6 initially and 33 during a staged procedure—with no difference in survival (15). Likewise, neither the surgical approach (laparoscopic versus open) nor the time to second operation had any effect on survival (8). Again, these results support referral to a hepatobiliary surgeon for staged resection when the initial surgeon is inexperienced in such procedures (15).

For the remainder of patients in whom gallbladder cancer is diagnosed preoperatively, extent of resection is dependent upon the depth of tumor invasion and stage of disease. When malignancy is suspected, an open procedure should be performed, preceded by a diagnostic laparoscopy to rule out occult metastatic disease to the liver and peritoneum (7). In two prospective series, this procedure prevented nontherapeutic laparotomy in 33–55% of patients with metastatic disease and was more sensitive than abdominal CT in detecting peritoneal metastases (16). If the laparoscopy is negative, attempt at curative resection is undertaken. Staged resections, following previous laparoscopic cholecystectomy, may be accompanied by resection of port-site tissue; the advantage of this procedure has not been studied (7). The role of lymphadenectomy in curative resections for advanced gallbladder cancer should be emphasized. Overall, the most important predictor of survival is lymph node involvement, suggesting that all curative operations must include lymphadenectomy to achieve accurate pathologic staging and to maximize the therapeutic benefit. In one series, R0 resection was possible in 45% of patients with Stage III disease; 15% of node-positive patients were surgically cured, compared to 81% with node-negative disease. This again emphasizes the importance of lymph node status as a prognostic factor as well as the fact that, although rare, some patients with nodal metastases can be salvaged by radical surgery. (7). Five-year survival rates as high as 31% have been reported for node-positive disease following resection with lymphadenectomy (15). Despite the potential benefits of lymphadenectomy, most studies have found especially dismal prognosis for disease involving nodes beyond the hepatoduodenal ligament (8).

The treatment of Stage IA disease, with tumors extending into the muscle layer (T1b), remains controversial. These tumors are associated with relatively high rates of lymph node involvement (16–20%), local invasion (13–28%), and recurrence after simple cholecystectomy (50–60%), suggesting that cholecystectomy alone is not sufficient treatment (8). Extended cholecystectomy consists of wedge resection or complete resection (central hepatectomy) of liver segments IVb and V (those adjacent to the gallbladder) and removal of the nodes in the hepatoduodenal ligament (cystic, pericholedochal, hilar). In some centers, additional nodes anterior and posterior to the pancreatic head, and those surrounding the hepatic artery up to its origin at the celiac axis, are also resected (8). In Stage I disease, resection of the extrahepatic bile duct confers no survival advantage and should be performed only to facilitate removal of the hepatoduodenal nodes (8, 15). A few retrospective reviews have failed to demonstrate any survival difference in patients undergoing simple versus extended cholecystectomy for this stage of disease (7). To date, no prospective evidence exists to guide treatment decisions, and surgical therapy for T1b tumors tends to be center-dependent. Stage IB disease, with tumor invasion of the perimuscular connective tissue (T2), is associated with even higher rates of lymph node involvement and recurrence, and several studies have demonstrated significantly improved survival after extended versus simple cholecystectomy (8). In a recent retrospective review of 410 patients at Memorial Sloan-Kettering, 5-year survival was 61 and 19% following radical resection and simple cholecystectomy, respectively, for T2 tumors (17). The survival advantage conferred by extensive resection is explained by the predilection of this tumor to spread via the lymphatics; one series documented positive nodes in 46% of patients with T2 tumors (15).

For Stage II disease (tumor invasion into the liver, T3, in most cases), extended resection results in improved outcomes when compared to simple cholecystectomy alone. In recent series, 5-year survival following extended resections has ranged from 49 to 59%, compared to 0% in patients undergoing simple cholecystectomy (8, 15). The extent of hepatic resection is controversial. Most authors suggest at least central hepatectomy (full resection of segments IVb and V). Others suggest central trisegmentectomy (resection of segments IV, V, and VIII) with or without caudate resection, or extended right hepatectomy (resection of segments IV, V, VI, VII, and VIII) (8). As with Stage I disease, lymphadenectomy of the hepatoduodenal ligament, at a minimum, should be performed. Some groups employ extended lymphadenectomy, removing celiac, superior mesenteric, and para-aortic lymph nodes as well, though there are inadequate data to evaluate any therapeutic benefit to this practice (8). Extrahepatic bile duct resection for Stage II disease has not been shown to improve survival (8, 15). Gross involvement of the hepatoduodenal ligament usually renders a tumor noncurable due to the high likelihood of microscopic invasion of the periductal soft tissues and/or vascular structures. Bile duct involvement significantly reduces the incidence of R0 resection due to perineural invasion within the hepatoduodenal ligament, resulting in a positive connective tissue margin; in one series,

<30% of resections of these tumors could be resected with tumor-free margins. In two Japanese studies of "advanced gallbladder cancer," which included T3 and T4 tumor involvement, hepatoduodenal ligament involvement was found to occur in 54–60% of patients, even though relatively few (18%) had jaundice. These data suggest that routine extrahepatic bile duct resection for Stage II disease may improve staging, but not survival (8).

Curative surgical therapy for Stage III disease, with T4 tumors involving the main portal vein, hepatic artery, or multiple extrahepatic structures, is rarely possible. Portal vein resection and reconstruction must be performed in most cases as part of an R0 resection; while this has been achieved, it is associated with a significantly increased operative mortality rate (8). In a retrospective review from one North American center, extended resection of Stage III disease conferred no survival advantage. However, the operations performed were limited to extended liver resections with lymphadenectomy, with or without extrahepatic bile duct resections (i.e., no portal vein reconstructions or pancreaticoduodenectomies occurred) (15). Japanese surgeons have approached advanced disease more aggressively. One small retrospective review concluded that portal vein resection did not improve survival in patients with T4 tumors (8). In Japan, hepatopancreaticoduodenectomy has been performed to achieve R0 resections of tumors involving the distal bile duct, pancreatic head, or duodenum, with mixed results. In the largest series of 24 patients, median survival was 12 months, and 20% of patients survived 2 years, but these operations were associated with profound morbidity and a 12% mortality rate. Hepatic failure contributed to most instances of morbidity and mortality (8). In general, aggressive operations for Stage III gallbladder cancer should be attempted only when R0 operations can be achieved, in patients with optimal preoperative health status. Stage IV disease, with distant hematogenous or lymphatic metastases, peritoneal seeding, or gross involvement of major vascular structures (celiac or superior mesenteric arteries, vena cava, and aorta), is an absolute contraindication to resection.

NONOPERATIVE THERAPY

Because of the relative rarity of gallbladder cancer, trials assessing the activity of chemoradiotherapy regimens against this tumor have been limited. To date, no chemotherapy or chemoradiotherapy regimen has been shown to improve survival in patients with gallbladder cancer, and surgical resection remains the only option for cure (5). In the 1980s and 1990s, 5-fluorouracil (5-FU) served as the basis of several trials, alone and in combination with other agents, with response rates of 12–30% and average response duration of 3–6 months. (18) More recently, response rates of 36–60% have been reported with gemcitabine in trials of patients with both gallbladder and other biliary tract cancers (18). Gemcitabine used in combination with cisplatin and capecitabine, an oral 5-FU analogue, have demonstrated even higher response rates (53–64%) (18). Because gallbladder cancer often spreads and recurs locally, several trials have also examined the role of radiation, typically with 5-FU as a chemotherapeutic sensitizer. In one study, 5-FU and radiation administered preoperatively did allow several patients with initially unresectable tumors to undergo resection, but in the end conferred no survival advantage over patients undergoing surgical resection primarily (no data was provided comparing these patients to those with initially unresectable tumors not undergoing resection). In two small studies, adjuvant use of 5-FU with radiation was found to confer a survival advantage over patients who underwent surgical resection alone; however, the sample sizes were too small to determine statistical significance (18). Future studies will likely elucidate the survival advantage (if any) of newer chemoradiotherapy regimens, clarify the different responses of gallbladder versus other biliary tumors, and focus on molecular tumor characteristics as therapeutic targets (5).

PROGNOSIS

The prognosis for patients diagnosed with gallbladder cancer remains poor (Table 16.3). An observational study of 724 patients performed in 1994 revealed a median survival of 3 months, with 5-year survival of 5%. However, more aggressive surgical therapy has recently yielded better results, with 5-year survival rates in the range of 35% following aggressive resections (15). Further advances in both hepatobiliary surgery and molecular chemotherapy will hopefully translate into improved outcomes for this aggressive malignancy.

TABLE 16.3
Gallbladder Cancer Survival by Stage

STAGE	1-YEAR	2-YEAR	3-YEAR	4-YEAR	5-YEAR
0	87	81	81	81	81
IA	77	66	59	54	50
IB	65	45	36	32	29
IIA	37	19	11	9	7
IIB	42	21	13	10	9
III	17	6	4	3	3
IV	11	4	2	2	2

Source: Adapted from Ref. 19.

References

1. National Cancer Data Base. Site by stage distribution of cases reported to the NCDB: Diagnosis year 2004. American College of Surgeons, June 16. 2007.https://web.facs.org/ncdbr/help/BMarks/Compare/Ver8/site_stage_2004.htm
2. Detailed guide: gallbladder cancer. What are the key statistics about gallbladder cancer? American Cancer Society, July 29, 2007. http://www.cancer.org/docroot/CRI/content/CRI_2_4_1X+_What_are_the_key_statistics_for_gall_bladder_cancer_68.asp?rnav=cri
3. Goodman MT, Yamamoto J. Descriptive study of gallbladder, extrahepatic bile duct, and ampullary cancers in the United States, 1997-2002. Cancer Causes Control 2007; 18(4): 415–422.
4. Randi G, Franceschi S, La Vecchia C. Gallbladder cancer worldwide: geographical distribution and risk factors. Int J Cancer 2006; 118(7):1591–1602.
5. Thomas MB. Biological characteristics of cancers in the gallbladder and biliary tract and targeted therapy. Crit Rev Oncol Hematol 2007; 61(1):44–51.
6. Roa I, de Aretxabala X, Araya JC, Roa J. Preneoplastic lesions in gallbladder cancer. J Surg Oncol 2006; 93(8):615–623.
7. Steinert R, Nestler G, Sagynaliev E, Muller J, Lippert H, Reymond M. Laparoscopic cholecystectomy and gallbladder cancer. J Surg Oncol 2006; 93(8):682–689.
8. Sikora SS, Singh RK. Surgical strategies in patients with gallbladder cancer: nihilism to optimism. J Surg Oncol 2006; 93(8):670–681.
9. Chan KM, Yu MC, Lee WC, Jan YY, Chen MF. Adenosquamous / squamous cell carcinoma of the gallbladder. J Surg Oncol 2007; 95(2):129–134.
10. Anjaneyulu V, Shankar-Swarnalatha G, Rao SC. Carcinoid tumor of the gallbladder. Ann Diagn Pathol 2007;11(2): 113–116.
11. Katz SC, Bowne WB, Wolchok JD, Busam KJ, Jaques DP, Coit DG. Surgical management of melanoma of the gallbladder: a report of 13 cases and review of the literature. Am J Surg 2007; 193(4):493–497.
12. Strom BL, Maislin G, West SL, et al. Serum CEA and CA 19-9: potential future diagnostic or screening tests for gallbladder cancer? Int J Cancer 1990; 45(5):821–824.
13. Chaube A, Tewari M, Singh U, Shukla HS. CA 125: a potential tumor marker for gallbladder cancer. J Surg Oncol 2006; 93(8):665–669.
14. Rodriguez-Fernandez A, Gomez-Rio M, Medina-Benitez A, et al. Application of modern imaging methods in diagnosis of gallbladder cancer. J Surg Oncol 2006; 93(8):650–664.
15. Shih SP, Schulick RD, Cameron JL, et al. Gallbladder cancer: the role of laparoscopy and radical resection. Ann Surg 2007; 245(6):893–901.
16. Choi EA, Rodgers SE, Ahmad SA, Abdalla EK. Hepatobiliary cancers. In: Feig BW, Berger DH, Fuhrman GM (eds.), The M.D. Anderson Surgical Oncology Handbook. 4th ed. Philadelphia: Lippincott, Williams & Wilkins, 2006:320–366.
17. Fong Y, Jarnagin W, Blumgart LH. Gallbladder cancer: comparison of patients presenting initially for definitive operation with those presenting after prior noncurative intervention. Ann Surg 2000; 232(4):557–569.
18. de Aretxabala X, Roa I, Berrios M, et al. Chemoradiotherapy in gallbladder cancer. J Surg Oncol 2006; 93(8):699–704.
19. Fong Y, Wagman L, Gonen M, et al. Evidence-based gallbladder cancer staging: changing cancer staging by analysis of data from the national cancer database. Ann Surg 2006; 243(6): 767–774.

17 Systemic Therapy for Biliary Tract Cancer

Bassel F. El-Rayes
Philip A. Philip

Biliary cancers arise from the epithelial lining of the gall bladder or extrahepatic or intrahepatic bile ducts. The annual incidence of these tumors is estimated at 7800 cases in the United States (1). The majority of these patients present with advanced disease, which precludes surgical resection, the only potentially curative therapy (2–4). Furthermore, the risk of systemic recurrence in patients who undergo complete resection remains high (5). Therefore, improvements in the outcome of biliary tumors are dependent on the development of more effective systemic therapy.

In the past four decades, several chemotherapeutic agents ranging from fluoropyrimidines to targeted drugs have been evaluated in clinical trials in biliary cancers (Table 17.1). Unfortunately, the impact of available systemic therapy remains at best modest, and therefore there is no effective standard of care in biliary tumors. The challenges that face clinical trials in this disease are many. First, biliary tumors are relatively resistant to conventional cytotoxic drugs and generally have an aggressive biologic behavior. Second, the low incidence of the disease limits the ability to conduct prospective, multiarm randomized trials. The rarity of biliary cancers also contributes to the lack of interest in the pharmaceutical industry and cooperative groups to support trials in these cancers. Therefore, treatment recommendations for early and advanced-stage disease are based on relatively small phase II trials. Third, the majority of clinical trials have included patients with tumors in the gallbladder and intra- and extrahepatic cholangiocarcinoma despite the differences between these cancers with respect to clinical behavior and molecular pathology. With the advent of targeted agents, the differences in the molecular pathology of biliary tumors will necessitate a more selective approach to the design of clinical trials in this disease. Fourth, the evaluation of response to therapy in biliary tumors by conventional cross-sectional imaging is complicated by the infiltrative nature of the disease and the frequent peritoneal metastases. Therefore, the primary endpoints used in several trials have been progression-free survival or overall survival. The evaluation of these endpoints in phase II trials is complicated by selection bias and the inclusion of patients with different baseline characteristics with respect to stage of disease (locally advanced and metastatic) and prior treatment. Finally, the administration of effective systemic therapy to patients with biliary tumors is frequently complicated by liver dysfunction as a result of biliary obstruction.

SINGLE-AGENT CHEMOTHERAPY

Several classes of cytotoxic agents have demonstrated modest single-agent activity in biliary cancers. The objective response rates for 5-FU in phase II trials were in the range of 10–13% (6, 7). Mitomycin C was eval-

TABLE 17.1
Results of Selected Systemic Therapy Trials in Biliary Cancer

AGENT	NO. OF CASES	RESPONSE RATE	SURVIVAL (MONTHS)	REF.
5-FU	30	10%	5	7
	23	13%	4	6
Gemcitabine	11	0	N/A	10
	19	16%	6.5	11
	40	17%	7.6	12
DX-8951f	42	4.9%	7	13
Cisplatin/ 5-FU	25	24%	N/A	17
Cisplatin/5-FU/Epirubicin	14	33%	N/A	18
Oxaliplatin/ 5-FU	21	14%	8.7	19
Oxaliplatin/ Capecitabine	21	19%	N/A	20
Gemcitabine/ Cisplatin	50	22%	7	22
	86	24%	N/A	24
Gemcitabine/5-FU	9	33%	9	26
Gemcitabine/Oxaliplatin/5-FU	38	45%	10	28
Gemcitabine/Capecitabine	34	11%	7.8	27
Gemcitabine/Irinotecan	13	18%	9.5	30
Erlotinib	42	8%	7.5	62
Lapatinib	19	0	N/A	46
Sorafenib	36	6%	6	61

uated in two phase II trials with response rates of 10 and 47% (8, 9). Gemcitabine has demonstrated a response rate and stable disease in 0–16% and 21–54%, respectively (10, 11). A recently reported multi-institutional phase II trial of single-agent gemcitabine in 40 patients revealed a response rate, median progression-free survival, and overall survival of 17%, 2.3 months, and 9.4 months, respectively (12). DX-8951f is a topoisomerase-1 inhibitor that in a phase II trial of 42 patients with biliary cancer demonstrated modest activity with a partial response rate and survival of 4.9% and 7.8 months, respectively (13). No activity has been documented for taxane group of drugs in this disease (14, 15). Given the widespread use of gemcitabine in patients with pancreatic cancer, it is now also given to patients with advanced biliary cancers. Unlike in pancreatic cancer, the efficacy of gemcitabine in biliary cancers has not been tested in randomized trials.

COMBINATION CHEMOTHERAPY

Based on the low response rates of single agents, several trials evaluated combination chemotherapy regimens in biliary tumors.

Fluoropyrimidine-Based Chemotherapy

The response rate of 5-FU and either streptozotocin or MeCCNU was 10% (7). Efficacy of platinum and 5-FU

combinations was reported in a series of small phase II trials. The response rates for cisplatin/5-FU in 25 patients (16), carboplatin/5-FU in 14 patients (17), and epirubicin/cisplatin/5-FU in 14 patients (18) were 24, 21, and 33%, respectively. Lim et.al. evaluated 5-FU and oxaliplatin (FOLFOX) in 21 patients with advanced biliary tumors (19). The observed response rate was 14%. The median progression-free survival and overall survival were 6.6 and 8.7 months, respectively. Similar results were observed in 21 patients with advanced biliary cancer treated with oxaliplatin and capecitabine (20). The overall response rate was 19%. Irinotecan and infusional 5-FU (FOLFIRI) regimen was evaluated in 30 patients with biliary tumors (21). The response rate was 10%, which was similar to the activity of single-agent 5-FU but with the added toxicities of irinotecan.

Gemcitabine-Based Chemotherapy

The combination of gemcitabine and platinum drugs was based on preclinical data suggesting synergism in a variety of human cancer cell lines. Furthermore, the regimen was clinically well tolerated and revealed promising activity in phase II trials in non–small-cell lung cancer and pancreatic cancer. Goldstein et al. reported on 50 patients with advanced biliary tumors treated with fixed-dose-rate gemcitabine and cisplatin. The response rate and one-year survival were 22 and 30%, respectively (22). Gemcitabine and oxaliplatin were evaluated in 31 patients with biliary tumors. The response rate and median overall survival were 26% and 10.4 months, respectively (23). Walle et.al. reported a randomized multi-institutional phase II trial of gemcitabine versus gemcitabine and cisplatin in 86 patients with advanced biliary cancer (24). The results indicated a superior response rate (24 vs. 15%) and progression-free survival (8.0 vs. 5.5 months) in favor of the combination. Lethargy and thrombocytopenia were higher in the combination arm. The trial was not powered for a statistical comparison of both arms. However, the results of this trial are similar to the reported results in pancreatic cancer where combination therapy resulted in an improvement in disease control (response rate), increased toxicity, but without a statistically significant improvement of overall survival (25).

Gemcitabine and fluoropyrimidine combinations have also been evaluated in biliary tumors. DeGusmao et al. reported a response rate of 33% in 9 patients treated with gemcitabine and 5-FU (26). The response rate and median time to progression for gemcitabine and capecitabine in 34 patients with advanced biliary cancer were 11% and 2.6 months, respectively (27). Wagner et al. reported the results of gemcitabine, oxaliplatin, and 5-FU in 38 patients (28). The median and one-year survival were 10 months and 45%, respectively.

Disappointing results have been recently reported with the combination of gemcitabine with pemetrexed or irinotecan. Pemetrexed is a multitargeted antifolate. The North Central Cancer Therapy Group reported on 58 patients treated with gemcitabine and pemetrexed (29). The median time to progression and survival were 3.8 and 6.3 months, respectively. Stieler et al. evaluated gemcitabine and irinotecan in 13 patients with biliary tumor (30). The response rate and median survival were 18% and 9.5 months, respectively.

Conclusion

Information on combination therapy for advanced biliary cancers is based on multiple pilot trials with a relatively small number of patients. These series had very heterogeneous groups of patients, and results are therefore difficult to interpret. Nevertheless, one may conclude that combination chemotherapy did not produce major responses or prolongations in progression or overall survival. The decision whether to treat a patient with a single drug such as gemcitabine or a combination based on a fluoropyrimidine or gemcitabine will largely depend on the ability of the patient to tolerate a combination. Patients with a good performance status, well-preserved organ function, including that of the liver, and who are motivated may be good candidates for combination therapy. Otherwise the standard of care at this time is to use a single agent such as gemcitabine for the palliation of patients with advanced biliary cancer. Given the low incidence of this cancer and the molecular heterogeneity, patients should be invited to participate in national or even international collaborative studies to test novel agents.

TARGETED THERAPIES

The prognosis of patients with bile duct tumors has remained poor because of the systemic nature of disease and lack of effective drug therapies. The role of cytotoxic therapy remains controversial because of the minimal impact on the disease and the toxicities associated with such therapies. Researchers therefore focus on new therapeutic strategies to develop more effective treatments for this disease. Advances in the understanding of the molecular mechanisms of cancer have identified dysregulated pathways in malignant cells, including those of the biliary cancer. These include abnormalities of proliferative signaling pathways, apoptosis, invasion, and angiogenesis. In general, two overlapping strategies were adopted in clinical development of targeted drugs for biliary cancer: (a) development of targeted agents to inhibit tumor growth and metastasis, and (b) strategies to sensitize tumor cells to conventional cytotoxic chemotherapy.

Targeting the ErbB Receptor

The ErbB tyrosine kinase receptor family includes the epidermal growth factor receptor (EGFR), HER2/neu (ErbB2), ErbB3, and ErbB4 (31,32). The ErbB receptors at the cell surface share a common structure composed of an extracellular ligand-binding domain, transmembrane segment, and an intracellular tyrosine kinase domain. In normal tissues, the ErbB receptors are activated by a variety of receptor specific ligands (32). After ligand binding the receptors form homo- or heterodimeric complexes activating the cytoplasmic tyrosine kinase domain, resulting in phosphorylation and activation of downstream signaling pathways leading to the modulation of gene transcription (31,33).

Mechanisms involved in the activation of the ErbB receptors in cancer cells include (a) receptor overexpression (34,35), (b) mutant receptors resulting in ligand-independent activation (35), (c) autocrine activation by overproduction of ligand (36), or (d) ligand-independent activation through other receptor systems such as the urokinase plasminogen receptor (37). Activation of the ErbB receptors is involved in malignant transformation and tumor growth through the inhibition of apoptosis, cellular proliferation, promotion of angiogenesis, and metastasis (38).

EGFR and HER2/neu are believed to be dysregulated in human biliary cancers. The frequency of EGFR overexpression by immunohistochemistry (IHC) ranges from 21 to 100% (39–41). Seventy-seven percent of bile duct tumors with overexpression of EGFR by IHC had amplification of *EGFR* by FISH (42). The overexpression of transforming growth factor (TGF)-α, a ligand of EGFR, and inhibition of proliferation of cholangiocarcinoma cell lines by EGFR inhibitors supported an important role for EGFR signaling in bile duct cancer. Based on these findings, trials evaluating targeted agents against the ErbB receptors have been initiated.

Philip et al. reported on 42 patients with bile duct cancer treated with erlotinib, which is a potent selective tyrosine kinase inhibitor of the EGFR (43). The primary endpoint was progression-free survival at 6 months. Fifty-seven percent of patients had received prior chemotherapy. The progression-free survival at 6 months was 17%, and the study achieved its primary endpoint. The overall response rate and median overall survival were 51% and 7.5 months, respectively. Erlotinib was well tolerated, and the most common toxicity was skin rash. Lapatinib is a dual receptor tyrosine kinase inhibitor of the EGFR and Her2neu receptors (44). In a phase II trial of lapatinib in 19 patients with bile duct cancer, no responses were observed and the median progression-free survival was 1.8 months (45).

Cetuximab is a chimeric monoclonal antibody against the extracellular domain EGFR (46). In colorectal cancer, patients resistant to irinotecan responded to cetuximab and irinotecan, suggesting that cetuximab can modulate chemoresistance to irinotecan (47). Paule et al. reported a retrospective series of nine patients in whom cetuximab was added to gemcitabine and oxaliplatin after progression on first-line chemotherapy with the same regimen (48). Results showed a partial response in three patients and stable disease in three. The median survival from initiation of cetuximab was 10 months. The results of this study, though limited by the retrospective nature and the small number of patients, raise an interesting question of potentation of chemotherapy effect with cetuximab.

Targeting the Cyclooxegynase-2 (COX-2) Pathway

The COX-2 enzyme is known to be overexpressed in bile duct cancers (49,50). Preclinical evidence suggests that COX-2 has a central role in carcinogenesis (51), proliferation (49), and angiogenesis (52,53). COX-2 activity has antiapoptotic effects leading to chemoresistance (53). Preliminary results of a trial of irinotecan, capecitabine, and celecoxib in 12 patients with bile duct cancer were encouraging (54). The response rate and median overall survival were 25% and 17 months, respectively.

Targeting Angiogenesis and raf Pathways

Sorafenib is a multi-targeted tyrosine kinase inhibitor of the c-Raf/b-Raf, vascular endothelial receptor (VEGFR) 2/3 and platelet-derived growth factor (PDGFR) (55). Activating mutations of ras (56, 57) and Raf (58, 59) are present in bile duct cancer. El-Khoueiry et al. reported on a phase II study conducted by the Southwest Oncology Group in 36 patients with advanced bile duct cancer treated with sorafenib (60). The response rate and median progression-free survival were 6% and 2 months, respectively. Although sorafenib was well tolerated, the antitumor activity was somewhat disappointing.

Summary

There are early attempts to test targeted agents in advanced biliary cancers. Results so far have shown very modest activity if any. None of the patients were selected on the basis of prevalent molecular abnormality in the tumor. Future studies with better selection are likely to demonstrate benefits to a number of agents tested.

ONGOING CLINICAL TRIALS

Targeting ErbB Receptor

Encouraged by the results of the activity of erlotinib in bile duct cancer, two trials are evaluating the benefit of combining erlotinib with either bevacizumab a monoclonal antibody against VEGF or docetaxel. Cetuximab is being evaluated in a randomized phase II trial of gemcitabine oxaliplatin versus gemcitabine oxaliplatin and cetuximab. Trastuzumab, a monoclonal antibody against HER2neu, is being evaluated in a phase II trial of patients with FISH-positive amplification of the *HER2neu* gene.

Cytotoxic Agents

Taxoprexin, a conjugate of paclitaxel with DHA (docosahexaenoic acid), has been shown to achieve higher tumor levels with no increase in systemic toxicity. Taxoprexin is currently being evaluated in a phase II trial in bile duct cancer. A phase III trial is comparing gemcitabine and gemcitabine cisplatin in advanced bile duct cancer.

Other Targeted Agents

AZD6244 is a selective MEK inhibitor. MEK has a central role in the EGFR/Ras/Raf signaling pathway. A phase II trial is currently evaluating the activity of AZD6244 in bile duct cancer. The proteasomes are involved in the degradation of proteins and, as such, regulate cell cycle and apoptosis. The pro-apoptotic effects of proteasome inhibition are attributed to inhibition of the NF-κB signaling pathway. Bortezomib, a proteosome inhibitor, is currently being evaluated as a single agent in bile duct cancer. Triapine is an inhibitor of the ribonuclotide reductase. Preclinical data indicate that triapine, an inhibitor of ribonucleotide reductase, can increase the intracellular uptake and activity of gemcitabine. Triapine in combination with gemcitabine is currently in a clinical trial in a number of solid tumors, including bile duct cancer.

CONCLUSION

There is no standard systemic therapy regimen in biliary tumors. Gemcitabine and fluoropyrimidines are the most commonly used agents, with most trials demonstrating a response rate of approximately 10% and overall survival of 6–9 months. Combination chemotherapy might improve response rates and at best have a modest impact on the disease, but at the cost of higher toxicity. Patients with good performance status and normal organ function being treated off clinical trials could be considered for combination chemotherapy. Among the targeted agents, erlotinib has shown promising activity. Ongoing trials are focused on identifying novel agents with activity against bile duct caner or on building on the observed activity of agents like erlotinib and gemcitabine. Given the small number of patients with this disease and the lack of a standard drug therapy, it is important to enroll patients with newly diagnosed disease into clinical trials.

References

1. Jemal A, Siegel R, Ward E, et al. Cancer statistics, 2007. CA Cancer J Clin 2007; 57:43–66.
2. Nagorney DM, Donohue JH, Farnell MB, et al. Outcomes after curative resections of cholangiocarcinoma. Arch Surg 1993; 128:871–877; discussion 877–879.
3. Berdah SV, Delpero JR, Garcia S, et al. A western surgical experience of peripheral cholangiocarcinoma. Br J Surg 1996; 83:1517–1521.
4. Farley DR, Weaver AL, Nagorney DM. "Natural history" of unresected cholangiocarcinoma: patient outcome after noncurative intervention. Mayo Clin Proc 1995; 70:425–429.
5. Nakeeb A, Pitt HA, Sohn TA, et al. Cholangiocarcinoma. A spectrum of intrahepatic, perihilar, and distal tumors. Ann Surg 1996; 224:463–473; discussion 473–475.
6. Davis HL, Jr., Ramirez G, Ansfield FJ. Adenocarcinomas of stomach, pancreas, liver, and biliary tracts. Survival of 328 patients treated with fluoropyrimidine therapy. Cancer 1974; 33:193–197.
7. Falkson G, MacIntyre JM, Moertel CG. Eastern Cooperative Oncology Group experience with chemotherapy for inoperable gallbladder and bile duct cancer. Cancer 1984; 54:965–969.
8. Crooke ST, Bradner WT. Mitomycin C: a review. Cancer Treat Rev 1976; 3:121–139.
9. Taal BG, Audisio RA, Bleiberg H, et al. Phase II trial of mitomycin C (MMC) in advanced gallbladder and biliary tree carcinoma. An EORTC Gastrointestinal Tract Cancer Cooperative Group Study. Ann Oncol 1993; 4:607–609.
10. Mezger J, et al. Phase II trial of gemcitabine in biliary tract cancer, Proc Am Soc Clin Oncol, Vol. 1, Abstract 1059, 1997.
11. Raderer M, Hejna MH, Valencak JB, et al. Two consecutive phase II studies of 5-fluorouracil/leucovorin/mitomycin C and of gemcitabine in patients with advanced biliary cancer. Oncology 1999; 56:177–180.
12. Okusaka T, Ishii H, Funakoshi A, et al. Phase II study of single-agent gemcitabine in patients with advanced biliary tract cancer. Cancer Chemother Pharmacol 2006; 57:647–653.
13. Abou-Alfa GK, Rowinsky EK, Patt YZ, et al. A Phase II study of intravenous exatecan administered daily for 5 days, every 3 weeks to patients with biliary tract cancers. Am J Clin Oncol 2005; 28:334–339.
14. Jones DV, Jr., Lozano R, Hoque A, et al. Phase II study of paclitaxel therapy for unresectable biliary tree carcinomas. J Clin Oncol 1996; 14:2306–2310.
15. Pazdur R, Royce ME, Rodriguez GI, et al. Phase II trial of docetaxel for cholangiocarcinoma. Am J Clin Oncol 1999; 22:78–81.
16. Ducreux M, Rougier P, Fandi A, et al. Effective treatment of advanced biliary tract carcinoma using 5-fluorouracil continuous infusion with cisplatin. Ann Oncol 1998; 9:653–656.
17. Sanz-Altamira PM, Ferrante K, Jenkins RL, et al. A phase II trial of 5-fluorouracil, leucovorin, and carboplatin in patients with unresectable biliary tree carcinoma. Cancer 1998; 82:2321–2325.
18. Di Lauro L, Carpano S, Campomolla E. Cisplatin, epirubicin, and 5-FU for advanced biliary tract carcinoma, Proc Am Soc Oncol, Vol. 1, Abstract 1021, 1997.
19. Lim JY, Cho JY, Paik YH, et al. Oxaliplatin combined with leucovorin plus 5-FU(FOLFOX) in patients with advanced/metastatic biliary tract carcinoma. Proc Am Soc Oncol, Atlanta, GA, June 2–6, 2006.
20. Glover KY, Thomas MB, Brown TD, et al. A phase II study of oxaliplatin and capecitabine (XELOX) in patients with unresectable cholangiocarcinoma, including carcinoma of the gallbladder and biliary tact.\, Proc Am Soc Oncol, Orlando, FL, May 13–17, 2005.
21. Feisthammel J, Schoppmeyer K, Mossner J, et al. Irinotecan with 5-FU/FA in advanced biliary tract adenocarcinomas: a multicenter phase II trial. Am J Clin Oncol 2007; 30: 319–324.
22. Goldstein D, Shannon J, Brown C, et al. ABC; An AGITG trial of fixed dose rate (FDR) gemcitabine (gem) and cisplatin for patients (pts) with advanced biliary tract cancer (ABC). Proc Am Soc Oncol. Chicago, June 1–5, 2007.
23. Harder J, Riecken B, Kummer O, et al. Outpatient chemotherapy with gemcitabine and oxaliplatin in patients with biliary tract cancer. Br J Cancer 2006; 95:848–852.
24. Valle JW, Wasan H, Johnson P, et al. Gemcitabine, alone or in combination with cisplatin, in patients with advanced or metastatic cholangiocarcinoma (CC) and other biliary tract tumors: a multicenter, randomized, phase II (the UK ABC-01) study, GI ASCO Symposium. San Francisco, January 26–28, 2006.
25. Adsay NV, El-Rayes BF, Philip PA. Pancreatic cancer: the evolving role of systemic therapy. Expert Opin Pharmacother 2001; 2:1939–1947.
26. Murad AM, Guimaraes RC, Aragao BC, et al. Phase II trial of the use of gemcitabine and 5-fluorouracil in the treatment of advanced pancreatic and biliary tract cancer. Am J Clin Oncol 2003; 26:151–154.
27. Chang H, Ryu M, Lee J, et al. Phase II trial of gemcitabine plus capecitabine in patients with advanced biliary tract cancer. Proc Am Soc Oncol, Orlando, FL, May 13–17, 2005.
28. Wagner A, Buechner-Steudel P, Wein A, et al. Gemcitabine, oxaliplatin and weekly high-dose 5-FU as a 24-hr-infusion in

chemonaive patients with advanced or metastatic biliary tree adenocarcinoma: preliminary results of a multicenter phase II-study. Proc Am Soc Oncol, Orlando, FL, May 13–17, 2005.

29. McWilliams RR, Foster NR, Quevedo FJ, et al. NCCTG phase I/II trial (N9943) of gemcitabine and pemetrexed in patients with biliary tract or gallbladder carcinoma: phase II results. Proc Am Soc Oncol, Chicago, June 1–5, 2007.

30. Stieler J, Roll L, Arning M, et al. Gemcitabine and irinotecan-a pilot study for patients with non-resectable cancer of the bile duct system. Proc Am Soc Oncol. Chicago, May 31–June 3, 2003.

31. Olayioye MA, Neve RM, Lane HA, et al. The ErbB signaling network: receptor heterodimerization in development and cancer. EMBO J 2000; 19:3159–3167.

32. Yarden Y, Sliwkowski MX. Untangling the ErbB signalling network. Nat Rev Mol Cell Biol 2001; 2:127–137.

33. Mendelsohn J, Baselga J. Status of epidermal growth factor receptor antagonists in the biology and treatment of cancer. J Clin Oncol 2003; 21:2787–2799.

34. Hirsch FR, Varella-Garcia M, Bunn PA, Jr., et al. Epidermal growth factor receptor in non-small-cell lung carcinomas: correlation between gene copy number and protein expression and impact on prognosis. J Clin Oncol 2003; 21:3798–3807.

35. Moscatello DK, Holgado-Madruga M, Godwin AK, et al. Frequent expression of a mutant epidermal growth factor receptor in multiple human tumors. Cancer Res 1995; 55:5536–5539.

36. Prenzel N, Zwick E, Daub H, et al. EGF receptor transactivation by G-protein-coupled receptors requires metalloproteinase cleavage of proHB-EGF. Nature 1999; 402:884–888.

37. Liu D, Aguirre Ghiso J, Estrada Y, et al. EGFR is a transducer of the urokinase receptor initiated signal that is required for in vivo growth of a human carcinoma. Cancer Cell 2002; 1:445–457.

38. El-Rayes BF, LoRusso PM. Targeting the epidermal growth factor receptor. Br J Cancer 2004; 91:418–424.

39. Nonomura A, Ohta G, Nakanuma Y, et al. Simultaneous detection of epidermal growth factor receptor (EGF-R), epidermal growth factor (EGF) and ras p21 in cholangiocarcinoma by an immunocytochemical method. Liver 1988; 8:157–166.

40. Lee CS, Pirdas A. Epidermal growth factor receptor immunoreactivity in gallbladder and extrahepatic biliary tract tumours. Pathol Res Pract 1995; 191:1087–1091.

41. Ito Y, Takeda T, Sasaki Y, et al. Expression and clinical significance of the erbB family in intrahepatic cholangiocellular carcinoma. Pathol Res Pract 2001; 197:95–100.

42. Nakazawa K, Dobashi Y, Suzuki S, et al. Amplification and overexpression of c-erbB-2, epidermal growth factor receptor, and c-met in biliary tract cancers. J Pathol 2005; 206:356–365.

43. Philip PA, Mahoney MR, Allmer C, et al. Phase II study of erlotinib in patients with advanced biliary cancer. J Clin Oncol 2006; 24:3069–3074.

44. Montemurro F, Valabrega G, Aglietta M: Lapatinib: a dual inhibitor of EGFR and HER2 tyrosine kinase activity. Expert Opin Biol Ther 2007; 7:257–268.

45. Ramanathan R, Belani C, Singh D, et al. Phase II study of lapatinib, a dual inhibitor of epidermal growth factor receptor (EGFR) tyrosine kinase 1 and 2 (Her2/Neu) in patients (pts)

with advanced biliary tree cancer (BTC) or hepatocellular cancer (HCC). A California Consortium (CCC-P) Trial. Proc Am Soc Oncol, Atlanta, GA, June 2–6, 2006.

46. Labianca R, La Verde N, Garassino MC. Development and clinical indications of cetuximab. Int J Biol Markers 2007; 22:S40–46.

47. Cunningham D, Humblet Y, Siena S, et al. Cetuximab monotherapy and cetuximab plus irinotecan in irinotecan-refractory metastatic colorectal cancer. N Engl J Med 2004; 351:337–345.

48. Paule B, Bralet M, Herelle M, et al. Cetuximab plus gemcitabine/oxaliplatin (GEMOX) for patients with unresectable/recurrent intrahepatic cholangiocarcinoma refractory to GEMOX. Proc Am Soc Oncol, Atlanta, GA, June 2–6; 2006.

49. Schmitz KJ, Lang H, Wohlschlaeger J, et al. Elevated expression of cyclooxygenase-2 is a negative prognostic factor for overall survival in intrahepatic cholangiocarcinoma. Virchows Arch 2007; 450:135–141.

50. Legan M, Luzar B, Marolt VF, et al. Expression of cyclooxygenase-2 is associated with p53 accumulation in premalignant and malignant gallbladder lesions. World J Gastroenterol 2006; 12:3425–3429.

51. Legan M, Luzar B, Ferlan-Marolt V, et al. Cyclooxygenase-2 expression determines neo-angiogenesis in gallbladder carcinomas. Bosn J Basic Med Sci 2006; 6:58–63.

52. Zhi YH, Liu RS, Song MM, et al. Cyclooxygenase-2 promotes angiogenesis by increasing vascular endothelial growth factor and predicts prognosis in gallbladder carcinoma. World J Gastroenterol 2005; 11:3724–3728.

53. El-Rayes BF, Ali S, Sarkar FH, et al. Cyclooxygenase-2-dependent and -independent effects of celecoxib in pancreatic cancer cell lines. Mol Cancer Ther 2004; 3:1421–1426.

54. Lee F, Roach M, Parasher G, et al. Combination irinotecan, capecitabine and celecoxib in patients with advanced biliary cancers. Proc Am Soc Oncol, Atlanta, GA, June 2–6, 2006.

55. Takimoto CH, Awada A. Safety and anti-tumor activity of sorafenib (Nexavar®) in combination with other anti-cancer agents: a review of clinical trials. Cancer Chemother Pharmacol, 2008; 61:535–548.

56. Yamaguchi K, Nakano K, Nagai E, et al. Ki-ras mutations in codon 12 and p53 mutations (biomarkers) and cytology in bile in patients with hepatobiliary-pancreatic carcinoma. Hepatogastroenterology 2005; 52:713–718.

57. Saetta AA. K-ras, p53 mutations, and microsatellite instability (MSI) in gallbladder cancer. J Surg Oncol 2006; 93:644–649.

58. Saetta AA, Papanastasiou P, Michalopoulos NV, et al. Mutational analysis of BRAF in gallbladder carcinomas in association with K-ras and p53 mutations and microsatellite instability. Virchows Arch 2004; 445:179–182.

59. Tannapfel A, Sommerer F, Benicke M, et al. Mutations of the BRAF gene in cholangiocarcinoma but not in hepatocellular carcinoma. Gut 2003; 52:706–712.

60. El-Khoueiry A, Rankin C, Lenz H, et al. SWOG 0514: a phase II study of sorafenib (BAY 43-9006) as single agent in patients (pts) with unresectable or metastatic gallbladder cancer or cholangiocarcinomas. Proc Am Soc Oncol, Chicago, June 1–5, 2007.

18 Radiation Therapy

Brian G. Czito
Clifton David Fuller

arcinomas of the gallbladder and biliary system are rare, with an estimated 9250 cases occurring in the United States in 2007 (1). Because the majority of patients with biliary cancers present with unresectable or metastatic disease, the overall 5-year survival rate is less than 10% (2, 3). Surgery is the only potentially curative treatment for patients with biliary carcinoma; however, only a minority of patients are candidates at presentation (4–6). In resected patients, outcome is closely associated with the pathologic findings of depth of tumor penetration and nodal metastases. Even for patients resected for cure, the prognosis remains poor, with high local failure rates with associated morbidity and mortality (7, 8). Given these poor outcomes, further therapy should be considered in management. However, the role of radiation therapy and chemotherapy in patients with cholangiocarcinoma is poorly defined given the rarity of this malignancy and physician's therapeutic nihilism.

LOCAL TUMOR CONTROL FOLLOWING RESECTION

Patients with primary carcinoma of the gallbladder and bile duct cancer are rarely cured with any treatment modality other than surgical resection. However, most patients will present with locally advanced or metastatic disease, with resectability rates ranging from 10 to 35%. Therefore, most patients with gallbladder and biliary carcinomas are approached with palliative intent, including the establishment and ongoing management of biliary drainage. Overall survival in all patients is poor, ranging from 2 to 3 months in patients receiving medical management alone, 6 to 12 months for those undergoing surgical palliation, and 12 to 22 months for resected patients. Overall 5-year survival remains dismal at less than 10% (9).

Of patients undergoing "curative" resection for biliary cancers, approximately 50% will experience local-regional recurrence, leading to death from biliary obstruction, sepsis, and liver failure (10). Reports describing patterns of failure following surgery for biliary cancers are limited. Available data suggest that local-regional recurrence is common and ultimately leads to death, usually from complications of biliary obstruction and liver failure. Literature review indicates local recurrence occurs in up to 86% of patients following cholecystectomy alone for gallbladder cancer. In long-term survivors following surgery, local recurrence rates remain high, even beyond 5 years (10-12). A likely explanation for this is because occult nodal involvement is common and localized invasion of the liver is not recognized and resected. This high incidence of residual microscopic disease has been reported in autopsy series (13). Even in patients treated with cholecystectomy with accompanying liver resection, local-regional recurrence has been reported to be as high as 75% (11). A large contemporary experience from Memorial Sloan-Kettering Cancer Center showed that in patients undergoing extended resection for gallbladder cancer, 31% of relapsing patients had some component of local-regional recurrence in follow-up (14). Similarly, the rate of local-regional recurrence in patients undergoing extended resection for hilar cholangiocarcinoma in this series was 58% (14). Korean investigators described 83 patients undergoing curative radical resection for extrahepatic bile duct tumors. Most patients had uninvolved nodes at resection. Despite uninvolved margins, over 50% experienced local-regional tumor relapse (15). In patients with distal common bile duct cancers undergoing radical resection alone, reported local recurrence rates have ranged from 35 to 74% (16, 17). This high incidence of local-regional failure may be overlooked once patients develop metastatic disease, likely underestimating the true incidence of local failure in many series, given not all patients undergo thorough posttreatment imaging or autopsy. In addition, the role persistent local-regional disease plays in the subsequent development of distant metastases remains uncertain. Given patterns of failure in biliary tract malignancies and morbidity and mortality associated with such, the use of radiation therapy is rational.

TOLERANCE OF THE HEPATOBILIARY TREE, LIVER, AND SURROUNDING STRUCTURES TO RADIATION THERAPY

When considering the use of radiotherapy in the treatment of different malignancies, normal tissue tolerance of surrounding organs and structures must be considered. Tolerance depends upon multiple factors, including volume of tissue irradiated, dose delivered per fraction, the use of concurrent chemotherapy, and other coexisting medical conditions. Potential dose-limiting organs adjacent to the hepatobiliary tree include liver, adjacent bile ducts, kidneys, small bowel, stomach, distal esophagus, and spinal cord. The risk of radiation-related complications has been estimated based upon dose per fraction, treatment volume, and the cumulative radiation dose (23). These data were derived empirically and not based on formal dose escalation studies. The tolerance dose defined as TD 5/5 represents the radiation dose that would result in a 5% risk of severe complications within 5 years following irradiation, while the TD 50/5 represents the radiation dose that would result in a 50% probability of developing severe complications with 5 years after treatment. Table 18.1 summarizes radiation tolerance of key organs in the abdomen (24).

TABLE 18.1

Normal Tissue Tolerance to External Irradiation (with Fractionated Dose of 1.8 Gy/day)

Structure	TD 5/5[a] (Gy)	TD 50/5[a] (Gy)
Whole liver	30	40
Partial liver	See text	See text
Bile duct	60	—
Duodenum	50	60
Small bowel	50	60
Esophagus	60	75
Stomach	50	55
Kidney	23	28
Spinal cord	50	60

[a] TD 5/5 represents the radiation dose that results in a 5% severe complication rate within 5 years following irradiation. TD 50/5 represents the radiation dose that results in a 50% severe complication rate within 5 years following irradiation.

There is general agreement that whole liver tolerance is approximately 30 Gy. Whole liver doses beyond this result in an increasing incidence of radiation-induced liver disease (RILD), which is characterized by hepatomegaly, ascites, and elevated liver function tests, generally occurring 2 weeks to 4 months following radiation completion. This condition may lead to progressive liver failure and death. The pathogenesis of RILD is thought to be secondary to small vessel veno-occlusive disease. Until recently, relatively few data existed regarding partial liver irradiation. Early estimates gauged the TD 5/5 and TD 50/5 for treatment of one third of the hepatic volume at 50 and 55 Gy, respectively. However, with the advent of three-dimensional planning and computer-aided volumetric analysis, the TD 5/5 and TD 50/5 have been estimated to be as high as 90 Gy and beyond depending on the volume irradiated. Additionally, recent literature suggests that TD 5/5 and TD 50/5 for two thirds of the liver volume range from 43 to 52 Gy and 61 to 75 Gy, respectively (25). With the administration of concurrent chemotherapy, these numbers may be less. Bile duct tolerance is thought to be approximately 60 Gy using conventional fractionation, including intrahepatic ducts, when treated to small volume. Reported complications include biliary fibrosis (9).

When kidneys are included in radiation treatment fields, a minimum of two thirds of one functional kidney should be excluded to reduce the risk of irreversible renal complications. Unilateral renal irradiation results in minimal-long term clinical sequelae, assuming baseline renal function in the contralateral kidney is normal (26). Strictly speaking, the dose to the "spared" kidney is often limited to 14–18 Gy using standard dose fractionation (1.8–2 Gy) to avoid irreversible damage, which is lower than the estimated TD 5/5. Tolerance of the spinal cord, small intestine, and stomach is approximately 45–50 Gy using standard dose fractionation.

The increasing use of brachytherapy (the temporary or permanent insertion of radioactive sources into a tumor and/or peritumoral tissues) and intraoperative radiotherapy (IORT) has also allowed better understanding of upper abdominal organ tolerance. IORT delivers a single large dose of radiotherapy in the operating room, allowing the extent of tumor and surrounding normal tissues to be directly visualized and direct normal tissue shielding. Figures 18.1 and 18.2 demonstrate the use of IORT with an iridium-192 source via a HAM applicator in the operating suite. Low-energy photons (e.g., Ir-192) or electrons are typically used for IORT, allowing rapid dose fall-off with increasing distance, resulting in minimal dose to the surrounding normal critical structures. Intraluminal transcatheter brachytherapy allows the delivery of radioactive sources such as Ir-192 to the tumor through a percutaneous transhepatic biliary drainage (PTBD) tube under fluoroscopic guidance or through catheters placed in the tumor bed during surgery. Figure 18.5 (page 228) depicts the placement of intraluminal Ir-192 seeds via a PTBD tube. In contrast to high-energy photons used for external beam radiation therapy (EBRT), IORT and brachytherapy allow administration of higher radiation doses without exceeding normal tissue tolerance by direct normal tissue shielding and rapid dose fall-off with distance. Dosewise, the incidence of complications from IORT is minimized if the dose is 20 Gy or less in a single fraction (27). Additionally, limiting the transcatheter brachytherapy dose to 20–30 Gy when combined with EBRT of 45–50 Gy in 25–28 fractions is associated with acceptable complication levels.

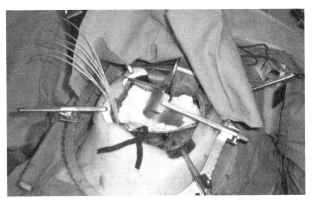

FIGURE 18.1

Treatment of biliary tract tumor using Harrison-Anderson-Mick (HAM) applicator and Ir-192 source. Applicator is held flush against tumor bed by suturing to adjacent tissues (note guide tubes on left, which connect to source housing).

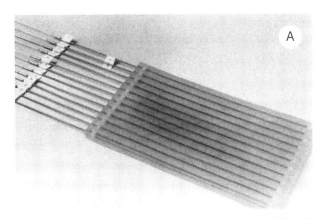

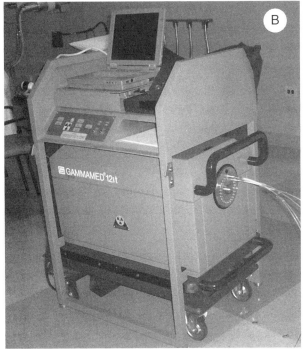

FIGURE 18.2

(A) HAM applicator used to guide Ir-192 source during IORT. (B) Source housing for Ir-192 source. This device allows computer-assisted remote-controlled treatment delivery of the radioactive source into the guide tubes during IORT. Using this high-activity radiation source, treatment can be completed within 30 minutes.

ANATOMY AND ROUTE OF SPREAD WITH REGARD TO RADIATION THERAPY PLANNING

Carcinoma of the gallbladder and bile duct spreads local-regionally by direct extension as well as lymphatic infiltration. Study of patterns of spread facilitates design of radiation fields. Local invasion of tumor into surrounding tissue and liver by gallbladder cancer is aided by the gallbladder's thin wall as well as continuum of perimuscular connective tissue with interlobular connective tissue of the liver (28). Hepatic infiltration has been reported in 60–70% of patients on collective review and autopsy series. Lymphatic spread by gallbladder cancer is also common. Regional nodal involvement has been reported in 40–80% of patients (2, 29). For patients with T2 lesions, the incidence of nodal metastases ranges from 40 to 62% (14, 30–32). When disease invades the covering serosa or adjacent organs, nodal metastases rates rise to 70–80% (31, 32). The primary draining nodal groups are along the cystic and common bile ducts. Retrograde spread to hilar nodes can occur, particularly in more advanced disease. (33). Secondary spread occurs to the pancreaticoduodenal nodes and later to the periaortic nodes. Similarly, bile duct carcinomas frequently invade adjacent structures by direct extension as well as by lymphatic invasion. Regional nodal metastases or adjacent organ involvement are found in up to 50% of patients (34). The incidence of a nodal involvement is believed to be higher in intrahepatic cholangiocarcinomas compared to extrahepatic biliary tumors. Common sites of nodal spread from proximal biliary tumors include hepatoduodenal ligament, left gastric, portal, pericholedochal, and peripancreatic lymph nodes. More distally, tumors are more likely to involve the pancreaticoduodenal, hepatoduodenal and common hepatic artery lymph nodes (35).

TREATMENT OF GALLBLADDER AND BILE DUCT TUMOR WITH RADIOTHERAPY: RADIATION DOSE RESPONSE

The optimal radiation dose in the adjuvant and "definitive" treatment of biliary malignancies is unknown. Published studies describing dose response are generally nonrandomized and single institutional experiences, subject to selection bias, with higher performance patients often receiving higher doses (36, 37). Mahe et al. reported on patients receiving external radiotherapy for bile duct carcinoma in the curative and palliative setting. Patients receiving doses of ≥40 Gy experienced median survivals of 22 months compared to 10 months in patients receiving ≤35 Gy (36). Mittal et al. found that patients receiving radiation doses of ≥45 Gy had improved median survival compared to those receiving <45 Gy (11 vs. 4.4 months) (38). Results of these and other reports are likely confounded by varying disease stages and patient performance status with respect to dose selection.

Researchers from Thomas Jefferson University Hospital evaluated patients who were treated with combined EBRT and Ir-192 brachytherapy. Patients were retrospectively stratified as receiving total radia-

tion dose ≤55 or >55 Gy. Median and 2-year survival rates were 6 and 24 months and 0 and 48%, respectively. Median survival tended to increase with increasing dose, with median survivals of 4.5, 9, 18, 25, and 24 months for patients receiving <45, 45–54, 55–65, 66–70, and >70 Gy, respectively (39). In contrast, investigators from the University of Amsterdam showed no obvious benefit of doses >55 Gy when compared to patients receiving <55 Gy (40). Similarly, investigators from M.D. Anderson Cancer Center found no significant differences in local control or survival using doses of 30, 36–50.4, or 54–85 Gy (41).

The optimal radiotherapy dosage in the treatment of biliary cancers remains unknown.

OPERABLE DISEASE

Postoperative Radiotherapy: Extrahepatic Bile Duct

The use of adjuvant radiotherapy in resected extrahepatic cholangiocarcinoma remains controversial. Patterns of failure data suggest that local-regional failure following resection is common and therefore the use of adjuvant radiation therapy is rational. Varying single institution series have examined the role of adjuvant radiotherapy following resection and are discussed here.

Kopelson et al. described 13 patients undergoing resection with curative intent. Three patients receiving radiation therapy following surgery had a longer median survival (32 months) compared with the entire cohort (13 months) (10). An EORTC (European Organization for Research and Treatment of Cancer) series retrospectively reviewed 112 patients with Klatskin tumors (tumors at the bifurcation of common hepatic duct) treated at seven centers and found a statistically improved survival in patients receiving resection and postoperative radiotherapy versus those with resection only (median survival 19 vs. 8.3 months; 3-year survival 31% vs. 10%) (42). Japanese investigators reported on 39 patients treated with adjuvant radiation therapy following resection of hilar cholangiocarcinoma (mean total dose 74 Gy). Some patients were treated with EBRT only to a mean dose of 37.5 Gy. No patients received chemotherapy. Three-year survival in patients receiving radiation therapy was 41% versus 33% in patients receiving surgery alone (p = NS). In patients with pathologic stage III–IVa disease, radiation therapy appeared to result in improved survival (3-year survival 50% vs. 0%, p = 0.04), although patient numbers were small (43). Another Japanese series described 59 patients receiving postoperative radiotherapy following resection using EBRT (16–80 Gy), brachytherapy (40–80 Gy), or both (48–80 Gy). No patients received concurrent chemotherapy. One- and 5-year survivals were 73 and 18%, respectively, with median survival of 21.5 months (44).

Investigators from Johns Hopkins Hospital reported the outcome results of 96 patients with proximal cholangiocarcinoma treated surgically (41% curative resection, 14% noncurative resection, 45% palliative stenting). Sixty-six percent of patients received postoperative radiation therapy. Patients undergoing gross total resection or major debulking surgery had improved survival versus those receiving stenting alone. The 1-, 3-, 5-, and 10-year survivals in the resection group were 66, 21, 8, and 4%, respectively, compared to 27, 6, 0, and 0%, respectively, in the stenting-alone group. Improved 2-year survival was observed in stented patients undergoing radiation therapy versus patients treated with stent only (10% vs. 0%). Additionally, 5-year survival in resected patients receiving adjuvant RT was 16% versus 0% with resection alone (NS), with all 5-year survivors in the resection group receiving adjuvant radiotherapy (45). A more recent series from Johns Hopkins Hospital analyzed the clinical course of 34 patients with distal common bile duct cancer receiving adjuvant chemoradiotherapy following pancreaticoduodenectomy. Median and 5-year survivals were 37 months and 35%, respectively. Compared to a histologically more favorable group of patients from the same institution undergoing pancreaticoduodenectomy alone, survival was significantly improved (median survival 37 months vs. 22 months, $p < 0.05$) (46). Investigators from Duke University treated 33 patients with resected extrahepatic cholangiocarcinoma with adjuvant radiotherapy to a median dose of 50.4 Gy. Patients received concurrent 5-fluorouracil based therapy. Three and five-year survivals were 35% and 23%, respectively. Five-year actuarial local control was 82%, with 5-year metastases free survival of 27% (105).

In a study from the University of Amsterdam, 112 patients underwent resection for hilar cholangiocarcinoma. In patients surviving the postoperative period, 20 had no additional treatment, 30 EBRT only, and 41 combined EBRT and brachytherapy. Patients receiving adjuvant radiotherapy had an improved median survival compared to no additional treatment (24 vs. 8 months). The authors concluded that radiotherapy following resection of hilar cholangiocarcinoma improved survival, although there was no obvious benefit of intraluminal brachytherapy (47). Korean investigators reported on 60 patients with resected biliary cancers receiving a median dose of 45 Gy EBRT, with a minority of patients receiving concurrent chemotherapy. Median survival was 19 months; however, despite adjuvant therapy, local-regional failure still occurred in 48 patients (48). Other Korean investigators reported on 84 patients receiving postoperative EBRT (40–45 Gy), most of whom received

concurrent chemotherapy administration. Five-year survival was 31%. The authors concluded that long-term survival can be achieved in patients undergoing resection and postoperative chemoradiation (49).

In contrast to previous observations, a report from Pitt et al. at Johns Hopkins described a prospective, nonrandomized study of patients with perihilar cholangiocarcinoma. Fifty nonmetastatic patients underwent resection or palliative decompression. The decision to deliver adjuvant RT was based on patient preference. In treated patients, mean radiation dose following curative resection was 54 and 51 Gy in palliative patients. Radiotherapy was delivered as EBRT only or EBRT plus Ir-192 implant. In patients undergoing curative resection, no difference in median survival was seen whether or not patients received RT (20 months in both groups). Additionally, no significant difference in median survival was seen with the addition of radiation in patients undergoing palliative surgery (8 vs. 12.5 months). The authors concluded that postoperative radiotherapy does not improve survival (50). Limitations of this study (and other studies) include small sample size, lack of concurrent chemotherapy administration, possible group imbalance with regard to extent of resection (R0 vs. R1 vs. R2) and adverse histologic features, and variable RT techniques. Given this significant heterogeneity among studies, the efficacy of postoperative RT is inconclusive. A summary of postoperative RT studies is compiled in Table 18.2.

SEER analyses regarding the benefit of adjuvant radiotherapy for extrahepatic cholangiocarcinoma are somewhat equivocal (21, 22). Analyses from population-based datasets have shown mixed evidence of a survival benefit from the addition of radiotherapy to surgical intervention (Figure 18.3). Specifically, examination of the survival outcomes in local-regional extrahepatic cholangiocarcinoma patients receiving surgery and radiotherapy demonstrates an early survival benefit, with 1- and 2-year survival for patients receiving adjuvant radiotherapy statistically superior to those receiving surgery alone. However, by 5 years or more postdiagnosis, survival outcomes for the adjuvant radiotherapy cohort are equivalent or worse than surgery alone. The interpretation of these findings, as with any SEER analysis, are limited by the lack of specificity and inherent limitations regarding radiotherapy data extraction from registry data; nonetheless, no institutional series is as robust. Consequently, the suggestion of even an early survival benefit makes the implementation of adjuvant radiation therapy reasonable for local-regional extrahepatic bile duct tumors. Population-based registry analysis lends credence to the evidence from institutional series and patterns of failure analyses which cumulatively suggest a beneficent effect of first-line adjuvant radiotherapy in selected biliary tract cancer patients.

TABLE 18.2

*Outcomes Following Surgery for Extrahepatic Bile Duct Cancers
with or Without Postoperative Radiotherapy (RT)*

AUTHOR (REF.)	N	RT	RT DOSE (GY)	MEDIAN SURVIVAL (MONTHS)	3-YEAR SURVIVAL (%)	LOCAL CONTROL (%)
Kopelson (10)	13	Yes	38–72.25	12.7[a]	—	—
Gerhards (47)	71	Yes	42/46[b]	24	36 (est)	—
	20	No	—	8	10 (est)	—
Cameron (45)	63	Yes	50–80[c]	—	21	—
	33	No	—	—	0	—
Pitt (50)	23	Yes	51/54[d]	20[e]	—	—
	27	No	—	20[e]	—	—
Hughes[g] (46)	34	Yes	40–54	37	35[f]	82
	30	No	—	22	27[f]	—
Sagawa (43)	39	Yes	37/38[b]	23	41[f]	—
	30	No	—	20	33[f]	—
Kamada (44)	59	Yes	16–80[c]	22	31	—
Oh (48)	60	Yes	40–55	19	25(est)	52
Kim (49)	84	Yes	40–45	—	38 (est)	53
Nelson[g] (105)	33	Yes	10.8–54	29	50	82

[a] 31.9 months for patients treated with a curative intent.
[b] Mean EBRT dose with /without Ir-192 treatment.
[c] EBRT, Ir-192, or both.
[d] Mean dose.
[e] Patients treated with a curative intent.
[f] 5-Year survival.
[g] Concurrent chemotherapy in most.

Postoperative Radiotherapy: Gallbladder

Given patterns of failure data and poor prognosis in resected gallbladder cancer, consideration of adjuvant treatments is appropriate. It is estimated that only 20% of patients receive radiotherapy or chemotherapy following resection, and fewer than 10% of all presenting patients undergo surgery, radiotherapy, and chemotherapy (6). Therefore, reports describing the use of adjuvant chemoradiotherapy in the setting of resected gallbladder carcinoma are limited. Recent series have suggested that local- regional control and possibly ultimate outcome can be improved with the use of adjuvant therapy.

Duke University investigators reported on 22 patients with primary and nonmetastatic gallbladder carcinoma treated with external radiation therapy following attempted curative resection. Patients appeared to benefit from an extended resection versus simple cholecystectomy. Estimated 5-year survival for the entire cohort was 37%, which compares favorably to reported surgery-alone results for locally advanced disease (51). Mayo Clinic investigators reported on 21 patients who underwent resection followed by adjuvant chemoradiotherapy with 5- fluorouracil (5-FU). They reported a 5-year survival rate of 33%, with a

5-year survival of 64% in patients undergoing margin negative resection followed by adjuvant chemoradiotherapy in a cohort consisting primarily of Stage III/IV patients (52). Treadwell et al. reviewed 41 cases of gallbladder cancer with 26 patients undergoing surgery alone and 15 patients treated with adjuvant radiation or chemotherapy. Adjuvantly treated patients experienced improved short-term survival; however, this benefit disappeared after 2-year follow-up (53). Institutional datsets are limited by the rarity of biliary tumor presentation. Thus, population-based datasets may shed some light on the potential benefit of adjuvant radiotherapy. The SEER (Survey of Epidemiology and End Results) dataset from the National Institutes of Health (NIH) has been mined repeatedly. One large National Cancer Database collective report has suggested that patients undergoing trimodality therapy may have a superior survival when compared to patients undergoing surgery alone (6). A study of the SEER database of over 3000 patients diagnosed with gallbladder cancer between 1992 and 2002 showed that patients receiving adjuvant radiation therapy had more advanced disease stage than those treated with surgery alone. Despite this, median survival was significantly improved (14 months vs. 8 months, $p < 0.001$) in patients receiving radiation ther-

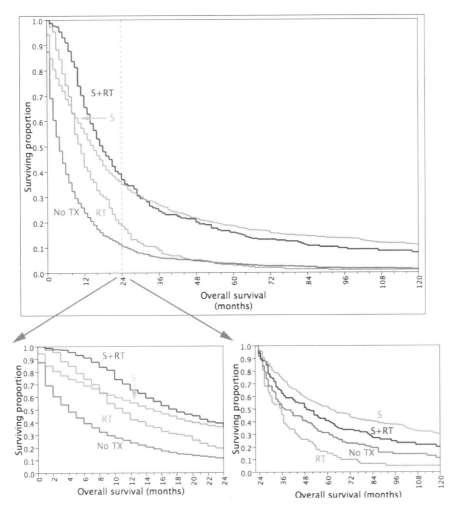

FIGURE 18.3

Kaplan-Meier plot of overall survival for locoregional extrahepatic cholangiocarcinoma from the SEER dataset (1973–1998) by treatment cohort (S, surgery alone; RT, RT alone; S+RT, adjuvant radiotherapy; No TX, no local/regional therapy reported). While early survival is improved, no advantage is observed for those surviving more than 24 months. Bottom shows survival partitioned by time span from diagnosis (0–24 months, left; >24 months, right).

apy. In patients with involved lymph nodes, this benefit was even greater (16 vs. 5 months, $p < 0.001$) and persisted despite the use of radical surgery (54). In another SEER-derived analysis, Wang et al. derived a risk model for estimation of the potential survival benefit for addition of radiotherapy postresection in historic gallbladder carcinoma cohorts (19) and generated a comparative nomogram (Figure 18.4) and online risk prediction tool using said data (19, 20).

Conceivably, such tools might afford identification of specific patient populations whose benefit from radiotherapy postoperatively for gallbladder carcinoma patients. A summary of institutional postoperative RT studies is shown in Table 18.3. These data suggest that an approach of radical resection followed by EBRT with radiosensitizing chemotherapy in patients with locally advanced, nonmetastatic gallbladder cancer may improve ultimate outcomes.

TABLE 18.3

Outcomes Following Surgery for Gallbladder Cancers with Postoperative Radiotherapy (RT)

AUTHOR	N	RT DOSE (GY)	MEDIAN SURVIVAL (MONTHS)	5-YEAR SURVIVAL (%)	LOCAL CONTROL (%)
Czito (51)	22	39.6–60	23	37%[a]	59%[b]
Kresl (52)	21	50.4–60.8	31	33%	73%
Treadwell (53)	15	10–45	—	47%[c]	—

[a] 46% in 18 patients receiving concurrent chemotherapy.
[b] 71% in 18 patients receiving concurrent chemotherapy.
[c] 1-year survival rates.

Preoperative Radiotherapy

Despite multimodality treatment with surgery, radiation, and chemotherapy, the risk of local-regional recurrence in cholangiocarcinomas remains high. This fact, along with a low percentage of potentially resectable patients, has led to investigation of novel treatment approaches in efforts to improve local control and survival. One

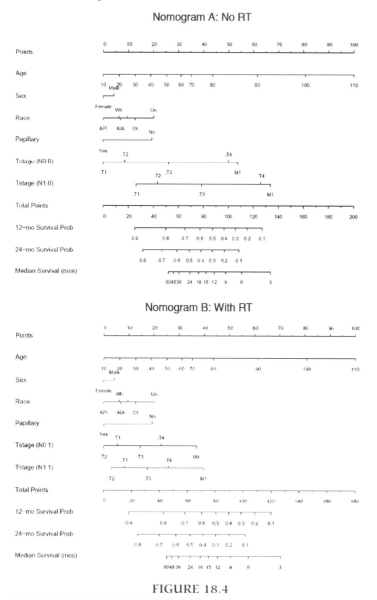

FIGURE 18.4

Nomograms for comparing the expected survival with and without adjuvant RT for cancer of the gallbladder. For an individual patient, first use nomogram **A** to calculate the expected survival without adjuvant RT, and then use nomogram **B** to calculate the expected survival with adjuvant RT. To use the nomogram, first draw a vertical line up to the top "Points" row to assign points for each variable. Then, add up the total points and drop a vertical line from the "Total Points" row to obtain the 12-month overall survival, 24-month overall survival, and median overall survival (in months). The difference between the two estimates is the expected net survival gain from adjuvant RT. (19,20)

such approach is delivering therapy neoadjuvantly. Although no randomized trial data exist on the use of preoperative versus postoperative radiation therapy in biliary tract malignancies, the former offers potential advantages. By postponing surgical resection until completion of chemoradiation, patients with disease that is rapidly progressive may avoid an unnecessary surgical procedure. Preoperative therapy may facilitate tumor downstaging and potentially convert unresectable tumors to resectable, facilitating resection with curative intent. Theoretically, preoperative therapy may reduce tumor seeding and dissemination at the time of resection, as well as allowing tumor irradiation with an intact vasculature. This may improve the therapeutic effect of both chemotherapy and radiotherapy via improved drug delivery and enhanced tumor oxygenation, which renders cells more sensitive to RT. Additionally, the morbidity and delayed recovery time associated with surgery may preclude the timely delivery of postoperative therapy in a high percentage of patients (55, 56).

The role of preoperative versus postoperative therapy has been evaluated in other gastrointestinal cancers. A large, randomized German trial in rectal cancer showed patients receiving neoadjuvant chemoradiation experienced significantly improved local control and less toxicity compared to patients receiving postoperative therapy (57). Duke University investigators reported on 12 patients who were treated neoadjuvantly, primarily because of borderline or unresectable disease as determined by imaging or exploratory laparotomy. Patients received a median dose of 50.4 Gy with concurrent fluoropyrimidine-based chemotherapy. Three of 12 patient experienced patholgoic complete response while the remaining nine showed varying degrees of histologic response; 11 of 12 (91%) achieved R0 resection. At pathologic analysis, no patients treated neoadjuvantly had lymph node metastases. Despite the clinical impression that neoadjuvantly treated patients had primarily borderline or unresectable disease, five-year survival was 53%. Median survival was 4.1 years, comparing favorably to adjuvantly treated patients over the same time period. Only one patient experienced local failure. Additionally, rates of grade 2/3 surgical morbidity were similar to patients treated in the adjuvant setting the over the same time period. (105) A report from M.D. Anderson Cancer Center described 9 patients (5 hilar and 4 distal common duct cholangio-carcinoma) treated with preoperative chemoradiotherapy. Patients received continuous infusion 5-FU at 300 mg/m²/day concurrent with EBRT. Three of 9 patients experienced a pathologic complete response and the remaining 6 varying degrees of histologic response. The rate of margin negative resection was 100% for the preoperative chemoradiation group, compared with 54% for patients receiving surgery alone ($p < 0.01$). Patients receiving preoperative treatment did not experience any treatment-related complications (58). Gerhards et al. described 21 patients with proximal cholangiocarcinoma undergoing low-dose preoperative irradiation (10.5 Gy delivered over three fractions). No patients receiving preoperative treatment developed implantation metastases versus a 20% rate of implant metastases development in similar patients undergoing surgery only (59). Chilean investigators described 14 patients undergoing cholecystectomy revealing transmural gall bladder cancer. Patients then received 45 Gy EBRT with continuous 5-FU followed by repeat resection. Seven patients had residual disease. At a median follow-up of 44 months, 5 (36%) are still alive (60). Japanese investigators reported on 9 patients receiving preoperative radiation therapy with intraluminal brachytherapy (40–94 Gy). No patients received concurrent chemotherapy. One- and 5- year survival rates were 33 and 11%, respectively, and median survival 8.4 months (44).

NONOPERABLE DISEASE

Unresectable Disease

Because the majority of patients with cholangiocarcinoma present with unresectable disease, palliative radiotherapy is an important consideration. For patients with unresectable disease, palliative irradiation following biliary bypass has been shown to prolong survival. A Mayo Clinic report analyzed the outcome of 103 patients with unresectable cholangiocarcinoma. Three-year survival of the entire group was 9%. Multivariate analysis suggested a significant survival benefit for patients receiving additional palliative therapy, including radiotherapy. No details were given (61). Grove et al. noted a survival advantage for locally advanced patients who received radiation therapy versus those who did not (median survival 12.2 vs. 2.2 months) (62). Veeze-Kuijpers et al. reported on 42 patients with unresectable EHBD carcinoma who received EBRT with or without an Ir-192 implant boost. These patients had a 14% 2-year survival and 10-month median survival. Patients undergoing subtotal resection followed by radiation experienced a longer

median survival than those receiving radiation alone (15 vs. 8 months) (63). Crane et al. reported on 52 patients with unresectable cholangiocarcinoma treated with radiation doses ranging from 30 to 85 Gy. Twenty–seven (52%) patients ultimately developed radiographic disease progression, with 20 (74%) of these experiencing local recurrence. The first site of disease progression was local in 72% of cases. Median survival for all patients was 10 months, with 1- and 2-year survival rates of 44% and 13%, respectively. Increasing radiation dose and use of concurrent chemotherapy did not impact any outcome parameters (41). Ghafoori et al. from Duke University reported on 37 patients receiving external beam radiation therapy, with or without brachytherapy, in patients with locally advanced extrahepatic cholangiocarcinoma. Two-year survival was 22% and two-year local control rate 61%. Two patients lived beyond five years without evidence of recurrence. The investigators concluded that most patients had local control of disease at the time of death. (106) Brunner et al. reported on 25 patients with locally advanced or recurrent biliary malignancies. With shrinking field techniques, patients received a median of EBRT dose of 51 Gy. Four patients with Klatskin tumors underwent brachytherapy, and 24 patients received concurrent chemotherapy. Median survival in all patients was 16.5 months versus 9.3 months in patients undergoing stenting alone (64). As mentioned above, limitations of these studies include small sample size, lack of concurrent chemotherapy administration in some patients, possible group imbalance with regard to extent of disease and adverse histologic features, and variable RT techniques. Given this significant heterogeneity among studies, no definitive conclusions as to the benefit, or lack thereof, of "definitive" RT can be reasonably drawn. A summary of studies describing outcomes in patients with unresectable disease is shown in Table 18.4.

Intraluminal Transcatheter Brachytherapy

Despite the addition of EBRT, most patients with gallbladder and bile duct cancer expire of disease-related local progression and obstruction of the biliary tree. This fact suggests that conventional doses of EBRT are insufficient to reliably eradicate all disease. Radiotherapy modalities such as intraluminal brachytherapy have been used alone or in conjunction with EBRT in the treatment of gallbladder and biliary carcinomas. Brachytherapy is the temporary or permanent insertion of radioactive sources into a tumor and/or peritumoral tissues. This permits focal dose escalation of the tumor and peritumoral tissues, resulting in higher effective doses of radiation therapy with sparing of surround-

TABLE 18.4

Results of Radiotherapy (RT) for Unresectable Biliary Cancers

Author	N	RT	RT dose (Gy)	Median survival (months)	3-Year survival (%)	Local control (%)
Farley (61)	103	Yes[a]	—	—	9	—
Grove (62)	19	Yes	12.6–64.0	12.2	10[b]	—
	9	No	—	2.2	—	—
Veeze-Kuijpers (63)	42	Yes	30–65	10	14[b]	—
Crane[f] (41)	52	Yes	30–85 Gy	10	13[b]	41[c]
Brunner[f] (64)	25	Yes	30.4–55.8[d]	16.5	—	—
	39	No	—	9.3	—	—
Kamada (44)	54	Yes	70–135	12.4	13	—
Ghafoori[f] (106)	37	Yes	25-81	14	22[b]	61[e]

[a] In some patients but details not given.
[b] 2-year survival rates.
[c] 1-year local control
[d] EBRT-only doses.
[e] 2-year local control
[f] Concurrent chemotherapy in most

ing normal tissues. This dose escalation should result in improved local control. Although a number of isotopes are available for brachytherapy, Ir-192 is the most widely used source in clinical practice given its high specific activity, short half-life, and ease in shielding.

Advantages of intraluminal brachytherapy include administration of high radiation doses with rapid dose fall-off over a short distance from the radioactive source, sparing adjacent normal tissues and localizing dose to the tumor and peritumoral tissues. Usually, brachytherapy treatments are delivered through a percutaneous transhepatic biliary drainage (PTBD) tube under fluoroscopic guidance or through catheters placed in the tumor bed during surgery. Typical doses delivered with intraluminal therapy range from 20 to 30 Gy prescribed to 0.5–1 cm from the Ir-192 source within the duct (low-dose rate). This treatment is often combined with a course of EBRT (45–50.4 Gy in 25–28 fractions).

Since the original report by Fletcher and coworkers describing the use of intraluminal brachytherapy with Ir-192, multiple studies have demonstrated the feasibility of using brachytherapy alone or in combination with EBRT for treating gallbladder and bile duct cancers (36, 37, 63, 65–72). Although there are no randomized trials comparing combined EBRT plus brachytherapy with either modality alone, some investigators have suggested improved survival among patients treated with combination treatment. Combined EBRT and intraluminal brachytherapy can also provide durable palliation (73–75). Occasional reports have described long-term survival in unresectable patients with the use of EBRT and transcatheter

brachytherapy boost. Foo et al. reported the Mayo Clinic experience of 24 patients with unresectable extrahepatic biliary cancer treated to a median EBRT dose of 50.4 Gy in 28 fractions and median brachytherapy boost of 20 Gy delivered at 1-cm radius. Median and 5-year survival for all patients was 12.8 months and 14%, respectively. At publication, three patients were still alive at 10, 6.9, and 8.2 years after diagnosis. It was recommended that Ir-192 catheter brachytherapy boost be limited to 20–30 Gy when combined with EBRT 45–50 Gy in 25–28 fractions (65). A small prospective study from the Czech Republic randomized 42 patients with cholangiocarcinoma with percutaneous stent to Ir-192 brachytherapy (mean dose 30 Gy) and EBRT (mean dose 50 Gy) or stent placement only. Significant improvement in survival (median 9.8 vs. 12.8 months, $p < 0.05$) was seen in patients receiving radiation therapy. Additionally, reintervention was required in only one patient treated with radiation therapy versus five patients treated with stenting alone. The authors concluded that intraluminal brachytherapy can significantly prolong survival in patients with unresectable disease treated with stent placement (76). Japanese investigators described 93 patients with unresectable extrahepatic bile duct carcinoma (including patients with metastatic disease) who received EBRT and Ir-192 boost. EBRT was delivered at 2 Gy per fraction to a total dose of 50 Gy followed by intraluminal boost to a mean dose of 39 Gy (range 20–50 Gy). Median survival for all patients was 12 months with 1- and 5-year survivals of 50 and 4%, respectively. Four patients survived longer than 5 years. Local regional failure rate was 44% and usually associated with distant metastases. No dose-response relationship to survival was observed (77). Other Japanese investigators reported on 54 patients with unresectable extrahepatic biliary cancers treated with primary radiation therapy (40–50 Gy EBRT) with intraluminal brachytherapy (≥25 Gy). No patients received concurrent chemotherapy. One- and 5- year survival rates were 56 and 6%, respectively with a median survival of 12.4 months (44).

Buskirk and coworkers reported the results of patients with subtotally or unresected disease treated with external beam radiation therapy with or without implant or IORT (intraoperative radiation therapy). Patients who received Ir-192 implant or IORT in addition to EBRT experienced survival longer than 18 months. Additionally, patients who received Ir-192 boost or IORT experienced lower rates of local failure than those who received EBRT alone (±5-FU chemotherapy) (73). Fields et al. reported on 20 patients treated with curative intent; those who received an Ir-192 implant in addition to EBRT exhibited an improved survival when compared to those patients who received EBRT alone (median survival 15 vs. 7 months) (70). Montemaggi and coworkers likewise concluded that the addition of intraluminal RT after biliary drainage prolongs survival (72). In contrast, Italian investigators analyzed the outcome of 22 patients with unresectable/residual extrahepatic biliary tumors receiving external beam radiation therapy, concurrent with 5-FU with or without intraluminal brachytherapy. In their series, brachytherapy had no significant impact on survival (78). Similarly, a study from M.D. Anderson Cancer Center also showed no benefit from the addition of brachytherapy (41).

In addition to potentially enhancing survival, the combination of EBRT and intraluminal brachytherapy may extend stent patency for patients with locally advanced biliary carcinoma. Eschelman et al. described a mean stent patency of 19.5 months and mean survival of 23 months for 11 patients with cholangiocarcinoma treated with EBRT with brachytherapy. This compared favorably to the surgical literature using stenting alone for malignant biliary obstruction (mean stent patency 5–10 months) (74). In a previously described Japanese series, 88 patients underwent metallic stenting followed by EBRT/Ir-192 brachytherapy for unresectable disease. Forty-nine percent of patients developed reobstruction at a mean duration of 11.6 months following treatment. In half of these patients, the cause was deemed to be tumor recurrence. Cumulative biliary patency rates at 1- and 3-years were 52 and 29%, respectively. In 20 patients undergoing autopsy, 17 showed no evidence of tumor-related obstruction. Nonmalignant causes of obstruction included debris, stones, and bleeding (77). External beam radiation therapy may also extend stent patency. Japanese investigators reported on 51 patients with unresectable (10 metastatic) hilar cholangiocarcinoma. Median survival in patients receiving stent plus EBRT (22–50 Gy) was significantly improved versus those receiving metallic expandable metal stent alone or PTBD (13 vs. 7.6 vs. 4.2 months). One-year survival was 57% in patients receiving radiation therapy alone versus 0% in patient undergoing stenting. Importantly, average performance scores were significantly higher in patients receiving radiation therapy, and only one patient receiving radiation therapy developed stent obstruction, with a significant improvement in mean stent patency noted following initial stenting with the addition of radiation therapy (10 months vs. 4 months, $p = 0.0002$). These authors concluded that EBRT combined with endoscopic stenting can increase the length and quality of survival and provide a definite palliative benefit in patients with unresectable hilar cholangiocarcinoma (79).

The most commonly used technique for intraluminal treatment of biliary cancer is low-dose-rate (LDR) brachytherapy. This technique typically delivers doses of 0.4–0.6 Gy/hr at 0.5–1.0 cm depth using Ir-192 sources. Prior to loading of the active sources, the PTBD catheter is typically changed over a wire for a larger 10 French Ford stent, which is more conducive to loading/accommodating an Ir-192 implant. Dummy sources are first inserted to aid in the treatment planning. After dummy source removal, active sources are loaded and accuracy of their placement is confirmed by orthogonal films. Dose calculations are performed and sources remain in place for duration sufficient to deliver the prescribed dose. A dose of 20–30 Gy is usually prescribed to 0.5-cm depth, delivered over approximately 30–50 hours. Following unloading of the implant, the Ford stent is again changed out over a wire for a PTBD catheter and the patient is typically discharged home the same day. Figure 18.5 depicts the placement of intraluminal Ir-192 seeds via PTBD tube.

In contrast to LDR brachytherapy, high-dose-rate (HDR) brachytherapy uses a high activity source, allowing rapid dose delivery (approximately 0.2 Gy/min) compared to LDR techniques. University of Miami investigators reported a phase I/II dose escalation trial utilizing HDR brachytherapy. Eighteen patients with unresectable or subtotally resected extrahepatic biliary duct carcinoma received 45 Gy EBRT with concurrent 5-FU chemotherapy and HDR brachytherapy, using either one, two, or three weekly fractions of 7 Gy delivered at 1-cm depth. Median and 2-year survivals were 12.2 months and 28%, respectively. Three patients survived longer than 5 years. Improved response was seen with increasing doses in the three groups (median survival 9 months vs. 12 months vs. 20 months). The authors concluded that

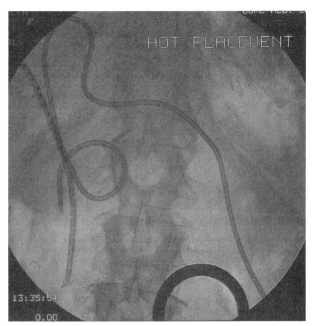

FIGURE 18.5

Placement of intraluminal Ir-192 seeds via a percutaneous transhepatic biliary drainage catheter. Varying pencil marks (left side of image) are used to identify radioactive seeds within the catheter. In contrast to the high-activity Ir-192 sources used in IORT, this low-activity source is usually left in place for 24–48 hours in order to deliver the prescribed dose of radiation.

HDR brachytherapy of 21 Gy in three divided weekly treatments with 45 Gy EBRT with 5-FU–based chemotherapy is well tolerated (80). At the University of Heidelberg, 30 patients undergoing palliative resection or with locally advanced tumors received HDR therapy using Ir-192. Most patients received weekly fraction sizes of 5–10 Gy, to a total dose of 20–45 Gy, along with EBRT to doses of 30–45 Gy. Median survival for the entire group was 10 months, with a 3-year

survival rate of 8%. Seven patients developed duodenal ulceration; however, there was only one case of such in patients receiving 20 Gy in 4 fractions. The authors concluded that a treatment schedule of 40 Gy EBRT along with 20 Gy (5 Gy × 4) by HDR brachytherapy was appropriate for treatment of cholangiocarcinoma (75). Shin et al. analyzed 31 patients with inoperable bile duct carcinoma. Seventeen patients received EBRT alone and 14 EBRT in combination with HDR brachytherapy boost. Median EBRT was 50.4 Gy (range 36–55 Gy). The brachytherapy dose was 15 Gy prescribed to 1.5-cm depth, delivered in 5-Gy fractions over 3 days. Median time to tumor recurrence was improved in patients receiving HDR treatment (5 months vs. 9 months) as was 2-year survival (0% vs. 21%).(81). The role of HDR brachytherapy in biliary cancers remains under investigation.

Given the caveats of patient selection (i.e., better-prognosis patients receiving brachytherapy) and other uncontrolled factors, retrospective data suggest improved survival for locally advanced patients receiving intraluminal brachytherapy. The addition of intraluminal radiotherapy to EBRT may be beneficial, likely due to the increased delivery of radiation dose to the primary tumor along the bile ducts, where the largest volume of gross disease exists. Table 18.5 summarizes the outcome of selected studies utilizing intraluminal therapy.

Intraoperative Radiotherapy

IORT is the delivery of a single high-dose irradiation treatment to the target at the time of operation while minimizing exposure of the surrounding normal tissues, achieving high effective doses. The most commonly used radiation techniques for IORT include electron beam as well as HDR Ir-192 therapy. IORT, in a general sense, has theoretical advantages over intraluminal brachytherapy. Small bowel, stomach, duodenum, and

TABLE 18.5
Outcome of External Beam Radiotherapy Plus Intraluminal Brachytherapy for Biliary Cancers

AUTHOR	N	BRACHYTHERAPY	MEDIAN SURVIVAL (MONTHS)	5-YEAR SURVIVAL (%)	LOCAL CONTROL (%)
Foo (65)	24	Yes	12.8	14	67
Fields (70)	8	Yes	15	—	—
	12	No	7	—	—
Montemaggi (72)	12	Yes	14	—	—
Eschelman (74)	11	Yes	—	22.6[a]	—
Fritz (75)	30	Yes	—	8	—
Takamura (77)	93	Yes	11.9	4	56

[a] 2-year survival rate with noncurative resection.

other normal structures can be directly shielded or displaced during the procedure, thus sparing these tissues. Additionally, tumor or tumor-bearing tissues outside the biliary system can be treated if clinically indicated. Typical IORT doses range from 10 to 20 Gy given as a single fraction. This is generally delivered preceding or following a course of EBRT of 45–50.4 Gy over 25–28 fractions.

The potential role of IORT in the treatment of bile duct cancer was first reported by Japanese physicians. Iwasaki et al. reported on the use of IORT alone or in conjunction with EBRT in 20 patients with biliary cancers. They described a 2-year survival rate of 17% in patients receiving IORT combined with noncurative resection, compared to 9% after noncurative resection alone (27). Deziel and coworkers reviewed the Rush-Presbyterian experience in nine patients with unresectable or partially resected proximal biliary tract cancer. These patients had a median survival of 13 months with the use of IORT, with or without EBRT. These survival figures were comparable to 13 contemporaneous patients treated with EBRT with or without Ir-192 brachytherapy at their institution (82). Busse et al. reported similar results for 15 (12 primary, 3 recurrent) patients treated with IORT with or without EBRT. Median survival of 12 patients with primary disease was 14 months, with disease control in the porta hepatis achieved in 5 of 10 evaluable patients (83). Monson et al. described similar results from the Mayo Clinic with IORT for unresectable cholangiocarcinoma. Thirteen patients experienced a median survival of 16.5 months (84). Todoroki et al. reported on 63 patients

with locally advanced cholangiocarcinoma. Following extended resection, 42 patients received adjuvant RT (12 IORT alone, 22 IORT plus EBRT, 8 EBRT only). Almost all (41/42) patients had microscopic or macroscopic residual disease. Patients receiving adjuvant radiotherapy for microscopic residual experienced improved 5-year survival (34%) versus resection alone (14%). Local-regional control rates were also significantly improved in patients receiving adjuvant RT versus resection alone (79% vs. 31%). The best survival rates were seen in patients who underwent IORT and EBRT (5-year survival 39%) (85). The results of IORT studies are also summarized in Table 18.6.

Radiosensitization with Chemotherapy

The role of chemotherapy alone or in combination with radiation therapy for gallbladder and bile duct carcinomas is unclear. The use of 5-FU–based chemotherapy in combination with radiation is extrapolated from the survival benefit demonstrated in other gastrointestinal malignancies, including pancreatic cancer (86–88). Multiple studies have reported the use of varying combinations of chemotherapy concurrent with RT, with or without surgery. However, the number of patients receiving such treatment is too small to draw definitive conclusions. With these caveats, preliminary results are encouraging.

In an early study, Kopelson et al. reported the feasibility and potential benefit of chemotherapy in addition to radiation (10). Minsky and coworkers reported

TABLE 18.6
Outcome of External Beam Radiotherapy Plus Intraoperative Radiotherapy for Biliary Cancers

Author	N	Boost	Median Survival (Months)	5-Year Survival (%)	Local Control (%)
Buskirk (66)	17	I/B[a]	___	30–43[b]	67–70[c]
	17	No	___	12	47
Iwasaki (27)	20	I	17[d]	___	___
	41	No	9[d]	___	___
Deziel (82)	9	I	14	___	50
Busse (83)	12	I	14	___	50
Monson (84)	13	I	16.5	___	50
Takamura (77)	93	I	11.9	4	56
Todoroki[e] (85)	28	I	32	34	80
	19	No	10	14	31

[a] I/B, some patients received IORT(I) while others received brachytherapy (B).
[b] 18-month survival rate: 30% brachytherapy, 43% IORT.
[c] 67% with IORT and 70% with brachytherapy.
[d] Mean survival.
[e] Includes 5 pts patients receiving EBRT alone; all pts patients underwent R1 resection; 5-year survival in patients receiving IORT with EBRT was 39%.

an aggressive combined modality treatment for biliary carcinoma in 12 patients using EBRT, brachytherapy boost, and concurrent 5-FU/mitomycin-C chemotherapy with or without a curative resection (68). Five patients underwent surgical decompression, and the remaining seven had a biopsy or subtotal resection of the tumor. Median survival for all patients was 17 months and 4-year survival 36%. Four patients had no evidence of disease at 16, 30, 40, and 64 months, respectively. Alden and colleagues described a similar aggressive approach in 19 patients with extrahepatic biliary duct cancer using EBRT, brachytherapy, and chemotherapy (5-FU alone or in combination with doxorubicin or mitomycin-C) (39). They observed a 2-year survival rate of 30%. Foo et al. reporting the Mayo Clinic experience in the treatment of extrahepatic bile duct carcinoma showed a nonstatistical improvement in survival in patients receiving concurrent 5-FU–based chemotherapy versus EBRT alone (65). Reports from the University of Michigan Medical Center at Ann Arbor described 22 patients with hepatobiliary cancers treated with concurrent intrahepatic arterial fluorodeoxyuridine and twice-daily (hyperfractionated) 3D-CRT to either 48 or 66 Gy (depending on the volume of liver irradiated) at 1.5–1.65 Gy per fraction. Median survival of all patients was 16 months with an actuarial 4-year survival of 20%. Overall freedom from hepatic progression at more than 2 years was about 50% (89–92). Crane et al. from M.D. Anderson Cancer Center showed no significant survival impact with the addition of 5-FU–based chemotherapy. However, based on the lack of significant added toxicity from chemotherapy in these studies and proven benefit in other gastrointestinal malignancies, these investigators judged that combined chemoradiation is indicated for biliary tract disease (41). A summary of selected studies in unresectable disease is listed in Table 18.7.

Intrahepatic Cholangiocarcinoma

Intrahepatic cholangiocarcinoma is a rare malignancy, estimated to account for 1% of all hepatic tumors (93). Literature review reveals no significant survival difference between intrahepatic and extrahepatic bile duct cancer, stage for stage, and the treatment philosophy is very similar. Altaee et al. reported a similar median survival of 12 months for 42 patients with intrahepatic cholangiocarcinoma and 70 patients with perihilar biliary cancers (94). Literature review suggests median survival for all patients undergoing radical resection for intrahepatic cholangiocarcinoma ranges from 5 to 26 months (98). Although limited data are available, recurrence in the liver remnant following resection occurs in 38–70% of patients. Local-regional lymph nodes are also a common site of failure (93). In one series of 123 patients with intrahepatic cholangiocarcinoma, 56 underwent curative resection. Recurrence was observed in 46 patients, primarily occurring in the liver, lymph nodes, and intraductal sites (95).

Ben-Josef et al. treated 46 patients with intrahepatic cholangiocarcinomas with high-dose conformal external radiation combined with hepatic arterial floxuridine. Median survival was 13.3 months, which compared favorably to historical controls. Increasing radiation dose was associated with improved prognosis, with patients receiving ≥75 Gy experiencing significantly improved survival versus those receiving lower doses. These results appear promising, notably in the setting of biliary carcinomas with a significant intrahepatic ductal component (96). Chen et al. reviewed 20 patients with intrahepatic cholangiocarcinoma who underwent curative or palliative surgery followed by intraluminal brachytherapy and chemotherapy. Median survival for all patients was 20.5 months, with four patients living more than 3 years and one patient alive at 5 years. This seemingly improved survival was judged to be due to early diagnosis in most patients

TABLE 18.7
Concurrent Chemoradiotherapy for Biliary Carcinomas

AUTHOR (REF.)	N	CHEMOTHERAPY	MEDIAN SURVIVAL (MONTHS)	SURVIVAL (%)
Minsky (68)	12	5-FU + mitomycin-C[a]	17	36[e]
Alden (39)	19	5-FU[b]	—	30[c]
Kopelson (10)	13	5-FU	12.7	—
Deodato (78)	22	5-FU	23[d]	41[c]

[a] 5-FU, 5-fluorouracil.
[b] 5-FU alone or in combination with doxorubicin or mitomycin-C.
[c] 2-year survival rate.
[d] One patient did not receive 5-FU.
[e] 4-year survival rate.

(97). Analysis of the SEER database of nearly 4000 patients showed that only 17% of patients with intrahepatic cholangiocarcinoma received radiation therapy, either alone or in combination with surgery. Median overall survival was 11, 6, 7, and 3 months for patients undergoing surgery with adjuvant radiation therapy, surgery alone, radiation therapy alone or no treatment. Survival was significantly improved in patients receiving surgery and adjuvant radiation therapy versus surgery alone, as well as with radiation therapy alone versus no treatment. The authors concluded that adjuvant and definitive radiation therapy prolongs survival in patients with intrahepatic cholangiocarcinoma (107). Because reports of radiation delivered either adjuvantly or in a "definitive" fashion for intrahepatic cholangiocarcinomas are limited, definitive conclusions about its role are difficult.

Radiotherapy with Hepatic Transplant

Because of the poor prognosis associated with cholangiocarcinoma, investigators have pursued novel treatment approaches to improve outcomes. One strategy has been to combine chemoradiotherapy with liver transplantation. At the University of Pittsburgh, 61 patients with biopsy proven cholangiocarcinoma received a median "preoperative" radiation dose of 49.5 Gy (range 5.4–85), including four patients who received brachytherapy. Concurrent chemotherapy was administered in 30 patients. Five-year survival for the entire cohort was 24%. Patients undergoing complete resection had a 54% 5-year survival. Seventeen patients with uninvolved lymph nodes undergoing orthotopic liver transplantation experienced a 5-year survival of 65%. This compared favorably to a 22% 4-year survival in a prior report from this group. The authors concluded that complete surgical resection in combination with combined modality therapy, with or without transplantation, can be curative in the majority of patients with biliary carcinoma (99, 100). A report from the Mayo Clinic described 56 patients undergoing neoadjuvant EBRT, brachytherapy, and 5-FU–based chemotherapy for early-stage perihilar cholangiocarcinoma. Patients received 45 Gy EBRT delivered in 30 fractions over 3 weeks (2 fractions per day) along with concurrent intravenous 5-FU. Patients then received a transluminal boost of 20–30 Gy with Ir-192 with concurrent 5-FU. Eligible patients then went on to undergo liver transplantation. Twenty-eight patients underwent transplantation, with seven (25%) showing pathologic complete response. Five-year survival for all patients was 54%. In patients undergoing transplantation, 5-year survival was 82%. The authors concluded that neoadjuvant chemoradiotherapy with transplantation

achieved excellent results for patients with localized, node negative hilar cholangiocarcinoma (101). A follow-up study from this group reported on 71 patients undergoing neoadjuvant chemoradiotherapy. Of these, 61 subsequently underwent operative staging, and 38 of these underwent transplantation. Sixteen of 38 (42%) patients showed no evidence of residual tumor, with a 5-year recurrence rate of 12%. Survival for all patients enrolled was 58% at 5 years, 66% for patients undergoing operative staging, and 82% for patients undergoing transplantation (102). These results suggest that cholangiocarcinoma (compared to pancreatic cancer) may be a relatively radiosensitive disease. Treatment strategies of chemoradiation with liver transplantation appear encouraging and are under active investigation.

Charged-Particle Radiotherapy

Charged particles such as protons and helium ions have also been used in the treatment of gallbladder and biliary cancers. In contrast to photons, the energy-deposition patterns from charged particles are highly localized. This is due to a disproportionate absorption of the majority of their energy at the end of their track range, the so-called Bragg peak. The dose unit of charged particles is the Gray equivalent (GyE). Figure 18.6 demonstrates the energy deposition patterns of 15 MV photons, 9 MeV electrons, 30 MeV neutrons, 160 MeV protons, and Ir-192 seeds.

Schoenthaler and coworkers at the University of California at San Francisco reviewed their experience of 129 patients with extrahepatic bile duct carcinoma. Sixty-two patients were treated with surgery alone, and of these, 24% underwent gross total resection. The remaining surgery-only patients underwent debulking,

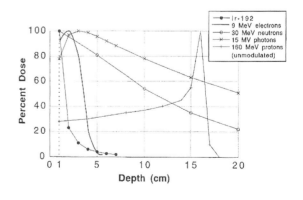

FIGURE 18.6

Relative dose deposition as a function of depth for varying radiation sources, including Ir-192 seeds, 9 MeV electrons, 30 MeV neutrons, 15 MV photons, and 160 MeV protons.

biopsy, or decompression alone. Sixty-seven patients received adjuvant radiotherapy, 45 with conventional EBRT and 22 with charged particles using helium and/or neon. Patients who underwent gross total resection or received greater than 45 Gy (E) after any surgical procedure were defined as treated with "curative intent." Fifty patients were treated with curative intent in the surgery-alone group, 35 in the surgery-plus-conventional-RT group, and 18 in the surgery-plus-charged particle group. Five patients in the conventional RT group also received Ir-192 brachytherapy. Improved survival was seen in patients undergoing gross total resection versus those undergoing debulking or decompression only. Patients with microscopic residual disease experienced an improved median survival with the addition of adjuvant irradiation, more so after charged particle therapy (p = 0.0005), but also with conventional RT (p = 0.01). Patients with gross residual disease had a less marked but still statistically significant improved survival after irradiation (p = 0.05 for conventional RT and p = 0.04 for charged-particle RT). Median survival with surgery alone, surgery plus conventional RT, and surgery plus charged particle therapy was 6.5, 11, and 14 months for the entire group, respectively, and 16, 16, and 23 months for patients treated with curative intent, respectively (p = 0.008) (103).

Metastases to the Hepatobiliary System

The treatment of hepatobiliary metastases from other primary cancers by irradiation is generally used for symptomatic relief of pain and obstructive symptoms. Generally, biliary stent placement (either endoscopically or percutaneously) is performed when possible. Radiation therapy is often used adjunctively in attempts to eradicate disease causing obstruction. Approximately two thirds of symptomatic patients experience relief of pain and obstructive symptoms, including pruritus and jaundice, though most patients also require stenting. EBRT doses ranging from 30 Gy in 10 fractions to 60 Gy in 30–33 fractions have been used. The most commonly used palliative RT dose to the whole liver is 21 Gy in 7 fractions. Small portions of the liver or extrahepatic biliary tract can be palliatively irradiated to a much higher dose as in many cases; however, doses must be individualized and normal tissue tolerance respected.

OTHER RARE MALIGNANCIES OF GALLBLADDER AND BILIARY SYSTEM

Rare malignancies of the gallbladder and bile duct such as anaplastic carcinoma, squamous cell carcinoma, and adenocanthoma are generally treated in a similar fashion as adenocarcinoma, though data are lacking. Primary biliary sarcoma is exceedingly rare, and the prognosis is poor in spite of treatment.

Lymphoma of the gallbladder and bile duct is rare and is generally treated with a combined modality approach with chemotherapy and low-dose irradiation. Typical radiation doses range from 25 to 40 Gy (at 1.8–2 Gy/fraction, 5 days/wk), usually given in series with chemotherapy, depending upon stage and histology of disease.

TOXICITIES AND COMPLICATIONS

Potential acute toxicities of EBRT and chemotherapy include nausea, vomiting, anorexia, dehydration, skin irritation, distal esophagitis, gastritis, duodenitis, fatigue, weight loss, asymptomatic elevation in liver function tests (usually alkaline phosphatase), and mild immunosuppression. In a series of 81 patients with extrahepatic cholangiocarcinoma receiving combined chemotherapy and radiation therapy, the incidence of acute nausea, fatigue, and diarrhea was 41, 31, and 16%, respectively. Five patients with hilar carcinoma developed late complications (ulcer formation, gastritis, liver veno-occlusive disease) at a median onset of 6 months (104).

Most acute symptoms resolve following treatment completion. Late-treatment–related complications of RT for biliary carcinomas include gastrointestinal bleeding (especially duodenal), biliary fibrosis and duct stricture, cholangitis, hepatitis, and small bowel obstruction. Complications related to radiotherapy may be difficult to define precisely as many patients do not survive long enough to exhibit such effects. Signs and symptoms suggesting treatment-related complication may be nonspecific and potentially related to tumor progression (i.e., gastrointestinal bleeding, biliary fibrosis and stricture, cholangitis, and hepatitis); additionally, many patients have undergone numerous therapeutic interventions that carry similar complications.

Nevertheless, when EBRT doses of >55 Gy are used in the treatment of gallbladder and biliary carcinoma, as many as 30–50% of patients will develop complications such as duodenal hemorrhage, ulceration, and obstruction (9). Care must always be taken to respect dose tolerance of surrounding normal structures (see Table 18.1). When treating with EBRT doses of 45–50 Gy at 1.8–2.0 Gy per fraction combined with the brachytherapy boost, gastrointestinal complications including bleeding and ulceration have been reported (37, 66, 73, 104). Therefore, LDR brachytherapy doses should be limited to 20–30 Gy or less when combined with "curative" EBRT doses of 45–50.4 Gy. In addition, it is important to ensure that implant sources not pass beyond the ampulla, reducing the risk

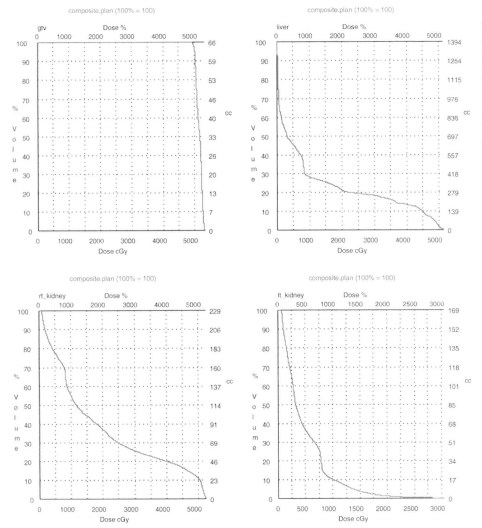

FIGURE 18.7

Dose volume histogram (DVH) for patient treated preoperatively for biliary cancer. GTV, gross tumor volume. Each curve displays the volume of tumor or normal organ receiving a specified radiation dose.

of resultant bleeding. When treating biliary carcinomas with IORT, doses in excess of 20 Gy have been associated with significant complications, including hepatic artery injury, and should generally be avoided. As above, efforts should be made to shield nontarget tissues from the treatment field by mobilization and shielding devices.

TREATMENT RECOMMENDATIONS

Based on patterns of failure in patients with resected biliary cancers, and the previously discussed data, EBRT concurrent with 5-FU–based chemotherapy should be considered in the pre- or postoperative setting. A similar approach is adopted in patients with locally advanced disease. Locally advanced patients treated neoadjuvantly are restaged following treatment and reevaluated for resection. Computed tomography–based treatment planning and multiple field techniques are used. Customized field shaping is

achieved using a computerized blocking system (multileaf collimation) to shield nontarget tissues. High-energy (≥6 MV) photons are used to treat all fields. Figure 18.7 demonstrates a dose-volume histogram (DVH) generated through three-dimensional planning. The DVH displays the volume of tumor and surrounding normal tissues/organs receiving a specified radiation dose level.

Recent innovations in radiation planning and delivery have been achieved through the use of computer-aided beam orientation and optimization, referred to as intensity-modulated radiotherapy (IMRT). This permits optimized dose distribution within the defined target as well as decreased normal tissue irradiation with a decrease in treatment-related side effects and should be considered in the treatment of these patients. Additionally, the use of "four-dimensional" treatment planning should be employed. These techniques account for the variable of organ/tumor motion using externally or internally placed fiducial markers which track the tumor during respiration and permit precise treatment delivery. In the preoperative or postoperative setting, doses generally ranging from 45 to 54 Gy are delivered at 1.8 Gy/fraction, 5 days per week using multiple fields. Final dose is selected individually for each case, depending on factors such as extent of resection, volume of normal tissues irradiated, etc. For patients with locally advanced/unresectable disease, "definitive" chemoradiation is utilized. Typically, patients receive EBRT to a dose of 50.4–54 Gy at 1.8 Gy per day, 5 days per week. As in potentially resectable patients, concurrent 5-FU–based chemotherapy is delivered. Selected patients with a good performance status may receive additional dose by Ir-192 implant (typically 20–30 Gy delivered at approximately 10 Gy/day, prescribed to 0.5 cm from the source).

CONCLUSIONS AND FUTURE DIRECTIONS

Gallbladder and bile duct cancers carry a poor prognosis. Innovative treatment strategies are mandatory to improve upon these poor results. Surgery, when feasible, remains the only curative treatment modality. Most patients undergoing resection are found to have adverse pathologic prognostic factors (lymphovascular invasion, involved lymph nodes, involved margins, etc.) and are often referred for adjuvant irradiation. RT (with or without chemotherapy) decreases the risk of local-regional recurrence and may improve survival. Given the rarity of malignancy, no randomized data exist proving a survival advantage. Patients receiving concurrent chemoradiation appear to have an improved survival compared to those receiving radiotherapy alone, possibly due to radiosensitization effect by chemotherapy. An aggressive multimodality approach should be considered in appropriate patients who are potentially resectable by combining surgery and EBRT with concurrent chemotherapy. Intraoperative radiotherapy and/or brachytherapy with Ir-192 may be useful for selected patients. For unresectable cancers, combined modality therapy with EBRT and chemotherapy is advised, followed by restaging and consideration of resection and IORT in select patients. Intraluminal brachytherapy may allow further dose escalation in patients not suitable for resection.

Despite these efforts, the majority of patients with biliary cancers will succumb to their disease. The integration of novel therapeutic strategies in this disease is indicated, including combined modality therapy with hepatic transplant as well as use of potential radiosensitizers such as epidermal growth factor receptor (EGFR) antagonist, receptor tyrosine kinase inhibitors, and vascular endothelial growth factor inhibitors. When combined with traditional chemotherapeutic agents and precision radiation techniques such as IMRT and four

dimensional treatment delivery, these strategies may improve local control and survival in these patients.

ACKNOWLEDGMENT

We would like to express great thanks to Wanda Lawrence for her assistance in preparation of this chapter.

*R*eferences

1. Jemal A, Siegel R, Ward E, et al. Cancer statistics, 2007. CA Cancer J Clin 2007; 57:43–66.
2. Piehler JM, Crichlow RW. Primary carcinoma of the gallbladder. Surg Gynecol Obstet 1978; 147:929–942.
3. Yee K, Sheppard BC, Domreis J, et al. Cancers of the gallbladder and biliary ducts. Oncology (Williston Park) 2002; 16:939–946, 949; discussion 949–950.
4. Daines WP, Rajagopalan V, Grossbard ML, et al. Gallbladder and biliary tract carcinoma: a comprehensive update, Part 2. Oncology (Williston Park) 2004; 18:1049–1059; discussion 1060, 1065–1068.
5. Mahe A, Stampfli C, Romestang P, et al. Primary carcinoma of the gallbladder: Potential for external radiation therapy. Radiother Oncol 1994; 33:204–208.
6. Donohue JH, Stewart K, Menck H. The National Cancer Data Base Report on carcinoma of the gallbladder, 1989–1995. Cancer 1998; 83:2618–2628.
7. Todoroki T, Gunderson L, Nagorney D. Biliary Tract IORT. Totowa, NJ: Humana Press, 1999.
8. Maibenco DC, Smith JL, Nava HR, et al. Carcinoma of the gallbladder. Cancer Invest 1998; 16:33–39.
9. Schoenthaler R. Hepatobiliary Carcinomas. Philadelphia: WB Saunders, 1998.
10. Kopelson G, Harisiadis L, Tretter P, et al. The role of radiation therapy in cancer of the extra-hepatic biliary system: an analysis of thirteen patients and a review of the literature of the effectiveness of surgery, chemotherapy and radiotherapy. Int J Radiat Oncol Biol Phys 1977; 2:883–894.
11. Kopelson G, Galdabini J, Warshaw AL, et al. Patterns of failure after curative surgery for extra-hepatic biliary tract carcinoma: implications for adjuvant therapy. Int J Radiat Oncol Biol Phys 1981; 7:413–417.
12. Cady B, McDonald J, Gunderson LL. Cancer of the Hepatobiliary System Philadelphia: Lippincott, 1985.
13. Vaittinen E. Carcinoma of the gallbladder: a study of 390 cases diagnosed in Finland 1953–1967. Ann Chir Gyn Fenn 1970; 168:1–81 suppl.
14. Jarnagin WR, Ruo L, Little SA, et al. Patterns of initial disease recurrence after resection of gallbladder carcinoma and hilar cholangiocarcinoma: implications for adjuvant therapeutic strategies. Cancer 2003; 98:1689–1700.
15. Park S, Park Y, Chung J, et al. Patterns and relevant factors of tumor recurrence for extrahepatic bile duct carcinoma after radical resection. Hepato-gastroenterology 2004; 51:1612–1618.
16. Kim JK, Ha HK, Han DJ, et al. CT analysis of postoperative tumor recurrence patterns in periampullary cancer. Abdom Imaging 2003; 28:384–391.
17. de Castro SM, Kuhlmann KF, van Heek NT, et al. Recurrent disease after microscopically radical (R0) resection of periampullary adenocarcinoma in patients without adjuvant therapy. J Gastrointest Surg 2004; 8:775–784; discussion 784.
18. Mojica P, Smith D, Ellenhorn J. Adjuvant radiation therapy is associated with improved survival for gallbladder carcinoma with regional metastatic disease. J Surg Oncol 2007; 96:8–13.
19. Wang SJ, Fuller CD, Sanghvi PR, et al. A regression model for predicting the survival benefit of adjuvant radiotherapy for gallbladder cancer. Int J Radiation Oncol Biol Physics 2007; 69:S550–S551.

20. Wang SJ, Fuller CD, Kim JS, Sittig DF, Thomas CR Jr, Ravdin PM. Prediction model for estimating the survival benefit of adjuvant radiotherapy for gallbladder cancer. J Clin Oncol. 2008 May 1;26(13):2112-7.

21. Shivnani AT, Lee CM, Tward JD, et al. Survival outcomes for adjuvant radiation therapy versus no radiation therapy in extrahepatic cholangiocarcinoma: a surveillance, epidemiology, and end results (SEER) analysis. Int J Radiation Oncol Biol Physics 2007; 69:S283.

22. Fuller CD, Thomas CR, Wang SJ. Adjuvant radiotherapy demonstrates improved survival for locoregional extrahepatic cholangiocarcinoma (EHCC): a population-based analysis. Int J Radiation Oncol Biol Physics 2007; 69:S279.

23. Rubin P, Cooper R, Phillips T. Radiation biology and radiation pathology syllabus. Chicago, 1975.

24. Rubin P, Constine L, Williams J. Late Effects of Cancer Treatment: Radiation and Drug Toxicity. 3rd ed. Philadelphia: Lippincott-Raven, 1998.

25. Dawson LA, Ten Haken RK, Lawrence TS. Partial irradiation of the liver. Semin Radiat Oncol. 2001 Jul; 11(3):240-6.

26. Willett CG, Tepper JE, Orlow EL, et al. Renal complications secondary to radiation treatment of upper abdominal malignancies. Int J Radiat Oncol Biol Phys 1986; 12:1601–1604.

27. Iwasaki Y, Todoroki T, Fukao K, et al. The role of intraoperative radiation therapy in the treatment of bile duct cancer. World J Surg 1988; 12:91–98.

28. Henson D, Albores-Saavedra J, Corre D, et al. Carcinoma of the gallbladder: histologic types, stage of disease, grade, and survival rates. Cancer 1992; 70:1493–1497.

29. Sons HU, Borchard F, Joel BS, et al. Carcinoma of the gallbladder: autopsy findings in 287 cases and review of the literature. J Surg Oncol 1985; 28:199–206.

30. Shamada H, Endo I, Togo S, et al. The role of lymph node dissection in the treatment of gallbladder carcinoma. Cancer 1997; 79:892–899.

31. Tsukada K, Korosaki I, Uchida K, et al. Lymph nodes spread from carcinoma of the gallbladder. Cancer 1997; 80:661–667.

32. Ogura Y, Mizumoto R, Isaji S, et al. Radical operations for carcinoma of the gallbladder: present status in Japan. World J Surg 1991; 15:337–343.

33. Fahim R, McDonald J, Richards J, et al. Carcinoma of the gallbladder: a study of its modes of spread. Ann Surg 1962; 156:114.

34. Cariaga F, Henson D. Liver, gallbladder, extrahepatic bile ducts, and pancreas. Cancer 1995; 75:171–190.

35. Cheng S, Huang A. Liver and hepatobiliary tract. In: Perez C, Brady LW, Halperin E, et al. (eds.). Principles and Practice of Radiation Oncology. Philadelphia: Lippincott Williams and Wilkins, 2004.

36. Mahe M, Romestaing P, Talon B, et al. Radiation therapy in extrahepatic bile duct carcinoma. Radiother Oncol 1991; 21:121–127.

37. Hayes J, Sapozink M, Miller F, et al. Definitive radiation therapy in bile duct cancer. Int J Radiat Oncol Biol Phys 1988; 15:735–744.

38. Mittal M, Romestaing P, Iwatsuki S, et al. Primary cancers of extrahepatic biliary passages. Int J Radiat Oncol Biol Phys 1985; 11:849–854.

39. Alden ME, Mohiuddin M. The impact of radiation dose in combined external beam and intraluminal Ir-192 brachytherapy for bile duct cancer. Int J Radiat Oncol Biol Phys 1994; 28:945–951.

40. Gonzalas Gonzalas D, Gouma D, Rauws E, et al. Role of radiotherapy, in particular intraluminal brachytherapy, in the treatment of proximal bile duct carcinoma. Ann Oncol 1999; 10:215–220.

41. Crane C, McDonald K, Bauthty J, et al. Limitations of conventional doses of chemoradiation for unresectable biliary cancer. Int J Radiat Oncol Biol Phys 2002; 53:969–974.

42. Gonzales Gonzales D, Gerard J, Maners A. Results of radiation therapy in carcinoma of the proximal bile duct (Klatskin tumor). Semin Liver Dis 1990; 10:131–141.

43. Sagawa N, Kondo S, Morikawa T, et al. Effectiveness of radiation therapy after surgery for hilar cholangiocarcinoma. Surg Today 2005; 35:548–552.

44. Kamada T, Saitou H, Takamura A, et al. The role of radiotherapy in the management of extrahepatic bile duct cancer: an analysis of 145 consecutive patients treated with intraluminal and/or external beam radiotherapy. Int J Radiat Oncol Biol Phys 1996; 34:767–774.

45. Cameron J, Pitt H, Zinner M, et al. Management of proximal cholangiocarcinomas by surgical resection and radiotherapy. Am J Surg 1990; 159:91–98.

46. Hughes MA, Frassica DA, Yeo CJ, et al. Adjuvant concurrent chemoradiation for adenocarcinoma of the distal common bile duct. Int J Radiat Oncol Biol Phys 2007; 68:178–182.

47. Gerhards M, Vangulik T, Gonzalez Gonzalez D, et al. Results of posteroperative radiotherapy for resectable hilar cholangiocarcinoma. World J Surg 2003; 27:173–179.

48. Oh D, Lim do H, Heo JS, et al. The role of adjuvant radiotherapy in microscopic tumor control after extrahepatic bile duct cancer surgery. Am J Clin Oncol 2007; 30:21–25.

49. Kim S, Kim S, Bang Y, et al. The role of postoperative radiotherapy in the management of extrahepatic bile duct cancer. Int J Rad Onc Biol Phys 2003; 54:414–419.

50. Pitt H, Nakeeb A, Abrams R, et al. Perihilar cholangiocarcinoma. Postoperative radiotherapy does not improve survival. Ann Surg 1995; 221:788–798.

51. Czito B, Hurwitz H, Clough R, et al. Adjuvant external beam radiotherapy with concurrent chemotherapy following resection of primary gallbladder carcinoma: a 23-year experience. Int J Rad Onc Biol Phys 2005; 62:1030–1034.

52. Kresl JJ, Schild SE, Henning GT, et al. Adjuvant external beam radiation therapy with concurrent chemotherapy in the management of gallbladder carcinoma. Int J Radiat Oncol Biol Phys 2002; 52:167–175.

53. Treadwell T, Hardin W. Primary carcinoma of the gallbladder. The role of adjunctive therapy in its treatment. Am J Surg 1976; 132:703–706.

54. Mojica P, Smith D, Ellenhorn J, et al. Adjuvant radiation therapy is associated with improved survival for gallbladder carcinoma with regional metastatic disease. J Surg Oncol 2007.

55. Sohn T, Yeo C, Cameron J, et al. Resected adenocarcinoma of the pancreas—616 patients: results, outcomes, and prognostic indicators. J Gastrointest Surg 2000; 4:567–579.

56. Spitz F, Abbruzzese J, Lee J, et al. Preoperative and postoperative chemoradiation strategies in patients treated with pancreaticoduodectomy for adenocarcinoma of the pancreas. J Clin Oncol 1997; 15:928–937.

57. Sauer R, Becker, H, Hohenberger W, et al. Preoperative versus postoperative chemoradiotherapy for rectal cancer. N Engl J Med 204;351:1731-40.

58. McMasters K, Tuttle T, Leach S, et al. Neoadjuvant chemoradiation enhances margin-negative resection rates for extrahepatic cholangiocarcinoma. Am J Surg 1997; 174:605–609.

59. Gerhards M, Gonzalez Gonzalez D, Hoopen-Neumann t, et al. Prevention of implantation metastases after resection of proximal bile duct tumors with pre-operative low dose radiation therapy. Eur J Surg Oncol 2000; 26:40–45.

60. de Aretxabala X, Roa I, Berrios M, et al. Chemoradiotherapy in gallbladder cancer. J Surg Oncol 2006; 93:699–704.

61. Farley D, Weaver A, Nagorney D. "Natural history" of unresected cholangiocarcinoma: patient outcome after noncurative intervention. Mayo Clin Proc 1995; 70:425–429.

62. Grove M, Hermann R, Vogt D, et al. Role of radiation after operative palliation in cancer of the proximal bile ducts. Am J Surg 1991; 161:454–458.

63. Veeze-Kuijpers B, Merrwaldt J, Mameris J, et al. The role of radiotherapy in the treatment of bile duct carcinoma. Int J Radiat Oncol Biol Phys 1990; 18:63–67.

64. Brunner T, Schwab D, Meyer T, et al. Chemoradiation may prolong survival of patients with non-bulky unresectable extrahepatic biliary carcinoma: A retrospective analysis. Strahlenther Onkol 2004; 180:751–757.

65. Foo ML, Gunderson LL, Bender CE, et al. External radiation therapy and transcatheter iridium in the treatment of extra-

hepatic bile duct carcinoma. Int J Radiat Oncol Biol Phys 1997; 39:929–935.

66. Buskirk SJ, Gunderson LL, Adson MA, et al. Analysis of failure following curative irradiation of gallbladder and extrahepatic bile duct carcinoma. Int J Radiat Oncol Biol Phys 1984; 10:2013–2023.

67. Fletcher M, Dawson J, Wheeler P, et al. Treatment of high bile duct carcinoma by internal radiotherapy with iridium-192 wire. Lancet 1981; 2:172–174.

68. Minsky B, Wesson M, Armstrong JG, et al. Combined modality therapy of extrahepatic biliary system cancer. Int J Radiat Oncol Biol Phys 1990; 18:1157–1163.

69. Minsky BD, Kemeny N, Armstrong JG, et al. Extrahepatric biliary system cancer: an update of a combined modality approach. Am J Clin Oncol 1991; 14:433–437.

70. Fields J, Emami B. Carcinoma of the extrahepatic biliary system—results of primary and adjuvant radiotherapy. Int J Radiat Oncol Biol Phys 1987; 13:331–338.

71. Johnson D, Safai C, Goffinet D. Malignant obstruction jaundice: treatment with external-beam and intracavitary radiotherapy. Int J Radiat Oncol Biol Phys 1985; 11:411–416.

72. Montemaggi O, Costamagna G, Dobelbower R, et al. Intraluminal brachytherapy in the treatment of pancreas and bile duct carcinoma. Int J Radiat Oncol Biol Phys 1995; 32:437–443.

73. Buskirk SJ, Gunderson LL, Schild S, et al. Analysis of failure after curative irradiation of extrahepatic bile duct carcinoma. Ann Surg 1991; 215:125–131.

74. Eschelman D, Shapiro M, Bonn J, et al. Malignant biliary duct obstruction: long-term experience with Gianturco stents and combined-modality radiation therapy. Radiology 1996; 200:717–724.

75. Fritz P, Branbs H, Schraube P, et al. Combined external beam radiotherapy in intralumenal high-dose-rate brachytherapy on bile duct carcinoma. Int J Radiat Oncol Biol Phys 1994; 29:855–861.

76. Valek V, Kysela P, Kala Z, et al. Brachytherapy and percutaneous stenting in the treatment of cholangiocarcinoma: a prospective randomised study. Eur J Radiol 2007; 62: 175–179.

77. Takamura A, Saito H, Camada T, et al. Intraluminal low-doserate Ir192 brachytherapy combined with external beam radiotherapy and biliary stenting for unresectable extrahepatic bile duct carcioma. Int J Radiat Oncol Biol Phys 2003; 1357–1365.

78. Deodata F, Clemente G, Mattiucci G, et al. Chemoradiation and brachytherapy in biliary tract carcinoma: long-term results. Int J Rad Oncol Biol Phys 2006; 64:683–688.

79. Shinchi H, Takao S, Nishida H, et al. Length and quality of survival following external beam radiotherapy combined with expandable metallic stent for unresectable hilar cholangiocarcinoma. J Surg Oncol 2000; 75:89–94.

80. Lu J, Baines Y, Abdel-Wahab M, et al. High-dose-rate remote after loading intracavitary brachytherapy for the treatment of extra hepatic biliary duct carcinoma. Cancer 2002; 8:74–78.

81. Shin H, Seong J, Kim W, et al. Combination of external beam irradiation in high-dose-rate intraluminal brachytherapy for inoperable carcinoma of the extrahepatic bile ducts. Int J Radiat Oncol Biol Phys 2003; 57:105–112.

82. Deziel D, Kiel K, Kranner T, et al. Intraoperative radiation therapy in biliary tract cancer. Am Surg 1988; 54:402–407.

83. Busse P, Stone M, Sheldon T. Intraopertive radiation therapy for biliary tract carcinoma: results of a 5-year experience. Surgery 1989; 105:724–733.

84. Monson JR, Donohue JH, Gunderson LL, et al. Intraoperative radiotherapy for unresectable cholangiocarcinoma—the Mayo Clinic experience. Surg Oncol 1992; 1:283–290.

85. Todoroki T, OHara K, Kawamoto T, et al. Benefits of adjuvant radiotherapy after radical resection of locally advanced main hepatic duct carcinoma. Int J Radiat Oncol Biol Phys 2000; 46:581–587.

86. Moertel C, Childs D, Reitmeier R, et al. Combined 5-fluorouracil and supervoltage radiation therapy of locally unresectable gastrointestinal cancer. Lancet 1969; 2:865–867.

87. Moertel C, Frytak S, Hahn R, et al. Therapy of locally unresectable pancreatic carcinoma: A randomomized comparison of high-dose (6000 rads) radiation alone, moderate dose radiation (4000 rads + 5-fluorouracil) and high-dose radiation plus 5-fluorouracil. Cancer 1981; 48:1705–1710.

88. Kalser M, Elenberg S. Pancreatic cancer: adjuvant combine radiation and chemotherapy following curative resection. Arch Surg 1985; 120:899–903.

89. Lawrence TS, Dworzanin L, Walker-Andrews S, et al. Treatment of cancers involving the liver and porta hepatis with external beam irradiation and intraarterial hepatic fluorodexoyuridine. Int J Radiat Oncol Biol Phys 1991; 20:555–561.

90. McGinn C, Lawrence TS. Clinical results of the combination of radiation and fluoropyrimidines in the treatment of intrahepatic cancer. Sem Rad Oncol 1997; 7:313–323.

91. Robertson J, McGinn C, Walker S, et al. Phase I trial of hepatic arterial bromodeoxyuridine and conformal radiation therapy for patients with primary hepatobiliary cancers or colorectal liver metastases. Int J Radiat Oncol Biol Phys 1997; 39:1087–1092.

92. Robertson J, Lawrence TS, Anderson J, et al. Long-term results of hepatic artery fluorodeoxyuridine and conformal radiation therapy for primary hepatobiliary cancers. Int J Radiat Oncol Biol Phys 1997; 37:325–330.

93. Martin R, Jarnagin W. Intrahepatic cholangiocarcinoma: current management. Minerva Chir 2003; 58:469–478.

94. Altaee M, Johnson P, Farrant M, et al. Etiologic and clinical characteristics of peripheral and hilar cholangiocarcinoma. Cancer 1991; 68:2051–2055.

95. Maymamoto M, Takasiki K, Otsubo T, et al. Recurrence after surgical resection of intrahepatic cholangiocarcinoma. J Hepatobiliary Pancreat Surg 2001; 8:154–157.

96. Ben-Josef E, Normolle D, Ensminger W, et al. Phase II trial of high-dose conformal radiation therapy with concurrent hepatic artery floxuridine for unresectable itrahepatic malignancies. J Clin Oncol 2005; 23:8739–8747.

97. Chen M, Jan Y, Wang C, et al. Clinical experience in 20 hepatic resections for peripheral cholangiocarcinoma. Cancer 1989; 64:2226–2232.

98. Shirabe K, Shimada M, Harimoto N, et al. Intrahepatic cholangiocarcinoma: Its mode of spreading and therapeutic modalities. Surg 2002; 131:159–164.

99. Flickinger J, Epstin A, Iwatzuki S, et al. Radiation therapy for primary carcinoma of the extrahepatic biliary system. Cancer 1991; 68:289–294.

100. Urego M, Flickinger J, Car B, et al. Radiotherapy and multimodality management of cholangiocarcinoma. Int J Radiat Oncol Biol Phys 1999; 44:121–126.

101. Heimbach J, Gores G, Haddock M, et al. Liver transplantation for unresectable perihilar cholangiocarcinoma. Sem Liver Dis 2004; 24:201–207.

102. Rea DJ, Heimbach JK, Rosen CB, et al. Liver transplantation with neoadjuvant chemoradiation is more effective than resection for hilar cholangiocarcinoma. Ann Surg 2005; 242:451–458; discussion 458–461.

103. Schoenthaler R, Phillips T, Castro J. Carcinoma of the extrahepatic bile ducts: UCSF experience. Ann Surg 1994; 219:267–274.

104. Ben-David MA, Griffith KA, Abu-Isa E, et al. External-beam radiotherapy for localized extrahepatic cholangiocarcinoma. Int J Radiat Oncol Biol Phys 2006; 66:772–779.

105 Nelson JW, Willet CG, Cough, R, et al. Concurrent chemoradiation for resectable extrahepatic cholangiocarcinoma. Int J Radiat Oncol Biol Phys 2007; 69:3S, 2183.

106 Ghafoori AP, Nelson, JW, Willett CG, et al. Chemoradiation for inoperable extrahepatic cholangiocarcinoma. 2008 Gastrointestinal Cancers Symposium Proceedings. 166, January 25-27, 2008, Orlando Fl.

107 Shinohara E, Mitra, N, Guo M, et al. Radiation therapy is associated with improved survival in the adjuvant and definitive treatment of intrahepatic cholangiocarcinoma. Int J Radiat Oncol Bio Phys 2008 (in press).

19 3D-Conformal and Intensity-Modulated Radiation Therapy

Joshua D. Lawson
Jerome C. Landry

ancers of the biliary tract have historically been treated with unsatisfactory results both from a disease-control standpoint as well as from a toxicity vantage. While those patients with early disease have been treated with surgery alone, patients presenting with more advanced or unresectable disease have a much inferior prognosis. The use of adjuvant radiation therapy has been shown to provide a local control benefit compared to surgery alone and has also shown a potential survival benefit, but radiation therapy has historically had a limited role in the treatment of these cancers (1–3). This is due, to at least some extent, to the proximity of organs at risk (OAR) and the appropriate required dosing constraints. The liver and kidneys, in particular, have known low whole-organ tolerances to radiation, limiting both the postoperative and definitive radiation dose that can be safely given.

Efforts at dose escalation have used intraoperative radiotherapy and intraluminal brachytherapy, either alone or in combination with external beam radiation therapy. Using a combination of techniques, definitive doses as high as 135 Gy have been safely delivered in patients with extrahepatic biliary cancer. As a component of combined modality treatment, doses of >55 Gy have been associated with improved survival over doses <55 Gy (4). In this series, 2-year survival was 48% for the higher-dose group versus 0% for those in the lower-dose group (4). However, other series have shown no significant dose response in patients treated with radical radiotherapy (5, 6).

THREE-DIMENSIONAL CONFORMAL RADIATION THERAPY (3D-CRT)

Using computed tomography (CT) simulation allows improved delineation of both target structures as well as OAR. Gross tumor volume (GTV) is defined as the radiographically or clinically evident extent of disease. The clinical target volume (CTV) encompasses the GTV as well as areas of potential microscopic disease. For intrahepatic cholangiocarcinoma, the three most common areas of lymphatic positivity are the hepatoduodenal, common hepatic, and para-aortic lymph node groups (7). A separate series of patients with hilar cholangiocarcinoma found pericholedochal, periportal, and common hepatic lymph node stations most frequently involved (8). Finally, a planning target volume (PTV) is generated by adding margin to the CTV to account for set-up uncertainty; improvements in both intra- and interfraction motion management may allow for a reduction in this requirement and are discussed more later in this chapter.

With the advent of 3D-CRT and the knowledge that death from disease is generally related to persistence of local disease, interest in dose escalation has increased (9). In a series from Michigan, total doses of 48 or 66 Gy were chosen based on fraction of normal liver receiving 50% of the prescribed dose. With median follow-up of 54 months, encouraging intrahepatic control of 50% was observed. There was no late hepatic dysfunction seen in any long-term survivor (10).

Using normal tissue complication probability (NTCP) modeling to predict radiation-induced liver disease (RILD), it was predicted that small volumes of liver could tolerate much higher radiation doses than previously thought (11). Phase I investigation included 27 patients with hepatobiliary cancer treated with split-course twice-daily radiotherapy to 28.5–90 Gy (median 61.5 Gy) along with hepatic artery floxuridine. Median tumor size for the patients with hepatobiliary cancer was $10 \times 10 \times 8$ cm. The response rate for these patients was 45%, with median time to progression of 3 months. For all patients, there was a significant delay in median time to progression for those patients treated to >70 Gy (22 months) versus <70 Gy (9 months). Progression-free and overall survival favored patients treated to higher radiation doses, independent of tumor volume. There was only one case of reversible grade 3 RILD (2).

A subsequent phase II trial including 46 cholangiocarcinoma patients substantiated the earlier experience (12). Treatments were designed to limit the predicted risk of RILD to 10–15%, generally sparing at least 10% of the normal liver. Patients received split-course twice-daily radiation treatment given with concurrent hepatic artery floxuridine; isocenter doses ranging from 40 to 90 Gy (median 60.75 Gy) were successfully delivered. Using this fractionation, the dose constraints to the duodenum/stomach and spinal cord were 68 and 37.5 Gy, respectively. In the event of >50% of one kidney receiving ≥20 Gy, <10% of the other kidney could be treated to >18 Gy. Of the 46 cholangiocarcinoma patients, 33 were evaluable for response. Of these, 12 (36%) showed complete or partial response to treatment and another 20 (61%) showed stable disease. Only one showed disease progression. Median survival for cholangiocarcinoma patients was 13.3 months, with an improvement in survival for increasing dose from 60 to 90Gy. For the whole group, patients in the highest dose range (>75 Gy) had median survival of 23.9 months versus 14.9 months for patients treated to lower doses. Patients treated for primary hepatobiliary tumors showed less extrahepatic progression overall, with 48.5% free of extrahepatic progression at 3 years. Grade 3/4 toxicity was observed in 30% of patients, with one death from RILD (12).

INTENSITY-MODULATED RADIATION THERAPY (IMRT)

With very sharp dose fall-off at the edge of target volumes, IMRT offers a potential advantage over other methods of radiation delivery for treatment of biliary tract tumors. Biliary tract tumors are situated in the midst of OAR, such as in the liver, stomach, spinal cord, small bowel, and kidneys, each of which can limit the feasibility of safely delivering tumoricidal radiation doses. With a tendency for local (intrahepatic) failure, interest in both IMRT and further dose escalation is high (13, 14). As yet, there are very few published reports on the use of IMRT in biliary tract malignancies.

Fuller et al. published a report of 10 patients with gallbladder tumors treated to a median of 59 Gy. Ultrasound image guidance was used, allowing for CTV to PTV expansions of 10–15 mm for the initial treatment volumes and 6–10 mm for the boost volumes. Median dose to the initial PTV was 50 Gy with a median boost dose of 14 Gy. Mean dose to liver, left kidney, right kidney, and spinal cord were 28.8, 8.9, 14.3, and 10.6 Gy, respectively. The authors compared the delivered IMRT plan to a plan generated using larger volume margins thought required in the absence of image guidance; the decreased margins gave a significant reduction in mean dose to the liver, spinal cord, and right kidney. Grade 3 or higher toxicity was observed in one patient. Survival estimates for 1 and 2 years were 76 and 39%, respectively (15).

A somewhat larger series from the University of Chicago included mainly patients with pancreatic tumors but did include several patients with biliary tract tumors. A total of 25 patients were treated, each using IMRT with seven to nine fields. In six cases, a comparison four-field non-IMRT plan was generated. Median prescribed dose in postoperative cases was 50.4 Gy with a median definitive radiotherapy dose of 59.4 Gy. Comparison of the four-field and IMRT plans showed a significant reduction in mean dose to the small bowel and the right kidney for the IMRT plan; the reduction in volume above a threshold dose was significant for the liver and both kidneys. Grade 3 and 4 acute gastrointestinal toxicities were observed in four and two patients, respectively. There was only one instance of late-grade 3/4 toxicity. Median survival for cholangiocarcinoma patients was 9.3 months, with 33% 1-year survival. Median metastasis-free survival was 5.7 months (13).

Shown in Figure 19.1 are representative samples of field arrangements for a patient treated with IMRT for locally recurrent adenocarcinoma of the gallbladder. This patient was initially found at cholecystectomy to have a 1.5-cm poorly differentiated adenocarcinoma with extension into pericystic adipose tissue and angiolymphatic invasion. There were no positive lymph nodes in this resection. The patient received no adjuvant treatment but was followed with serial imaging. Seventeen months after surgery the patient developed abdominal pain and jaundice and was found to have a

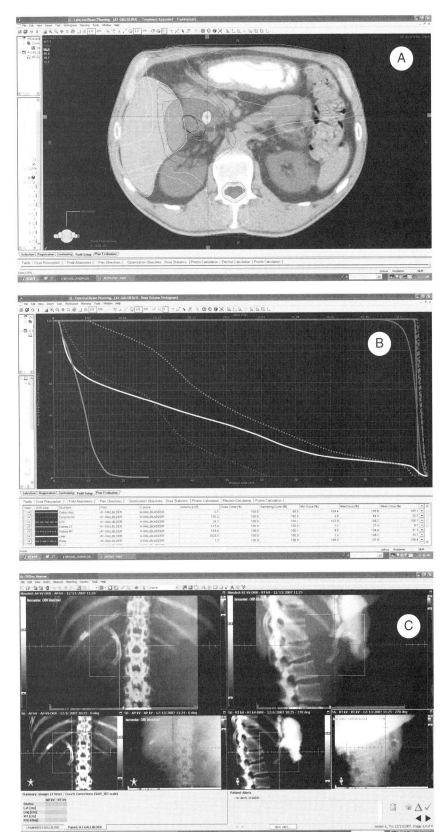

FIGURE 19.1

(A) Sample axial image with isodose distributions. (B) Dose-volume histogram for patient treated with IMRT. (C) Representative imaging from treatment session using kv-kv matching prior to treatment delivery. The graticule is shown in green on digitally reconstructed radiographs (DRR) from CT simulation and shown in red on kV images obtained just before treatment delivery. The top frame in each series shows the overlay of the two images, indicating an appropriate anatomic match.

2.9-cm mass of locally recurrent adenocarcinoma. This was not thought to be amenable to surgical resection so the patient was treated with concurrent capecitabine and IMRT to 50.4 Gy using daily image guidance. Targeted structures were the residual mass, as defined by both PET and CT imaging with a modified 2.5-cm margin, the celiac axis, and the porta hepatis. Together these structures comprised the PTV. Standard target and organ-at-risk constraints are shown in Table 19.1. This patient also is being considered for an 18-Gy single-fraction image-guided boost.

Overall, the body of work exploring the use of IMRT in biliary tract cancers is quite small. Still, there is strong interest as reflected by a recent survey, and there is a growing body of experience with IMRT in various other intra-abdominal sites. Multiple series have shown potential advantage for IMRT in reduction of dose to critical OAR (13, 15–17). While it is unlikely that a randomized comparison of radiation techniques will ever be completed, there are strong potential advantages for IMRT which warrant further investigation.

TABLE 19.1
Standard Target and Organ-at-Risk Constraints

ORGAN/TARGET	VOLUME	CONSTRAINT
GTV	100%	50.4 Gy minimum
PTV	100%	50.4 Gy minimum
Small bowel	100%	45 Gy maximum
	75%	48 Gy maximum
	50%	50 Gy maximum
	25%	55 Gy maximum
R kidney	50%	18 Gy maximum
	25%	20 Gy maximum
L kdney	50%	10 Gy maximum
	25%	15 Gy maximum
Liver	50%	30 Gy maximum
	25%	35 Gy maximum
Spinal cord + 0.5 cm	100%	43 Gy maximum

References

1. Todoroki T, et al. Benefits of adjuvant radiotherapy after radical resection of locally advanced main hepatic duct carcinoma. Int J Radiation Oncol Biol Physics 2000; 46(3):581–587.
2. Dawson LA, et al. Escalated focal liver radiation and concurrent hepatic artery fluorodeoxyuridine for unresectable intrahepatic malignancies. J Clin Oncol 2000; 18(11):2210–2218.
3. Gonzalez Gonzalez D, et al. Results of radiation therapy in carcinoma of the proximal bile duct (Klatskin tumor). Semin Liver Dis 1990; 10(2):131–141.
4. Alden ME, Mohiuddin M. The impact of radiation dose in combined external beam and intraluminal Ir-192 brachytherapy for bile duct cancer. Int J Radiat Oncol Biol Phys 1994; 28(4):945–951.
5. Kamada T, et al. The role of radiotherapy in the management of extrahepatic bile duct cancer: An analysis of 145 consecutive patients treated with intraluminal and/or external beam radiotherapy. Int J Radiation Oncol Biol Physics 1996; 34(4):767–774.
6. Vallis KA, et al. External beam and intraluminal radiotherapy for locally advanced bile duct cancer: role and tolerability. Radiother Oncol 1996; 41(1):61–66.
7. Tsuji T, et al. Lymphatic spreading pattern of intrahepatic cholangiocarcinoma. Surgery 2001; 129(4):401–407.
8. Kitagawa YMD, et al. Lymph node metastasis from hilar cholangiocarcinoma: audit of 110 patients who underwent regional and paraaortic node dissection. Ann Surg 2001; 233(3):385–392.
9. Gunderson LL, et al. Conformal irradiation for hepatobiliary malignancies. Ann Oncol 1999; 10(0):221–225.
10. Robertson JM, et al. Long-term results of hepatic artery fluorodeoxyuridine and conformal radiation therapy for primary hepatobiliary cancers. Int J Radiation Oncol Biol Physics 1997; 37(2):325–330.
11. Dawson LA, et al. Analysis of radiation-induced liver disease using the Lyman NTCP model. Int J Radiation Oncol Biol Physics 2002; 53(4):810–821.
12. Ben-Josef E, et al. Phase II trial of high-dose conformal radiation therapy with concurrent hepatic artery floxuridine for unresectable intrahepatic malignancies. J Clin Oncol 2005; 23(34):8739–8747.
13. Milano MT, et al. Intensity-modulated radiotherapy in treatment of pancreatic and bile duct malignancies: toxicity and clinical outcome. Int J Radiation Oncol Biol Physics 2004; 59(2):445–453.
14. Loren K, Mell A. Intensity-modulated radiation therapy use in the U.S., 2004. Cancer 2005; 104(6):1296–1303.
15. Fuller CD, et al. Image-guided intensity-modulated radiation therapy for gallbladder carcinoma. Radiother Oncol 2006; 81(1):65–72.
16. Hong L, et al. IMRT of large fields: whole-abdomen irradiation. Int J Radiation Oncol Biol Physics 2002; 54(1):278–289.
17. Landry JC, et al. Treatment of pancreatic cancer tumors with intensity-modulated radiation therapy (IMRT) using the volume at risk approach (VARA): employing dose-volume histogram (DVH) and normal tissue complication probability (NTCP) to evaluate small bowel toxicity. Med Dosim 2002; 27(2):121–129.

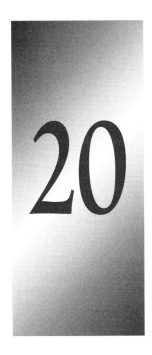

20 Brachytherapy

Subir Nag
Kevin Forsythe
Andrew Kennedy

The definitive treatment for hepatobiliary malignancies is primarily surgical. However, a majority of patients with hepatobiliary malignancies are not suitable for surgical intervention (1–8), either because of comorbid conditions or because of tumor involvement with critical structures such as vasculature or the presence of distant disease at the time of the patient's diagnosis. Therefore, radiation therapy assumes an important role in the treatment of hepatobiliary malignancies.

In the treatment of malignant disease with radiation, a distinction is made based on the method of delivery. When radiation is delivered in the form of an external beam that is generated from a device located some distance away from the target, it is referred to as "teletherapy" (from the Greek root *tele-*, meaning distant). A linear accelerator is generally used to deliver teletherapy radiation. In contrast, when radiation is delivered from sources placed inside of or close to the tumor within the patient's body, it is referred to as brachytherapy (from the Greek root *brachy-*, meaning short). Examples of brachytherapy include the use of intracavitary (placed within a body cavity like the vagina), intraluminal (placed within an organ lumen like the bile duct), interstitial (placed within tumor tissue), and surface radioactive implants (e.g., skin surface molds). While brachytherapy techniques are generally used to treat discrete, localized tumors and high-risk areas, brachytherapy can also be employed

for more diffuse tumors by the systemic administration of radioactive substances. Examples of this latter type of brachytherapy include the use of radioactive strontium for the palliation of metastatic bony disease and the use of radioactive microparticles that can preferentially home in on metastatic tumors in the liver.

Both teletherapy and brachytherapy have their own relative advantages and disadvantages, and the decision to use one or the other (or both) in the treatment of a patient is determined by the clinical judgment of the radiation oncologist. One advantage that brachytherapy offers over teletherapy is that when radioactive sources are placed very close to or within a tumor, the radiation produced attenuates rapidly as the distance from the source increases. This phenomenon is described by the "inverse square law," which simply states that the intensity of radiation is inversely proportional to the square of the distance from the source of the radiation. Brachytherapy can also utilize types of radiation that have short-distance tissue penetration that would not reach the target site if the radiation were originating from outside of the patient. Together, these properties of brachytherapy allow for the delivery of higher doses of radiation to a tumor while the radiation exposure of the surrounding normal tissues remains minimal, thereby minimizing the morbidity of radiation therapy. However, brachytherapy has limitations and drawbacks as well: there is some degree of procedural trauma risk associated with brachytherapy, and it is generally not suitable for treating large volumes such as bulky tumors or regional lymphatic networks.

In treating hepatobiliary malignancies, the ability of brachytherapy to deliver high doses of radiation to discrete tumor areas is invaluable because the liver is extremely sensitive to radiation. While the whole liver can tolerate about 30–35 Gy (9–14), doses in excess of 60–70 Gy are generally required to definitively treat these tumors (15). Hence, external beam radiation therapy (EBRT) is often used in conjunction with brachytherapy, rather than as a stand-alone therapy in the treatment of hepatobiliary malignancies. When used in conjunction with brachytherapy, EBRT doses typically range from 45 to 50 Gy, and the brachytherapy doses from about 15 to 25 Gy (measured at 1 cm from the source) (7, 16–30). As brachytherapy is inherently limited to the treatment of tumors of a limited size, brachytherapy is not commonly employed as a stand-alone therapy in the definitive treatment of hepatobiliary malignancies. More commonly, brachytherapy is used after surgical resection, with or without EBRT. In palliative therapy, however, brachytherapy can be employed as a stand-alone treatment. When brachytherapy was first used over 100 years ago, radioactive ("hot") sources were implanted directly into tumors and left in place for several days to deliver continuous radiation at a low dose rate (LDR). This subjected the patient's families and caregivers to radiation hazards. Brachytherapy is therefore commonly given today using high dose rate (HDR) remote afterloading techniques. In HDR brachytherapy, hollow applicators are first placed within or close to tumors and then connected by means transfer tubes to a high-intensity radioactive source that is housed in a shielded container. The radioactive source is remotely transferred from the HDR machine into the patient and delivers the treatment within a few minutes. This eliminates the radiation exposure hazards to the caregivers and also allows for brachytherapy to be given on an outpatient basis.

INTRALUMINAL BILIARY BRACHYTHERAPY

Patients with obstructing biliary tumors often require the placement of intraluminal catheters to drain bile and relieve their jaundice. Once placed, these catheters can also be used to deliver brachytherapy to the tumor (19, 31–36). This approach allows for the delivery of brachytherapy in a relatively fast, simple, and accurate manner.

Methods

The placement of a transhepatic biliary catheter is performed by an interventional radiologist and entails placing a needle percutaneously, and then transhepatically, into a dilated bile duct. The location and extent of the cancer is then characterized by a transhepatic cholangiography (THC). Once the obstruction has been identified, a thin guidewire is passed through the needle, past the obstructing tumor, and into the duodenum. A small catheter is then advanced over the guidewire into the duodenum. If the catheter cannot be passed through the obstructing tumor initially, then it may be left in place to drain bile externally via the proximal end of the catheter; after 2–4 days of such decompression, it is often easy to pass the catheter into the duodenum due to decreased tissue edema. Passing a catheter through an obstruction can also be facilitated by reducing the obstruction with a course of intraluminal brachytherapy (37, 38). Catheters placed in this manner allow for both internal and external drainage of bile via the distal and proximal ends of the catheter (37, 39–41).

To deliver brachytherapy through the catheter, a "Tuohy" sidearm adaptor is first fixed to the external end of the catheter. This adaptor simultaneously accommodates external biliary drainage and delivery of brachytherapy. A blind-ended afterloading nylon catheter, with a stainless steel wire inside it to prevent kinking, is then inserted into the larger-diameter drainage catheter and is advanced to the desired position under fluoroscopy. An orthogonal radiograph or computed tomography (CT) scan is obtained to confirm placement and is used for radiation dosimetry calculations. During the actual delivery of brachytherapy, the catheter is connected to the HDR machine (in HDR brachytherapy), or the iridium sources are inserted into the tube (in LDR brachytherapy). Once the prescribed dose of radiation has been administered, the source is removed and the drainage catheter is flushed. A permanent indwelling biliary stent is kept in place to prevent stricture and fibrosis of the bile duct. Doses for LDR (at 1 cm from the source) have been about 20–30 Gy as a boost and 40–50 Gy as sole modality given over 1–3 days. HDR doses (at 1 cm from the source) of 15–20 Gy in three to four fractions are generally given as a boost; 30–40 Gy in five to eight fractions, given twice a day, can be used as a sole modality. After the procedure, patients should be given antibiotics to reduce the risk of infection.

It is important to note that the biliary drainage catheter must have a sufficient diameter to allow for placement of a brachytherapy catheter inside it. LDR sources have usually required a 8-10 Fr catheter; HDR sources require a 8-14 Fr catheter, depending on the type of HDR source and catheter used. The Varisource® machine has a narrow source; the Gamma-Med® and Nucletron® machines have a wider-diameter source. Further, soft drainage catheters, which are more comfortable for patients than hard drainage catheters, require larger diameters because they have higher internal friction. Hence, it is good practice to insert the afterloading catheter into the drainage catheter and ensure easy passage before the performing the procedure.

The catheters for brachytherapy can also be placed transnasally using an endoscopic technique at the time of ERCP (42–56). This approach allows for internal drainage of bile after sphincterotomy and placement of stents and avoids the complications associated with puncturing the liver as in the transhepatic approach described above. This approach requires a longer catheter and is not used often, because the HDR source may encounter difficulty in negotiating sharp curves.

Results

Published results on the use of intraluminal brachytherapy suggest that this treatment technique can prolong the relief from obstruction and prolong survival as well. Wheeler et al. published a series demonstrating that surgical drainage improved survival (median survival 9 months *vs.* 3 months) and that the addition of radiation further improved this survival advantage (32, 36). Fletcher, Karani, and Nunnerley have also shown the increased survival benefits of biliary drainage combined with intraluminal brachytherapy (41, 57, 58).

When combined with surgical resection, postoperative intraluminal brachytherapy can also increase survival when compared to surgery alone, as reported by Gonzalez et al. (44) and Verbeek et al. (27). Median survival for surgery alone was 8.25 months; with postoperative brachytherapy the median survival increased to 19 months. One-, 2-, and 3-year survival rates for surgery alone were 36, 18, and 10%, respectively; with the addition of postoperative brachytherapy, these rates increased to 85, 42, and 31%, respectively ($p = 0.0005$). Surgical resection with postoperative brachytherapy was also shown to be superior to biliary drainage with brachytherapy, this latter group having a median survival of 12.3 months and 1-, 2-, and 3-year survivals of 46, 15, and 12%, respectively.

For patients not suited for surgical resection and patients with positive margins, intraluminal brachytherapy combined with external beam radiation has been reported by Kadama et al. to increase survival (29).

Not all published reports on the use of adjuvant brachytherapy have shown such clear support for the use of postoperative radiation. Cameron et al. reported noting a significant increase in survival for patients undergoing palliative stenting with radiation, but they did not note such benefits for patients undergoing surgical resection with postoperative radiation (16). Pitt et al. found no survival benefit with adjuvant radiation (24). Kraybill et al. did note a trend of increased survival for those patients who received adjuvant postoperative radiation; however, this trend was not found to be statistically significant (28). Vallis et al. similarly noted a trend supporting adjuvant radiation, but this observation did not fulfill the requirements for statistical significance. Montemaggi et al. reported that using both external beam radiation and intraluminal brachytherapy improved locoregional control, but the survival rates did not show a statistically significant improvement (49, 50).

INTERSTITIAL BRACHYTHERAPY

In addition to the intraluminal approach described above, brachytherapy can also be administered interstitially. This is typically done intraoperatively by the placement of permanent radioactive ^{125}I seeds or temporary HDR delivered via needles or catheters. These approaches offer the advantage of direct visualization of the site to which the radiation will be delivered, thus increasing the likelihood that the prescribed radiation dose is delivered to its intended target.

Methods

Small, localized, unresectable liver tumors can be implanted with permanent ^{125}I seeds. The activity and number of seeds to be used is typically determined by using a nomograph, such as the Memorial Sloan-Kettering nomograph (61). The target volume is first defined, and then interstitial needles are inserted into the target area evenly spaced about 1 cm apart. Intraoperative ultrasound can be used when placing the needles to localize the tumor and avoid puncturing large blood vessels. If and when bleeding occurs, simple pressure can often stop the bleeding. When all of the interstitial needles are placed, a "Mick" applicator is attached to the end of each needle; this device deposits the ^{125}I seeds in the target volume, spaced approximately 1 cm apart along the needle track. The needles are removed after depositing the seeds. Follow-up CT scans are performed for dosimetry and to verify the position of the seeds in relation to surrounding structures. Doses of 140–160 Gy are usually prescribed with ^{125}I seeds.

Alternatively, if the tumor has been resected with close margins (usually adjacent to large vessels), the ^{125}I seeds can be affixed to two-dimensional substrate and used as a surface implant to deliver brachytherapy to the tumor bed. The radioactive seeds are placed 1 cm apart on a gelfoam sheet trimmed to the dimension of the tumor bed and covered with vicryl mesh or surgicel to prevent seed displacement. This gelfoam implant is then sutured directly onto the tumor bed. Whenever possible, omental pedicle flaps should be used to cover the implanted area to reduce the radiation dose to the surrounding bowel.

Unresectable liver tumors can also be implanted using intraoperative techniques and ultrasound guidance during laparotomy to place interstitial needles or catheters to deliver doses of about 20–30 Gy HDR brachytherapy in a single fraction to the periphery of the tumor (62). Alternatively, after surgical resection, tumor beds with close surgical margins can be irradiated with HDR brachytherapy using surface applicators to deliver 10–20 Gy to the tumor bed.

Results

Nag et al. reported their results using permanent ^{125}I interstitial implants in a relatively large retrospective study of 64 patients with intrahepatic malignancies that were either unresectable or were incompletely resected. In this study, 58 patients had hepatic metastases from colorectal carcinoma, 4 patients had intrahepatic cholangiocarcinoma, and 2 patients had hepatic metastases from noncolorectal cancers. Plans were designed for a minimum peripheral dose of 160 Gy. The 1-, 3-, and 5-year actuarial control rates for liver disease in these patients were 44, 22, and 22%, respectively, and the median time to liver recurrence was 9 months (95% CI, 6–12 months). The overall liver recurrence rate was 75%, and these were isolated recurrences in 55% of the patients. Overall, control rates of liver disease correlated to the number of liver metastases: patients with solitary metastases had a 38% 5-year control of liver disease; patients with three or fewer metastases had a 32% 5-year control of liver disease; and patients with four or more metastases had an 8% 5-year control of liver disease. Median times to liver recurrence in these subgroups were 17 months (95% CI 3–31), 12 months (95% CI 2–22), and 6 months (95% CI 5–7), respectively. Analysis of the number of implants, implant volume, and MPD failed to show any significant correlation to the control of liver disease. The 1-, 3-, and 5-year survival rates for all patients in this study were 73, 23, and 5%, respectively, and the median survival time was 20 months (95% CI 16–24). The overall 5-year survival rate with no liver metastases was 3%. Overall survival was found to correlate inversely to the size of the implant volume (p = 0.049); patients with implant volumes of ≤20 cc, 21–64 cc, and ≥65 cc had median survival times of 25 months (95% CI 20–30), 14 months (95% CI 5–23), and 7 months (95% CI 1–13), respectively. Complications in this study were reported in only 6 patients (9%). There were 2 deaths (3%) within the 30-day postoperative period; one patient developed a small-bowel fistula distant from the implanted area and died of multiorgan failure, and the

second patient died of aspiration pneumonia. Other complications included a small-bowel obstruction, a small-bowel perforation, a liver abscess, and a wound abscess related to seed implantation.

Thomas et al. reported their experience with intraoperative HDR brachytherapy in patients with hepatic metastases from colorectal carcinoma (62). In this study, 22 patients with unresectable disease underwent HDR brachytherapy during laparotomy. As measured by CT or magnetic resonance imaging (MRI) scans, local control at 26 months was 25% and median time to progression was 8 months. No acute or chronic radiation toxicity was noted in this study.

RADIOEMBOLIZATION (^{90}Y MICROSPHERES)

Radioembolization of liver cancers takes advantage of the unique vascular system of the liver. In normal liver tissue, approximately 70–80% of the organ's blood flow is supplied by the portal vein, and the hepatic artery accounts for the rest. This contrasts with both hepatocellular carcinoma (HCC) and metastatic tumors in the liver, in which the hepatic artery supplies approximately 80–100% of the blood flow (63–65). This difference in perfusion is exploited by the technique known as radioembolization, whereby radioactive microspheres embedded with a β-emitting isotope, ^{90}Y, are used to both embolize and irradiate tumors in the liver by delivering the microspheres through the hepatic artery to selectively target malignant disease. Since this is a new and upcoming modality, an independent group of international experts from the fields of interventional radiology, radiation oncology, nuclear medicine, medical oncology, and surgical oncology involved with ^{90}Y microsphere therapy, the Radioembolization Brachytherapy Oncology Consortium (REBOC), has recently issued clinical guidelines for ^{90}Y microsphere brachytherapy (66).

The use of radioactive vascular-borne microparticles in the treatment of cancer dates back to the 1940s. In the early years, primarily ^{63}Zn, ^{198}Au, or radioactive carbon microparticles were used (67–69). Nowadays, use of ^{90}Y microspheres is favored; these are available in two forms: ^{90}Y-bound resin microspheres (SIR-Spheres, Sirtex Medical, Australia) and ^{90}Y-imbedded glass microspheres (TheraSpheres, MDS Nordion, Canada). ^{90}Y is an ideal isotope because it has a short half-life (approximately 2.5 days) and produces radiation as it decays to stable zirconium. Both of the commercially available microspheres contain ^{90}Y, which is produced either by bombarding ^{89}Y in the microspheres with neutrons in a nuclear reactor or using free ^{90}Y to bind to the microsphere. The "hot" radioactive micros-

TABLE 20.1

Properties of Resin and Glass Y90 Microspheres

PARAMETER	RESIN	GLASS
Trade Name	SIR-Spheres®	TheraSpheres®
Manufacturer	Sirtex Medical Lane Cove, Australia	MDS Nordion Kanata, Canada
Diameter	20–60 microns*	20–30 microns**
Specific Gravity	1.6 g/dl	3.6 g/dl
Activity per Particle	50 Bq	2500 Bq
Number of microspheres per 3 GBq vial	40–80 million	1.2 million
Material	Resin with bound yttrium	Glass with yttrium in matrix

*SirSpheres, Package insert, Sirtex Medical, Inc., Lane Cove, Australia

**TheraSphere, Package insert, MDS Nordion, Kanata, Canada

pheres are delivered to the facility where the treatment is to be performed either on the day of the procedure (resin) or days earlier (glass). Resin microspheres gained premarket approval from the U.S. Food and Drug Administration (FDA) in 2002 for the treatment, with concurrent fluorodeoxyuridine chemotherapy, of hepatic metastases from colorectal adenocarcinoma. Glass microspheres have been approved under humanitarian device exemption for the treatment of unresectable HCC. Table 20.1 outlines the characteristics of each type of microsphere.

Methods

Guidelines regarding the use of ^{90}Y microspheres have recently been published by the Radioembolization Brachytherapy Oncology Consortium (REBOC) and are summarized here (66). Because this multidisciplinary technology has been developed by and involves the skill sets of the fields of radiation oncology, interventional radiology, and nuclear medicine, it is strongly recommended that a multidisciplinary team be established that includes individuals with the expertise needed to safely and successfully conduct radioembolization procedures. The team should be able to assume the overall medical management of a cancer patient, perform vascular catheterization, perform and interpret radiologic scans, assume responsibility for the delivery of the ^{90}Y microspheres and be an authorized user, and monitor radiation safety. Typically, institutions have achieved this by combining personnel from various disciplines, including: interventional radiology, radiation oncology, nuclear medicine, medical physics,

hepatology, surgical oncology, medical oncology, and radiation safety.

Patients should always be evaluated for surgical resection before being considered for ^{90}Y microsphere radioembolization. In addition, the patient's hepatic disease should represent the bulk of their disease, and they should have a life expectancy of at least 3 months. Relative contraindications include limited hepatic reserve, irreversible hyperbilirubinemia (>2 mg/mL), compromised portal vein (unless selective radioembolization can be performed), and previous radiation to the liver. It is unclear whether capecitabine chemotherapy represents a contraindication to the use of ^{90}Y microspheres. Goin et al. have published a risk stratification analysis for the use of ^{90}Y glass microspheres in 121 patients with unresectable HCC that divided patients into low- and high-risk groups for 3-month survival (70). Seven risk variables were identified as associated with 3-month mortality and were classified as either liver reserve risk factors or non–liver reserve risk factors. The five liver reserve risk factors included: bulky disease (tumor volume ≥70%, or tumors too numerous to count), infiltrative disease (indistinct tumor/liver interface, exhibiting high degree of vascular infiltration on contrast CT), serum transaminase levels greater than five times the normal limit, bilirubin levels ≥2 mg/dL, and tumor volume ≥50% with serum albumin levels <3 g/dL. The two non–liver reserve risk factors included: lung dose >30 Gy and a diagnosis of non-HCC disease. Patients included in the low-risk group according to this schema had improved survival compared with that of patients at high risk (median survival 466 days vs. 108 days).

Prior to treatment with ^{90}Y microspheres, several important studies and procedures should be performed. To evaluate hepatic and renal function, the standard serum laboratory values should be obtained. A three-phase contrast CT and/or a gadolinium-enhanced MRI scan should be performed to evaluate portal vein patency and the hepatic and extrahepatic disease burden. A PET scan may also be useful in measuring hepatic and extrahepatic disease burden. Arteriograms of the aorta, superior mesenteric, celiac, and right and left hepatic arteries should be performed to evaluate the patient for any anatomic variations in vasculature and to document the perfusion characteristics of the areas of interest. For these studies, percutaneous catheterization is generally preferred over the use of indwelling arterial catheter devices. In order to reduce the risk of unwanted reflux of microspheres into the gastrointestinal tract, it is also recommended that the gastroduodenal artery and right gastric artery be embolized. As revascularization can occur in a short period of time, repeat arteriograms should be performed immediately before the actual administration of ^{90}Y microspheres to make sure that revascularization has occurred. A 99mTc macro-aggregated albumin (MAA) scan should be performed to evaluate the extent of any extrahepatic shunting; results suggesting radiation exposure to the lungs or gastrointestinal tract ≥30 Gy represent a contraindication to radioembolization with microspheres. When the MAA scan is performed, catheter position and flow rates that are used should be representative of the anticipated catheter position and flow rates of the ^{90}Y infusion. Scintigraphy should be performed within 1 hour of MAA administration to prevent false-positive extrahepatic activity due to free technetium. Once the results of these studies are reviewed and approved by the treating team and there is consensus regarding the planning tumor volume, proposed activity, and optimal catheter placement, treatment with ^{90}Y microspheres may safely proceed.

Whole liver or uni-lobar administrations are both acceptable approaches for ^{90}Y microspheres, and the decision between the two depends on the location and characteristics of each patient's disease. Treating the entire liver in one session is called *whole liver delivery*, and treating a single lobe is called *lobar delivery*. Sometimes the entire liver will be treated one lobe at a time, which is referred to as *sequential delivery*. In sequential treatments, a 30- to 45-day interval between treatments is generally observed (71–73). The dosage, number of microspheres, and volumes to be infused will vary for each individual patient and will differ depending on the types of microspheres being used (Table 20.1). Resin microspheres are received in bulk, and the individual medical centers extract the desired activity from a 3-GBq source vial that arrives on the day of treatment. This process differs from that for glass microspheres, which arrive a few days prior to the procedure and all of which (i.e., the entire contents of the vial containing the spheres) are delivered to the tumor.

When choosing an activity, the significant physical differences between the two spheres must be considered:

1. *Activity per microsphere:* Glass microspheres contain 2500 Bq/sphere; thus only 1–2 million spheres are delivered for the typical patient. This number of glass spheres is not sufficient to cause significant embolization in the main hepatic arteries. Resin microspheres contain approximately 50 Bq/sphere; thus an average treatment contains 40–60 million spheres, a number that can cause embolic effects in the arteries.

2. *Embolic effect on dose delivery:* The total number of glass spheres in the vial is not sufficient to cause significant embolization in the main hepatic arteries; hence, the entire prescribed dose of glass microsphere is completely infused. In contrast, because of reduced antegrade hepatic arterial flow, the prescribed activity of resin spheres cannot always be infused. When delivery of resin spheres is stopped earlier than planned, the residual activity in the delivery vial is measured and deducted from the activity present at the beginning of the procedure to obtain the amount infused.

Because the microspheres are designed to embolize the hepatic arterial vasculature, it is important to monitor the rate of anterograde flow in the vasculature that is being embolized so that microsphere administration can be stopped before vascular stasis occurs, thereby preventing reflux of the microspheres into unintended vasculature. For this reason, termination of microsphere infusion before the intended activity has been delivered is acceptable when reduced anterograde blood flow is noticed during the procedure. A Bremsstrahlung scan should be obtained within 24 hours after the delivery of microspheres has concluded to confirm and evaluate the distribution of the ^{90}Y microspheres. Radiologic studies performed after microsphere treatment to assess response must be interpreted with care, as liver edema, congestion, and micro-infarctions will decrease attenuation on CT scan; these changes are reversible and can be erroneously mistaken for tumor response. PET scans may be able to demonstrate decreased metabolic activity suggesting tumor response, even though this may be discordant with findings by CT (72). When the tumor marker carcinoembryonic antigen (CEA) has been used to track tumor response after treatment with microspheres, a nadir has been observed at about 12 weeks posttreatment; this maximal response time has been noted by CT scan as well (71).

Results

More than 3000 patients have been treated with ^{90}Y microspheres in over 80 medical centers worldwide, but at this time no large-scale prospective clinical studies have been conducted. Nevertheless, substantial evidence has been published demonstrating the safety and efficacy of ^{90}Y microspheres in the treatment of primary and metastatic liver cancers.

Considerable experience using ^{90}Y microspheres for HCC has been published demonstrating their efficacy. One report by Carr studied the use of ^{90}Y glass microspheres in 65 patients with biopsy-proven unresectable HCC and made comparisons to historical controls (74). In this report, 42 patients (64.6%) had a substantial decrease in tumor vascularity in response to therapy, and 25 patients (38.4%) had a partial response by CT scan. Median survival for Okuda stage I patients (*n* = 42) and Okuda stage II patients (*n* = 23) was 649 days and 302 days, respectively. Historical controls for these two groups are estimated to be 244 and 64 days, respectively. Clinical toxicities included nine episodes of abdominal pain and two episodes of acute cholecystitis requiring cholecystectomy. The main lab toxicity was elevated bilirubin, which increased by more than 200% in 25 patients (30.5%) during 6 months of therapy, but 18 of these patients had only transient elevation. A prominent finding was prolonged and profound (>70%) lymphopenia in more than 75% of the patients, but these were regarded to lack clinical significance.

In another study by Dancey et al., 20 patients with HCC receiving ^{90}Y microspheres were evaluated for treatment efficacy (75). The median dose delivered was 104 Gy (range 46–145 Gy), and response rate was 20%. Nine patients were Okuda stage I, and 11 were Okuda stage II. The median duration of response was 127 weeks, and the median survival was 54 weeks. Every patient in the study experienced at least one adverse event, and the most common were elevations in liver enzymes and bilirubin and upper gastrointestinal tract ulceration. Multivariate analysis suggested that a dose of >104 Gy ($p = 0.06$), tumor-to-liver activity uptake ratio of >2 ($p = 0.06$), and Okuda stage I ($p = 0.07$) were associated with longer survival.

In a report by Geschwind et al. of 80 patients with HCC receiving ^{90}Y microspheres delivering liver doses ranging from 47 to 270 Gy, 54 patients with Okuda stage I and 26 patients with Okuda stage II had median survival durations and 1-year survival rates of 628 days and 63%, and 384 days and 51%, respectively ($p = 0.02$). One patient died of liver failure judged as possibly related to the treatment (76).

Kim et al. have published a case report describing use of ^{90}Y microsphere treatment as a bridge to transplantation in a patient with end-stage liver disease secondary to hepatitis C and HCC (77). This patient was not initially a candidate for transplantation because the size of his tumor exceeded the Milan criteria. After two treatments with ^{90}Y microspheres, the patient's tumor shrank; his AFP returned to the normal range, and he subsequently received a liver transplant. He was tumor-free with normal AFP levels 2 years posttransplant. Kulik et al. also published a case report in which a patient with an unresectable T3 HCC was downstaged to T2 disease after being treated with ^{90}Y microspheres. The patient received a liver transplant 42 days after treatment; pathology showed complete necrosis of the target tumor (78).

Kulik et al. also reported using ^{90}Y microspheres in 35 patients with unresectable UNOS stage T3 HCC with the specific intent of downstaging to enable resection, radiofrequency ablation (RFA), or liver transplantation (79). Overall, 19 patients (56%) were successfully downstaged from T3 to T2 following

treatment, and 11 patients (32%) were downstaged to target lesions measuring 3.0 cm or less. Also, 23 patients (66%) were downstaged to either T2 status, lesion <3.0 cm (RFA candidate), or resection. A total of 17 patients (50%) had an objective tumor response by World Health Organization (WHO) criteria, and 8 patients (23%) were successfully downstaged and subsequently underwent liver transplant. One, 2-, and 3-year survival was 84, 54, and 27%, respectively; median survival for the entire cohort was 800 days.

The acute and late side effects of using ^{90}Y microspheres in HCC have been well characterized in the literature (11, 70, 80–84). Commonly, patients experience a mild postembolization syndrome on the day of and up to 3 days posttreatment, and symptoms include fatigue, nausea, and abdominal pain. Damage to nontarget organs can also include gastrointestinal ulcers, pancreatitis, and radiation pneumonitis, but observing the recommended preventative pretreatment guidelines can minimize this risk. One potential serious late side effect is radiation-induced liver disease (RILD), also known as radiation hepatitis. Fatal radiation pneumonitis is not common, and observing the radiation dose limit of <30 Gy to the lungs can prevent this complication (85).

In addition to treating HCC, ^{90}Y microspheres have been used to treat metastatic disease in the liver. Kennedy et al. published a retrospective study from seven centers in the united States that examined the use of microspheres in patients with chemorefractory metastatic colorectal cancer with liver-predominant disease (71). In this study, more than two thirds of the patients responded to treatment despite a significant history of previous chemotherapy treatments. In patients who responded to the microspheres, median survival was 10.5 months compared to 4.5 months for nonresponders. There were no cases of grade 4 or 5 toxicity, veno-occlusive disease, or RILD. The most common side effects were fatigue, brief nausea, and transient elevation of liver enzymes. Maximal response occurred at 12 weeks as measured by CT scan and the nadir of the tumor maker CEA.

Prospective clinical trials have also shown promising results for the use of ^{90}Y microspheres. One such study, published by Gray et al. (86), was a phase III trial studying the use of resin ^{90}Y microspheres in chemotherapy-naive colorectal cancer patients with metastases to the liver. Patients were randomized to hepatic artery infusion of FUDR alone or FUDR plus a single whole liver treatment of microspheres. Each arm of the study included 32 patients, and partial or complete tumor response rates were higher for the patients receiving the microspheres (44% vs. 17.6%; $p = 0.01$). The median time to progression in the liver was longer for the patients receiving microspheres (15.9

months vs. 9.7 months, $p = 0.04$), and survival was also improved for the patients receiving microspheres (5-year survival: 3.5% vs. 0%). Quality of life and toxicity was found to be similar for the two groups.

The use of ^{90}Y microspheres for neuroendocrine primary tumors in the liver has been examined retrospectively by 10 institutions, and the results have been reported by Kennedy et al. (87). A total of 148 patients were treated with 185 separate procedures. The median age was 58 years (26–95 years) at treatment with median performance status of ECOG (0). There were no acute or delayed toxicity of common toxicity criteria (CTC) 3.0 grade 3 in 67% of patients, with fatigue (6.5%) being the most common side effect. Imaging response was stable in 22.7%, partial response in 60.5%, complete in 2.7%, and progressive disease in 4.9%. No radiation liver failure occurred. The median survival was 70 months. The authors reviewed published experiences with local therapy in the liver, including surgery, embolization, and radiation (systemic and external beam), and concluded that ^{90}Y microspheres compared very favorably to these other treatments. They also found that microsphere therapy to the whole liver or lobe with single or multiple fractions was safe and produced high response rates, even with extensive tumor replacement of normal liver and/or heavy pretreatment.

CONCLUSIONS

Brachytherapy is a very useful modality in the treatment of unresectable liver tumors. Solitary or a limited number of localized tumors can be treated with interstitial permanent ^{125}I seeds, HDR brachytherapy, or intraluminal ^{192}Ir to the unresected tumor or to the tumor bed after surgical resection. Diffuse liver tumors can be palliated with ^{90}Y glass or resin microspheres. The role of these therapies must be investigated further in controlled clinical trials to integrate and quantify the benefit when combined with other therapies.

ACKNOWLEDGMENT

The authors wish to express their gratitude to Mr. David Carpenter for editorial assistance.

References

1. Belli G, D'Agostino A, Ciciliano F, et al. Liver resection for hepatic metastases: 15 years of experience. J Hepatobiliary Pancreat Surg 2002; 9(5):607–613.
2. Nakamura S, Suzuki S, Konno H. Resection of hepatic metastases of colorectal carcinoma: 20 years' experience. J Hepatobiliary Pancreat Surg 1999; 6(1):16–22.
3. Harmon KE, Ryan JA, Jr., Biehl TR, et al. Benefits and safety of hepatic resection for colorectal metastases. Am J Surg 1999; 177(5):402–404.
4. Fuhrman GM, Curley SA, Hohn DC, et al. Improved survival after resection of colorectal liver metastases. Ann Surg Oncol 1995; 2(6):537–541.
5. Rodgers MS, McCall JL. Surgery for colorectal liver metastases with hepatic lymph node involvement: a systematic review. Br J Surg 2000; 87(9):1142–1155.
6. Kopelson G, Gunderson LL. Primary and adjuvant radiation therapy in gallbladder and extrahepatic biliary tract carcinoma. J Clin Gastroenterol 1983; 5(1):43–50.
7. Chitwood WR, Jr., Meyers WC, Heaston DK, et al. Diagnosis and treatment of primary extrahepatic bile duct tumors. Am J Surg 1982; 143(1):99–106.
8. Cameron JL. Proximal cholangiocarcinomas. Br J Surg 1988; 75(12):1155–1156.
9. Austin-Seymour MM, Chen GT, Castro JR. Dose volume histogram analysis of liver radiation tolerance. J Radiat Oncol Biol Phys 1986; 12:31–35.
10. Dawson LA, Ten Haken RK, Lawrence TS. Partial irradiation of the liver. Semin Radiat Oncol 2001; 11(3):240–246.
11. Ingold J, Reed G, Kaplan H. Radiation hepatitis. Am J Roentgenol 1965; 93:200–208.
12. Lawrence TS, Robertson JM, Anscher MS, et al. Hepatic toxicity resulting from cancer treatment. Int J Radiat Oncol Biol Phys 1995; 31(5):1237–1248.
13. Lawrence TS, Ten Haken RK, Kessler ML, et al. The use of 3-D dose volume analysis to predict radiation hepatitis. Int J Radiat Oncol Biol Phys 1992; 23(4):781–788.
14. Ogata K, Hizawa K, Yoshida M. Hepatic injury following irradiation: a morphologic study. Tukushima J Exp Med 1963; 9:240–251.
15. Dawson LA, McGinn CJ, Normolle D, et al. Escalated focal liver radiation and concurrent hepatic artery fluorodeoxyuridine for unresectable intrahepatic malignancies. J Clin Oncol 2000; 18(11):2210–2218.
16. Cameron JL, Pitt HA, Zinner MJ, et al. Management of proximal cholangiocarcinomas by surgical resection and radiotherapy. Am J Surg 1990; 159(1):91–97; discussion 97–98.
17. Fields JN, Emami B. Carcinoma of the extrahepatic biliary system—results of primary and adjuvant radiotherapy. Int J Radiat Oncol Biol Phys 1987; 13(3):331–338.
18. Flickinger JC, Epstein AH, Iwatsuki S, et al. Radiation therapy for primary carcinoma of the extrahepatic biliary system. An analysis of 63 cases. Cancer 1991; 68(2):289–294.
19. Herskovic A, Heaston D, Engler MJ, et al. Irradiation of biliary carcinoma. Radiology 1981; 139(1):219–222.
20. Kurisu K, Hishikawa Y, Taniguchi M, et al. High-dose-rate intraluminal brachytherapy for bile duct carcinoma after surgery. Radiother Oncol 1991; 21(1):65–66.
21. Mahe M, Romestaing P, Talon B, et al. Radiation therapy in extrahepatic bile duct carcinoma. Radiother Oncol 1991; 21(2):121–127.
22. Meyers WC, Jones RS. Internal radiation for bile duct cancer. World J Surg 1988; 12(1):99–104.
23. Mornex F, Ardiet JM, Bret P, et al. Radiotherapy of high bile duct carcinoma using intra-catheter iridium 192 wire. Cancer 1984; 54(10):2069–2073.
24. Pitt HA, Nakeeb A, Abrams RA, et al. Perihilar cholangiocarcinoma. Postoperative radiotherapy does not improve survival. Ann Surg 1995; 221(6):788–797; discussion 797–788.
25. Tasker DG, Jones MR. Jaundice, ultrasound and percutaneous transhepatic cholangiography—a surgical appraisal. Br J Clin Pract 1983; 37(10):333–335, 358.
26. Veeze-Kuijpers B, Meerwaldt JH, Lameris JS, et al. The role of radiotherapy in the treatment of bile duct carcinoma. Int J Radiat Oncol Biol Phys 1990; 18(1):63–67.
27. Verbeek PC, Van Leeuwen DJ, Van Der Heyde MN, et al. Does additive radiotherapy after hilar resection improve survival of cholangiocarcinoma? An analysis in sixty-four patients. Ann Chir 1991; 45(4):350–354.
28. Kraybill WG, Lee H, Picus J, et al. Multidisciplinary treatment of biliary tract cancers. J Surg Oncol 1994; 55(4):239–245.

29. Kamada T, Saitou H, Takamura A, et al. The role of radiotherapy in the management of extrahepatic bile duct cancer: an analysis of 145 consecutive patients treated with intraluminal and/or external beam radiotherapy. Int J Radiat Oncol Biol Phys 1996; 34(4):767–774.

30. Hejna M, Pruckmayer M, Raderer M. The role of chemotherapy and radiation in the management of biliary cancer: a review of the literature. Eur J Cancer 1998; 34(7):977–986.

31. Conroy RM, Shahbazian AA, Edwards KC, et al. A new method for treating carcinomatous biliary obstruction with intracatheter radium. Cancer 1982; 49(7):1321–1327.

32. Fletcher MS, Brinkley D, Dawson JL, et al. Treatment of high bileduct carcinoma by internal radiotherapy with iridium-192 wire. Lancet 1981; 2(8239):172–174.

33. Loigman BI, Mattern RF, Healey RF, et al. Nonsurgical evaluation and management of malignant biliary tract obstruction. J Med Soc N J 1981; 78(13):883–886.

34. McLean GK, Ring EJ, Freiman DB. Therapeutic alternatives in the treatment of intrahepatic biliary obstruction. Radiology 1982; 145(2):289–295.

35. Mornex F, Gerard JP, Bret P, et al. Iridium wire radiotherapy for high bileduct carcinoma. Lancet 1981; 2(8244):479.

36. Wheeler PG, Dawson JL, Nunnerley H, et al. Newer techniques in the diagnosis and treatment of proximal bile duct carcinoma—an analysis of 41 consecutive patients. Q J Med 1981; 50(199):247–258.

37. Nag S, Tai DL, Gold RE. Biliary tract neoplasms: a simple management technique. South Med J 1984; 77(5):593–595.

38. Pennington L, Kaufman S, Cameron JL. Intrahepatic abscess as a complication of long-term percutaneous internal biliary drainage. Surgery 1982; 91(6):642–645.

39. Ikeda H, Kuroda C, Uchida H, et al. (Intraluminal irradiation with iridium-192 wires for extrahepatic bile duct carcinoma—a preliminary report [author's transl]). Nippon Igaku Hoshasen Gakkai Zasshi 1979; 39(12):1356–1358.

40. Koster R, Schmidt H, Greuel H. (Afterloading method for the irradiation of malignant bile duct obstructions). Strahlentherapie 1982; 158(11):678–680.

41. Nunnerley HB, Karani JB. Interventional radiology of the biliary tract. Intraductal radiation. Radiol Clin North Am 1990; 28(6):1237–1240.

42. Bowling TE, Galbraith SM, Hatfield AR, et al. A retrospective comparison of endoscopic stenting alone with stenting and radiotherapy in non-resectable cholangiocarcinoma. Gut 1996; 39(6):852–855.

43. Ede RJ, Williams SJ, Hatfield AR, et al. Endoscopic management of inoperable cholangiocarcinoma using iridium-192. Br J Surg 1989; 76(8):867–869.

44. Gonzalez Gonzalez D, Gerard JP, Maners AW, et al. Results of radiation therapy in carcinoma of the proximal bile duct (Klatskin tumor). Semin Liver Dis 1990; 10(2):131–141.

45. Levitt MD, Laurence BH, Cameron F, et al. Transpapillary iridium-192 wire in the treatment of malignant bile duct obstruction. Gut 1988; 29(2):149–152.

46. Pakisch B, Klein GE, Stucklschweiger G, et al. (Metallic mesh endoprosthesis and intraluminal high dose rate 192Ir brachytherapy in the palliative treatment of malignant bile duct obstruction. Initial results). Rofo 1992; 156(6):592–595.

47. Trodella L, Mantini G, Barina M, et al. External and intracavitary radiotherapy in the management of carcinoma of extrahepatic biliary tract. Rays 1991; 16(1):71–75.

48. Urban MS, Siegel JH, Pavlou W, et al. Treatment of malignant biliary obstruction with a high-dose rate remote afterloading device using a 10 F nasobiliary tube. Gastrointest Endosc 1990; 36(3):292–296.

49. Montemaggi P, Costamagna G, Dobelbower RR, et al. Intraluminal brachytherapy in the treatment of pancreas and bile duct carcinoma. Int J Radiat Oncol Biol Phys 1995; 32(2):437–443.

50. Montemaggi P, Morganti AG, Dobelbower RR, Jr., et al. Role of intraluminal brachytherapy in extrahepatic bile duct and pancreatic cancers: is it just for palliation? Radiology 1996; 199(3):861–866.

51. Morganti AG, Trodella L, Valentini V, et al. Combined modality treatment in unresectable extrahepatic biliary carcinoma. Int J Radiat Oncol Biol Phys 2000; 46(4):913–919.

52. Prempree T, Cox EF, Sewchand W, et al. Cholangiocarcinoma. A place for brachytherapy. Acta Radiol Oncol 1983; 22(5):353–359.

53. Siegel JH, Lichtenstein JL, Pullano WE, et al. Treatment of malignant biliary obstruction by endoscopic implantation of iridium 192 using a new double lumen endoprosthesis. Gastrointest Endosc 1988; 34(4):301–306.

54. Phillip J, Hagenmuller F, Manegold K, et al. (Endoscopic intraductal radiotherapy of high bile-duct carcinoma). Dtsch Med Wochenschr 1984; 109(11):422–426.

55. Classen M, Hagenmuller F. Endoprosthesis and local irradiation in the treatment of biliary malignancies. Endoscopy 1987; 19(suppl 1):25–30.

56. Venu RP, Geenen JE, Hogan WJ, et al. Intraluminal radiation therapy for biliary tract malignancy—an endoscopic approach. Gastrointest Endosc 1987; 33(3):236–238.

57. Fletcher MS, Brinkley D, Dawson JL, et al. Treatment of hilar carcinoma by bile drainage combined with internal radiotherapy using 192iridium wire. Br J Surg 1983; 70(12):733–735.

58. Karani J, Fletcher M, Brinkley D, et al. Internal biliary drainage and local radiotherapy with iridium-192 wire in treatment of hilar cholangiocarcinoma. Clin Radiol 1985; 36(6):603–606.

59. Fritz P, Brambs HJ, Schraube P, et al. Combined external beam radiotherapy and intraluminal high dose rate brachytherapy on bile duct carcinomas. Int J Radiat Oncol Biol Phys 1994; 29(4):855–861.

60. Vallis KA, Benjamin IS, Munro AJ, et al. External beam and intraluminal radiotherapy for locally advanced bile duct cancer: role and tolerability. Radiother Oncol 1996; 41(1):61–66.

61. Anderson LL. Spacing nomograph for interstitial implants of 125I seeds. Med Phys 1976; 3(1):48–51.

62. Thomas DS, Nauta RJ, Rodgers JE, et al. Intraoperative high-dose rate interstitial irradiation of hepatic metastases from colorectal carcinoma. Results of a phase I-II trial. Cancer 1993; 71(6):1977–1981.

63. Ackerman NB, Lien WM, Kondi ES, et al. The blood supply of experimental liver metastases I: The distribution of hepatic artery and portal vein blood to "small" and "large" tumors. Surgery 1970; 66(6):1067–1072.

64. Breedis C, Young G. The blood supply of neoplasms in the liver. Am J Pathol 1954; 30:969–984.

65. Lien WM, Ackerman NB. The blood supply of experimental liver metastases II: A microcirculatory study of the normal and tumor vessels of the liver with the use of perfused silicone rubber. Surgery 1970; 68(2):334–340.

66. Kennedy A, Nag S, Salem R, et al. Recommendations for radioembolization of hepatic malignancies using yttrium-90 microsphere brachytherapy: a consensus panel report from the radioembolization brachytherapy oncology consortium. Int J Radiat Oncol Biol Phys 2007; 68(1):13–23.

67. Di Matteo G, Gennarelli L, Lenti R. Una nuova metodica per la fissazione elettiva dell' Au198 adsorbio su carbonio in terriori lobari e sublobari. Gazz Intern Med Chir 1962; 67:1875.

68. Muller JH, Rossier PH. Treatment of cancer of the lungs by artificial radioactivity. Experientia 1947; 3:75.

69. Muller JH, Rossier PH. A new method for the treatment of cancer of the lungs by means of artificial radioactivity (Zn63 and Au198). Acta Radiol 1951; 35:449–468.

70. Goin JE, Salem R, Carr BI, et al. Treatment of unresectable hepatocellular carcinoma with intrahepatic yttrium 90 microspheres: a risk-stratification analysis. J Vasc Interv Radiol 2005; 16(2 Pt 1):195–203.

71. Kennedy AS, Coldwell D, Nutting C, et al. Resin 90Y-microsphere brachytherapy for unresectable colorectal liver metastases: modern USA experience. Int J Radiat Oncol Biol Phys 2006; 65(2):412–425.

72. Lewandowski RJ, Thurston KG, Goin JE, et al. 90Y microsphere (TheraSphere) treatment for unresectable colorectal cancer metastases of the liver: response to treatment at targeted doses of 135-150 Gy as measured by [18F]fluorodeoxyglucose

positron emission tomography and computed tomographic imaging. J Vasc Interv Radiol 2005; 16(12):1641–1651.

73. Salem R, Lewandowski RJ, Atassi B, et al. Treatment of unresectable hepatocellular carcinoma with use of ^{90}Y microspheres (TheraSphere): safety, tumor response, and survival. J Vasc Interv Radiol 2005; 16(12):1627–1639.

74. Carr BI. Hepatic arterial 90Yttrium glass microspheres (Therasphere) for unresectable hepatocellular carcinoma: interim safety and survival data on 65 patients. Liver Transpl 2004; 10(2 Suppl 1):S107–110.

75. Dancey JE, Shepherd FA, Paul K, et al. Treatment of nonresectable hepatocellular carcinoma with intrahepatic ^{90}Y-microspheres. J Nucl Med 2000; 41(10):1673–1681.

76. Geschwind JF, Salem R, Carr BI, et al. Yttrium-90 microspheres for the treatment of hepatocellular carcinoma. Gastroenterology 2004; 127(5 suppl 1):S194–205.

77. Kim DY, Kwon DS, Salem R, et al. Successful embolization of hepatocelluar carcinoma with yttrium-90 glass microspheres prior to liver transplantation. J Gastrointest Surg 2006; 10(3):413–416.

78. Kulik LM, Mulcahy MF, Hunter RD, et al. Use of yttrium-90 microspheres (TheraSphere) in a patient with unresectable hepatocellular carcinoma leading to liver transplantation: a case report. Liver Transpl 2005; 11(9):1127–1131.

79. Kulik LM, Atassi B, van Holsbeeck L, et al. Yttrium-90 microspheres (TheraSphere) treatment of unresectable hepatocellular carcinoma: downstaging to resection, RFA and bridge to transplantation. J Surg Oncol 2006; 94(7):572–586.

80. Goin JE, Dancey JE, Roberts CA, et al. Comparison of post-embolization syndrome in the treatment of patients with unresectable hepatocellular carcinoma: trans-catheter arterial chemo-embolization versus yttrium-90 glass microspheres. World J Nucl Med 2004; 3(1):49–56.

81. Goin JE, Salem R, Carr BI, et al. Treatment of unresectable hepatocellular carcinoma with intrahepatic yttrium 90 microspheres: factors associated with liver toxicities. J Vasc Interv Radiol 2005; 16(2 pt 1):205–213.

82. Ho S, Lau WY, Leung TW, et al. Partition model for estimating radiation doses from yttrium-90 microspheres in treating hepatic tumours. Eur J Nucl Med 1996; 23(8):947–952.

83. Steel J, Baum A, Carr B. Quality of life in patients diagnosed with primary hepatocellular carcinoma: hepatic arterial infusion of cisplatin versus 90-yttrium microspheres (Therasphere). Psychooncology 2004; 13(2):73–79.

84. Thamboo T, Tan KB, Wang SC, et al. Extra-hepatic embolisation of Y-90 microspheres from selective internal radiation therapy (SIRT) of the liver. Pathology 2003; 35(4):351–353.

85. Leung TW, Lau WY, Ho SK, et al. Radiation pneumonitis after selective internal radiation treatment with intraarterial 90yttrium-microspheres for inoperable hepatic tumors. Int J Radiat Oncol Biol Phys 1995; 33(4):919–924.

86. Gray BN, Van Hazel G, Hope M, et al. Randomised trial of SIR-spheres plus chemotherapy vs. chemotherapy alone for treating patients with liver metastases from primary large bowel cancer. Ann Oncol 2001; 12(12):1711–1720.

87. Kennedy, A.S., Dezam WA, McNellie P, et al. Radioembolization for unresectable neuroendocrine hepatic metastases using resin ^{90}Y-microspheres: early results in 148 patients. Am J Clin Oncol, in press, March 2008; 31(3):271–279.

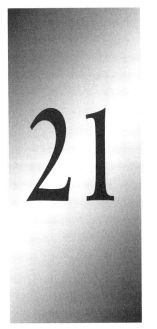

21 Image-Guided Radiation Therapy and Stereotactic Body Radiation Therapy

Laura A. Dawson
Martin Fuss

Local and regional recurrences are the most common pattern of relapse in biliary tract and gallbladder cancers, providing a rationale to use radiation therapy (RT) in the management of these cancers to reduce the risk of local-regional recurrence or as definitive therapy either on its own or with concurrent or sequential chemotherapy. However, challenges in defining the target volume required to be irradiated and in delivering radiation therapy safely have hampered the routine use. Also, randomized trials investigating the role of radiation therapy in these uncommon cancers have not feasible. Furthermore, the low whole liver tolerance to radiation and proximity of biliary tract tumors to the stomach and small bowel has made delivery of radiation therapy to these cancers challenging. Dose-limiting toxicities that have traditionally limited the role of radiation therapy in this setting are summarized below.

Emerging techniques in imaging and in high-precision radiation therapy make it possible for radiation therapy to be used more effectively in biliary track and gallbladder cancers, with improved target definition and improved quality of radiation planning and delivery. Image-guided radiation therapy (IGRT) (including both imaging at the time of radiation planning and delivery) and stereotactic body radiation therapy (SBRT), the topics of this chapter, are two developing technologies in radiation oncology that should lead to

improvements in the use of radiation for biliary tract and gallbladder cancer.

POTENTIAL RADIATION THERAPY TOXICITIE

Liver Toxicity

There is a 5% risk of radiation-induced liver toxicity following uniform whole liver radiation of 28 and 32 Gy in 2 Gy per fraction for liver metastases and primary liver cancer, respectively (1). While these doses exhaust the liver radiation tolerance, they are far lower than doses required for sustained tumor control or cure in solid tumors. The most common liver toxicity observed in North America is radiation-induced liver disease (RILD), a clinical syndrome of anicteric hepatomegaly, ascites and elevated liver enzymes (particularly serum alkaline phosphatase) occurring 2 weeks to 3 months following external beam radiation. Treatment for RILD consists of supportive measures. Diuretics and steroids are often used, although there is no evidence that they change the natural history of RILD. Most cases resolve with conservative treatment, but some cases lead to irreversible liver failure and occasionally death. RILD has been observed 1.5 and 2.5 months following SBRT (45 and 30 Gy in three fractions of 15 and 10 Gy, respectively) (2). Although whole liver radiation therapy is not expected to be associated with sustained control of tumors, high tumoricidal doses of radiation therapy can be delivered safely if they are directed focally to liver tumors. For example, doses up to 90 Gy in 1.5-Gy fractions delivered twice daily can be delivered safely to less than 25% of the liver using highly conformal radiation therapy (3). The University of Michigan group summarized the partial liver tolerance for RILD and concluded that the mean liver dose was strongly associated with probability of developing RILD. The mean liver doses associated with a 5 and 50% risk of RILD was 32 and 40 Gy, respectively, in 1.5 Gy per fraction, for patients with primary liver cancer (including patients with intrahepatic cholangiocarcinoma) (1).

Also relevant to the treatment of hepato-biliary tumors is reactivation of viral hepatitis and precipitation of underlying liver disease observed following radiation therapy for hepatocellular carcinoma (4).

In liver cancer SBRT series, where high doses of radiation therapy are delivered in few fractions, several different criteria have been used to avoid liver toxicity. It has been recommended that at least 700 cm³ of uninvolved liver receive less than a cumulative dose of 15 Gy in three fractions (5). Herfarth et al. recommended that no more than 50% of the liver receive more than 15 Gy in three fractions (or 7 Gy in one fraction), and doses to 30% do not exceed 21 Gy in three fractions (or 12 Gy in one fraction) (6). Hoyer reported a single incident of early post-SBRT hepatic failure following administration of 45 Gy in three fractions (7). It was noted that in this particular case, over 60% of the normal liver was exposed to more than 10 Gy, with a mean total liver dose of 14.4 Gy, in one fraction.

Following SBRT, there is the potential for different hepatobiliary toxicities to occur, including biliary sclerosis and hepatic subcapsular injury. A subcapsular bleed was observed 2 weeks following SBRT in a patient with two anterior tumors, both treated with high-dose SBRT (2). In one report from Japan, when the dose per fraction was greater than 4 Gy, late biliary toxicity was observed 29 and 38 months following irradiation (8).

Nonhepatic Toxicities

Although small volumes of the liver can be irradiated to very high doses safely, very high doses to small volumes of luminal gastrointestinal (GI) tissues can cause serious toxicity such as a bleed, fistula, stenosis, or obstruction. In their early report on SBRT, Blomgren reported a case of hemorrhagic gastritis; dose exposure to the gastric wall was 14 Gy in two fractions (9). Herfarth et al. restricted single doses to stomach and small bowel to maximally 12 Gy in a phase I–II trial assessing safety and efficacy of single dose liver SBRT. While

no data were provided on actual stomach and bowel dose exposure, no related toxicities were observed (10). Following liver SBRT, Hoyer et al. observed three cases of colonic and duodenal perforation following focal dose exposure to 30 Gy or higher in three fractions (7).

Acute and late GI toxicity has also been observed following pancreatic cancer SBRT. The majority of patients treated in Denmark with 15 Gy in three fractions for unresectable pancreatic cancer developed pronounced acute GI toxicity despite the use of prophylactic proton pump inhibitors (11). Four of 22 patients (18%) developed late gastritis, GI ulceration and/or perforation, highlighting the caution that needs to be used when high doses are delivered to tumors adjacent to the stomach, duodenum, and small bowel. Interestingly, another study of SBRT for pancreas cancer reported on 15 patients treated with 15–25 Gy single-fraction SRS, with a small volume of duodenum receiving up to 22.5 Gy without development of substantial GI toxicity (12).

More patients are required to be treated with SBRT to have better confidence in the tolerances of the luminal GI structures to high doses per fraction of RT, but these tissues needs to be carefully considered in all RT planning for biliary tract and gallbladder cancers.

IMAGE-GUIDED RADIATION THERAPY (IGRT)

Imaging for Radiation Planning

At the time of simulation, decisions are made regarding the most appropriate patient positioning, immobilization, and the type of imaging required to define appropriate radiation target volumes. A computed tomography (CT) scan is generally used to create a model of the patients upon which a radiation plan can be created. This simulation CT scan may also serve as the reference image dataset for image-guided setup throughout the course of radiation delivery.

CT scanning parameters, including the use of intravenous (IV) contrast media, the phase of IV contrast, CT slice thickness, and whether other imaging modalities (magnetic resonance imaging [MRI], positron emission tomography [PET]) are required at the time of radiation therapy planning, need to be defined.

While MRI is used in select institutions for staging of liver malignancies, its use for radiation therapy target volume delineation is not well established. While image quality may depend on the degree of liver respiratory motion and bowel peristalsis, MRI can aid in detecting extent of hepatic invasion of gallbladder cancer (13,14). Cholangiocarcinoma typically appears hypointense com-

Non contrast CT   Contrast MR   Fused CT and MR

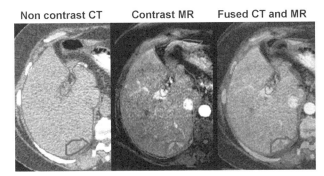

FIGURE 21.1

Intrahepatic cholangiocarcinoma in a patient with a contraindication to IV CT contrast. A dynamic MR displayed the tumor. The fused images with overlaying liver volumes allowed the gross tumor volume (GTV) to be contoured on the planning CT dataset.

pared with normal liver on T1-weighted and moderately hyperintense in T2-weighted sequences (15). Tumors may show heterogeneous contrast enhancement, with peripheral enhancement in early arterial studies, and late central fill-in, and contrast media retention in delayed gadolinium-enhanced image studies (Figure 21.1). The value of functional MRI sequences assessing liver and tumor perfusion and the utility of diffusion weighted imaging to differentiate between normal liver and tumor for target volume delineation will need to be assessed in clinical studies. Magnetic resonance cholangiopancreatography (MRCP) can depict tumor extent as an occlusion of bile ducts above and below a stricture.

PET may be useful for both detection and localization of cholangiocarcinoma. However, its use for gallbladder and cholangiocarcinoma has been predominantly studied to assess nodal staging of disease

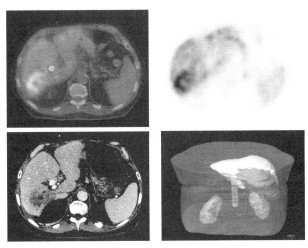

FIGURE 21.2

Integration of CT-PET imaging for IMRT radiation therapy planning for a cholangiocarcinoma. The upper two figures display CT-PET fusion and PET imaging; the lower right figure represents the contrast enhanced simulation CT. The lower left figure is a 3D reconstruction of the ITV derived from 4DCT and PET uptake information, as well as organs at risk (liver, kidneys, spinal cord).

(16–19). No general recommendation can be made at this point in time regarding the usefulness of PET to establish tumor extent for target volume delineation. Figure 21.2 depicts a radiation simulation FDG-PET study of a patient with biopsy-confirmed cholangiocarcinoma. The FDG uptake area was used to aid in target volume delineation. A follow-up PET scan, 5 months following conventionally fractionated IMRT, documented widely disseminated disease in the liver not detected earlier, indicating the potential limitations of metabolic radiolabeled glucose imaging.

Free breathing   MIP   Breath-hold

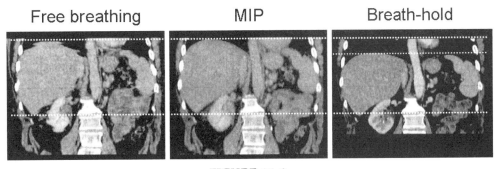

FIGURE 21.3

Typical CT simulation imaging and the respective impact on target and organ-at-risk delineation. The left figure depicts a standard free-breathing CT with waving artifacts appreciated on the outlines of both liver and right kidney. The middle figure represents a maximum intensity projection (MIP) reconstruction of a 4DCT acquired immediately following the free-breathing simulation study. Here the outlines of the organs are smooth; this study best renders the motion envelope of the organs during a cycle of respiration—organs are likely represented larger than their true anatomy. The right figure depicts an inspiration breath hold scan during contrast administration. Note the significant caudal displacement of liver and kidney.

Breathing Motion Management

Organ motion due to breathing can be substantial, with up to 3–5 cm of motion possible in the gallbladder, liver, and biliary tract. Strategies to compensate for breathing motion include the use of abdominal pressure, voluntary shallow breathing, voluntary deep inspiration, voluntary breath holds at variable phases of the respiratory cycle, active breathing control (ABC), gated radiotherapy, and real-time tumor tracking.

Organ motion in the upper abdomen second to breathing can introduce imaging artifacts, typically waving artifacts changing organ shapes (Figure 21.3). Such aliasing may have an impact on the accurate assessment of tumor extent and normal tissue definition. Thus, target and organ at-risk definition based on free-breathing simulation imaging can lead to incorrect estimates of tumor control probability and normal tissue complication probabilities, unless significant planning target volume safety margins are used. One generally employed method to account for breathing-related organ motion is to eliminate it, for example, with a breath-hold scan. Diagnostic breath hold scans are often obtained in the inhale position, which may not correspond to the treatment-delivery situation during which patients continue to breathe (Figure 21.3). A protocol of respiratory organ motion assessment for radiation therapy simulation may include a free-breathing CT as well as scans acquired during inhale and exhale. Planning on the inhale or exhale dataset with asymmetric margins to account for breathing and planning using the mean tumor position are options to account for breathing motion (20).

Although voluntary breath holds may be beneficial for some patients, there is potential for leaking air and patient error. ABC refers to organ immobilization with breath holds that are controlled, triggered, and monitored by a caregiver. In 60–80% of patients with liver cancer, ABC can be used successfully, with excellent reproducibility of the liver position during breath hold relative to the vertebral bodies within the time period of one radiation fraction (intrafraction reproducibility, standard deviation [s]) of the liver relative to the vertebral bodies: 1.5–2.5 mm (21,22). However, with ABC, from day to day the position of the immobilized liver varies relative to the bones (interfraction reproducibility, s 3.4–4.4 mm), providing rationale for daily imaging of the internal soft tissue anatomy with image guidance when ABC is used to immobilize the liver.

Today, the utilization of four-dimensional CT (4DCT) is increasing. Here, multiple images are acquired over one slice location during the respiratory cycle and reconstructed or sorted into multiple CT datasets representing different phases of the breathing cycle (23,24). Thus, the full range of respiration-dependent motion of an organ or the target can be assessed and an according internal target volume (ITV) representing the motion envelope of the target can be developed (Figure 21.4). Challenges to the acquisition of 4DCT imaging for planning of hepatobiliary tumors include the relatively slow acquisition process that may make timing of an optimal contrast phase difficult and the fact that the required image dose setting to achieve sufficient soft tissue contrast may exceed the tube heat tolerance of the respective CT scanner, potentially resulting in qualitatively inferior CT data.

Gated radiotherapy, with the beam triggered to be on only during a predetermined phase of the respira-

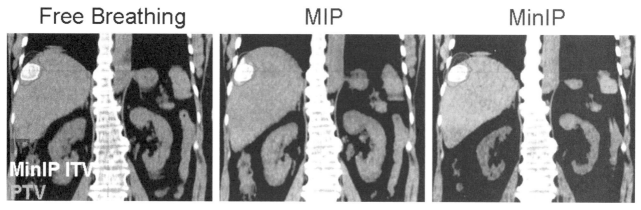

FIGURE 21.4

Target volume generation for SBRT planning of a small hepatocellular carcinoma. Free-breathing and 4DCT reconstructed MIP scan allow one to define the motion envelop (ITV). The PTV was created by adding symmetric margins of 5 mm over the ITV. A MinIP ITV represents the motion overlap area of the target during respiration, the area that always contains components of the target during a respiratory cycle. A differential (higher) dose can be prescribed to this target volume during SBRT planning.

tory cycle, most often refers to the use of an external surrogate for tumor position (as opposed to direct tumor imaging) to gate the radiation. This can be used to reduce the volume of normal tissue irradiated. Similar to breath hold, changes in baseline organ position can occur from day to day, and thus image guidance is important to avoid geographic misses.

Tumor tracking is another approach to reduce adverse effects of organ motion. An elegant real-time tumor tracking system consisting of fluoroscopic x-ray tubes in the treatment room allowing visualization of radio-opaque markers in tumors was first described by Shirato et al. The linear accelerator is turned on only when the marker is located within the planned treatment region (25). As an alternative to turning the radiation beam off when the tumor moves outside treatment region, multileaf collimators, the couch position or the entire accelerator on a robotic arm may move with the tumor to ensure adequate tumor coverage (e.g., CyberKnife image-guided radiosurgery system, Accuray, Sunnyvale, CA).

There are advantages to gating, breath hold, and tracking in exhalation phase of the respiratory breathing cycle versus inhalation. These include the fact that exhale tends to be more reproducible, and is longer than inhalation, so that treatment during exhalation reduces duty time.

Imaging for Radiation Delivery Guidance

Image-Guided Radiation Therapy (IGRT) Rationale

Historically, surrogates for the target have been used in guiding the placement of treatment fields. For example, skin marks and in-room laser beams are still used to initially set up patients prior to radiation delivery. This does not work very well for upper abdominal cancer localization, as the internal organs including the biliary system can move day to day as a function of respiration, as described above, and filling of hollow organs such as bowel and stomach. Potential fluctuations in the degree of ascites, if present, will also affect the liver and, thus, target location, relative to the surface of the patient. The use of bony anatomy with electronic portal imaging is another common practice in radiation therapy. However, the bones are also not well correlated with the liver position. Options for locating internal anatomy include the use of implanted radio-opaque fiducial markers as surrogates for the target, biliary stents that may be present in biliary tract tumors, and/or soft tissues adjacent to the tumor or the tumor itself. Inserted fiducial markers may also be used to measure organ motion and or track/gate the beam.

IGRT Strategies

Two primary correction strategies that may be used to reduce setup errors using image guidance are an *online* approach and an *offline* approach. The online approach refers to the use of imaging daily immediately prior to the delivery of the respective radiation fraction with comparison with a reference imaging study and correction for offsets in position greater than a predefined threshold. An offline approach refers to either an acquisition of image data with analysis after the patient was treated, analogous to a review of weekly port films, combined with subsequent setup corrections for the next radiation fraction, or the collection of imaging data with high frequency at the beginning of therapy (e.g., first five fractions), followed by an offline analysis to determine the patients systematic (mean offset) and random (standard deviation, s) setup errors. A correction in position is made to consider the systematic error, with possible replanning based on the initial setup data.

Online correction strategies reduce both systematic and random setup errors, with a greater error reduction compared to the offline approach, generally at the expense of more time and cost. While online correction strategies are mandatory for hypofractionated regimens such as SBRT, the optimal frequency of online image guidance for conventionally fractionated treatment courses is subject to discussion. Recently published data analyzing scheduling of image guidance for head and neck cancer indicate that daily schedules provide the largest benefit to optimal treatment setup (26), a finding that likely can be extrapolated to the treatment of gallbladder and hepatobiliary cancer.

Goals for IGRT

A goal of all radiotherapy treatments is that radiation be delivered to the target volumes as planned. Imaging at the time of radiation treatments with repositioning the patient relative to the treatment beams (i.e., IGRT) increases the confidence with which this occurs. IGRT improves setup accuracy and allows for reduction of PTV margins required to be used without sacrificing local tumor control. Any reduction in PTV margins consequently affords reducing the volume of normal tissue irradiated. Thus, image guidance can facilitate safe dose escalation, lead to reductions in normal tissue complication probabilities, and, hence, potentially increase the overall therapeutic ratio.

Since image-guidance technologies provide confidence in the dose placement, the actual delivered doses can be verified and documented, effectively reducing variability in dose delivery across a population. By these virtues, IGRT, if appropriately employed, should improve interpretation of future clinical trials and our understanding of dose-tumor control and dose–normal tissue toxicity relationships.

IGRT Technologies

2D IMAGE GUIDANCE Orthogonal MV portal films and, more recently, images from electronic portal imaging devices (EPIDs) have traditionally been used for image guidance and may be appropriate for targets in close relationship with the bony anatomy. These images can be used not only to guide therapy, but also to verify shape and orientation of the treatment fields. Unfortunately, many tumors are not well visualized with megavoltage (MV) imaging and are not in direct continuity with bones, and some soft tissues can move considerably relative to the bones. If radio-opaque fiducial markers are inserted in or near the tumor, the fiducial markers themselves may be used for guidance. Other alternatives for guidance include using surrogates that are in close proximity to the tumor, for example, the diaphragm as a surrogate for liver tumors (27). Using the diaphragm as a surrogate for liver cancers immobilized with breath hold, the accuracy of liver positioning was investigated by obtaining volumetric imaging following orthogonal MV IGRT. In 72 fractions of liver SBRT following orthogonal MV imaging using the diaphragm for superior-inferior positioning and the vertebral bodies for medial lateral and anterior posterior positioning, kV cone beam CT was obtained to verify the liver position. The whole liver was within 5 mm in all directions in the great majority of patients. Population random setup errors (s) in liver position were 2.7 mm (superior inferior), 2.3 mm (medial lateral), and 3.0 mm (anterior posterior), and systematic errors (S) were all less than 2 mm (28). In biliary tract tumors, internal or external biliary stents may also be used as surrogates for the tumor.

Due to the low contrast of MV radiographs and the doses delivered with repeat MV imaging, orthogonal kV radiographs and kV fluoroscopy were developed for image guidance of tumors and/or fiducial markers, either immediately prior to each radiation fraction (29) or throughout radiation delivery (25). Kilo-voltage x-ray tubes may be ceiling or wall mounted or attached to the linear accelerator. Real-time kV fluoroscopy is used in a tumor-tracking approach developed by Shirato et al. (25), where tumors that move due to breathing are exposed to radiation only when the markers are located within a predefined volume. Alternative approaches involve tracking the tumor with moving collimators to chase the tumor or dynamically controlling the couch or the accelerator movement to follow the markers (30).

3D VOLUMETRIC IMAGE GUIDANCE Technological advances allowing volumetric imaging in the RT treatment room allow image guidance immediately prior to treatment using the tumor directly or the outlines of the organ harboring the tumor (in the case of cholangiocarcinoma, the liver), rather than bony anatomy. Volumetric image guidance can also utilize implanted fiducial markers. Advantages of volumetric imaging systems include visualizion of adjacent normal organs for more accurate avoidance of critical structures.

Volumetric image guidance is afforded by diagnostic grade CT imaging using an in-room linear accelerator-linked CT unit, MVCT as afforded on a helical tomotherapy unit, or kV cone-beam CT (CBCT) available on conventional C-arm linear accelerators. Should systematic changes from the simulation setup be assessed during IGRT imaging, both diagnostic CT and MVCT could be used as the basis for adaptive radiation treatment adjustments based on accurate rendering of tissue densities. The utility and resulting dosimetric accuracy of adaptive planning for abdominal targets based on CBCT datasets is not established for clinical use at this time.

The placement of a diagnostic CT scanner in the treatment room is realized with a known geometric relationship to the linear accelerator. While conceptually not necessarily required, all installed systems place the CT scanner in close proximity to the linear accelerator, allowing a shared couch for both the imaging and treatment device. For image guidance, the table top is rotated from the treatment position to the imaging position, in a typical arrangement by 180 degrees. The CT scanner gantry is translated on rails during acquisition; no active couch motion is required.

Advantages of in-room CT include that state of the art diagnostic quality CT can be used for optimal image quality and robustness. Ideally, the exact parameters of the simulation CT are replicated; resulting in imaging that fully matches the simulation imaging quality. Since imaging and treatment isocenter are not coincident, quality assurance measures have to be developed and tested on an established schedule. Because the table with the patient is rotated or moved between two devices, organ motion or setup changes between imaging and delivery are at least theoretical concerns. In-room CT has been used to monitor volumetric change and for guidance in upper abdominal malignancies (31).

Helical MVCT scans can be obtained using a helical tomotherapy treatment unit (TomoTherapy, Madison, WI), which allows the MV treatment beam to rotate around the patient while the couch moves through the bore. Single slice or volumetric MV images of the irradiated region can be constructed. While soft tissue contrast cannot match the quality achieved with in-room CT imaging, and the matrix of image reconstruction is reduced to 256 × 256, the resulting images are suitable for abdominal image-guidance (32). However, the utility of MVCT for image guidance of small SBRT liver lesions may be limited, as small lesion may not be discriminated from the surrounding normal liver tissue owing to a lack of sufficient soft tissue contrast (33).

Cone-beam CT (CBCT) refers to tomographic reconstruction from a series of 2D radiographs obtained in a single rotation of source and detector about the patient. Kilo-voltage CBCT systems integrate a kV tube and a flat panel detector mounted on a linear accelerator. The same axis of rotation is shared between the kV imaging and MV treatment beams, and the central axis of the kV beam is oriented perpendicular to (Elekta Synergy and Varian OBI) or parallel to (Siemens Artiste) the treatment MV beam. Hundreds of projections are acquired over a 30- to 240-second interval, while the volumetric reconstruction proceeds in parallel. Doses delivered to obtain kV cone beam CT scans typically range from 0.5 to 2 cGy, which is substantially less than the dose from MV orthogonal images. Routine clinical experience in the use of CBCT for cholangiocarcinoma is limited. Feasibility and acceptable soft-tissue definition of organs in the upper abdomen for IGRT have been reported by McBain (34) and Hawkins (28). Breathing motion and motion of the GI contents during imaging can introduce artifacts to

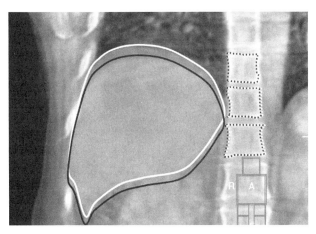

FIGURE 21.5

Registration of vertebral bodies from kV cone beam CT acquired at the time of radiation treatment to the CT acquired at the time of radiation planning in a patient imaged and treated with repeat exhale breath holds to immobilize the liver. Despite good alignment of the vertebral bodies, the liver position has changed between the two imaging sessions, providing rationale for image guidance to account for day-to-day positional variability. The liver itself can be used for image guidance and positioning.

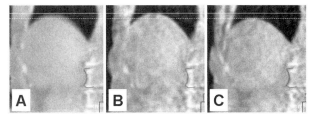

FIGURE 21.6

kV cone beam CT reconstructions from imaging acquiring in a patient treated during shallow breathing. The first panel (A) demonstrates the reconstruction of all projections obtained during free breathing, creating an image of a "blurred" liver. The second and third panels show respiratory sorted reconstructions made from projections only obtained during exhale (B) and inhale (C). Vertebral bodies from each reconstruction are aligned.

the CBCT scans, and the use of oral contrast can improve conspicuity of tissues. Using kV and MV CBCT without IV contrast, the tumor itself is not visible, and surrogates for IGRT such as the whole liver have been used for image guidance.

Kilo-voltage CBCT scans can be acquired in breath hold when patients are to be treated in breath hold (28,35). Breath-hold CBCT is associated with fewer artifacts than CBCTs acquired during free breathing and allows direct liver-to-liver image registration and positioning. Examples of a liver image acquired with the Elekta CBCT system is shown in Figure 21.5. Breath-hold CBCT is not yet routinely available on commercial systems.

While also not yet routinely available, respiratory-sorted CBCT scans (referring to volumetric imaging acquired at different phases of the respiratory cycle, or 4D CBCT) allow the changes in tumor and normal position due to breathing to be measured (36) (Figure 21.6).

CBCT systems can also produce kV fluoroscopic images from any gantry position, and they have the potential for real-time (i.e., concurrent with the MV radiotherapy treatment) fluoroscopic tumor monitoring and tracking, capabilities that are under current clinical investigation.

CBCT using the MV beam (MV-CBCT) requires less modification to a conventional linear accelerator compared to kV CBCT. The MV beam itself is used to construct a CBCT, in a similar manner as kV CBCT scans are obtained, with a single rotation around the patient. MV-CBCT image guidance has been particularly useful for IGRT of paraspinal tumors with orthopedic hardware in place that can cause artifacts on kV CT scans. A similar advantage should exist for metallic biliary stents that may be used in biliary tract cancers.

More advanced IGRT technologies are rapidly being developed, including a ring-gantry system that offers CBCT imaging along with a tilting treatment head for tumor tracking using kV fluoroscopy (37) and development of MR-guided RT systems.

ULTRASOUND-BASED IMAGE GUIDANCE

Ultrasound is a nonionizing modality also useful for image guidance for upper abdominal tumors including gallbladder cancer and cholangiocarcinoma (38,39). Initially developed to provide for image guidance for prostate cancer external beam radiation, the feasibility of using a 2D ultrasound system for abdominal tumor image guidance has been tested and validated in comparison with CT imaging (39). Intrahepatic tumor location and nonobese body habit of the patients was found to facilitate ultrasound-based image guidance. The accuracy of ultrasound image guidance as validated by CT-CT comparison does suggest meaningful improvement in target setup. Clinical experience in a series of 10 patients treated for gallbladder cancer by IMRT suggested the feasibility of using daily ultrasound-based image guidance and documented favorable outcomes (38). Ultrasound-based IGRT afforded PTV volume reduction of 41.4% for initial target volume treated to 45 Gy, and 62.2% for boost target treated to mean total doses of 59 Gy, respectively, compared to more conventional PTV definitions. This PTV margin reduction also enabled statistically significant organ-at-risk dose sparing, with the reduction of the mean liver dose (28.8 Gy vs. 39.6 Gy) being most relevant in the context of this publication. It is unclear if similar feasibility can be confirmed for 3D ultrasound guidance systems as organ motion during image acquisition will cause aliasing of the resulting 3D reconstructed ultrasound image data set. Similar to breath-hold CBCT, acquisition of 3D ultrasound data during breath hold should be feasible and may aid in overcoming such obstacles.

STEREOTACTIC BODY RADIOTHERAPY (SBRT)

Definition

The advances in imaging described in the first section of this chapter—to better define biliary and gallbladder cancers, assess their motion and improve accuracy and precision of radiation delivery with image-guided radiation therapy (IGRT)—along with advances in conformal radiation planning facilitate the delivery of high radiation doses that conform tightly around the target volume and fall off steeply around the target volume. This makes it possible for very potent doses of radiation to be delivered to small target volumes safely.

Although high-dose radiation may be delivered in a single fraction— referred to as extracranial stereotactic radiosurgery (SRS)—more often high precision radiation is delivered in more than one fraction, leading to the concept of SBRT.

SBRT refers to the use of a limited number of high-dose fractions delivered very conformally to targets with high accuracy, using biologic doses of radiation far higher than those used in standard fractionation. The term "stereotactic" refers to the use of a reference coordinate system (i.e., stereotactic frame/body immobilization system with integrated or attached localizer system) to aid in localizing the tumor. As the fraction-by-fraction positions of biliary and gallbladder cancers are not well correlated with the bones or an external reference system, as discussed above, daily online image-guided targeting of the tumor or adjacent soft tissues is required for precise localization.

SBRT as a valid treatment concept has found broad adaptation, as evidenced by an ASTRO consensus document on SBRT (40) and the development of a specialized Medicare billing code for SBRT in the United States. While SBRT is today defined in the United States as comprising treatments between one and five fractions of high radiation doses, SBRT is clearly an evolving technology, and definitions may change with time. In the peer-reviewed literature, extracranial hypofractionated stereotactic treatment concepts delivered in 6–10 fractions are also commonly reported as SBRT.

In SBRT, multiple static or dynamic beams in a variety of beam arrangements, with or without segments or intensity modulation, or dynamic conformal arc arrangements including serial and helical tomotherapy can be used to produce a dose distribution in which isodose lines tightly conform to the target volume. Although most reports on SBRT refer to MV photon irradiation, protons may be used. Inhomogeneity within the target volume is typically accepted; significant dose inhomogeneities approaching or even exceeding maximal doses of 150% of the dose prescribed to the periphery of a target are encouraged to increase the chance of tumor ablation (33,41). Doses are generally prescribed to an isodose line covering the planning target volume with very steep dose gradients outside the target volume.

Rationale for SBRT

For biliary tract and gallbladder cancer, local recurrence remains the predominant pattern of disease recurrence following surgery and conventional radiation therapy, providing a rationale to study innovations that may improve local control, hopefully improving overall survival. Local recurrences are often associated with sub-

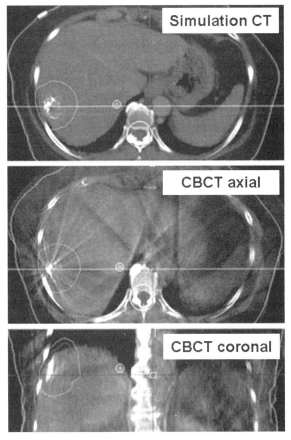

FIGURE 21.7

Use of lipiodol tumor staining for SBRT image guidance. The upper figure (simulation CT) documents tumor lipiodol retention. The middle and lower figures document kV CBCT image guidance; the lipiodol stain is well visualized and can be used to optimize target setup for treatment.

stantial morbidity, chronic requirement for stents, and their associated morbidities. Escalated dose with standard fractionation is associated with very long treatment times, and thus SBRT has the potential to deliver very high biologic equivalent doses in a far shorter time.

SBRT per se is a noninvasive, outpatient intervention, generally completed within 1–2 weeks. While the placement of radio-opaque fiducial markers, or prior tumor staining by intra-arterial tumorembolization (with or without a chemoembolization component, TACE), constitutes moderately invasive procedures, such internal markers can serve as surrogates to determine treatment tumor location during image guidance (Figure 21.7). The short radiation treatment time and high dose per fraction in SBRT may have potential radiobiologic therapeutic advantages compared with conventional fractionation, owing to the ability to overcome tumor radiation resistance constituted by tumor hypoxia, tumor repopulation, and repair. Furthermore, the shorter SBRT treatment times

are more convenient for patients and may have resource utilization advantages.

Advancements outside of radiation oncology also provide rationale for SBRT. Ablative therapies such as photo-dynamic therapy for peri-hilar tumors, radiofrequency ablation (RFA), and transarterial chemoembolization are used to treat focal primary liver tumors including cholangiocarcinoma in ablative intent (42–44). Furthermore, improvements in systemic therapy more likely to control micro-metastases provide rationale for improving local therapies, such as SBRT, to reduce macroscopic foci of tumor burden.

SBRT Radiation Planning

Because of steeper dose gradients and ablative dose prescription with SBRT, the consequences of error in tumor delineation, and errors introduced by dosimetry and geometric uncertainties may be more deleterious. Thus, all aspects of treatment planning that are important in conformal radiation planning are even more crucial in SBRT, especially for tumors in close proximity to critical normal tissues, where any systematic error could lead to permanent serious toxicity if the normal tissue planned to be spared from the high-dose region of the radiation dose distribution is irradiated to the high doses planned for the tumor.

Sometimes, noncoplanar beams or arcs are used if required to reduce the dose to normal tissues. One strat-

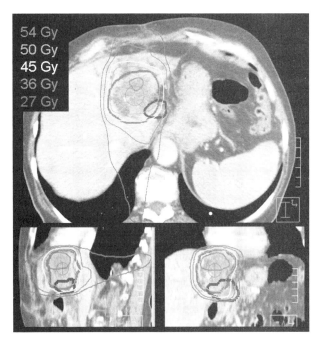

FIGURE 21.8

SBRT plan for intrahepatic cholangiocarcinoma planning target volume (PTV), treated with 45 Gy in six fractions over 2 weeks.

egy to obtain very steep dose gradients at the edge of the PTV is to close the aperture of the beams to coincide or be within the PTV outline, not leaving a gap for penumbra as usually done for conformal radiation therapy. Resultant high doses/hotspots occur in the center of the PTV, ideally depositing the highest dose to the center of a hypoxic target volume, although the clinical benefit of such a strategy is unproven (Figure 21.8). The use of segments within the beams can adjust the dose distribution to ensure that the hot spot is within the tumor, while reducing the overall integral dose to the liver and other normal tissues. Alternatively, using 4DCT data as the basis for dose planning, doses can be prescribed to the periphery of a PTV derived from the ITV, with differential dose prescription to a minimum intensity projection (MinIP) derived target volume, representing the motion overlap area always containing tumor during the respiratory cycle (Figure 21.2). Thus, defined dose heterogeneity to central parts of the ITV can be achieved (Figure 21.9).

Typical prescription doses for SBRT range from the delivery of 5 Gy for 10 fractions to 20 Gy for 3 fractions. One to 5 fractions are most often used, with a dose per fraction usually greater than 6 Gy. The feature common to most of the SBRT fractionation schemes is that they are biologically potent. Multiple fraction regimens have some theoretical radiobiologic advantages over single fraction SBRT. While proximity of the target to normal tissues that function serially (e.g., small bowel) may require fractionated delivery to minimize the risk of toxicity, randomized data to support multifraction regimens over single treatments are not available. Also, there exists a lack of clinical data to provide guidance for optimal prescription doses and dose

scheduling for each clinical scenario. In clinical use, most regimens are delivery in 48- to 72-hour increments (i.e., every other day, or twice weekly).

Clinical Experience with SBRT

Although there is little published experience in SBRT for biliary tract cancers, there is a growing literature of SBRT for liver metastases and hepatocellular carcinoma. The liver cancer SBRT series have sometimes included cholangiocarcinoma patients. These clinical series are summarized here.

Blomgren et al. from the Karolinska Institute in Sweden provided the first reported outcomes following SBRT for liver cancers. Twenty to 45 Gy in one to four fractions were used to treat 29 liver tumors in 23 patients (8 patients with hepatocellular carcinoma, one with intrahepatic cholangiocarcinoma, and 14 with metastases) (2). Radiographic responses were observed in 29 and 43% of evaluable patients with primary and metastatic liver cancer, respectively. Complete responses occurred quickly for small tumors, but the time to maximal response was prolonged for larger tumors. Using this approach, the mean liver dose generally ranged from 1 to 8 Gy, with a maximum of 18 Gy delivered in three fractions for one patient. Several serious toxicities were seen following hepatocellular carcinoma SBRT, including one sudden death 2 days after 30 Gy in one fraction to a large tumor, two cases of radiation induced liver disease (RILD) 1.5 and 2.5 months following SBRT (45 and 30 Gy in three fractions, respectively), and one subcapsular bleed 2 weeks following SBRT.

At the Princess Margaret Hospital in Toronto, a phase I study of a six-fraction regimen of SBRT in 41

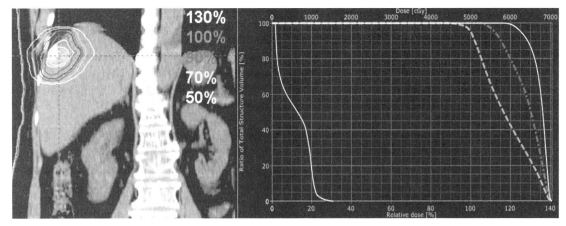

FIGURE 21.9

Differential SBRT dose prescription based on ITV/MinIP ITV target volume delineation derived from 4DCT simulation imaging. Doses were prescribed so that 95% of the PTV received a dose of 50 Gy in five fractions; the small motion overlap area (MinIP ITV) was prescribed to receive 130% of the prescribed dose. Thus a potentially hypoxic core of the target volume receives a higher dose than the periphery of the PTV.

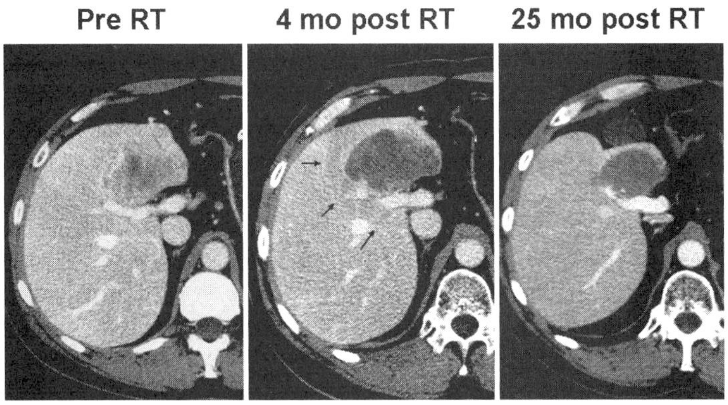

Pre RT   **4 mo post RT**   **25 mo post RT**

FIGURE 21.10

Intrahepatic cholangiocarcinoma treated with 33 Gy in six fractions over 2 weeks. CT scan at 4 months following SBRT shows a decrease in attenuation in high-dose liver volume surrounding the tumor and reduction in density of tumor. At 25 months post-SBRT the tumor is more cystic with little enhancement. The liver irradiated to high doses has contracted.

patients with unresectable intrahepatic cholangiocarcinoma (10 patients) or hepatocellular carcinoma (31 patients) was completed (45). An individualized treatment approach was used in this study in which the prescribed tumor dose was dependent on volume of liver irradiated. The median dose delivered was 32.5 Gy in six fractions with a range from 28 to 48 Gy. The cholangiocarcinoma patients were refractory to prior chemotherapy and/or not suitable for chemotherapy. Their median volume was 172 cm³, with a range from 10 to 465 cm³, respectively. At least 800 cm³ of uninvolved liver was required, and the mean liver doses were less than 22 Gy in six fractions. The maximal permitted dose to 0.5 cm3 of the esophagus, stomach, duodenum, or other bowel was 30 Gy. IGRT was used for target positioning prior to delivery of each radiation fraction (27, 28). No radiation-induced liver disease (RILD) or treatment-related grade 4/5 toxicity was seen within 3 months following SBRT. Two patients (5%) with cholangiocarcioma developed transient biliary obstruction following the first few fractions, leading to a policy of pretreatment steroids for subsequent patients with central tumors, with no further biliary obstruction observed. Seven patients (five hepatocellular carcinoma, two cholangiocarcinoma) developed a decline in liver function from Child-Pugh class A to B within 3 months following SBRT. Both cholangiocarcinoma patients had rapid tumor progression that likely contributed to the decline in liver function. Another cholangiocarcinoma developed a small bowel obstruction 17 months after SBRT requiring bypass surgery, at which time extrahepatic progressive disease was detected. Local control of the irradiated tumor was common, but hepatic and extrahepatic recurrences outside the irradiated fields occurred, providing rationale for combining SBRT with systemic therapies. The median survival of cholangiocarcinoma patients treated with this SBRT approach was 15.0 months (95% CI 6.5–29.0) (45). Typical response to SBRT is documented in Figure 21.10.

Other series of SBRT for liver metastases and hepatocellular carcinoma have shown the safety of different SBRT fractionations. Herfarth et al. used single fraction SRS to treat 60 liver tumors in 37 patients (4 primary and 56 metastases). The median tumor size was 10 cm³ (1–132 cm³), with an upper maximum diameter of 6 cm. The single dose was safely escalated from 14 to 26 Gy, and a maximal tolerated dose was not found (6, 10). With a median follow-up of 5.7 months, there was no major toxicity. Ninety-eight percent of all tumors were locally controlled after 6 weeks, with complete and partial responses seen in 4 and 28 patients, respectively. Actuarial local tumor control was 81% 18 months after therapy. Normal tissue constraints restricted dose exposure of no more than 30 and 50% of the liver to less than 12 and 7 Gy, respectively, and maximal doses to esophagus and stomach of 14 and 12 Gy, respectively.

Wulf et al. from the University of Wurzburg used SBRT delivered in three fractions (30 Gy total) to treat 23 patients with solitary liver tumors. No grade 3 toxicity was observed. Crude local control was 76 and 61% at 1 and 2 years, respectively (46).

Schefter et al. reported on a multi-institutional trial of three fraction SBRT for liver cancer (5). Twenty-five tumors in 18 patients with a variety of diagnoses (16 metastases, 2 hepatocellular carcinomas) were treated with 36–60 Gy, in three fractions delivered within 14 days. At least 700 cm³ of uninvolved liver had to receive less than 15 Gy in three fractions. Most patients were given prophylactic antiemetic therapy with or without dexamethasone. The average tumor volume was 17.8 cm³ (3–98 cm³). No dose-limiting toxicity was seen. A tumor equivalent uniform dose (EUD) of more than 54 Gy in three fractions was associated with improved local control compared to an EUD of less than 54 Gy in 3 fractions (47).

CONCLUSIONS

Advances in imaging and in image guidance of radiation therapy allow radiation therapy to be delivered conformally to biliary tract and gallbladder cancers with more accuracy and precision than previously possible, allowing dose escalation and reduced doses to normal tissues. IGRT increases awareness of geometric change occurring during radiation therapy and provides the ability to confirm that the dose is delivered as planned.

However, IGRT is particularly challenging in the upper abdomen, and quality of imaging and efficiency continue to rapidly improve. There is not one ideal IGRT technology or strategy most suitable for all biliary tract and gallbladder cancers. Nonetheless, IGRT brings with it the opportunity to investigate adaptive radiation therapy and facilitates hypo-fractionation and SBRT. Future efforts in IGRT are needed to efficiently archive, analyze, and correlate large volumes of imaging data with clinical, biologic, and outcome data.

SBRT is an exciting clinically applicable emerging technology of radiation oncology that brings together many of the technological advancements that have occurred recently in radiation oncology. SBRT requires utilization of high-quality imaging for target definition, immobilization, high-precision planning, and delivery under daily image guidance. Using these technological advancements, potent radiobiologic doses can be delivered in convenient fractionation schemes, generally ranging from one to five fractions. Preliminary data suggest that SBRT can be delivered safely to liver cancers with a high likelihood of local control and an acceptable safety profile. However, clinical experience in SBRT for biliary tract tumors is limited. Outcomes are expected to be improved further if SBRT can be safely combined with other systemic and regional therapies. Serious acute and early delayed toxicities have been reported in the early SBRT experience, including radiation-induced liver injury and GI bleeding. However, late sequelae from of SBRT may not manifest until many years following therapy. As experience in SBRT in biliary tract cancer SBRT increases, the efficacy and safety of SBRT should become better defined. Optimal fractionation, potential, and limitations of image guidance and appropriate application of SBRT in biliary tract and potentially also gallbladder cancers are not well established at this time. It is recommended that SBRT be used for the treatment of biliary and gallbladder cancers only in the context of clinical trials, as published experience in this site are limited.

References

1. Dawson LA, Normolle D, Balter JM, et al. Analysis of radiation-induced liver disease using the Lyman NTCP model. Int J Radiat Oncol Biol Phys 2002; 53:810–821.
2. Blomgren H, Lax I, Naslund I, et al. Stereotactic high dose fraction radiation therapy of extracranial tumors using an accelerator. Clinical experience of the first thirty-one patients. Acta Oncol 1995; 34:861–870.
3. Ben-Josef E, Normolle D, Ensminger WD, et al. Phase II trial of high-dose conformal radiation therapy with concurrent hepatic artery floxuridine for unresectable intrahepatic malignancies. J Clin Oncol 2005; 23:8739–8747.
4. Cheng JC, Wu JK, Lee PC, et al. Biologic susceptibility of hepatocellular carcinoma patients treated with radiotherapy to radiation-induced liver disease. Int J Radiat Oncol Biol Phys 2004; 60:1502–1509.
5. Schefter TE, Kavanagh BD, Timmerman RD, et al. A phase I trial of stereotactic body radiation therapy (SBRT) for liver metastases. Int J Radiat Oncol Biol Phys 2005; 62:1371–1378.
6. Herfarth KK, Debus J, Wannenmacher M. Stereotactic radiation therapy of liver metastases: update of the initial phase-I/II trial. Front Radiat Ther Oncol 2004; 38:100–105.
7. Hoyer M, Roed H, Traberg Hansen A, et al. Phase II study on stereotactic body radiotherapy of colorectal metastases. Acta Oncol 2006; 45:823–830.
8. Chiba T, Tokuuye K, Matsuzaki Y, et al. Proton beam therapy for hepatocellular carcinoma: a retrospective review of 162 patients. Clin Cancer Res 2005; 11:3799–3805.
9. Blomgren H, Lax I, Goranson H, et al. Radiosurgery for tumors in the body: Clinical experience using a new method. J Radiosurg 1998; 1:63–74.
10. Herfarth KK, Debus J, Lohr F, et al. Stereotactic single-dose radiation therapy of liver tumors: results of a phase I/II trial. J Clin Oncol 2001; 19:164–170.
11. Hoyer M, Roed H, Sengelov L, et al. Phase-II study on stereotactic radiotherapy of locally advanced pancreatic carcinoma. Radiother Oncol 2005; 76:48–53.
12. Koong AC, Le QT, Ho A, et al. Phase I study of stereotactic radiosurgery in patients with locally advanced pancreatic cancer. Int J Radiat Oncol Biol Phys 2004; 58:1017–1021.
13. Schwartz LH, Black J, Fong Y, et al. Gallbladder carcinoma: findings at MR imaging with MR cholangiopancreatography. J Comput Assist Tomogr 2002; 26:405–410.
14. Tseng JH, Wan YL, Hung CF, et al. Diagnosis and staging of gallbladder carcinoma. Evaluation with dynamic MR imaging. Clin Imaging 2002; 26:177–182.
15. Manfredi R, Barbaro B, Masselli G, et al. Magnetic resonance imaging of cholangiocarcinoma. Semin Liver Dis 2004; 24:155–164.
16. Fritscher-Ravens A, Bohuslavizki KH, Broering DC, et al. FDG PET in the diagnosis of hilar cholangiocarcinoma. Nucl Med Commun 2001; 22:1277–1285.
17. Kim YJ, Yun M, Lee WJ, et al. Usefulness of 18F-FDG PET in intrahepatic cholangiocarcinoma. Eur J Nucl Med Mol Imaging 2003; 30:1467–1472.
18. Kluge R, Schmidt F, Caca K, et al. Positron emission tomography with [(18)F]fluoro-2-deoxy-D-glucose for diagnosis and staging of bile duct cancer. Hepatology 2001; 33:1029–1035.
19. Rodriguez-Fernandez A, Gomez-Rio M, Llamas-Elvira JM, et al. Positron-emission tomography with fluorine-18-fluoro-2-deoxy-D-glucose for gallbladder cancer diagnosis. Am J Surg 2004; 188:171–175.
20. Balter JM, Lam KL, McGinn CJ, et al. Improvement of CT-based treatment-planning models of abdominal targets using static exhale imaging. Int J Radiat Oncol Biol Phys 1998; 41:939–943.
21. Dawson LA, Brock KK, Kazanjian S, et al. The reproducibility of organ position using active breathing control (ABC) during liver radiotherapy. Int J Radiat Oncol Biol Phys 2001; 51:1410–1421.
22. Eccles CL, Brock KK, Hawkins M, et al. Reproducibility of liver position using active breathing coordinator for liver cancer radiotherapy. Int J Radiat Oncol Biol Phys 2005; 64:751–759.
23. Pan T, Lee TY, Rietzel E, et al. 4D-CT imaging of a volume influenced by respiratory motion on multi-slice CT. Med Phys 2004; 31:333–340.
24. Rietzel E, Pan T, Chen GT. Four-dimensional computed tomography: image formation and clinical protocol. Med Phys 2005; 32:874–889.

25. Shirato H, Shimizu S, Kitamura K, et al. Four-dimensional treatment planning and fluoroscopic real-time tumor tracking radiotherapy for moving tumor. Int J Radiat Oncol Biol Phys 2000; 48:435–442.

26. Kupelian PA, Choonik L, Langen KM, et al. Evaluation of image-guidance strategies in the treatment of head and neck cancers. Int J Radiat Oncol Biol Phys 2007; 67(3):670–677.

27. Dawson LA, Eccles C, Bissonnette JP, et al. Accuracy of daily image guidance for hypofractionated liver radiotherapy with active breathing control. Int J Radiat Oncol Biol Phys 2005; 62:1247–1252.

28. Hawkins M, Brock K, Eccles C, et al. Assessment of residual error in liver position using kV cone-beam CT for liver cancer high precision radiation therapy. Int J Radiat Oncol Biol Phys 2006; 66:610–619.

29. Beddar AS, Kainz K, Briere TM, et al. Correlation between internal fiducial tumor motion and external marker motion for liver tumors imaged with 4D-CT. Int J Radiat Oncol Biol Phys 2007; 67:630–638.

30. Keall P, Joshi S, Vedam S, et al. Four-dimensional radiotherapy planning for DMLC-based respiratory motion tracking. Med Phys 2005; 32:942–951.

31. Uematsu M, Fukui T, Shioda A, et al. A dual computed tomography linear accelerator unit for stereotactic radiation therapy: a new approach without cranially fixated stereotactic frames. Int J Radiat Oncol Biol Phys 1996; 35:587–592.

32. Li XA, Qi XS, Pitterle M, et al. Interfractional variations in patient setup and anatomic change assessed by daily computed tomography. Int J Radiat Oncol Biol Phys 2007; 68:581–591.

33. Fuss M, Shi C, Papanikolaou N. Tomotherapeutic stereotactic body radiation therapy: techniques and comparison between modalities. Acta Oncol 2006; 45:953–960.

34. McBain CA, Henry AM, Sykes J, et al. X-ray volumetric imaging in image-guided radiotherapy: the new standard in on-treatment imaging. Int J Radiat Oncol Biol Phys 2006; 64:625–634.

35. Duggan DM, Ding GX, Coffey CW, 2nd, et al. Deep-inspiration breath-hold kilovoltage cone-beam CT for setup of stereotactic body radiation therapy for lung tumors: initial experience. Lung Cancer 2007; 56:77–88.

36. Sonke JJ, Zijp L, Remeijer P, et al. Respiratory correlated cone beam CT. Med Phys 2005; 32:1176–1186.

37. Kamino Y, Takayama K, Kokubo M, et al. Development of a four-dimensional image-guided radiotherapy system with a gimbaled X-ray head. Int J Radiat Oncol Biol Physics 2006; 66:271–278.

38. Fuller CD, Thomas CR, Jr., Wong A, et al. Image-guided intensity-modulated radiation therapy for gallbladder carcinoma. Radiother Oncol 2006; 81:65–72.

39. Fuss M, Salter BJ, Cavanaugh SX, et al. Daily ultrasound-based image-guided targeting for radiotherapy of upper abdominal malignancies. Int J Radiat Oncol Biol Phys 2004; 59:1245–1256.

40. Potters L, Steinberg M, Rose C, et al. American Society for Therapeutic Radiology and Oncology and American College of Radiology practice guideline for the performance of stereotactic body radiation therapy. Int J Radiat Oncol Biol Phys 2004; 60:1026–1032.

41. Lax I, Blomgren H, Naslund I, et al. Stereotactic radiotherapy of malignancies in the abdomen. Methodological aspects. Acta Oncol 1994; 33:677–683.

42. Berr F. Photodynamic therapy for cholangiocarcinoma. Semin Liver Dis 2004; 24:177–187.

43. Burger I, Hong K, Schulick R, et al. Transcatheter arterial chemoembolization in unresectable cholangiocarcinoma: initial experience in a single institution. J Vasc Interv Radiol 2005; 16:353–361.

44. Chiou YY, Hwang JI, Chou YH, et al. Percutaneous ultrasound-guided radiofrequency ablation of intrahepatic cholangiocarcinoma. Kaohsiung J Med Sci 2005; 21:304–309.

45. Tse R, Hawkins M, Lockwood G, et al. Phase I study of individualized stereotactic body radiotherapy for hepatocellular carcinoma and intrahepatic cholangiocarcinoma. J Clin Oncol 2006; 45 (no 7): 848-855.

46. Wulf J, Hadinger U, Oppitz U, et al. Stereotactic radiotherapy of targets in the lung and liver. Strahlenther Oncol 2001; 177:645–655.

47. Kavanagh BD, Schefter TE, Cardenes HR, et al. Interim analysis of a prospective phase I/II trial of SBRT for liver metastases. Acta Oncol 2006; 45:848–855.

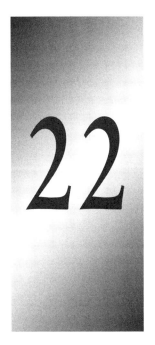

22 Symptom Management and Palliation

Eduardo da Silveira
Douglas O. Faigel
M. Brian Fennerty

Bile is an important vehicle for absorption of nutrients and the excretion of products of normal metabolism and toxic substances. If biliary excretion is impaired, retention of bile salts and other bile constituents such as bilirubin and cholesterol occurs (cholestasis). The reflux of these constituents into the systemic circulation and the decreased amount of bile salts reaching the intestine are associated with a wide spectrum of clinical manifestations such as jaundice, pruritus, malabsorption, hypocoagulation, immunologic changes, and renal dysfunction (1-3).

Malignancies of the biliary and pancreatic systems are common causes of biliary obstruction. Together they are among the 10 most common cancers in North America and Europe (4). For instance, it is estimated that more than 31,000 new cases of pancreatic cancer occurred in the United States in 2004 (4, 5). The most common causes of malignant biliary obstruction are tumors originating from of the head of the pancreas or the ampulla of Vater, and they obstruct the biliary system at its most distal portion where the common bile duct traverses the head of the pancreas and enters the duodenum. However, primary cancers of the liver and the biliary system as well as tumors from outside the gastrointestinal tract can also obstruct the biliary system at more proximal locations.

There are various approaches to the management of patients with distal malignant biliary obstruction, and optimal management often requires the combined involvement of a wide variety of specialists, including gastroenterologists, radiologists, surgeons, and/or medical and radiation oncologists. While a number of methods for palliation of biliary obstruction exist, cure of primary pancreaticobiliary cancers can only be achieved if surgical resection is performed at early stages of disease. Unfortunately, the natural history of pancreatic and biliary malignancies is such that they usually become clinically apparent only when the disease is either widespread or has locally invaded vascular structures, precluding curative surgical procedures (6, 7). Following staging, the majority of patients are determined to be not curable or are found not suitable candidates to undergo a surgical curative procedure; hence, palliative treatment of the biliary obstruction is indicated. While re-establishment of the normal bile flow has no impact on survival (8), it has been shown to prevent complications related to the biliary obstruction and to improve quality of life (9–11).

As histologic confirmation of malignancy resulting in biliary obstruction is not always feasible, a presumptive diagnosis and empirical management of biliary and pancreatic malignancies commonly relies upon imaging study results. There is no ideal diagnostic procedure for the evaluation of these malignancies, but advances in radiologic imaging over the last few decades have permitted better visualization of the biliary and pancreatic systems and consequently often led to the avoidance of unnecessary surgical procedures. Transabdominal ultrasound is often used as the initial method to differentiate obstructive jaundice from other forms of cholestasis, as it is inexpensive and noninvasive, and its sensitivity and specificity are excellent in the presence of jaundice (12). Helical computed tomography (CT) is the single most useful imaging test because not only can it adequately visualize most local organs of interest, but it can also assess the existence of distant metastatic disease. Newer generation CT scanners can also provide even more highly detailed, tridimensional images. Endoscopy ultrasound (EUS) offers the advantage of being able to detect small lesions, lymph nodes, and regional vascular invasion often not detectable by other modalities while allowing for tissue sampling during the same procedure (8, 13–15). In the majority of cases, the combination of these imaging modalities is sufficient to make an accurate diagnosis and appropriately stage a tumor. More invasive diagnostic procedures such as diagnostic laparoscopy, which was indicated in the past to exclude peritoneal and liver metastases, is no longer indicated for staging of disease considered resectable by conventional imaging (16–18).

MANAGEMENT

Pain

Abdominal discomfort is present in approximately 75% of patients with pancreatic cancer at diagnosis and over 90% in advanced stages. Pain is more commonly seen in tumor involving the body and tail of the pancreas due to its proximity to the celiac plexus. Usually this pain is described as dull, constant, in the epigastric region, and with radiation to the back. Associated symptoms such as nausea, vomiting, postprandial fullness, and sitiofobia can also be encountered. In contrast, tumors of the head, which account for the majority of the cases, are usually asymptomatic until involvement of adjacent organs or dilation of the biliary system occurs (19). Assessment of the possible sources of pain is important as specific treatment options exist. When duodenal obstruction is present, endoscopic stenting or gastric bypass surgery should be utilized to ameliorate the discomfort and the obstructive symptoms and improve quality of life (20).

The standard approach to pain management is based on the World Health Organization (WHO) three-step ladder, beginning with nonopioid analgesics (e.g., nonsteroidal anti-inflammatory drugs [NSAIDs] or acetaminophen), followed by weak opioids, and finally, strong opioids as necessary (21, 22). However, malignant pain can be difficult to control or refractory to treatment in many patients. Under these circumstances, alternative strategies such as patient controlled anesthesia, radiation therapy, and celiac plexus neurolysis (CPN) have to be considered (23). Although the terms "celiac plexus" and "splanchnic nerves" are often used interchangeably, these are anatomically distinct structures. The splanchnic nerves are located above the diaphragm (retro-crural) and are typically anterior to the 12th thoracic vertebra. The celiac plexus, however, is situated below the diaphragm (antecrural), surrounding the basis of the celiac trunk. This plexus is composed of a dense network of sympathetic and parasympathetic fibers and is the target of CPN, a chemical splanchnicectomy of the celiac plexus, which aims to preferentially ablate the sympathetic afferent nerve fibers that transmit pain from intra-abdominal viscera. Different approaches (retrocrural, anterocrural, and neurolysis of the splanchnic nerves) and methods (surgical, percutaneous, and endoscopic) of CPN have been applied (24–28). Due to rare cases of paraplegia with percutaneous fluoroscopy-guided CPN, EUS and CT-guided "anterior" approaches have become the preferred techniques for CPN. CPN is achieved with injection of absolute alcohol, but mixture with bupivacaine 0.25% is often utilized to decrease the immediate discomfort due to subsequent tissue necrosis. Analgesic responses are moderate (>50%) with a wide range of duration of effect (27, 29). However, these observations are based on uncontrolled and retrospective analysis subject to bias and confounding. Moreover, the studies are small, have heterogeneous patient populations, and have not used standardized scales for assessments of pain. No prospective controlled trials have been done comparing conventional opiates to neurolytic regimens for controlling pain secondary to pancreaticobiliary malignancy.

Duodenal Obstruction

Obstruction of the stomach or duodenum due to biliopancreatic malignancies is a late event that results in nausea, vomiting, malnutrition, and progressive deterioration in patients' quality of life. Surgical palliation is an available option, but the morbidity and mortality related to the procedures are high, and, unfortunately, control of symptoms is achieved in about only half of the patients treated (30, 31). Endoscopically placed self-expandable metallic stents (SEMS) is an alternative strategy which has also been used to palliate obstructive symptoms. However, recurrent stenosis of the stent either because of progressive tumor ingrowth or overgrowth has been a problem (32–34). Most studies have included only a small number of patients, but overall, recurrent stenosis rates range between 8 and 46% at intervals of 2–21 weeks (32–34). Although no large, controlled trials have been performed, published data suggest that SEMS are a safe and effective nonsurgical alternative treatment for inoperable cases (34–40).

Biliary Obstruction

Patients with bilio-pancreatic cancer and no evidence of metastatic disease or local vascular invasion should be considered for curative surgical resection. Unfortunately these patients account for only 10–20% of all cases (7). In addition, many elderly patients are not referred for consideration of surgery as they are judged unfit for operation due to advanced age or unrelated comorbidities. Despite an extensive preoperative workup, 11–53% of patients with pancreatic cancer thought to be surgical candidates are found to be unresectable at the time of laparotomy, and the prospect for patients with cholangiocarcinoma and gallbladder cancer is worse. Thus, for most patients with malignant pancreaticobiliary obstruction, palliative therapy directed at their primary symptom will be indicated. Many will experience symptomatic biliary obstruction that requires either a surgical bypass or placement of a biliary stent (41).

SURGERY

Historically, surgical procedures were used for the palliation of obstructive jaundice until effective, less invasive techniques became more widely available (42). Thirty-day mortality after surgical palliation for pancreatic cancer and cholangiocarcinoma may occur in up to one third of cases; with the risk being even more pronounced in individuals either above 60 years of age or with metastatic disease (43). Except for underdeveloped countries where endoscopic and radiologic expertise is not readily available, as well as for patients with concomitant gastric outlet obstruction, surgical palliative techniques are now rarely used in the management of obstructive jaundice; they have been replaced by percutaneous and endoscopic insertion of stents (44, 45).

Although endoscopic stenting is the most common management strategy for the palliation of biliary obstructions, the need for repetitive reinterventions often raises the question of surgery as a valid alternative. Three prospective randomized trials have compared open surgery with endoscopic stenting (46–48). Smith and colleagues randomized 203 patients to 10-French (Fr) Amsterdam plastic stent or biliary bypass (choledocoduodenostomy and choledocojejunostomy). Patients who underwent stent placement had fewer procedure-related and major complication rates as well as shorter hospital stays than the surgical group. Shepherd and Andersen conducted smaller studies that showed

similar results (46, 48). While overall survival did not differ between treatments, these studies demonstrated that endoscopic stenting had a lower rate of short-term complication than surgical treatment. Although patients in the endoscopy group had more obstructions and needed more reinterventions, the total number of days in-hospital was higher in the surgical group. A meta-anaylsis performed with these three studies confirmed a higher likelihood of intervention in the stent group (49).

While performed more than 10 years ago, before the advent of newer technologies for stents (SEMS) and less invasive surgical procedures, these studies suggest that palliation of pancreaticobiliary malignancy with endoscopic stents is as effective as and less costly than surgery. A recent single-center retrospective cost analysis in the United States also revealed a striking difference between endoscopic palliation and surgery despite the need for repetitive interventions and readmissions in the endoscopic group (50). However, surgical bypass remains an acceptable strategy in patients with unresectable disease at the time of laparotomy and for those requiring concomitant gastrointestinal bypass and/or celiac nerve block for management of chronic pain (18, 41). Whether prophylactic gastrointestinal bypass should be offered to patients with malignant obstructive jaundice is unknown (51–53). Recent studies have shown that gastrojejunostomy in addition to biliary bypass may decrease the incidence of late gastric outlet obstruction without higher morbidity or mortality for the initial surgery (41, 54). The impact of emerging minimally invasive surgical techniques will have in the management of these patients is still unknown and randomized clinical trials as well as cost-effectiveness analyses are needed (55).

PERCUTANEOUS APPROACH

A variety of nonoperative methods to relieve distal biliary malignant obstruction exist. Percutaneous drainage was the preferred palliative method in patients with malignant obstruction until several years ago. When compared to endoscopic placement of plastic stents, the percutaneous approach permits insertion of plastic drains with larger diameters. The consequent benefit of a longer stent patency represented a significant advantage over the plastic stents inserted by endoscopic retrograde cholangiopancreatography (ERCP), which was limited by the size of the accessory channel of duodenoscopes. Percutaneous insertion of stents appeared to be as effective as biliary bypass and still had some inherent advantages. Bornman et al. found the overall survival to be similar in both surgical and percutaneous groups, and indeed percutaneous drainage was associated with a lower procedure-related complication and 30-day mortality rate (56).

This procedure entails sterile catheterization of a peripheral biliary radical after percutaneous puncture. The technique has evolved over the years, and currently insertion of an indwelling catheter without external drainage is possible. The disadvantages of external biliary drainage included the risk of spontaneous catheter dislodgment, inflammation and pain around the puncture site, leak of ascitic fluid and bile around the catheter, and loss of fluid and electrolytes (57). In addition, the amount of resources utilized is higher. Unlike endoscopic insertion, which is routinely done as a single outpatient procedure, percutaneous stenting is a two-step procedure and requires follow-up interventions.

The advent of SEMS and larger size accessory channels in duodenoscopes has changed the prior management of pancreaticobiliary malignancy. Speer and colleagues conducted a prospective randomized study comparing percutaneous and endoscopic drainage in patients with malignant biliary obstruction (58). While overall survival was not different between both arms, 30-day mortality both by intention-to-treat and per-protocol analysis was significant lower in the endoscopy group and justified the early termination of the study. The authors found that complications associated with the percutaneous procedure accounted for the difference in mortality and that endoscopic insertion of a stent was safer and more likely to succeed (58). A collection of published series done by Coene et al. supports the superiority of an endoscopic versus a percutaneous approach with regards to early complication, 30-day mortality and successful drainage (59). However, a recent RCT showed that patients undergoing percutaneous drainage had longer survival than those in the endoscopy group, which conflicts with results from trials performed 2 decades ago (60). The authors argued that advances in radiologic techniques have led to a reduction in complication rates and that the results from "old" studies do not reflect current practice. However, this study included not only patients with unresectable distal biliary obstruction but also subjects with more proximal obstruction including hilar tumors. This difference in inclusion criteria could explain the low success rate of plastic stent insertion by endoscopy (58%), which in turn accounted for the suboptimal efficacy observed in this group.

Thus, the predominance of evidence in the literature advocates the use of endoscopy as first-line therapy (59). Nevertheless, the percutaneous approach remains a preferred option for management of hilar tumors, patients undergoing palliative brachytherapy, and distal malignant biliary obstruction not successfully treated by ERCP (61).

ENDOSCOPIC PALLIATION

A number of endoprostheses are commercially available under different brand names that can be separated in two main categories: (a) plastic polyethylene (PE) stents (Figure 22.1) (b) and self-expandable metal stents (SEMS) (Figure 22.2), which can be either uncovered (U-SEMS) or covered (C-SEMS). All three stent types have been shown to be effective in the relief of obstruction and re-establishing patency of the biliary tree, but they differ in several aspects, including physical characteristics, price, and average duration of patency (62–64).

Plastic Endoprosthesis

Endoscopic placement of plastic biliary stents were first described by Soehendra and Reynders-Frederix as an alternative to choledocoduodenostomy in high-risk and inoperable cancer patients (65). Plastic stents have several inherent advantages in patients with malignant biliary obstruction. First they are inexpensive compared to metal stents and surgical bypass, are easy to insert, and can be removed if necessary. The main disadvantage to plastic stents is their duration of patency, which can be shorter than the patient's life expectancy (66, 67). Because stent dysfunction occurs on average after 3–4 months and a significant proportion of patients survive beyond this period of time, stent exchange is needed in approximately 30–60% (47, 64). Consequently, patients are at risk of experiencing recurrent jaundice and or cholangitis due to stent obstruction and may require a repeated procedure and stent replacement (68).

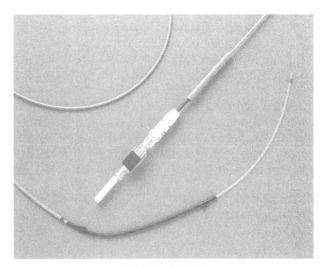

FIGURE 22.1

Plastic polyethylene (PE) biliary stent mounted on a rapid exchange (RX) system. (With permission of Boston Scientific®)

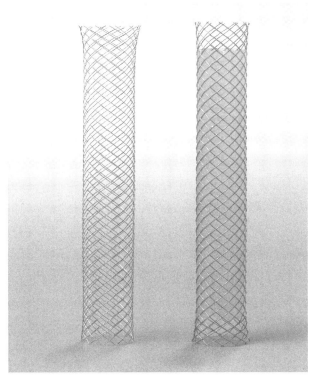

FIGURE 22.2

Uncovered (left) and covered (right) self-expandable metal stent (SEMS). (With permission of Boston Scientific®)

Plastic stents become obstructed by biofilm, a sludge-like material, which has no similarities with the sludge implicated in the pathogenesis of gallbladder stones. In contrast to gallbladder sludge, stent sludge is comprised primarily of protein, bilirubin, and crystals and has almost no cholesterol within it (69). The protein found in the obstructed stent is of unknown origin, but it has been postulated to arise from bacterial products, given that stents perfused with sterile bile do not to accumulate sludge (70). When bacteria reflux up the endoprosthesis (as the stent bridges the papilla and is exposed to the duodenal environment), bacterial enzymes such as β-glucoronidases degrade bilirubin glucoronides and liberate glucuronic acid and bilirubinate, which is then precipitated into a bacterial glycocalyx. The bacteria themselves attach to the stent surface and multiply within the formed glycocalyx, subsequently forming a biofilm. This biofilm permits the bacteria to adhere firmly to the stent despite the shearing forces created by the bile flow. Continuous deposition of bacterial degradation products and growth of bacterial colonies can eventually lead to complete occlusion of the stent (69, 71).

A large variety of plastic biliary stents are available with internal diameters ranging from 5 to 11.5 French (Fr) gauge with lengths varying from 5 to 15 cm.

Straight plastic stents with flaps in both extremities and side holes are the most common type of stent used. The presence of flaps minimizes the risk of stent migration which is even less likely to occur in pigtail stents due to their physical characteristic that allow greater anchoring inside the CBD and duodenum. Animal studies suggest that straight stents may provide better bile drainage than pigtail stents (72, 73). When compared to pigtail stents of equivalent diameters in either normal or dilated common bile duct, straight stents demonstrated a greater bile flow rate, which may decrease the risk of bile stasis, consequent biofilm formation (72), and subsequent stent clogging. Understanding the mechanisms involved in the occlusion has motivated studies aiming to improve the patency of these stents. The following measures have been evaluated in different clinical studies:

1. *Size of internal stent diameter.* Rodkiewicz et al. have shown that bile flow in a rigid tube behaves like a Newtonian fluid and the flow is thus laminar under physiologic conditions (74). The flow of bile through a stent is directly proportional to the internal diameter and the difference in pressure across the stent and inversely proportional to the viscosity of the fluid and the length of the stent ($Q = \pi.D^4.\Delta P/ 128.n.L$, where D is the internal diameter, P is the pressure across the stent, n is the viscosity of the fluid, and L the length of the stent). Therefore, at least under physiologic conditions, stents with larger internal diameters should improve the laminar flow and decrease the chance of stent clogging. The calculated flow capacity for an 11.5 Fr stent is 270 and 520% greater than a 10 and 8 Fr stent, respectively. Although flow capacity in 8, 10, and 11.5 Fr stents are much above the daily bile production, this may not be applicable to "real life" conditions such as biliary obstruction. In this scenario, not only are the amount to be drained (retained bile above the obstruction) and the viscosity of bile greater than normal, but the presence of stones and debris can also disrupt the pattern of flow seen under physiologic conditions. Thus, the bile flow rate can be markedly reduced to a point that a small-caliber stent has no safety margin of spare flow capacity.

   The hypothesis that increments in internal diameter of biliary stents improve patency rates was investigated in four nonrandomized retrospective studies—two comparing 10 Fr to 7 Fr and 8.5 Fr stents (75, 76) and two comparing 10 Fr to 11.5 Fr stents (77, 78). These studies have supported the current practice of inserting 10 Fr stents in the management of malignant biliary obstruction. In the absence of prospective evaluations of different sizes of plastic stents, retrospective studies suggest that 10 Fr and 11.5 Fr plastic stents are equally effective in providing drainage in patients with malignant obstruction. However, it remains unclear if 10 Fr stents are superior to 7 Fr or 8 Fr stents.

2. *Presence of side holes.* Side holes located at both extremities of PE stents are designed to permit bile drainage into the stent in case the cephalad orifice becomes occluded or abuts against the bile duct wall. However, in vitro studies suggested that side holes can also accelerate sludge formation presumably because of turbulence of the bile flow stream generated by the noncontiguous surface at the orifice (59). Coene and colleagues performed an in vitro and a pilot clinical study with plastic stents of different designs and materials. The in vitro analysis revealed that presence of side holes significantly increased the amount of sludge irrespective of the type of plastic material used (59). This finding was subsequently tested in 40 patients with distal biliary malignant obstruction. PE stents with and without side holes were inserted in a total of 40 patients and removed for analysis after 2 months. Although all stents were patent on eye examination at removal, a quantitative sludge analysis demonstrated that stents without side holes had a significantly lower amount of sludge that was distributed along the entire inner surface; in contrast, sludge accumulation was greatest at the rims of the side holes (59, 70). There has been only one RCT comparing stents of similar material with and without side holes (79). Sung et al. randomized 70 individuals with benign and malignant biliary obstruction to receive 10 Fr PE stents with versus without side holes. The number of stents found to be occluded, the median time to occlusion, and the amount of sludge within the stents were similar in both groups (79). These findings suggest that once colonization of bacteria into the inner surface of the stent occurs, adhesion is perpetuated regardless of the presence of side holes.

3. *Modification of stent surface.* In addition to PE, other polymers such as Teflon, hydrophilic-coated polyurethane (HCP), and double layer stent (DLS) have been investigated. These materials have been shown in vitro to have a lower coefficient of friction. Consequently, they reduce bacterial adhesion and biofilm formation, hopefully leading to prolonged stent patency. Teflon stents are commercially available as Teflon Tannenbaum (TT) and differ from PE stents in the material itself and the absence of side holes. Therefore trials comparing PE and TT stents evaluate the effect of two independent parameters which, at least in vitro, are known to influence the patency of plastic stents (80–84). However, the randomized controlled trials comparing Teflon to PE stents have not demonstrated superior effectiveness of Teflon stents as observed in the original case series by Binmoller and colleagues (85). HCP stents have the same design as the conventional PE stents, but the outer hydrophilic layer has an ultrasmooth surface, which greatly reduces bacterial colonization in vitro (86). Like the Teflon stents, HCP stents have not demonstrated superiority over PE stents despite promising in vitro results (87). DLS stents are constructed without side holes and consist of three layers. The inner layer is made of smoothed Teflon, which results in a flatter surface and prevents bacterial adhesion. The middle layer is made of stainless steel and not only provides elasticity but also helps to bond the inner to the outer layer. The outer layer is made of a polyamide elastomer that gives sufficient stiffness to the stent to withstand the pressure from a strictured bile duct. The only RCT comparing PE to DLS revealed that patients who received DLS instead of PE stents were more likely to have a patent stent at time of death. The mean time to occlusion was shorter, and the proportion of patients with stent occlusion was higher in the PE group (88). However, the DLS stent is not currently available in the United States or Canada.

4. *Position of the stent.* Although the biliary tract does not normally harbor microorganisms, transient incursions of bacteria into the biliary tree can occur in healthy individuals (89). Therefore, placement of the distal end of the stent above the sphincter of Oddi (inside-stent approach) was postulated to preserve the mechanical barrier to microbes, decrease the likelihood of duodenal reflux and bacterial contamination of the stent and consequently prolong the patency of stents. Pedersen and colleagues compared the patency of straight PE stents placed above and across the sphincter of Oddi (90). Median survival of stents and the proportion of stents exchanged were not significantly different. However, the causes of stent dysfunction were different between the two groups. Occlusion was the reason for most dysfunctions seen in patients with stents inserted by the conventional approach, while stent migration accounted for most cases of dysfunction in patients with stents placed above the sphincter of Oddi. The results suggest that an improvement in stent effectiveness might be achieved if stent migration could be avoided in patients with stents inserted above the sphincter of Oddi. However, the observed high rate of stent

dysfunction due to migration and associated complications speaks in favor the use of the conventional placement technique.

5. *Administration of choleretic agents and/or antibiotics.* A variety of agents have been shown in vitro to interfere with the mechanism of stent clogging (47). The earliest report was on the use of aspirin to reduce mucin secretion and doxycycline to inhibit bacterial colonization, an important process in the initial step of stent occlusion (91). Although the amount of sludge was significantly lower in both treatment groups after 2 months from the initial insertion, this interval was not sufficient to document differences in occlusion rate if there is a true difference. Libby et al. demonstrated that ciprofloxacin significantly reduced bacterial adherence to PE both in vitro and in an animal model (92). Hydrophobic bile salts such as deoxycholic and taurodeoxycholic acid are the strongest known inhibitors of bacterial adhesion to stent material, and could reduce bacterial adhesion on plastic 100- to 1000-fold (79). However, their cytopathic effects and the associated gastrointestinal side effects make them more poorly tolerated than the hydrophilic bile acids such as UDCA, which have little effect on bacterial adherence.

The results of randomized controlled trials evaluating antibiotics and hydrophilic bile salts have been controversial (Table 22.1). Five studies evaluating the role of antibiotics either alone, with ursodeoxycholic acid (UDCA), or with a choleretic agent (Rowachol) failed to demonstrate any advantage over placebo or UDCA alone (93–97).

In summary, randomized controlled trials comparing different plastic stent materials (PE, TT, and polyurethane), designs (with and without side holes) and adjuvant therapies have failed to demonstrate significant difference in terms of patency, and the choice of stent used should be based on operator experience with the device (Table 22.2).

Self-Expandable Metal Stents

The problems associated with PE stent dysfunction were at least partially overcome with the advent of SEMS (Figure 22.3). Once fully deployed, SEMS reaches an internal diameter approximately three times that of PE stents and is less likely to be clogged by bile plugs and biofilm (62). Instead, SEMS become obstructed by tumor ingrowth and overgrowth, which occurs on average 8–9 months after placement (62, 98, 99). The lower obstruction rate of SEMS is advantageous since the median patency is not only longer than PE stents, but also exceeds the average median survival time of patients with malignant biliary obstruction. The extended patency of SEMS is associated with several benefits, including (1) a better quality of life for patients not only because of avoidance of additional procedures but also due to increased symptom-free period (9–11), (b) improved survival (100), and (c) lower costs because of avoidance of repeated ERCP.

TABLE 22.1
Prospective Studies Evaluating the Effect of Oral Antibiotics and Choleretic Agents on Patency of Plastic Stents

COMPARISON	STENT PATENCY	SURVIVAL	N	REF.
Cyclic antibiotic and UDCA (median, weeks)	26	ND	70	94
No intervention (median, weeks)	28			
Norfloxacin + UDCA (median, weeks)	49*	67*		
No intervention (median, weeks)	6	18	20	108
Ciprofloxacin (median, weeks)	11.6	ND	58	97
No intervention (median, weeks)	11.9			
Ciprofloxacin and Rowachol (median, weeks)	23	ND	40	96
No intervention (median, weeks)	21			
Norfloxacin and UDCA (median, days)	149	ND	62	93
No intervention (median, days)	100			
Ofloxacin and UDCA (median, days)	95	ND	52	95
UDCA (median, days)	101			

UDCA, ursodeoxycholic acid; NS, not statistically significant.
*$p < 0.005$.

TABLE 22.2
Prospective Studies Comparing Different Plastic Technologies in Patients with Malignant Biliary Obstruction

COMPARISON	STENT PATENCY	SURVIVAL	N	REF.
PE with SH (median, weeks)	7.8	NS	70	79
PE without SH (median, weeks)	7.9			
TT (median, days)	83	NS	84	84
PE (median, days)	80			
TT (median, days)	96	NS	57	83
PE (median, days)	76			
TT (median, days)	181	NS	134	47
PE (median, days)	133			
HcPU (median, days)	103	NS	83	87
PE (median, days)	68			
TT (occlusion, %)	67	NS	106	81
PE (occlusion, %)	73			

PE, polyethylene; TT, Teflon Tannenbaum; HcPU, polyurethane; SH, side hole; NS, not statistically significant.

The insertion of expandable stents has been applied to strictures of the biliary tree as in blood vessels (101). Self-expandable metal stents are braided in the form a tubular mesh from surgical grade steel alloy. The elastic properties of the material allow the stent to adopt different configurations according to the site and intensity of force applied. SEMS are delivered into the bile duct while constrained by a sheath, allowing its insertion as a small-circumference delivery system. As the constraining sheath is progressively retracted from its more distal end, the intrinsic expansile forces of the stent make it regain its original configuration. After the sheath is completely withdrawn, the end result is an expanded stent which accommodates the shape of normal (if the diameter of the bile duct is smaller than the maximal stent diameter) and strictured bile duct by maintaining constant radial pressure against its wall (Figure 22.3). Since its first use in patients with biliary malignancies, a variety of SEMS types have been released. SEMS differ in regard to the type of delivery system, structural composition, design, length, and diameter (Table 22.3), and all achieve a much larger internal diameter and longer patency rate compared to the plastic stents.

Five RCT have clearly shown U-SEMS survive longer than plastic stents (Table 22.4) (62, 98, 102–104). The Wallstent Study Group multicenter trial is the largest comparative study to date, but was published in abstract form only. The study included 163 patients with either a hilar (*n* = 48) or common duct (*n* = 115) malignant obstruction who were randomly assigned to placement of either a 10–11.5 Fr plastic stent or a Wallstent®. Details regarding initial stent placement and timing were not included. Of note, 30% of all patients previously had had an initial plastic stent placed and were returning for stent replacement. Although the number of patients who developed stent occlusion before death or at the last follow-up was equal for both groups, median time to obstruction was shorter with plastic stents than SEMS. The 30-day mortality rate did not differ between groups (102). Similar results were obtained by the other RCTs. However, a retrospective study involving 156 patients with unresectable malignant extrahepatic obstruction (72%) and intrahepatic or hilar obstruction (28%) found that SEMS not only offered a longer stent patency than plas-

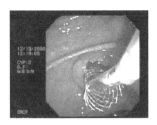
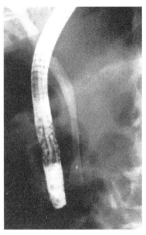

FIGURE 22.3

Endoscopic (left) and fluoroscopic (right) view of a SEMS after deployment. (With permission of Boston Scientific®)

TABLE 22.3

Self-Expandable Metal Stents (SEMS)

FEATURES NAME	DELIVERY SYSTEM (F)	METAL AND DESIGN	DEPLOYED LENGTH (CM)	DEPLOYED DIAMETER (MM)
Wallstent	7.5	Steel wire mesh	4, 6, 8	8
			4.2, 6.8, 8	10
Spiral Z-stent	8.5	Stainless steel, open wire mesh	5.7, 7.5	10
Za stent	8.5	Nitinol open wire mesh	4, 6, 8	10
Memotherm	7.5	Nitinol mesh	4, 6, 8, 10	8, 10
Diamond Ultraflex	9.25	Open wire nitinol mesh	4, 6, 8	10

tic stents, but also was associated with a significant survival advantage. It is unclear if the better patient compliance in the SEMS group was the reason for the improved patient survival. (100).

More recently, C-SEMS have been introduced as an attempt to prevent tumor ingrowth and stent-induced biliary epithelial hyperplasia. While both SEMS are built in a similar manner and achieve the same diameter when fully deployed, C-SEMS differs from its uncovered counterpart in that there is a Permalume membrane positioned over the alloy mesh. This property confers a theoretical advantage of prolonging patency by decreasing obstruction from tumor ingrowth. Initial poorly controlled studies comparing uncovered to covered SEMS not only failed to demonstrate any benefit of covered SEMS, but also suggested a higher rate of stent-related complications such as migration, cholecystitis, and pancreatitis (105, 106). To date one RCT comparing covered to uncovered SEMS has been performed (107). Isayama et al. randomized 112 patients with unresectable distal biliary malignant obstruction to receive a covered polyurethane ($n = 57$) or an uncovered polyurethane diamond stent ($n = 55$). All patients underwent stricture dilation and subsequent drainage with nasobiliary or plastic drainage before insertion of the metal stent. Percutaneous insertion after unsuccessful endoscopic deployment was utilized in 12/57 (21%) and 9/55 (16.3%) of patients with covered and uncovered SEMS, respectively. Stent occlusion, which was significantly different between groups, occurred in 14% of patients in the covered group and 38% in the uncovered group at a mean follow-up of 304 and 166 days, respectively. The patency duration of C-SEMS was superior to the uncovered, but no difference in patient survival was noted. The study also demonstrated a higher incidence of complications in the covered (4.8% of cholecystitis and 8.7% of pancreatitis) versus the uncovered group (no cholecystitis and 1.8% pancreatitis), although not formally compared statistically. The authors concluded that covered dia-

TABLE 22.4

Comparison of SEMS and Plastic Stents

STENT TECHNOLOGY	STENT PATENCY	SURVIVAL	N	REF.
SEMS (median, days)	273*	ND	105	62
PE (median, days)	126			
SEMS (occlusion, %)	22*	ND	62	98
PE (occlusion, %)	46			
SEMS (occlusion, %)	60*	ND	20	109[a]
PE (occlusion, %)	18			
SEMS (median, days)	272*	ND	101	110[b]
PE (median, days)	92			
SEMS (median, months)	4.8*	ND	67	111
PE (median, months)	3.2			

12/62 patients had percutaneous insertion of stents.
[a] Included patients with hilar tumors.
[b] Stents inserted percutaneously.
NS, not statistically significant.
*$p < 0.05$.

mond stents were superior to uncovered ones in preventing tumor ingrowth but carried a higher risk of complications not previously observed with U-SEMS.

SUMMARY

Tumors are a common cause of biliary obstruction. Unfortunately, most of these malignancies are not curable at the time of diagnosis, but improvements in endoscopic technology and the advent of biliary endoprosthesis have permitted delivery of effective methods of palliation using less invasive techniques at lower costs. Although palliation of malignant biliary obstruction can be successfully achieved with any one of the existing surgical, radiologic, or endoscopic techniques available, endoscopic palliation is the preferred approach to manage nonsurgical candidates. This approach is not only associated with a lower complication and mortality rate, but also more cost-effective than competing alternatives. A wide variety of biliary stents are currently available, and numerous studies have validated their efficacy. Among them, SEMS is certainly the most effective and probably the most cost-effective, depending on patient survival. Endoscopic insertion of biliary stents will remain the method of choice for palliation of obstruction for the next few years. New approaches using Natural Orifice Transluminal Endoscopy Surgery (NOTES) are currently under investigation, and their role in management of malignant biliary obstruction is still unclear. A significant amount of uncertainty remains, and more studies are needed before a formal algorithm can be substantiated.

References

1. Atkinson M, Nordin BE, Sherlock S. Malabsorption and bone disease in prolonged obstructive jaundice. Q J Med 1956; 25(99):299–312.
2. Cahill CJ, Pain JA. Obstructive jaundice. Renal failure and other endotoxin-related complications. Surg Annu 1988; 20:17–37.
3. O'Connor MJ. Mechanical biliary obstruction. A review of the multisystemic consequences of obstructive jaundice and their impact on perioperative morbidity and mortality. Am Surg 1985; 51(5):245–251.
4. Jemal A, Tiwari RC, Murray T, et al. Cancer statistics, 2004; CA Cancer J Clin 2004; 54(1):8–29.
5. Shaib Y, El-Serag HB. The epidemiology of cholangiocarcinoma. Semin Liver Dix 2004; 24(2):115–125.
6. Warshaw AL, Fernandez-del Castillo C. Pancreatic carcinoma. N Engl J Med 1992; 326(7):455–465.
7. Rosewicz S, Wiedenmann B. Pancreatic carcinoma. Lancet 1997; 349(9050):485–489.
8. Haycox A, Lombard M, Neoptolemos J, et al. Review article: current treatment and optimal patient management in pancreatic cancer. Aliment Pharmacol Ther 1998; 12(10):949–964.
9. Ballinger AB, McHugh M, Catnach SM, et al. Symptom relief and quality of life after stenting for malignant bile duct obstruction. Gut 1994; 35(4):467–470.
10. Abraham NS, Barkun JS, Barkun AN. Palliation of malignant biliary obstruction: a prospective trial examining impact on quality of life. Gastrointest Endosc 2002; 56(6):835–841.
11. Luman W, Cull A, Palmer KR. Quality of life in patients stented for malignant biliary obstructions. Eur J Gastroenterol Hepatol 1997; 9(5):481–484.
12. Schiff ER. Cholestatic evaluation. Lab Res Methods Biol Med 1983. 7:517–528.
13. Freeny PC. Computed tomography in the diagnosis and staging of cholangiocarcinoma and pancreatic carcinoma. Ann Oncol1999; 10(suppl 4):12–17.
14. Yoon JH, Gores GJ. Diagnosis, Staging, and Treatment of Cholangiocarcinoma. Curr Treat Options Gastroenterol 2003; 6(2):105–112.
15. Hunt GC, Faigel DO. Assessment of EUS for diagnosing, staging, and determining resectability of pancreatic cancer: a review. Gastrointest Endosc 2002; 55(2):232–237.
16. Hennig R, Tempia-Caliera AA, Hartel M, et al. Staging laparoscopy and its indications in pancreatic cancer patients. Dig Surg 2002; 19(6):484–488.
17. Pisters PW, Lee JE, Vauthey JN, et al. Laparoscopy in the staging of pancreatic cancer. Br J Surg 2001; 88(3):325–337.
18. Nieveen van Dijkum EJ, Romijn MG, Terwee CB, et al. Laparoscopic staging and subsequent palliation in patients with peripancreatic carcinoma. Ann Surg 2003; 237(1): 66–73.
19. Lindsay TH, Jonas BM, Sevcik MA, et al. Pancreatic cancer pain and its correlation with changes in tumor vasculature, macrophage infiltration, neuronal innervation, body weight and disease progression. Pain 2005; 119(1–3):233–246.
20. Soetikno RM, Lichtenstein DR, Vandervoort J, et al. Palliation of malignant gastric outlet obstruction using an endoscopically placed Wallstent. Gastrointest Endosc 1998; 47(3):267–270.
21. Lohri A, Herrmann R. (Palliative pain therapy in terminally ill tumor patients). Schweiz Rundsch Med Prax 1996; 85(9): 261–267.
22. Wiedemann B, Funke C. (Therapy of tumor pain). Z Arztl Fortbild Qualitatssich 1998; 92(1):23–28.
23. Cano JM, Salazar R, Estrany L. (Peroperative neurolysis of the celiac plexus in the control of intractable pain caused by carcinoma of the pancreas). Rev Esp Anestesiol Reanim 1987; 34(5):396.
24. Singler RC. An improved technique for alcohol neurolysis of the celiac plexus. Anesthesiology 1982; 56(2):137–141.
25. Buy JN, Moss AA, Singler RC. CT guided celiac plexus and splanchnic nerve neurolysis. J Comput Assist Tomogr 1982; 6(2):315–319.
26. Greiner L. (Puncture-sonographic alcohol neurolysis of the celiac plexus. A new technic for the therapy of severe chronic upper abdominal pain). Dtsch Med Wochenschr 1985; 110(21):833–836.
27. Wiersema MJ, Wiersema LM. Endosonography-guided celiac plexus neurolysis. Gastrointest Endosc 1996; 44(6):656–662.
28. Kretzschmar M, Krause J, Palutke I, et al. (Intraoperative neurolysis of the celiac plexus in patients with unresectable pancreatic cancer). Zentralbl Chir 2003; 128(5):419–423.
29. Gunaratnam NT, Sarma AV, Norton ID, et al. A prospective study of EUS-guided celiac plexus neurolysis for pancreatic cancer pain. Gastrointest Endosc 2001; 54(3):316–324.
30. Monson JR, Donohue JH, McIlrath DC, et al. Total gastrectomy for advanced cancer. A worthwhile palliative procedure. Cancer 1991; 68(9):1863–1868.
31. Meijer S, De Bakker OJ, Hoitsma HF. Palliative resection in gastric cancer. J Surg Oncol 1983; 23(2):77–80.
32. Pinto IT. Malignant gastric and duodenal stenosis: palliation by peroral implantation of a self-expanding metallic stent. Cardiovasc Intervent Radiol 1997; 20(6):431–434.
33. Bethge N, Breitkreutz C, Vakil N. Metal stents for the palliation of inoperable upper gastrointestinal stenoses. Am J Gastroenterol 1998; 93(4):643–645.
34. Feretis C, Benakis P, Dimopoulos C, et al. Palliation of malignant gastric outlet obstruction with self-expanding metal stents. Endoscopy 1996; 28(2):225–228.

35. Binkert CA, Jost R, Steiner A, et al. Benign and malignant stenoses of the stomach and duodenum: treatment with self-expanding metallic endoprostheses. Radiology 1996; 199(2):335–338.

36. Strecker EP, Boos I, Husfeldt KJ. Malignant duodenal stenosis: palliation with peroral implantation of a self-expanding nitinol stent. Radiology 1995; 196(2):349–351.

37. Maetani I, Inoue H, Sato M, et al. Peroral insertion techniques of self-expanding metal stents for malignant gastric outlet and duodenal stenoses. Gastrointest Endosc 1996; 44(4):468–471.

38. el-Shabrawi A, Cerwenka H, Bacher H, et al. (Endoscopic palliation of malignant gastric outlet obstruction by self-expanding metal stents). Wien Klin Wochenschr 2003; 115(23): 840–845.

39. Adler DG, Baron TH. Endoscopic palliation of malignant gastric outlet obstruction using self-expanding metal stents: experience in 36 patients. Am J Gastroenterol 2002; 97(1):72–78.

40. Truong S, Bohndorf V, Geller H, et al. Self-expanding metal stents for palliation of malignant gastric outlet obstruction. Endoscopy 1992; 24(5):433–435.

41. Kuhlmann KF, De Castro SM, Gouma DJ. Surgical palliation in pancreatic cancer. Minerva Chir 2004; 59(2):137–149.

42. Longmire WP, Jr., McArthur MMM. The management of extrahepatic bile duct carcinoma. Jpn J Surg 1973; 3(1):1–8.

43. Sarr MG, Cameron JL. Surgical palliation of unresectable carcinoma of the pancreas. World J Surg 1984; 8(6):906–918.

44. Sharma D, Bhansali M, Raina VK. Surgical bypass is still relevant in the palliation of malignant obstructive jaundice. Trop Doct 2002; 32(4):216–219.

45. Levy MJ, Baron TH, Gostout CJ, et al. Palliation of malignant extrahepatic biliary obstruction with plastic versus expandable metal stents: An evidence-based approach. Clin Gastroenterol Hepatol 2004; 2(4):273–285.

46. Andersen JR, Sorensen SM, Kruse A, et al. Randomised trial of endoscopic endoprosthesis versus operative bypass in malignant obstructive jaundice. Gut 1989; 30(8):1132–1135.

47. England RE, Martin DF, Morris J, et al. A prospective randomised multicentre trial comparing 10 Fr Teflon Tannenbaum stents with 10 Fr polyethylene Cotton-Leung stents in patients with malignant common duct strictures. Gut 2000; 46(3):395–400.

48. Shepherd HA, Royle G, Ross AP, et al. Endoscopic biliary endoprosthesis in the palliation of malignant obstruction of the distal common bile duct: a randomized trial. Br J Surg 1988; 75(12):1166–1168.

49. Taylor MC, McLeod RS, Langer B. Biliary stenting versus bypass surgery for the palliation of malignant distal bile duct obstruction: a meta-analysis. Liver Transpl 2000; 6(3): 302–308.

50. Martin RC, 2nd, Vitale GC, Reed DN, et al. Cost comparison of endoscopic stenting vs surgical treatment for unresectable cholangiocarcinoma. Surg Endosc 2002; 16(4): 667–670.

51. Van Heek NT, De Castro SM, van Eijck CH, et al. The need for a prophylactic gastrojejunostomy for unresectable periampullary cancer: a prospective randomized multicenter trial with special focus on assessment of quality of life. Ann Surg 2003; 238(6):894–902; discussion 902–905.

52. Lillemoe KD, Cameron JL, Hardacre JM, et al. Is prophylactic gastrojejunostomy indicated for unresectable periampullary cancer? A prospective randomized trial. Ann Surg 1999; 230(3):322–328; discussion 328–330.

53. Blievernicht SW, Neifeld JP, Terz JJ, et al. The role of prophylactic gastrojejunostomy for unresectable periampullary carcinoma. Surg Gynecol Obstet 1980; 151(6):794–796.

54. Lillemoe KD, Grosfeld JL. Addition of prophylactic gastrojejunostomy to hepaticojejunostomy significantly reduces gastric outlet obstruction in people with unresectable periampullary cancer. Cancer Treat Rev 2004; 30(4):389–393.

55. Giraudo G, Kazemier G, Van Eijck CH, et al. Endoscopic palliative treatment of advanced pancreatic cancer: thoracoscopic splanchnicectomy and laparoscopic gastrojejunostomy. Ann Oncol 1999; 10(suppl 4):278–280.

56. Bornman PC, Harries-Jones EP, Tobias R, et al. Prospective controlled trial of transhepatic biliary endoprosthesis versus bypass surgery for incurable carcinoma of head of pancreas. Lancet 1986; 1(8472):69–71.

57. Hoevels J. (Results of percutaneous transhepatic portography (author's transl)). Rofo 1978; 128(4):432–442.

58. Speer AG, Cotton PB, Russell RC, et al. Randomised trial of endoscopic versus percutaneous stent insertion in malignant obstructive jaundice. Lancet 1987; 2(8550):57–62.

59. Coene PP. Endoscopic Biliary Stenting: Mechanisms and Possible Solutions of the Clogging Phenomenon. In Meppel Krips Repro 1990; 13–50

60. Pinol V, Castells A, Bordas JM, et al. Percutaneous self-expanding metal stents versus endoscopic polyethylene endoprostheses for treating malignant biliary obstruction: randomized clinical trial. Radiology 2002; 225(1):27–34.

61. Hii MW, Gibson RN, Speer AG, et al. Role of radiology in the treatment of malignant hilar biliary strictures 2: 10 years of single-institution experience with percutaneous treatment. Australas Radiol 2003; 47(4):393–403.

62. Davids PH, Groen AK, Rauws EA, et al. Randomised trial of self-expanding metal stents versus polyethylene stents for distal malignant biliary obstruction. Lancet 1992; 340 (8834–8835):1488–1492.

63. Huibregtse K. Plastic or expandable biliary endoprostheses? Scand J Gastroenterol Suppl 1993; 200:3–7.

64. Costamagna G, Pandolfi M. Endoscopic stenting for biliary and pancreatic malignancies. J Clin Gastroenterol 2004; 38(1):59–67.

65. Soehendra N, Reynders-Frederix V. Palliative bile duct drainage—a new endoscopic method of introducing a transpapillary drain. Endoscopy 1980; 12(1):8–11.

66. Miura Y, Endo I, Togo S, et al. Adjuvant therapies using biliary stenting for malignant biliary obstruction. J Hepatobiliary Pancreat Surg 2001; 8(2):113–117.

67. Harris J, Bruckner H. Adjuvant and neoadjuvant therapies of pancreatic cancer: a review. Int J Pancreatol 2001; 29(1):1–7.

68. Frakes JT, Johanson JF, Stake JJ. Optimal timing for stent replacement in malignant biliary tract obstruction. Gastrointest Endosc 1993; 39(2):164–167.

69. Groen AK, Out T, Huibregtse K, et al. Characterization of the content of occluded biliary endoprostheses. Endoscopy 1987; 19(2):57–59.

70. Dowidar N, Kolmos HJ, Matzen P. Experimental clogging of biliary endoprostheses. Role of bacteria, endoprosthesis material, and design. Scand J Gastroenterol 1992; 27(1):77–80.

71. Libby ED, Leung JW. Prevention of biliary stent clogging: a clinical review. Am J Gastroenterol 1996; 91(7):1301–1308.

72. Scheeres D, O'Brien W, Ponsky L, et al. Endoscopic stent configuration and bile flow rates in a variable diameter bile duct model. Surg Endosc 1990. 4(2):91–93.

73. Rey JF, Maupetit P, Greff M. Experimental study of biliary endoprosthesis efficiency. Endoscopy 1985; 17(4):145–148.

74. Rodkiewicz CM, Otto WJ. On the Newtonian behavior of bile. J Biomech 1979; 12(8):609–612.

75. Speer AG, Cotton PB, MacRae KD. Endoscopic management of malignant biliary obstruction: stents of 10 French gauge are preferable to stents of 8 French gauge. Gastrointest Endosc 1988; 34(5):412–417.

76. Pedersen FM. Endoscopic management of malignant biliary obstruction. Is stent size of 10 French gauge better than 7 French gauge? Scand J Gastroenterol 1993; 28(2):185–189.

77. Pereira-Lima JC, Jakobs R, Maier M, et al. Endoscopic biliary stenting for the palliation of pancreatic cancer: results, survival predictive factors, and comparison of 10-French with 11.5-French gauge stents. Am J Gastroenterol 1996; 91(10): 2179–2184.

78. Kadakia SC, Starnes E. Comparison of 10 French gauge stent with 11.5 French gauge stent in patients with biliary tract diseases. Gastrointest Endosc 1992; 38(4):454–459.

79. Sung JJ, Chung SC, Tsui CP, et al. Omitting side-holes in biliary stents does not improve drainage of the obstructed biliary system: a prospective randomized trial. Gastrointest Endosc 1994; 40(3):321–325.

80. Schilling D, Rink G, Arnold JC, et al. Prospective, randomized, single-center trial comparing 3 different 10F plastic stents in malignant mid and distal bile duct strictures. Gastrointest Endosc 2003; 58(1):54–58.

81. Catalano MF, Geenen JE, Lehman GA, et al. "Tannenbaum" Teflon stents versus traditional polyethylene stents for treatment of malignant biliary stricture. Gastrointest Endosc 2002; 55(3):354–358.

82. Briggs AH. Handling uncertainty in cost-effectiveness models. Pharmacoeconomics 2000; 17(5):479–500.

83. Terruzzi V, Comin U, De Grazia F, et al. Prospective randomized trial comparing Tannenbaum Teflon and standard polyethylene stents in distal malignant biliary stenosis. Gastrointest Endosc 2000; 51(1):23–27.

84. van Berkel AM, Boland C, Redekop WK, et al. A prospective randomized trial of Teflon versus polyethylene stents for distal malignant biliary obstruction. Endoscopy 1998; 30(8): 681–686.

85. Binmoeller KF, Seitz U, Seifert H, et al. The Tannenbaum stent: a new plastic biliary stent without side holes. Am J Gastroenterol 1995; 90(10):1764–1768.

86. Jansen B, Goodman LP, Ruiten D. Bacterial adherence to hydrophilic polymer-coated polyurethane stents. Gastrointest Endosc 1993; 39(5):670–673.

87. Costamagna G, Mutignani M, Rotondano G, et al. Hydrophilic hydromer-coated polyurethane stents versus uncoated stents in malignant biliary obstruction: a randomized trial. Gastrointest Endosc 2000; 51(1):8–11.

88. Tringali A, Mutignani M, Perri V, et al. A prospective, randomized multicenter trial comparing DoubleLayer and polyethylene stents for malignant distal common bile duct strictures. Endoscopy 2003; 35(12):992–997.

89. Dye M, MacDonald A, Smith G. The bacterial flora of the biliary tract and liver in man. Br J Surg 1978. 65(4):285–287.

90. Pedersen FM, Lassen AT, Schaffalitzky de Muckadell OB. Randomized trial of stent placed above and across the sphincter of Oddi in malignant bile duct obstruction. Gastrointest Endosc 1998; 48(6):574–579.

91. Smit JM, Out MM, Groen AK, et al. A placebo-controlled study on the efficacy of aspirin and doxycycline in preventing clogging of biliary endoprostheses. Gastrointest Endosc 1989; 35(6):485–489.

92. Libby ED, Coimbre A, Leung JW. Early treatment with antibiotics prevent adherence of biliary biofilm. Gastrointest Endosc 1994; 40:A744.

93. De Ledinghen V, Person B, Legoux JL, et al. Prevention of biliary stent occlusion by ursodeoxycholic acid plus norfloxacin: a multicenter randomized trial. Dig Dis Sci 2000; 45(1): 145–150.

94. Ghosh S, Palmer KR. Prevention of biliary stent occlusion using cyclical antibiotics and ursodeoxycholic acid. Gut, 1994; 35(12):1757–1759.

95. Halm U, Schiefke I, Fleig WE, et al. Ofloxacin and ursodeoxycholic acid versus ursodeoxycholic acid alone to prevent occlusion of biliary stents: a prospective, randomized trial. Endoscopy 2001; 33(6):491–494.

96. Luman W, Ghosh S, Palmer KR. A combination of ciprofloxacin and Rowachol does not prevent biliary stent occlusion. Gastrointest Endosc 1999; 49(3 pt 1):316–321.

97. Sung JJ, Sollano JD, Lai CW, et al. Long-term ciprofloxacin treatment for the prevention of biliary stent blockage: a prospective randomized study. Am J Gastroenterol 1999; 94(11):3197–3201.

98. Knyrim K, Wagner HJ, Pausch J, et al. A prospective, randomized, controlled trial of metal stents for malignant obstruction of the common bile duct. Endoscopy 1993; 25(3): 207–212.

99. O'Brien S, Hatfield AR, Craig PI, et al. A three year follow up of self expanding metal stents in the endoscopic palliation of longterm survivors with malignant biliary obstruction. Gut 1995; 36(4):618–621.

100. Schmassmann A, von Gunten E, Knuchel J, et al. Wallstents versus plastic stents in malignant biliary obstruction: effects of stent patency of the first and second stent on patient compliance and survival. Am J Gastroenterol 1996; 91(4):654–659.

101. Rousseau H, Puel J, Joffre F, et al. Self-expanding endovascular prosthesis: an experimental study. Radiology 1987; 164(3):709–714.

102. Carr-Locke DL, Ball TJ, Connors PJ, et al. Multicenter, randomized trial of wallstent biliary endoprosthesis versus plastic stents. Gastrointest Endosc 1993; 39:310A.

103. Kaassis M, Boyer J, Dumas R, et al. Plastic or metal stents for malignant stricture of the common bile duct? Results of a randomized prospective study. Gastrointest Endosc 2003; 57(2):178–182.

104. Prat F, Chapat O, Ducot B, et al. Predictive factors for survival of patients with inoperable malignant distal biliary strictures: a practical management guideline. Gut 1998; 42(1):76–80.

105. Born P, Neuhaus H, Rosch T, et al. Initial experience with a new, partially covered Wallstent for malignant biliary obstruction. Endoscopy 1996; 28(8):699–702.

106. Yasumori K, Mahmoudi N, Wright KC, et al. Placement of covered self-expanding metallic stents in the common bile duct: a feasibility study. J Vasc Interv Radiol 1993; 4(6):773–778.

107. Isayama H, Komatsu Y, Tsujino T, et al. A prospective randomised study of "covered" versus "uncovered" diamond stents for the management of distal malignant biliary obstruction. Gut 2004; 53(5):729–734.

108. Barrioz T, Ingrand P, Besson I, et al. Randomised trial of prevention of biliary stent occlusion by ursodeoxycholic acid plus norfloxacin. Lancet 1994; 344(8922):581–582.

109. Wagner HJ, Knyrim K, Vakil N, et al. Plastic endoprostheses versus metal stents in the palliative treatment of malignant hilar biliary obstruction. A prospective and randomized trial. Endoscopy 1993; 25(3):213–218.

110. Lammer J, Hausegger KA, Fluckiger F, et al. Common bile duct obstruction due to malignancy: treatment with plastic versus metal stents. Radiology 1996; 201(1):167–172.

111. Prat F, Chapat O, Ducot B, et al. A randomized trial of endoscopic drainage methods for inoperable malignant strictures of the common bile duct. Gastrointest Endosc 1998; 47(1):1–7.

IV

SUMMARY

23 Future Directions

Clifton David Fuller
Charles R. Thomas

The history of biliary tract cancers reaches back more than three centuries. In 1777, Viennese surgeon Maxmilian de Stoll made the first report of cancer of the gallbladder (1, 2) in his text, *Rationis medendi in nosocomio practico vindobonensi* (Figures 23.1 and 23.2). In 1840, Charles Louise Maxime Durand-Fardel made the first credited report of cholangiocarcinoma (Figure 23.3) (3). Then, as now, the disease was insidious and deadly. In the intervening centuries, great technological progress has been made, with resultant benefits primarily in surgical practice. Additionally, the imaging, chemotherapeutic, radiotherapeutic, genomic, and epidemiologic tools available to the clinician scientist of today would have exceeded the dreams of Stoll and Durand-Fardel.

Nonetheless, while technical and technological advances provide pride to modern clinicians (and justify creation of textbooks), they are poor solace to the tens of thousands of patients killed by biliary tract cancers annually. Can we be proud of the progress made when single-digit 5-year survival is the norm? Is cancer of the biliary tract destined to remain an orphan, too rare for large-scale interest, just a question on a board examination for most practitioners? What must change if we are to combat the nihilistic prognosis this diagnosis entails? How many case reports and institutional series are enough?

Thus, it is evident that in the modern era several key tasks must be undertaken to advance the status of the field. While the typical section on "Future Directions" focuses on the latest basic science discoveries, technological advances just over the horizon, or silver bullet therapeutic agent, in most cases there can be no such easy answers. Rather, it is imperative that, as researchers and clinician, we must instead focus on the incremental gains that cumulatively grind away at seemingly intractable illnesses one study at a time. If we hope within the next decades to outpace the last two centuries of gains, which is neither a high bar nor a small task, there are a few new collective efforts that the authors of this text feel are the key to optimizing outcomes and minimizing delay in the advance against biliary tract cancers. While some individuals and research groups are modernizing the biliary tract research enterprise, the following goals must be stressed as collective responsibilities:

1. Large-scale collaborative dataset development and risk-cohort identification.
2. Identification of specific epidemiologic risk factors and development of preventive trials.
3. Compilation of multisite retrospective data for pretherapy risk stratification.
4. Translational investigation of targets derived from basic research.
5. Aggressive enrollment in clinical trials.

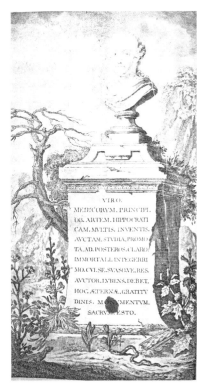

FIGURE 23.1

Frontcover of the first edition of *Rationis medendi in nosocomio practico vindobonensi,* by Maximillian de Stoll, which contains the first credited description of gallbladder cancer. (Courtesy of the P.I. Nixon Medical Historical Library at the University of Texas Health Science Center–San Antonio, San Antonio, TX)

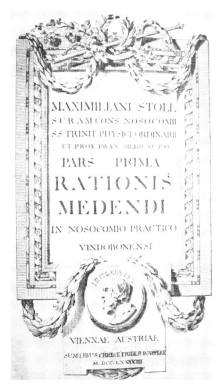

FIGURE 23.2

Title page of *Rationis medendi in nosocomio practico vindobonensi,* by Maximillian de Stoll. (Courtesy of the P.I. Nixon Medical Historical Library at the University of Texas Health Science Center–San Antonio, San Antonio, TX)

LARGE-SCALE COLLABORATIVE DATASET DEVELOPMENT AND RISK-COHORT IDENTIFICATION

Collaborative data sharing represents a key principle in combating rare cancers and should be extended to include not just large-scale population based registries (4) or federal programs (5, 6), but also institutional and international datasets (7). Despite a number of epidemiologic publications, until recently, reliable open-access population-based datasets have been largely unavailable. The numerical rarity of biliary tract cancers in most countries means that in order to identify large-scale risk factors and cohorts at risk, robust epidemiologic biliary tract cancer datasets will be required. "Unlocking" datasets to allow low-cost public access is a first step to building collaborative studies with enough statistical power to generate meaningful testable hypotheses. Currently open-access datasets, such as the United States National Cancer Institute's Survey of Epidemiology- End Results (SEER) (4), and the International Agency for Research on Cancer's Can-

cer Incidence on Five Continents (CIC) (7), represent some of the best meaningful steps in this direction. However, SEER and CIC have inherent limitations in terms of the structure and nature of data collected. Consequently, there is great need to offer, at minimal or no cost, access to other, more developed datasets from other countries. Additionally, determining how to provide reduced cost methods to link datasets (such as the SEER-Medicare linked dataset [8], which provides markedly more detail that SEER alone, but is comparatively and often prohibitively expensive) would substantially increase interaction. While these datasets take great time and cost to collect, and dissemination of data necessitates a relinquishing of central control, even modest costs are enough to deter researchers from developing countries, or even the impoverished graduate student, from choosing a rare cancer such as the gallbladder or bile duct neoplasms as a research interest. Similarly, collective efforts should support data collection and sharing with/from developing nations (Figure 23.4). There are already examples of this approach, such as the multinational case-control data from Mexico and Bolivia presented by Strom et al. (9, 10) Further, by allowing access to disparate data, identification

ANAT. PATHOL. DE LA VÉSICULE ET DES CANAUX BILIAIRES. 167

RECHERCHES ANATOMICO-PATHOLOGIQUES SUR LA VÉSICULE ET LES CANAUX BILIAIRES;

Par MAX. DURAND-FARDEL, *ex-interne des hôpitaux.*

1re PARTIE.—*Cancer de la vésicule biliaire et du canal cholédoque.*

On n'a jamais décrit, que je sache, dans l'histoire des maladies de l'appareil biliaire, le cancer de la vésicule du fiel, limité à cette poche, sans altération organique du foie lui-même. Cependant, cette circonstance a dû se présenter plusieurs fois à l'observation, puisque, dans un assez court espace de temps, j'ai rencontré trois fois une affection cancéreuse de la vésicule biliaire, et une fois du canal cholédoque, développée primitivement dans ces parties, et sans que la structure du foie fût aucunement altérée. Dans les divers passages des auteurs, où il est spécialement question de la dégénérescence carcinomateuse de la vésicule, j'ai toujours vu mentionner la participation du foie à cette dernière altération. Ainsi, M. Littré, dans un article sur les maladies de la vésicule biliaire, se contente de dire, au chapitre intitulé *Tubercules cancéreux*: « Baillie rapporte un exemple de cette altération de la vésicule. Les tuniques avaient, dans ce cas, un quart de pouce d'épaisseur, et étaient remplies en même temps de tubercules gros et durs; le foie était affecté de la même maladie. On les a vus de la grosseur d'un œuf de pigeon, et en pleine suppuration (1) ». Je n'ai pu, du reste, retrouver cette citation dans la traduction française de l'anatomie pathologique de Baillie. Cet auteur y parle seulement d'affection tuberculeuse de la vésicule, affection qui a été signalée par d'autres auteurs, bien que M. Littré l'ait passée sous silence. M. Cruveilhier, cité par le docteur Heyfelder (2),

(1) *Dict. de méd.*, t. V, p. 231, deuxième édit.
(2) *Archives*, décembre 1839.

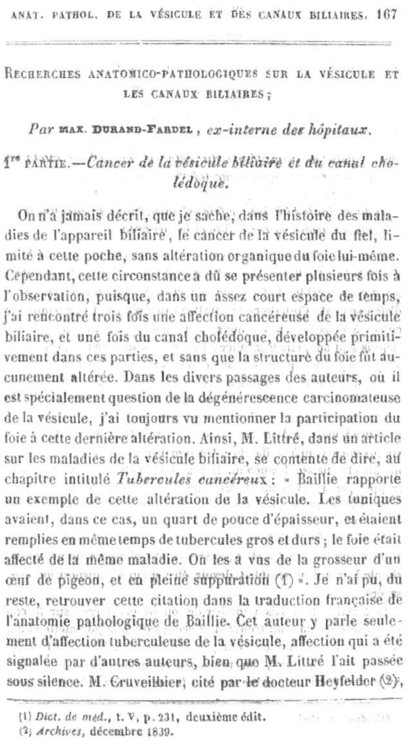

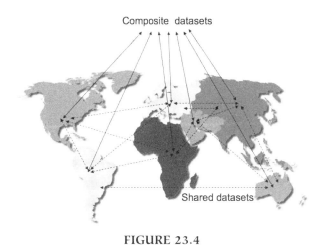

FIGURE 23.3

First page of *Cancer de la vesicule biliaire et du canal choledoque*, the first modern description of cholangiocarcinoma, by Maxime Durand-Fardel. (Courtesy of Bibliothèque interuniversitaire de Médecine [BIUM], Paris)

FIGURE 23.4

Collaborative data sharing and cross national database construction.

of new epidemiologic features and confirmation of previous hypotheses may be readily undertaken. For instance, when the same researchers are able to present data from both Danish (11) and U.S datasets (12), or U.S. and Bolivian data comparatively (13), we glimpse what the future might hold. By opening and compiling datasets, collected but otherwise untouched data may be fully implemented (Figure 23.5).

However, to stop such efforts at population-level research would be shortsighted. How many more small series retrospective publications will change the paradigm of biliary disease? If a continued reliance on single institution datasets for clinical hypotheses is maintained, we can only proceed as fast as the accrual and resources of the largest cancer centers or those centers in regions with enclaves of high incidence afford. However, by sharing and linking data, it might be possible to gradually accrue from a smattering of cases a large enough dataset to generate legitimate testable hypotheses for clinical trials. Such efforts are not without risk. By sharing data, each individual's control over his or her data is reduced, and academic credit (in the form of publications) must be shared. Thus, it might be proposed that some avenue be created

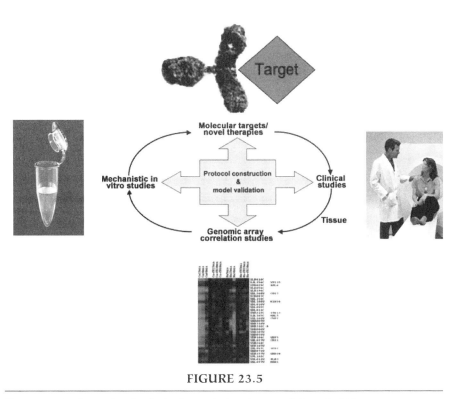

FIGURE 23.5

Conceptual schematic of a desired translational research loop in biliary tract cancer.

to collate and archive *published* data from retrospective clinical series already presented within the literature. Such efforts are not unknown. For instance, the Meta-Analyses of Chemotherapy in Head and Neck Cancer (MACH-NC) (14) group has presented cumulative data, many from published trials, which together afford much greater statistical power than extant trials could generate individually. While retrospective dataare, by nature, subject to limitations not evident in compilations of high-quality trial data such as MACH-NC, nonetheless an attempt to create a large clinical composite dataset could be a first window into defining the right questions for clinical trial development.

IDENTIFICATION OF SPECIFIC EPIDEMIOLOGIC RISK FACTORS AND DEVELOPMENT OF PREVENTIVE TRIALS

These proposed large-scale epidemiologic and clinical datasets would, among other features, also allow risk stratification of specific cohorts. With regard to epidemiologic datasets, this would be envisioned as specific demographic, environmental, or genetic features associated with risk of mortality from biliary tract cancers. For instance, specific immigrant populations in the United States have demonstrated a higher risk of biliary tract cancers than the standard population (15, 16). Ideally, such populations might be enrolled in specific screening protocols or low-risk population-based prospective trials, such as micronutrient supplementation (17) or daily aspirin (18). By selecting populations with the greatest potential to evidence gain, greater gains might be made than by casting too wide a net. Again, support of researchers in developing nations would be a crucial step to undertaking such efforts and in the long-term may be more cost-effective than attempting to undertake similar studies in low-incidence but wealthier Western nations (19).

COMPILATION OF MULTISITE RETROSPECTIVE DATA FOR PRETHERAPY RISK STRATIFICATION

For clinical series, this would entail exploration of specific subgroups within clinical populations. For instance, even today it is difficult to say with any conviction which groups might benefit most from external beam radiotherapy for microscopically positive margin disease. At present, SEER data is one of the few easily accessed resources large enough to afford the opportunity to model complex risk interaction (20). However, if sufficiently large composite datasets could be created, it

might conceivably be possible to determine whether investigatory trials would even be logically feasible.

TRANSLATIONAL INVESTIGATION OF TARGETS DERIVED FROM BASIC AND DLINICAL STUDIES

Of the proposed future directions listed herein, this is the area with perhaps more momentum at present. As basic research into the mechanistic processes involved in the development and progression of biliary tract cancers advances, not only does our fundamental knowledge advance, but potential therapeutic targets are also discovered. As with most cancers, there is some degree of overlap between specific molecular pathways/targets and those pathways/targets successfully explored in other organ sites. The recent phase II trial by Philip et al. demonstrating the activity of erlotinib in biliary tract cancers (21), and the data from Paule et al. regarding cetuximab plus gemcitabine-oxaliplatin in patients with refractory advanced intrahepatic cholangiocarcinoma (22) are not only significant and laudable as clinical trials, but also as the application of previously demonstrated in vitro evidence of epidermal growth factor receptor as a modulator of activity in biliary tract cell lines (23–27). Extant in vitro literature suggests that several existing agents, such as imatinib mesylate (28) or celecoxib (29–31), could also show efficacy against biliary malignancies, as could readily developable poten-

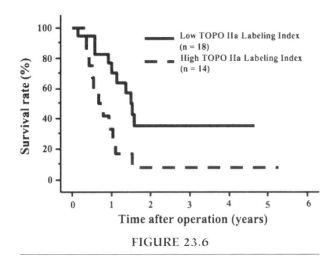

FIGURE 23.6

Results of analysis of TOPO IIa, a DNA microarray-derived postential chemotherapeutic target, by Washiro et al. (33): "Patient survival of advanced gallbladder carcinoma after surgical resection according to immunohistochemical labeling indices of TOPO IIα expression, excluding patients with R2-resection. Survival among patients with a high TOPO IIα labeling index (*n* = 14) was significantly worse than among patients with a low TOPO IIα labeling index (*n* = 18; *p* < 0.05)."

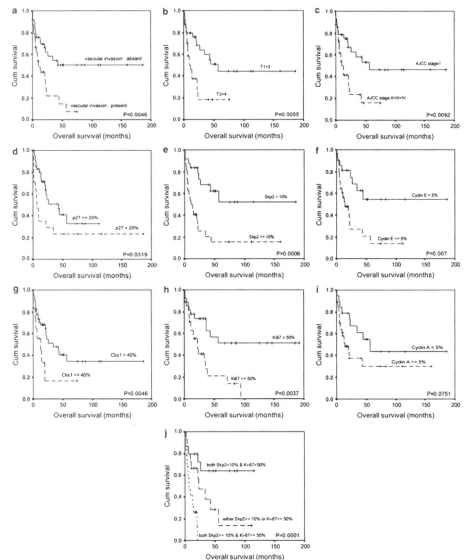

FIGURE 23.7

Results of analysis of prognostic clinical and tissue microarray features of gallbladder carcinoma by Li et al. (34): "By log-rank tests, OS of patients with gallbladder carcinoma were significantly associated with the status of vascular invasion (a), T stage (b), AJCC stage (c), and expression levels of p27Kip1 (d), Skp2 (e), cyclin E (f), Cks1 (g), and Ki-67 (h) the combination of Skp2 and Ki-67 (j) effectively classify three prognostically different groups of patients with gallbladder carcinoma."

tial molecular targeted agents. Realistically, it is likely that few industry sponsors would seek development of agents specifically for gallbladder and bile duct cancer alone; however, it is reasonable that exploration of approved or pipeline drugs with identified potential could represent a means of developing great leaps forward in a modicum of time. While the "home-run drug" which redefines the prognosis of disease is exceedingly infrequent, such phenomena are known to occur (32).

In addition to deriving protocols from basic science data, data from clinical series should be mined for potential targets through cross-correlation of pathologic and genomic markers with clinical data. The price of genomic microarray methods is now within reach for institutions in most industrialized nations. Excellent examples of the approach include recent studies by Washiro et al. (33) (Figure 23.6) and Li et al. (34) (Figure 23.7), who utilized microarray screening of tissue

samples from gallbladder cancer patients to derive not only potential histologic markers of survival and chemotherapy response, but also potential future biologic targets for clinical trials. Ideally, such efforts would result in a positive feedback loop, where clinical and basic data might be used to serial refine and expand usable hypotheses for clinical trials, which would then serve as a means of model validation (Figure 23.3).

AGGRESSIVE ENROLLMENT IN CLINICAL TRIALS

The final step is committed support for multi-institutional trials. This is perhaps the most difficult step, as opening and enrolling patients in trials is often time-consuming. As a field, we must become devoted to developing and accruing patients to novel clinical trials. However, in an era of limited resources, even cooperative groups may be leery of devoting substantial resources to a "rare" cancer. Nonetheless, without the efforts of committed researchers, retrospective and preclinical data will pave a road to nowhere. Already useful results are being demonstrated in phase I or II trials for multiagent chemotherapy regimens; the impetus must be on the research and clinical community to develop a "highway" for patient enrollment in similar studies, but also to develop robust phase III trials (35) for identified risk-cohorts. A recent search of the NIH clinical trial clearinghouse revealed 90 open trials for "gallbladder cancer"(36), with 47 for "cholangiocarcinoma"(37) and 87 open for "bile duct cancer"(38). Consequently, it is not difficult to find an open trial, but rather difficult to convince caregivers to take on the extra time and effort to enroll patients. Thus, we must steel our resolve and, besides enrolling patients ourselves, educate and advocate our colleagues to do the same. Though there is a loss of control in "handing over" patients in our care to a trial, the alternative in many cases is to subject patients to therapeutic courses whose benefits remain empirical, rather than demonstrated.

CONCLUSION

While significant progress has been made in a piecemeal fashion regarding biliary tract neoplasms, a concerted focus by interested physicians and scientists could potentially speed innovation and improve clinical outcomes. By developing collaborative efforts to pool resources and maximize participation by disparate research groups, it is possible that those afflicted with this morbid and deadly disease in the future might have greater hope than those diagnosed today.

References

1. Stoll M. Rationis medendi in nosocomio practico vindobonensi. Vienna: Bernardus; 1777.
2. Stoll M. Médecine pratique de Maximilien Stoll. Paris: J.A. Brosson; 1800.
3. Durand Fardel M. Mémoires et observations. Juin 1840. Recherches anatomico-pathologiques sur la vésicule et les canaux biliaires. Par Max Durand-Fardel... 1re Partie. Cancer de la vésicule biliaire et du canal cholédoque. Paris, 1840.
4. Surveillance, Epidemiology, and End Results (SEER) Program (www.seer.cancer.gov) SEER*Stat Database: Incidence - SEER 17 RegsLimited Use, Nov 2006 Sub (1973–2004 varying), National Cancer Institute, DCCPS, Surveillance Research Program, Cancer Statistics Branch, released April 2003, based on the November 2006 submission. 2007.
5. Oster S, Langella S, Hastings S, et al. caGrid 1.0: An enterprise grid Infrastructure for biomedical research. J Am Med Inform Assoc 2007.
6. Saltz J, Oster S, Hastings S, et al. caGrid: design and implementation of the core architecture of the cancer biomedical informatics grid. Bioinformatics 2006; 22:1910–1916.
7. Parkin DM, Whelan SL, Ferlay J, et al. Cancer Incidence in Five Continents, Volumes I to VIII. IARC CancerBase No. 7, 2005.
8. Warren JL, Klabunde CN, Schrag D, et al. Overview of the SEER-Medicare data: content, research applications, and generalizability to the United States elderly population. Med Care 2002; 40:IV-3–18.
9. Strom BL, Soloway RD, Rios-Dalenz J, et al. Biochemical epidemiology of gallbladder cancer. Hepatology 1996; 23:1402–1411.
10. Strom BL, Soloway RD, Rios-Dalenz JL, et al. Risk factors for gallbladder cancer. An international collaborative case-control study. Cancer 1995; 76:1747–1756.
11. Welzel TM, Mellemkjaer L, Gloria G, et al. Risk factors for intrahepatic cholangiocarcinoma in a low-risk population: a nationwide case-control study. Int J Cancer 2007; 120:638–641.
12. Welzel TM, Graubard BI, El-Serag HB, et al. Risk factors for intrahepatic and extrahepatic cholangiocarcinoma in the United States: a population-based case-control study. Clin Gastroenterol Hepatol 2007; 5:1221–1228.
13. Rios-Dalenz J, Takabayashi A, Henson DE, et al. The epidemiology of cancer of the extra-hepatic biliary tract in Bolivia. Int J Epidemiol 1983; 12:156–160.
14. Pignon JP, le Maitre A, Bourhis J. Meta-Analyses of Chemotherapy in Head and Neck Cancer (MACH-NC): an update. Int J Radiat Oncol Biol Phys 2007; 69:S112–114.
15. Menck HR, Henderson BE, Pike MC, et al. Cancer incidence in the Mexican-American. J Natl Cancer Inst 1975; 55:531–536.
16. Stellman SD, Wang QS. Cancer mortality in Chinese immigrants to New York City. Comparison with Chinese in Tianjin and with United States-born whites. Cancer 1994; 73:1270–1275.
17. Shukla VK, Adukia TK, Singh SP, et al. Micronutrients, antioxidants, and carcinoma of the gallbladder. J Surg Oncol 2003; 84:31–35.
18. Liu E, Sakoda LC, Gao YT, et al. Aspirin use and risk of biliary tract cancer: a population-based study in Shanghai, China. Cancer Epidemiol Biomarkers Prev 2005; 14:1315–1318.
19. Serra I. [Has gallbladder cancer mortality decrease in Chile?]. Rev Med Chil 2001; 129:1079–1084.
20. Wang SJ, Fuller CD, Kim JS, et al. A prediction model for estimating the survival benefit of adjuvant radiotherapy for gallbladder cancer. J Clin Oncol 2008;
21. Philip PA, Mahoney MR, Allmer C, et al. Phase II study of erlotinib in patients with advanced biliary cancer. J Clin Oncol 2006; 24:3069–3074.
22. Paule B, Herelle MO, Rage E, et al. Cetuximab plus gemcitabine-oxaliplatin (GEMOX) in patients with refractory advanced intrahepatic cholangiocarcinomas. Oncology 2007; 72:105–110.
23. Eckel F, Schmid RM. Emerging drugs for biliary cancer. Expert Opin Emerg Drugs 2007; 12:571–589.
24. Lee CS, Pirdas A. Epidermal growth factor receptor immunoreactivity in gallbladder and extrahepatic biliary tract tumours. Pathol Res Pract 1995; 191:1087–1091.
25. Leone F, Pignochino Y, Cavalloni G, et al. Targeting of epidermal growth factor receptor in patients affected by biliary tract carcinoma. J Clin Oncol 2007; 25:1145; author reply 1145–1146.
26. Malhi H, Gores GJ. Cholangiocarcinoma: modern advances in understanding a deadly old disease. J Hepatol 2006; 45:856–867.
27. Malik IA. Gallbladder cancer: current status. Expert Opin Pharmacother 2004; 5:1271–1277.
28. Wiedmann M, Kreth F, Feisthammel J, et al. Imatinib mesylate (STI571; Glivec)—a new approach in the treatment of biliary tract cancer? Anticancer Drugs 2003; 14:751–760.
29. Han C, Leng J, Demetris AJ, et al. Cyclooxygenase-2 promotes human cholangiocarcinoma growth: evidence for cyclooxygenase-2-independent mechanism in celecoxib-mediated induction of p21waf1/cip1 and p27kip1 and cell cycle arrest. Cancer Res 2004;64:1369–1376.
30. Wu GS, Zou SQ, Liu ZR, et al. Celecoxib inhibits proliferation and induces apoptosis via prostaglandin E2 pathway in human cholangiocarcinoma cell lines. World J Gastroenterol 2003; 9:1302–1306.

31. Zhang Z, Lai GH, Sirica AE. Celecoxib-induced apoptosis in rat cholangiocarcinoma cells mediated by Akt inactivation and Bax translocation. Hepatology 2004; 39:1028–1037.

32. Druker BJ, Talpaz M, Resta DJ, et al. Efficacy and safety of a specific inhibitor of the BCR-ABL tyrosine kinase in chronic myeloid leukemia. N Engl J Med 2001; 344:1031–1037.

33. Washiro M, Ohtsuka M, Kimura F, et al. Upregulation of topoisomerase IIalpha expression in advanced gallbladder carcinoma: a potential chemotherapeutic target. J Cancer Res Clin Oncol 2008.

34. Li SH, Li CF, Sung MT, et al. Skp2 is an independent prognosticator of gallbladder carcinoma among p27(Kip1)-interacting cell cycle regulators: an immunohistochemical study of 62 cases by tissue microarray. Mod Pathol 2007; 20:497–507.

35. Takada T, Amano H, Yasuda H, et al. Is postoperative adjuvant chemotherapy useful for gallbladder carcinoma? A phase III multicenter prospective randomized controlled trial in patients with resected pancreaticobiliary carcinoma. Cancer 2002; 95:1685–1695.

36. ClinicalTrials.gov : Gallbladder cancer. 2008.

37. ClinicalTrials.gov : Cholangiocarcinoma. 2008.

38. ClinicalTrials.gov : Bile duct cancer. 2008.

Index